Lovenox Fr
Novio
Lovenox

# Tarascon Pocket Pharmacopoeia®

W9-AQB-956

Amma
Zofran
Mylanta

2009 Deluxe Lab-Coat Pocket Edition

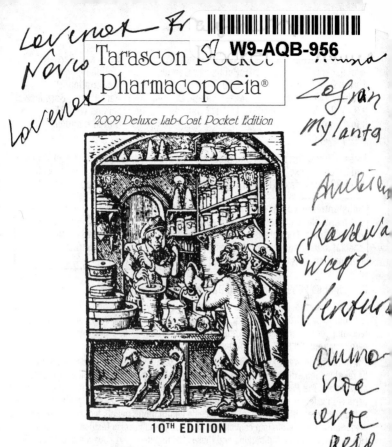

American
Hardware
wage
Venture
ammo
noe
erse
acid
savely

## 10TH EDITION

*"Desire to take medicines ... distinguishes man from animals."*
—Sir William Osler

Editor in Chief
**Richard J. Hamilton, MD, FAAEM, FACMT**
Chair, Department of Emergency Medicine
Drexel University College of Medicine
Philadelphia, PA

JONES AND BARTLETT PUBLISHERS
*Sudbury, Massachusetts*
BOSTON    TORONTO    LONDON    SINGAPORE

**World Headquarters**

Jones and Bartlett
  Publishers
40 Tall Pine Drive
Sudbury, MA 01776
978-443-5000
info@jbpub.com
www.jbpub.com

Jones and Bartlett
  Publishers Canada
6339 Ormindale Way
Mississauga, Ontario
L5V 1J2 Canada

Jones and Bartlett
  Publishers
  International
Barb House, Barb Mews
London W6 7PA
United Kingdom

Jones and Bartlett's books and products are available through most bookstores and online booksellers. To contact Jones and Bartlett Publishers directly, call 800-832-0034, fax 978-443-8000, or visit our website www.jbpub.com.

Substantial discounts on bulk quantities of Jones and Bartlett's publications are available to corporations, professional associations, and other qualified organizations. For details and specific discount information, contact the special sales department at Jones and Bartlett via the above contact information or send an email to specialsales@jbpub.com.

6048

Printed in the United States of America

12 11 10 09 08    10 9 8 7 6 5 4 3 2 1

## Production Credits

Chief Executive Officer: Clayton Jones

Chief Operating Officer: Don W. Jones, Jr.

President, Higher Education and Professional Publishing: Robert W. Holland, Jr.

V.P., Sales and Marketing: William J. Kane

V.P., Design and Production: Anne Spencer

V.P., Manufacturing and Inventory Control: Therese Connell

Publisher: Christopher Davis

Senior Acquisitions Editor: Nancy Anastasi Duffy

Editorial Assistant: Jessica Acox

Production Editor: Wendy Swanson

Associate Marketing Manager: Ilana Goddess

Composition: Newgen

Cover Design: Anne Spencer

Printing and Binding: Malloy

Cover Printing: Malloy

If you obtained your Pocket Pharmacopoeia from a bookstore, please send your address to info@tarascon.com. This allows you to be the first to hear of updates! (We don't sell or distribute our mailing lists, by the way.) To order extra copies, please go the the last page of this book.

The cover woodcut is *The Apothecary* by Jost Amman, Frankfurt, 1574. Many of you knew that The Well of Souls were the dark continent walls adorned with otherwordly caricatures of protocol and cleverness, hearkening to far away and long ago. We will send a free copy of next year's edition to the first 25 who can solve this puzzle: A pill bottle contains one pill, either clonazepam or clonidine. A clonidine pill is placed into the bottle, the bottle is shaken, and a clonidine pill is removed. What are the chances that a clonazepam pill remains? Pretty easy, right? Think, think, think, think.

*Tarascon Pocket Pharmacopeia 2009 Deluxe Lab-Coat Pocket Edition*
ISBN-13: 978-0-7637-6573-6

*Tarascon Pharmacopeia 2009 Library Edition* ISBN-13: 978-0-7637-7228-4

*Tarascon Pharmacopeia 2009 Professional Desk Reference Edition*
ISBN-13: 978-0-7637-7257-4

# CONTENTS

---

## PAGE INDEX FOR TABLES

# TARASCON POCKET PHARMACOPOEIA EDITORIAL STAFF*

# PREFACE TO THE TARASCON POCKET PHARMACOPOEIA®

The *Tarascon Pocket Pharmacopoeia* arranges drugs by clinical class with a comprehensive index in the back. Trade names are italicized and CAPITALIZED. Drug doses shown in mg/kg are generally intended for children, while fixed doses represent typical adult recommendations. Brackets indicate currently available formulations, although not all pharmacies stock all formulations. The availability of generic, over-the-counter, and scored formulations are mentioned. Codes are as follows:

▶ **METABOLISM & EXCRETION:** **L** = primarily liver, **K** = primarily kidney, **LK** = both, but liver > kidney, **KL** = both, but kidney

♀ **SAFETY IN PREGNANCY: A** = Safety established using human studies, **B** = Presumed safety based on animal studies, **C** = Uncertain safety; no humanstudies and animal studies show an adverse effect, **D** = Unsafe — evidence of risk that may in certain clinical circumstances be justifiable, **X** = Highly unsafe — risk of use outweighs any possible benefit. For drugs which have not been assigned a category: **+** Generally accepted as safe, **?** Safety unknown or controversial, **−** Generally regarded as unsafe.

▶ **SAFETY IN LACTATION: +** Generally accepted as safe, **?** Safety unknown or controversial, **−** Generally regarded as unsafe. Many of our "+" listings are from the AAP policy "The Transfer of Drugs and Other Chemicals Into Human Milk" (see www.aap.org) and may differ from those recommended by the manufacturer.

© **DEA CONTROLLED SUBSTANCES: I** = High abuse potential, no accepted use (eg, heroin, marijuana), **II** = High abuse potential and severe dependence liability (eg, morphine, codeine, hydromorphone, cocaine, amphetamines, methylphenidate, secobarbital). Some states require triplicates. **III** = Moderate dependence liability (eg, *Tylenol #3, Vicodin*), **IV** = Limited dependence liability (benzodiazepines, propoxyphene, phentermine), **V** = Limited abuse potential (eg, *Lomotil*).

$ **RELATIVE COST:** Cost codes used are "per month" of maintenance therapy (eg, antihypertensives) or "per course" of short-term therapy (eg, antibiotics). Codes are calculated using average wholesale prices (at press time in US dollars) for the most common indication and route of each drug at a typical adult dosage. For maintenance therapy, costs are calculated based upon a 30 day supply or the quantity that might typically be used in a

| Code | Cost |
|------|------|
| $ | < $25 |
| $$ | $25 to $49 |
| $$$ | $50 to $99 |
| $$$$ | $100 to $199 |
| $$$$$ | ≥ $200 |

given month. For short-term therapy (ie, 10 days or less), costs are calculated on a single treatment course. When multiple forms are available (eg, generics), these codes reflect the least expensive generally available product. When drugs don't neatly fit into the classification scheme above, we have assigned codes based upon the relative cost of other similar drugs. *These codes should be used as a rough guide only*, as (1) they reflect cost, not charges, (2) pricing often varies substantially from location to location and time to time, and (3) HMOs, Medicaid, and buying groups often negotiate quite different pricing. Check with your local pharmacy if you have any questions.

🍁 CANADIAN TRADE NAMES: Unique common Canadian trade names not used in the US are listed after a maple leaf symbol. Trade names used in both nations or only in the US are displayed without such notation.

If you obtained your Pocket Pharmacopoeia from a bookstore, please send us your address (info@tarascon.com). This allows you to be the first to hear of updates! (We don't sell or distribute our mailing lists, by the way.) The cover woodcut is *The Apothecary* by Jost Amman, Frankfurt, 1574. Congratulations to those who knew that The Blob is the sliding gliding splotchy blotch that should be feared. We will send a free copy of next year's edition to the first 25 who can tell us why the following sentence is more than meets the eye: Test argon release: acid soaked cleivite over night.

## CONVERSIONS

| Temperature | Liquid | Weight | |
|---|---|---|---|
| $F = (1.8)C + 32$ | 1 fluid ounce = 30 mL | | 1kg = 2.2 lbs |
| $C = (F - 32)/(1.8)$ | 1 teaspoon = 5 mL | | 1 ounce = 30 g |
| | 1 tablespoon = 15 mL | | 1 grain = 65 mg |

## FORMULAS

*Alveolar-arterial oxygen gradient* = A-a = 148 - 1.2(PaCO2) - PaO2
[normal = 10-20 mmHg, breathing room air at sea level]

*Calculated osmolality* = 2Na + glucose/18 + BUN/2.8 + ethanol/4.6
[norm 280-295 meq/L. Na in meq/L; all others in mg/dL]

*Pediatric IV maintenance fluids* (see table on page 302)
    4 ml/kg/hr or 100 ml/kg/day for first 10 kg, plus
    2 ml/kg/hr or 50 ml/kg/day for second 10 kg, plus
    1 ml/kg/hr or 20 ml/kg/day for all further kg

$$mcg/kg/min = \frac{16.7 \times \text{drug conc [mg/ml]} \times \text{infusion rate [ml/h]}}{\text{weight [kg]}}$$

$$\text{Infusion rate [ml/h]} = \frac{\text{desired mcg/kg/min} \times \text{weight [kg]} \times 60}{\text{drug concentration [mcg/ml]}}$$

*Fractional excretion of sodium* = $\dfrac{\text{urine Na / plasma Na}}{\text{urine creat / plasma creat}} \times 100\%$
[Pre-renal, etc <1%; ATN, etc >1%]

*Anion gap* = Na − (Cl + HCO3)    [normal = 10-14 meq/L]

*Creatinine clearance* = $\dfrac{\text{(lean kg)}(140 - \text{age})(0.85 \text{ if female})}{(72)(\text{stable creatinine [mg/dL]})}$
[normal >80]

*Glomerular filtration rate* using MDRD equation (ml/min/1.73 m$^2$)
= $186 \times (\text{creatinine})^{-1.154} \times (\text{age})^{-0.203} \times (0.742 \text{ if } ♀) \times (1.210 \text{ if African American})$

*Body surface area* (BSA) = square root of: $\sqrt{\dfrac{\text{height (cm)} \times \text{weight (kg)}}{3600}}$
[in m$^2$]

x

## ABBREVIATIONS IN TEXT

AAP - American Academy of Pediatrics
ac - before meals
ADHD - attention deficit & hyperactivity disorder
AHA - American Heart Association
ANC - absolute neutrophil count
ASA – aspirin
AUC – area under curve
bid - twice per day
BP - blood pressure
BPH - benign prostatic hyperplasia
CAD - coronary artery disease
cap - capsule
CMV - cytomegalovirus
CNS - central nervous system
COPD - chronic obstructive pulmonary disease
CrCl - creatinine clearance
CVA – stroke
d - day
D5W - 5% dextrose
DPI - dry powder inhaler
ET - endotracheal
EPS - extrapyramidal symptoms
g - gram
gtts - drops
GERD - gastroesophageal reflux dz
GU - genitourinary
h - hour
HAART - highly active antiretroviral therapy
HCTZ - hydrochlorothiazide
HSV - herpes simplex virus
HTN - hypertension
IM - intramuscular
INR - international normalized ratio
IU - international units
IV - intravenous
JRA - juvenile rheumatoid arthritis
kg - kilogram

LFTs - liver fxn tests
LV - left ventricular
mcg - microgram
MDI - metered dose inhaler
mEq - milliequivalent
mg - milligram
MI - myocardial infarction
min - minute
mL - milliliter
mo - months old
ng - nanogram
NHLBI – National Heart, Lung, and Blood Institute
NS - normal saline
NYHA - New York Heart Association
N/V -nausea/vomiting
OA - osteoarthritis
pc - after meals
PO - by mouth
PR - by rectum
prn - as needed
q - every
qhs - at bedtime
qid - four times/day
qod - every other day
q pm - every evening
RA - rheumatoid arthritis
SC - subcutaneous
soln - solution
supp - suppository
susp - suspension
tab - tablet
TB - tuberculosis
TCAs - tricyclic antidepressants
tid - 3 times/day
TNF - tumor necrosis factor
tiw - 3 times/week
UTI - urinary tract infection
wk - week
yo - years old

## ANALGESICS: Antirheumatic Agents—Biologic Response Modifiers

**NOTE:** Death, sepsis, and serious infections (eg, TB) have been reported. Do not start if current serious infection, discontinue if serious infection develops, and closely monitor for any new infection. Screening for latent TB infection is recommended. Use caution if history of recurring infections or with underlying conditions (eg, DM) that predispose to infections. Combination use of these drugs increases the risk of serious infection and is contraindicated.

**ABATACEPT (*Orencia*)** ▶Serum ♀C ▶? $$$$$
WARNING - Do not use with TNF-blocking drugs such as adalimumab, etanercept or infliximab or the IL-1 receptor antagonist anakinra.
ADULT - RA: Specialized dosing.
PEDS - Juvenile idiopathic arthritis ≥6 yo: Specialized dosing.
NOTES - Monitor patients with COPD for exacerbation and pulmonary infections. Avoid live vaccines.

**ADALIMUMAB (*Humira*)** ▶Serum ♀B ▶- $$$$$
WARNING - Hypersensitivity. Combination use with other immunomodulators increases the risk of serious infections. Aplastic anemia, thrombocytopenia & leukopenia. Rare CNS disorders (eg, multiple sclerosis, myelitis, optic neuritis) have been reported. May worsen heart failure; monitor signs/symptoms of heart failure.
ADULT - RA, psoriatic arthritis, ankylosing spondylitis: 40 mg SC q2 wk, alone or in combination with methotrexate or other disease-modifying antirheumatic drugs (DMARDs). May increase frequency to q wk if not on methotrexate. Crohn's disease: 160 mg SC at wk 0, 80 mg at wk 2, then 40 mg every other wk starting with wk 4.
PEDS - Not approved in children.
FORMS - Trade only: 40 mg pre-filled glass syringes or vials with needles, 2 per pack.
NOTES - Monitor CBC. Refrigerate & protect from light. Avoid live vaccines. Do not use in combination with anakinra.

**ANAKINRA (*Kineret*)** ▶K ♀B ▶? $$$$$
WARNING - Increased incidence of serious infections. Do not use in active infection or with other immunomodulators.
ADULT - RA: 100 mg SC daily, alone or in combination with other disease-modifying antirheumatic drugs (DMARDs) except TNF inhibitors.
PEDS - Not approved in children.
FORMS - Trade only: 100 mg pre-filled glass syringes with needles, 7 or 28 per box.
NOTES - Monitor for neutropenia. Refrigerate & protect from light. Avoid live vaccines.

**ETANERCEPT (*Enbrel*)** ▶Serum ♀B ▶- $$$$$
WARNING - Combination use with other immunomodulators increases the risk of serious infections. Rare nervous system disorders (eg, multiple sclerosis, myelitis, optic neuritis) have

been reported. May worsen heart failure; monitor closely.
ADULT - RA, psoriatic arthritis, ankylosing spondylitis: 50 mg SC q wk, alone or in combination with methotrexate. Plaque psoriasis: 50 mg SC twice weekly × 3 mo, then 50 mg SC q wk.
PEDS - JRA 4–17 yo: 0.8 mg/kg SC q wk, to max single dose of 50 mg.
UNAPPROVED PEDS - Plaque psoriasis 4–17 yo: 0.8 mg/kg SC q wk, to max single dose of 50 mg.
FORMS - Supplied in a carton containing four dose trays and as single-use prefilled syringes. Each dose tray contains one 25 mg single-use vial of etanercept, one syringe (1 mL sterile bacteriostatic water for injection, containing 0.9% benzyl alcohol), one plunger, and two alcohol swabs. Single-use syringes contain 50 mg/mL.
NOTES - Appropriate SC injection sites are thigh, abdomen & upper arm. Rotate injection sites. Refrigerate. Avoid live vaccines. The needle cover contains latex; caution if allergy.

**INFLIXIMAB (*Remicade*)** ▶Serum ♀B ▶? $$$$$
WARNING - May worsen heart failure; monitor signs/symptoms of heart failure. May increase risk of lymphoma; caution if history of malignancy or if malignancy develops during treatment. Hypersensitivity reactions may occur. Combination use with other immunomodulators increases the risk of serious infections. Rare CNS disorders (eg, multiple sclerosis, myelitis, optic neuritis) have been reported.
ADULT - RA: 3 mg/kg IV in combination with methotrexate at 0, 2 and 6 wk. Give q8 wk thereafter. May increase up to 10 mg/kg or q4 wk if incomplete response. Ankylosing spondylitis: 5 mg/kg IV at 0, 2 and 6 wk. Give q6 wk thereafter. Plaque psoriasis; psoriatic arthritis; moderately to severely active Crohn's disease, ulcerative colitis, or fistulizing disease: 5 mg/kg IV infusion at 0, 2, and 6 wk, then every 8 wk.
PEDS - Moderately to severely active Crohn's disease or fistulizing disease: 5 mg/kg IV infusion at 0, 2 and 6 wk then every 8 wk.
UNAPPROVED ADULT - Moderate to severe ulcerative colitis: Same dose as for Crohn's disease.
NOTES - Headache, dyspnea, urticaria, nausea, infections, abdominal pain, & fever. Avoid live vaccines. 3 cases of toxic optic neuropathy reported. Refrigerate.

## ANALGESICS: Antirheumatic Agents—Disease Modifying Antirheumatic Drugs (DMARDs)

**AURANOFIN (*Ridaura*)** ▶K ♀C ▶+ $$$$$
  WARNING - Gold toxicity may manifest as marrow suppression, proteinuria, hematuria, pruritus, rash, stomatitis or persistent diarrhea. Monitor CBC and urinary protein q 4–12 wk (oral) or q 1–2 wk (injectable) due to the risk of myelosuppression and proteinuria.
  ADULT - RA: Initial 3 mg PO bid or 6 mg PO daily. May increase to 3 mg PO tid after 6 mo.
  PEDS - RA: 0.1–0.15 mg/kg/d PO. Max dose 0.2 mg/kg/d. May be given daily or divided bid.
  UNAPPROVED ADULT - Psoriatic arthritis: 3 mg PO bid or 6 mg PO daily.
  FORMS - Trade only: Caps 3 mg.
  NOTES - Contraindicated in patients with a history of any of the following gold-induced disorders: anaphylactic reactions, necrotizing enterocolitis, pulmonary fibrosis, exfoliative dermatitis, bone marrow suppression. Not recommended in pregnancy. Proteinuria has developed in 3%-9% of patients. Diarrhea, rash, stomatitis, chrysiasis (gray-to-blue pigmentation of skin) may occur. Minimize exposure to sunlight or artificial UV light. Auranofin may increase phenytoin levels.

**AZATHIOPRINE (*Azasan, Imuran, +Immunoprin, Uprisine*)** ▶LK ♀D ▶- $$$
  WARNING - Chronic immunosuppression with azathioprine increases the risk of neoplasia. May cause marrow suppression or GI hypersensitivity reaction characterized by severe N/V.
  ADULT - Severe RA: Initial dose 1 mg/kg (50–100 mg) PO daily or divided bid. Increase by 0.5 mg/kg/d at 6–8 wk; if no serious toxicity and if initial response is unsatisfactory can then increase thereafter at 4-wk intervals. Max dose 2.5 mg/kg/d. In patients with clinical response, use the lowest effective dose for maintenance therapy.
  PEDS - Not approved in children.
  UNAPPROVED ADULT - Crohn's disease: 75–100 mg PO daily. Myasthenia gravis: 2–3 mg/kg/d PO. Behcet's syndrome, SLE: 2.5 mg/kg/d PO. Vasculitis: 2 mg/kg/d PO.
  UNAPPROVED PEDS - JRA: Initial: 1 mg/kg/d PO. Increase by 0.5 mg/kg/d every 4 wk until response or max dose of 2.5–3 mg/kg/d.
  FORMS - Generic/Trade: Tabs 50 mg, scored. Trade only (Azasan): 75, 100 mg, scored.
  NOTES - Monitor CBC q 1–2 wk with dose changes, then q 1–3 mo. ACE inhibitors, allopurinol, & methotrexate may increase activity & toxicity. Azathioprine may decrease the activity of anticoagulants, cyclosporine, & neuromuscular blockers.

**GOLD SODIUM THIOMALATE (*Myochrysine*)** ▶K ♀C ▶+ $$$$$
  WARNING - Gold toxicity may manifest as marrow suppression, proteinuria, hematuria, pruritus, rash, stomatitis or persistent diarrhea. Monitor CBC and urinary protein q 4–12 wk (oral) or q 1–2 wk (injectable) due to the risk of myelosuppression and proteinuria.
  ADULT - RA: weekly IM injections: 1st dose, 10 mg. 2nd dose, 25 mg. 3rd & subsequent doses, 25–50 mg. Continue the 25–50 mg dose weekly to a cumulative dose of 0.8–1 g. If improvement seen w/o toxicity, 25–50 mg every other wk for 2–20 wk. If stable, lengthen dosing intervals to q 3–4 wk.
  PEDS - RA: test dose 10 mg IM, then 1 mg/kg, not to exceed 50 mg for a single injection. Continue this dose weekly to a cumulative dose of 0.8–1 g. If improvement seen w/o toxicity, dose every other wk for 2–20 wk. If stable, lengthen dosing intervals to q 3–4 wk.
  UNAPPROVED ADULT - Load as per approved, but then continue weekly up to 1 yr.
  NOTES - Administer only IM, preferably intragluteally. Have patient remain recumbent for approximately 10 min after injection. Contraindicated in pregnancy & in patients who have uncontrolled DM, severe debilitation, renal disease, hepatic dysfunction or hepatitis, marked HTN, uncontrolled heart failure, SLE, blood dyscrasias, patients recently radiated & those with severe toxicity from previous exposure to gold or other heavy metals, urticaria, eczema & colitis. Arthralgia & dermatitis may occur.

**HYDROXYCHLOROQUINE (*Plaquenil*)** ▶K ♀C ▶+ $
  ADULT - RA: 400–600 mg PO daily to start, taken with food or milk. After clinical response, decrease to 200–400 mg PO daily. Discontinue if no objective improvement within 6 mo. SLE: 400 mg PO daily-bid to start. Decrease to 200–400 mg PO daily for prolonged maintenance.
  PEDS - Not approved in children.
  UNAPPROVED PEDS - JRA or SLE: 3–5 mg/kg/d, up to a max of 400 mg/d PO daily or divided bid. Max dose 7 mg/kg/d. Take with food or milk.
  FORMS - Generic/Trade: Tabs 200 mg, scored.
  NOTES - May exacerbate psoriasis or porphyria. Irreversible retinal damage possible with longterm or high dosage (>6.5 mg/kg/d). Baseline & periodic eye exams recommended. Anorexia, N/V may occur. May increase digoxin and metoprolol levels.

**LEFLUNOMIDE (*Arava*)** ▶LK ♀X ▶- $$$$$
  WARNING - Hepatotoxicity, interstitial lung disease. Rare reports of lymphoma, pancytopenia, agranulocytosis, thrombocytopenia, Stevens-Johnson Syndrome, cutaneous necrotizing vasculitis & severe HTN. Exclude pregnancy before starting. Women of childbearing potential must use reliable contraception.
  ADULT - RA: 100 mg PO daily × 3 d. Maintenance: 10–20 mg PO daily.
  PEDS - Not approved in children.
  UNAPPROVED ADULT - Psoriatic arthritis: Initial: 100 mg PO daily × 3 d. Maintenance: 10–20 mg PO daily.

**LEFLUNOMIDE** *(cont.)*
FORMS - Generic/Trade: Tabs 10, 20 mg. Trade only: Tab 100 mg.
NOTES - Avoid in hepatic or renal insufficiency, severe immunodeficiency, bone marrow dysplasia, or severe infections. Consider interruption of therapy if serious infection occurs & administer cholestyramine (see below). Monitor LFTs, CBC & creatinine monthly until stable, then q 1–2 mo. Avoid in men wishing to father children or with concurrent live vaccines. May increase INR if on warfarin; check INR within 1–2 d of initiation, then weekly for 2–3 wk & adjust the dose accordingly. Rifampin increases and cholestyramine decreases leflunomide levels. Give charcoal or cholestyramine in cases of overdose or drug toxicity. Cholestyramine: 8 g PO tid for up to 11 d. Administration on consecutive d is not necessary unless rapid elimination desired.

**METHOTREXATE** *(Rheumatrex, Trexall)* ▶LK ♀X ▶- $$
WARNING - Deaths have occurred from hepatotoxicity, pulmonary disease, intestinal perforation and marrow suppression. According to the manufacturer, use is restricted to patients with severe, recalcitrant, disabling rheumatic disease unresponsive to other therapy. Use with extreme caution in renal insufficiency. May see diarrhea. Folate deficiency states may increase toxicity. The American College of Rheumatology recommends supplementation with 1 mg/d of folic acid.

ADULT - Severe RA, psoriasis: 7.5 mg/wk PO single dose or 2.5 mg PO q12h × 3 doses given as a course once weekly. May be increased gradually to a max weekly dose of 20 mg. After clinical response, reduce to lowest effective dose. Psoriasis: 10–25 mg weekly IV/IM until response, then decrease to lowest effective dose. Supplement with 1 mg/d of folic acid. Chemotherapy doses vary by indication. Gestational trophoblastic tumors. ALL, treatment & prophylaxis of meningeal leukemia. Burkitt's lymphoma. Breast cancer. Head & neck cancer. Advanced mycosis fungoides. Squamous cell & small cell lung cancer. Advanced-stage non-Hodgkin's lymphomas, in combination regimens. Non-metastatic osteosarcoma w/leucovorin rescue.
PEDS - Severe JRA: 10 mg/meters squared PO q wk. Chemotherapy doses vary by indication. ALL, treatment & prophylaxis of meningeal leukemia.
UNAPPROVED ADULT - Severe RA, psoriasis: 25 mg PO q wk. After clinical response, reduce to lowest effective dose. Supplement with 1 mg/d of folic acid. Non-metastatic osteosarcoma with leucovorin rescue.
FORMS - Trade only (Trexall): Tabs 5, 7.5, 10, 15 mg. Dose Pak (Rheumatrex) 2.5 mg (#8,12,16,20,24's). Generic/Trade: Tabs 2.5 mg, scored.
NOTES - Contraindicated in pregnant & lactating women, alcoholism, liver disease, immunodeficiency, blood dyscrasias. Avoid ethanol. Monitor CBC q mo, liver & renal function q 1–3 mo.

## ANALGESICS: Muscle Relaxants

**NOTE:** May cause drowsiness and/or sedation, which may be enhanced by alcohol and other CNS depressants.

**BACLOFEN** *(Lioresal, Kemstro)* ▶K ♀C ▶+ $$
WARNING - Abrupt discontinuation of intrathecal baclofen has been associated with life-threatening sequelae and/or death.
ADULT - Spasticity related to MS or spinal cord disease/injury: 5 mg PO tid × 3 d, 10 mg PO tid × 3 d, 15 mg PO tid × 3 d, then 20 mg PO tid × 3 d. Max dose: 20 mg PO qid. Spasticity related to spinal cord disease/injury, unresponsive to oral therapy: Specialized dosing via implantable intrathecal pump.
PEDS - Spasticity related to spinal cord disease/injury: Specialized dosing via implantable intrathecal pump.
UNAPPROVED ADULT - Trigeminal neuralgia: 30–80 mg/d PO divided tid-qid. Tardive dyskinesia: 40–60 mg/d PO divided tid-qid. Intractable hiccoughs: 15–45 mg PO divided tid.
UNAPPROVED PEDS - Spasticity: ⩾2 yo: 10–15 mg/d PO divided q8h. Max doses 40 mg/d for 2–7 yo, 60 mg/d for ⩾8 yo.
FORMS - Generic only: Tabs 10, 20 mg. Trade only: (Kemstro) Tabs-orally disintegrating 10, 20 mg.
NOTES - Hallucinations & seizures with abrupt withdrawal. Administer with caution if impaired renal function. Efficacy not established for rheumatic disorders, stroke, cerebral palsy, or Parkinson's disease.

**CARISOPRODOL** *(Soma)* ▶LK ♀? ▶- $
ADULT - Acute musculoskeletal pain: 350 mg PO tid-qid with meals and qhs.
PEDS - Not approved in children.
FORMS - Generic/Trade: Tabs 350 mg. Trade only: Tabs 250 mg.
NOTES - Contraindicated in porphyria, caution in renal or hepatic insufficiency. Abuse potential. Use with caution if addiction-prone. Withdrawal and possible seizures with abrupt discontinuation.

**CHLORZOXAZONE** *(Parafon Forte DSC)* ▶LK ♀C ▶? $
WARNING - If signs/symptoms of liver dysfunction are observed, discontinue use.
ADULT - Musculoskeletal pain: Start 500 mg PO tid-qid, increase prn to 750 mg tid-qid. After clinical improvement, decrease to 250 mg PO tid-qid.
PEDS - Not approved in children.
UNAPPROVED PEDS - Musculoskeletal pain: 125–500 mg PO tid-qid or 20 mg/kg/d divided tid-qid depending on age & weight.
FORMS - Generic/Trade: Tabs 250 & 500 mg (Parafon Forte DSC 500 mg tabs scored).
NOTES - Use with caution in patients with history of drug allergies. Discontinue if allergic drug reactions occur or for signs/symptoms of liver dysfunction. May turn urine orange or purple-red.

**CYCLOBENZAPRINE (Amrix, Flexeril, Fexmid)** ▶LK ♀B ▶? $
  ADULT - Musculoskeletal pain: 5–10 mg PO tid up to max dose of 30 mg/d or 15–30 mg (extended release) PO daily. Not recommended in elderly or for use >2–3 wk.
  PEDS - Not approved in children.
  FORMS - Generic/Trade: Tab 5, 10 mg. Generic only: Tab 7.5 mg. Trade only: (Amrix) Extended-release caps 15, 30 mg.
  NOTES - Contraindicated with recent or concomitant MAO inhibitor use, immediately post-MI, in patients with arrhythmias, conduction disturbances, heart failure, & hyperthyroidism. Not effective for cerebral or spinal cord disease or in children with cerebral palsy. May have similar adverse effects & drug interactions as TCAs. Caution with urinary retention, angle-closure glaucoma, increased intraocular pressure.

**DANTROLENE (Dantrium)** ▶LK ♀C ▶- $$$$
  WARNING - Hepatotoxicity, monitor LFTs. Use the lowest possible effective dose.
  ADULT - Chronic spasticity related to spinal cord injury, stroke, cerebral palsy, MS: 25 mg PO daily to start, increase to 25 mg bid-qid, then by 25 mg up to max of 100 mg bid-qid if necessary. Maintain each dosage level for 4–7 d to determine response. Use the lowest possible effective dose. Malignant hyperthermia: 2.5 mg/kg rapid IV push q 5–10 min continuing until symptoms subside or to a max 10 mg/kg/dose. Doses of up to 40 mg/kg have been used. Follow with 4–8 mg/kg/d PO divided tid-qid × 1–3 d to prevent recurrence.
  PEDS - Chronic spasticity: 0.5 mg/kg PO bid to start; increase to 0.5 mg/kg tid-qid, then by increments of 0.5 mg/kg up to 3 mg/kg bid-qid. Max dose 100 mg PO qid. Malignant hyperthermia: use adult dose.
  UNAPPROVED ADULT - Neuroleptic malignant syndrome, heat stroke: 1–3 mg/kg/d PO/IV divided qid.
  FORMS - Generic/Trade: Caps 25, 50, 100 mg.
  NOTES - Photosensitization may occur. Warfarin may decrease protein binding of dantrolene & increase dantrolene's effect. The following website may be useful for malignant hyperthermia: www.mhaus.org

**METAXALONE (Skelaxin)** ▶LK ♀? ▶? $$$
  ADULT - Musculoskeletal pain: 800 mg PO tid-qid.
  PEDS - >12 yo: use adult dose.
  FORMS - Trade only: Tabs 800 mg, scored.

NOTES - Contraindicated in serious renal or hepatic insufficiency or history of drug-induced hemolytic or other anemia. Beware of hypersensitivity reactions, leukopenia, hemolytic anemia, & jaundice. Monitor LFTs. Coadministration with food, especially a high fat meal, enhances absorption significantly and may increase CNS depression.

**METHOCARBAMOL (Robaxin, Robaxin-750)** ▶LK ♀C ▶? $$
  ADULT - Musculoskeletal pain, acute relief: 1500 mg PO qid or 1000 mg IM/IV tid × 48–72h. Maintenance: 1000 mg PO qid, 750 mg PO q4h, or 1500 mg PO tid. Tetanus: specialized dosing.
  PEDS - Tetanus: Specialized dosing.
  FORMS - Generic/Trade: Tabs 500 & 750 mg. OTC in Canada.
  NOTES - Max IV rate 3 mL/min to avoid syncope, hypotension, & bradycardia. Total parenteral dosage should not exceed 3 g/d for >3 consecutive d, except in the treatment of tetanus. Urine may turn brown, black or green.

**ORPHENADRINE (Norflex)** ▶LK ♀C ▶? $$
  ADULT - Musculoskeletal pain: 100 mg PO bid. 60 mg IV/IM bid.
  PEDS - Not approved in children.
  UNAPPROVED ADULT - Leg cramps: 100 mg PO qhs.
  FORMS - Generic only: 100 mg extended release. OTC in Canada.
  NOTES - Contraindicated in glaucoma, pyloric or duodenal obstruction, BPH, & myasthenia gravis. Some products contain sulfites, which may cause allergic reactions. May increase anticholinergic effects of amantadine & decrease therapeutic effects of phenothiazines. Side effects include dry mouth, urinary retention and hesitancy, constipation, headache & GI upset.

**TIZANIDINE (Zanaflex)** ▶LK ♀C ▶? $$$$
  ADULT - Muscle spasticity due to MS or spinal cord injury: 4–8 mg PO q6–8h prn, max dose 36 mg/d.
  PEDS - Not approved in children.
  FORMS - Generic/Trade: Tabs 4 mg, scored. Trade only: Caps 2, 4, 6 mg. Generic only: Tabs 2 mg.
  NOTES - Monitor LFTs. Avoid with hepatic or renal insufficiency. Alcohol, oral contraceptives, fluvoxamine & ciprofloxacin increase tizanidine levels; may cause significant decreases in BP & increased drowsiness and psychomotor impairment. Concurrent antihypertensives may exacerbate hypotension. Dry mouth, somnolence, sedation, asthenia & dizziness most common side effects.

## ANALGESICS: Non-Opioid Analgesic Combinations

**NOTE:** Refer to individual components for further information. Carisoprodol and butalbital may be habit-forming; butalbital contraindicated with porphyria. May cause drowsiness and/or sedation, which may be enhanced by alcohol & other CNS depressants. Avoid exceeding 4 g/d of acetaminophen in combination products. Caution people who drink ≥3 alcoholic drinks/d to limit acetaminophen use to 2.5 g/d to additive liver toxicity.

**ASCRIPTIN (aspirin + aluminum hydroxide + magnesium hydroxide + calcium carbonate) (Aspir-Mox)** ▶K ♀D ▶? $
  WARNING - Multiple strengths; see FORMS.

ADULT - Pain: 1–2 tabs PO q4h.
PEDS - Not approved in children.
FORMS - OTC: Trade only: Tabs 325 mg ASA/50 mg Mg hydroxide/50 mg Al hydroxide/50 mg

**ASCRIPTIN** (*cont.*)

Ca carbonate (Ascriptin & Aspir-Mox). 500 mg ASA/33 mg Mg hydroxide/33 mg Al hydroxide/237 mg Ca carbonate (Ascriptin Max Strength).

NOTES - See warning: NSAIDs - Salicylic Acid subclass.

**BUFFERIN** (aspirin + calcium carbonate + magnesium oxide + magnesium carbonate) ►K ♀D ▶? $

ADULT - Pain: 1–2 tabs/caplets PO q4h while symptoms persist. Max 12 in 24 h.

PEDS - Not approved in children.

FORMS - OTC: Trade only: Tabs/caplets 325 mg ASA/158 mg Ca carbonate/63 mg of Mg oxide/34 mg of Mg carbonate. Bufferin ES: 500 mg ASA/222.3 mg Ca carbonate/88.9 mg of Mg oxide/55.6 mg of Mg carbonate

NOTES - See warning: NSAIDs - Salicylic Acid subclass.

**ESGIC** (acetaminophen + butalbital + caffeine) ►LK ♀C ▶? $

WARNING - Multiple strengths; see FORMS & write specific product on Rx.

ADULT - Tension or muscle contraction headache: 1–2 tabs or caps PO q4h. Max 6 in 24 h.

PEDS - Not approved in children.

FORMS - Generic only: Tabs/caps, 325 mg acetaminophen/50 mg butalbital/40 mg caffeine. Oral soln 325/50/40 mg per 15 mL. Generic/Trade: Tabs, Esgic Plus is 500/50/40 mg.

**EXCEDRIN MIGRAINE** (acetaminophen + aspirin + caffeine) ►LK ♀D ▶? $

ADULT - Migraine headache: 2 tabs/caps/geltabs PO q6h while symptoms persist. Max 8 in 24 h.

PEDS - ≥12 yo: Use adult dose.

FORMS - OTC/Generic/Trade: Tabs/caplets/geltabs acetaminophen 250 mg/ASA 250 mg/caffeine 65 mg.

NOTES - See NSAIDs - Salicylic Acid subclass warning. Avoid concomitant use of other acetaminophen-containing products.

**FIORICET** (acetaminophen + butalbital + caffeine) ►LK ♀C ▶? $

ADULT - Tension or muscle contraction headache: 1–2 tabs PO q4h. Max 6 in 24 h.

PEDS - Not approved in children.

FORMS - Generic/Trade: Tab 325 mg acetaminophen/50 mg butalbital/40 mg caffeine.

**FIORINAL** (aspirin + butalbital + caffeine) (✚Tecnal, Trianal) ►KL ♀D ▶- ©III $

ADULT - Tension or muscle contraction headache: 1–2 tabs PO q4h. Max 6 tabs in 24 h.

PEDS - Not approved in children.

FORMS - Generic/Trade: Cap 325 mg aspirin/50 mg butalbital/40 mg caffeine.

NOTES - See warning: NSAIDs - Salicylic Acid subclass.

**GOODY'S EXTRA STRENGTH HEADACHE POWDER** (acetaminophen + aspirin + caffeine) ►LK ♀D ▶? $

ADULT - Headache: Place one powder on tongue and follow with liquid, or stir powder into a glass of water or other liquid. Repeat in 4–6 h prn. Max 4 powders in 24 h.

PEDS - ≥12 yo: Use adult dose.

FORMS - OTC trade only: 260 mg acetaminophen/520 mg ASA/32.5 mg caffeine per powder paper.

NOTES - See warning: NSAIDs - Salicylic Acid subclass.

**NORGESIC** (orphenadrine + aspirin + caffeine) ►KL ♀D ▶? $$

WARNING - Multiple strengths; see FORMS & write specific product on Rx.

ADULT - Musculoskeletal pain: Norgesic: 1–2 tabs PO tid-qid. Norgesic Forte: 1 tab PO tid-qid.

PEDS - Not approved in children.

FORMS - Generic/Trade: Tabs Norgesic 25 mg orphenadrine/385 mg aspirin/30 mg caffeine. Norgesic Forte 50/770/60 mg.

NOTES - See warning: NSAIDs - Salicylic Acid subclass.

**PHRENILIN** (acetaminophen + butalbital) ►LK ♀C ▶? $

WARNING - Multiple strengths; see FORMS & write specific product on Rx.

ADULT - Tension or muscle contraction headache: Phrenilin: 1–2 tabs PO q4h. Phrenilin Forte: 1 cap PO q4h. Max 6 in 24 h.

PEDS - Not approved in children.

FORMS - Generic/Trade: Tabs, Phrenilin 325 mg acetaminophen/50 mg butalbital. Caps, Phrenilin Forte 650/50 mg.

**SEDAPAP** (acetaminophen + butalbital) ►LK ♀C ▶? $

ADULT - Tension or muscle contraction headache: 1–2 tabs PO q4h. Max 6 tabs in 24 h.

PEDS - Not approved in children.

FORMS - Generic only: Tab 650 mg acetaminophen/50 mg butalbital.

**SOMA COMPOUND** (carisoprodol + aspirin) ►LK ♀D ▶- $$$

ADULT - Musculoskeletal pain: 1–2 tabs PO qid.

PEDS - Not approved in children.

FORMS - Generic/Trade: Tab 200 mg carisoprodol/325 mg ASA.

NOTES - See NSAIDs - Salicylic acid subclass warning. Carisoprodol may be habit forming. Withdrawal with abrupt discontinuation.

**ULTRACET** (tramadol + acetaminophen) (✚Tramacet) ►KL ♀C ▶- $$

ADULT - Acute pain: 2 tabs PO q4–6h prn, max 8 tabs/d for no more than 5 d. If CrCl <30 mL/min, increase the dosing interval to 12 h. Consider a similar adjustment in elderly patients and in cirrhosis.

PEDS - Not approved in children.

FORMS - Generic/Trade: Tab 37.5 mg tramadol/325 mg acetaminophen.

NOTES - Do not use with other acetaminophen-containing drugs due to potential for hepatotoxicity. Contraindicated in acute intoxication with alcohol, hypnotics, centrally-acting analgesics, opioids or psychotropic drugs. Seizures may occur with concurrent antidepressants or with seizure disorder. Use with great caution with MAO inhibitors or in combination with SSRIs due to potential **(cont.)**

**ULTRACET (cont.)**
for serotonin syndrome; dose adjustment may be needed. Withdrawal symptoms may occur in patients dependent on opioids or with abrupt discontinuation. Overdose treated with naloxone may increase seizure risk. The most frequent side effects are somnolence & constipation.

## ANALGESICS: Nonsteroidal Anti-Inflammatories—COX-2 Inhibitors

**NOTE:** The risk of serious cardiovascular events and GI bleeding may be increased in patients taking long-term, high-dose NSAIDs, both COX-2 inhibitors as well as non-selective agents. All NSAIDs and COX-2 inhibitors are contraindicated immediately post-CABG surgery. The FDA advises evaluating alternative therapy or using the lowest effective dose of these drugs. Fewer GI side effects than 1st generation NSAIDs & no effect on platelets, but other NSAID-related side effects (renal dysfunction, fluid retention, CNS) are possible. May cause fluid retention or exacerbate heart failure. May elevate BP or blunt effects of antihypertensives & loop diuretics. Not substitutes for aspirin for cardiovascular prophylaxis due to lack of antiplatelet effects. Monitor INR with warfarin. May increase lithium levels. Caution in aspirin-sensitive asthma. Use around the time of conception appears to increase the risk of miscarriage (use acetaminophen instead).

**CELECOXIB (Celebrex)** ▶L ♀C (D in 3rd trimester) ▶?
$$$$$
WARNING - Increases the risk of serious cardiovascular events and GI bleeding. Contraindicated immediately post-CABG surgery.
ADULT - OA, ankylosing spondylitis: 200 mg PO daily or 100 mg PO bid. RA: 100–200 mg PO bid. Familial adenomatous polyposis (FAP), as an adjunct to usual care: 400 mg PO bid with food. Acute pain, dysmenorrhea: 400 mg × 1,

then 200 mg PO bid. May take an additional 200 mg on d 1.
PEDS - JRA: 2–17 yo: 10–25 kg: 50 mg PO bid. >25 kg: 100 mg PO bid.
FORMS - Trade only: Caps 50, 100, 200, 400 mg.
NOTES - Contraindicated in sulfonamide allergy. Decrease dose by 50% with hepatic dysfunction. Capsules may be opened and sprinkled into one teaspoon of apple sauce & taken immediately with water.

## ANALGESICS: Nonsteroidal Anti-Inflammatories—Salicylic Acid Derivatives

**NOTE:** The risk of serious cardiovascular events and GI bleeding may be increased in patients taking long-term, high-dose NSAIDs, both COX-2 inhibitors as well as non-selective agents (excluding aspirin). All NSAIDs and COX-2 inhibitors are contraindicated immediately post-CABG surgery. The FDA advises evaluating alternative therapy or using the lowest effective dose of these drugs. Avoid in ASA allergy, and in children and teenagers <17 yo with chickenpox or flu due to association with Reye's syndrome. May potentiate warfarin, heparin, valproic acid, methotrexate. Unlike aspirin, derivatives may have less GI toxicity & negligible effects on platelet aggregation & renal prostaglandins. Caution in aspirin-sensitive asthma. Ibuprofen and possibly other NSAIDs may antagonize antiplatelet effects of aspirin if given simultaneously. Use around the time of conception appears to increase the risk of miscarriage (use acetaminophen instead).

**ASPIRIN (Ecotrin, Empirin, Halfprin, Bayer, Anacin, Zorprin, ASA, ✦Asaphen, Entrophen, Novasen)** ▶K ♀D ▶? $
ADULT - Mild to moderate pain, fever: 325–650 mg PO/PR q4h prn. Acute rheumatic fever: 5–8 g/d, initially. RA/OA: 3.2–6 g/d in divided doses. Platelet aggregation inhibition: 81–325 mg PO daily.
PEDS - Mild to moderate pain, fever: 10–15 mg/kg/dose PO q4–6h not to exceed 60–80 mg/kg/d. JRA: 60–100 mg/kg/d PO divided q6–8h. Acute rheumatic fever: 100 mg/kg/d PO/PR × 2 wk, then 75 mg/kg/d × 4–6 wk. Kawasaki disease 80–100 mg/kg/d divided qid PO/PR until fever resolves, then 3–5 mg/kg/d PO qam × 7 wk or longer if there is ECG evidence of coronary artery abnormalities.
UNAPPROVED ADULT - Primary prevention of cardiovascular events (10-yr CHD risk >6–10% based on Framingham risk scoring): 75–325 mg PO daily. Post ST-elevation MI: 162–325 mg PO on d 1, continue indefinitely at 75–162 mg/d. Post Non-ST-elevation MI: 162–325 mg PO on d 1,

continue indefinitely at 75–162 mg/d. Long-term antithrombotic therapy for chronic atrial fib/flutter in patients with low-moderate risk of stroke (<75 yr without risk factors): 325 mg PO daily. Percutaneous coronary intervention pretreatment: Already taking daily ASA therapy: 75–325 mg PO before procedure. Not already taking daily ASA therapy: 300–325 mg PO at least 2–24 h before procedure. Post percutaneous coronary intervention: 325 mg daily in combination with clopidogrel for ≥1 mo after bare metal stent placement, ≥3–6 mo after drug-eluting-stent placement; then 75–162 mg PO daily indefinitely. Post percutaneous coronary brachytherapy: 75–325 mg daily in combination with clopidogrel indefinitely.
FORMS - Generic/Trade (OTC): tabs, 325, 500 mg; chewable 81 mg; enteric-coated 81,162 mg (Halfprin); 81,325,500 mg (Ecotrin), 650, 975 mg. Trade only: tabs, controlled-release 650, 800 mg (ZORprin, Rx). Generic only (OTC): susp 60, 120, 200, 300, 600 mg.

**ASPIRIN** (cont.)

NOTES - Consider discontinuation 1 wk prior to surgery (except coronary bypass or in first yr post-coronary stent implantation) because of the possibility of postoperative bleeding. Aspirin intolerance occurs in 4–19% of asthmatics. Use caution in liver damage, renal insufficiency, peptic ulcer or bleeding tendencies. Crush or chew tabs (including enteric-coated products) in first dose with acute MI. Higher doses of aspirin (1.3 g/d) have not been shown to be superior to low doses in preventing TIAs and strokes.

**CHOLINE MAGNESIUM TRISALICYLATE** (*Trilisate*) ▶K ♀C (D in 3rd trimester) ▶? $$

ADULT - RA/OA: 1500 mg PO bid. Mild to moderate pain, fever: 1000–1500 mg PO bid.

PEDS - RA, mild to moderate pain: 50 mg/kg/d (up to 37 kg) PO divided bid.

FORMS - Generic only: Tabs 500, 750, 1000 mg. Solution 500 mg/5mL.

**DIFLUNISAL** (*Dolobid*) ▶K ♀C (D in 3rd trimester) ▶- $$$

ADULT - Mild to moderate pain: Initially: 500 mg-1 g PO, then 250–500 mg PO q8–12h. RA/OA: 500 mg-1 g PO divided bid. Max dose 1.5 g/d.

PEDS - Not approved in children.

FORMS - Generic/Trade: Tabs 250 & 500 mg.

NOTES - Do not crush or chew tabs. Increases acetaminophen levels.

**SALSALATE** (*Salflex, Disalcid, Amigesic*) ▶K ♀C (D in 3rd trimester) ▶? $$

ADULT - RA/OA: 3000 mg/d PO divided q8–12h.

PEDS - Not approved in children.

FORMS - Generic only: Tabs 500 & 750 mg, scored.

## ANALGESICS: Nonsteroidal Anti-Inflammatories—Other

**NOTE:** The risk of serious cardiovascular events & GI bleeding may be increased in patients taking long-term, high-dose NSAIDs, both COX-2 inhibitors as well as non-selective agents. All NSAIDs and COX-2 inhibitors are contraindicated immediately post-CABG surgery. The FDA advises evaluating alternative therapy or using the lowest effective dose of these drugs. Chronic use associated with renal insufficiency, gastritis, peptic ulcer disease, GI bleeds. Caution in liver disease. May cause fluid retention or exacerbate heart failure. May elevate BP or blunt effects of antihypertensives & loop diuretics. May increase levels of methotrexate, lithium, phenytoin, digoxin & cyclosporine. May potentiate warfarin. Caution in aspirin-sensitive asthma. Ibuprofen or other NSAIDs may antagonize antiplatelet effects of aspirin if given simultaneously. Use around the time of conception appears to increase the risk of miscarriage (use acetaminophen instead).

**ARTHROTEC** (diclofenac + misoprostol) ▶LK ♀X ▶- $$$$$

WARNING - Because of the abortifacient property of the misoprostol component, it is contraindicated in women who are pregnant. Caution in women with childbearing potential; effective contraception is essential.

ADULT - OA: one 50/200 PO tid. RA: one 50/200 PO tid-qid. If intolerant, may use 50/200 or 75/200 PO bid.

PEDS - Not approved in children.

FORMS - Trade only: Tabs 50/200 mg, 75/200 mg diclofenac/mcg misoprostol.

NOTES - Refer to individual components. Abdominal pain & diarrhea may occur. Check LFTs at baseline then periodically. Do not crush or chew tabs.

**DICLOFENAC** (*Voltaren, Voltaren XR, Cataflam, Flector, ◆Voltaren Rapide*) ▶L ♀B (D in 3rd trimester) ▶- $$$

WARNING - Multiple strengths; see FORMS & write specific product on Rx.

ADULT - OA: immediate or delayed release 50 mg PO bid-tid or 75 mg bid. Extended release 100 mg PO daily. Gel: Apply 4 g to knees or 2 g to hands qid using enclosed dosing card. RA: immediate or delayed release 50 mg PO tid-qid or 75 mg bid. Extended release 100 mg PO daily-bid. Ankylosing spondylitis: immediate or delayed release 25 mg PO qid & hs. Analgesia & primary dysmenorrhea: immediate or delayed release 50 mg PO tid. Acute pain of strains, sprains or contusions: Apply one patch to painful area bid.

PEDS - Not approved in children.

UNAPPROVED PEDS - JRA: 2–3 mg/kg/d PO.

FORMS - Generic/Trade: Tabs, immediate-release (Cataflam) 50 mg, extended-release (Voltaren XR) 100 mg. Generic only: Tabs, delayed-release 25, 50, 75 mg. Trade only: Patch (Flector) 1.3% diclofenac epolamine. Topical gel (Voltaren) 1% 100 g tube.

NOTES - Check LFTs at baseline then periodically. Do not apply patch to damaged or non-intact skin. Wash hands and avoid eye contact when handling the patch. Do not wear patch while bathing or showering.

**ETODOLAC** (◆*Ultradol*) ▶L ♀C (D in 3rd trimester) ▶- $$$

WARNING - Multiple strengths; write specific product on Rx.

ADULT - OA: 400 mg PO bid-tid. 300 mg PO bid-qid. 200 mg tid-qid. Extended release 400–1200 mg PO daily. Mild to moderate pain: 200–400 mg q6–8h. Max dose 1200 mg/d or if ≤60 kg, 20 mg/kg/d.

PEDS - Not approved in children.

UNAPPROVED ADULT - RA, ankylosing spondylitis: 300–400 mg PO bid. Tendinitis, bursitis & acute gout: 300–400 mg PO bid-qid then taper.

FORMS - Generic only: Caps immediate-release 200, 300 mg, Tabs immediate-release 400, 500 mg, Tabs extended-release 400, 500, 600 mg.

NOTES - Brand name Lodine no longer marketed.

**FENOPROFEN (*Nalfon*)** ▶L ♀C (D in 3rd trimester) ▶- $

WARNING - Appears to represent a greater nephrotoxicity risk than other NSAIDs.

ADULT - RA/OA: 300–600 mg PO tid-qid. Max dose: 3,200 mg/d. Mild to moderate pain: 200 mg PO q 4–6h prn.

PEDS - Not approved in children.

FORMS - Generic/Trade: Caps 200 & 300 mg. Generic only: Tab 600 mg.

**FLURBIPROFEN (*Ansaid*, *✦Froben, Froben SR*)** ▶L ♀B (D in 3rd trimester) ▶+ $$$

ADULT - RA/OA: 200–300 mg/d PO divided bid-qid. Max single dose 100 mg.

PEDS - Not approved in children.

UNAPPROVED ADULT - Ankylosing spondylitis: 150–300 mg/d PO divided bid-qid. Mild to moderate pain: 50 mg PO q6h. Primary dysmenorrhea: 50 mg PO daily at onset, d/c when pain subsides. Tendinitis, bursitis, acute gout, acute migraine: 100 mg PO at onset, then 50 mg PO qid, then taper.

UNAPPROVED PEDS - JRA: 4 mg/kg/d PO.

FORMS - Generic/Trade: Tabs immediate-release 50 & 100 mg.

**IBUPROFEN (*Motrin, Advil, Nuprin, Rufen, Neoprofen*)** ▶L ♀B (D in 3rd trimester) ▶+ $

ADULT - RA/OA: 200–800 mg PO tid-qid. Mild to moderate pain: 400 mg PO q4–6h. Primary dysmenorrhea: 400 mg PO q4h prn. Fever: 200 mg PO q4–6h prn. Migraine pain: 200–400 mg PO not to exceed 400 mg in 24 h unless directed by a physician (OTC dosing). Max dose 3.2 g/d.

PEDS - JRA: 30–50 mg/kg/d PO divided q6h. Max dose 2400 mg/24h. 20 mg/kg/d may be adequate for milder disease. Analgesic/antipyretic >6 mo: 5–10 mg/kg PO q6–8h, prn. Max dose 40 mg/kg/d. Patent ductus arteriosus in neonates ≤32 wk gestational age weighing 500–1500 g (NeoProfen): Specialized dosing.

FORMS - OTC: Cap/Liqui-Gel Cap 200 mg. Tabs 100, 200 mg. Chewable tabs 50, 100 mg. Suspension (infant drops) 50 mg/1.25 mL (with calibrated dropper) & 100 mg/5 mL. Rx Generic/Trade: Tabs 300, 400, 600, 800 mg.

NOTES - May antagonize antiplatelet effects of aspirin if given simultaneously. Take aspirin 2 h prior to ibuprofen.

**INDOMETHACIN (*Indocin, Indocin SR, Indocin IV, ✦Indocid-P.D.A.*)** ▶L ♀B (D in 3rd trimester) ▶+ $

WARNING - Multiple strengths; see FORMS & write specific product on Rx. Use during labor increases risk of fetal and maternal complications: premature closure of the ductus arteriosus, fetal pulmonary hypertension, oligohydramnios, higher rate of postpartum hemorrhage.

ADULT - RA/OA, ankylosing spondylitis: 25 mg PO bid-tid to start. Increase incrementally to a total daily dose of 150–200 mg. Bursitis/tendinitis: 75–150 mg/d PO divided tid-qid. Acute gout: 50

mg PO tid until pain tolerable, rapidly taper dose to D/C. Sustained release: 75 mg PO daily-bid.

PEDS - Closure of patent ductus arteriosus in neonates: Initial dose 0.2 mg/kg IV, if additional doses necessary, dose and frequency (q12h or q24h) based on neonate's age and urine output.

UNAPPROVED ADULT - Primary dysmenorrhea: 25 mg PO tid-qid. Cluster headache: 75–150 mg SR PO daily. Polyhydramnios: 2.2–3.0 mg/kg/d PO based on maternal weight; premature closure of the ductus arteriosus has been reported. Preterm labor: initial 50–100 mg PO followed by 25 mg PO q6–12h up to 48 h.

UNAPPROVED PEDS - JRA: 1–3 mg/kg/d tid-qid to start. Increase prn to max dose of 4 mg/kg/d or 200 mg/d, whichever is less.

FORMS - Generic/Trade: Cap, sustained-release 75 mg. Generic only: Caps, immediate-release 25, 50 mg, Supp 50 mg. Trade only: Oral susp 25 mg/5 mL (237 mL).

NOTES - May aggravate depression or other psychiatric disturbances. Do not crush sustained release cap.

**KETOPROFEN (*Orudis, Orudis KT, Actron, Oruvail, ✦Orudis SR*)** ▶L ♀B (D in 3rd trimester) ▶- $$$

ADULT - RA/OA: 75 mg PO tid or 50 mg PO qid. Extended release 200 mg PO daily. Mild to moderate pain, primary dysmenorrhea: 25–50 mg PO q6–8h prn.

PEDS - Not approved in children.

UNAPPROVED PEDS - JRA: 100–200 mg/m²/d PO. Max dose 320 mg/d.

FORMS - OTC: Tab, immediate-release 12.5 mg. Rx Generic only: Caps, extended-release 100, 150, 200 mg, Caps, immediate-release 25, 50, 75 mg.

**KETOROLAC (*Toradol*)** ▶L ♀C (D in 3rd trimester) ▶+ $

WARNING - Indicated for short-term (up to 5 d) therapy only. Ketorolac is a potent NSAID and can cause serious GI and renal adverse effects. It may also increase the risk of bleeding by inhibiting platelet function. Contraindicated in patients with active peptic ulcer disease, recent GI bleeding or perforation, a history of peptic ulcer disease or GI bleeding, and advanced renal impairment.

ADULT - Moderately severe, acute pain, single-dose treatment: 30–60 mg IM or 15–30 mg IV. Multiple-dose treatment: 15–30 mg IV/IM q6h. IV/IM doses are not to exceed 60 mg/d in patients ≥65 yo, <50 kg, & for patients with moderately elevated serum creatinine. Oral continuation therapy: 10 mg PO q4–6h prn, max dose 40 mg/d. Combined duration IV/IM and PO is not to exceed 5 d.

PEDS - Not approved in children.

UNAPPROVED PEDS - Pain: 0.5 mg/kg/dose IM/IV q6h not to exceed 30 mg q6h or 120 mg/d. >50 kg: 10 mg PO q6h prn not to exceed 40 mg/d.

FORMS - Generic only: Tab 10 mg.

**MECLOFENAMATE** ▶L ♀B (D in 3rd trimester) ▶- $$$
  ADULT - Mild to moderate pain: 50 mg PO q4–6h prn. Max dose 400 mg/d. Menorrhagia & primary dysmenorrhea: 100 mg PO tid for up to 6 d. RA/OA: 200–400 mg/d PO divided tid-qid.
  PEDS - Not approved in children.
  UNAPPROVED PEDS - JRA: 3–7.5 mg/kg/d PO. Max dose 300 mg/d.
  FORMS - Generic only: Caps 50 & 100 mg.
  NOTES - Reversible autoimmune hemolytic anemia with use for >12 mo.

**MEFENAMIC ACID (*Ponstel, ✦Ponstan*)** ▶L ♀D ▶- $$$$
  ADULT - Mild to moderate pain, primary dysmenorrhea: 500 mg PO initially, then 250 mg PO q6h prn for ≤1 wk.
  PEDS - >14 yo: use adult dose.
  FORMS - Trade only: Cap 250 mg.

**MELOXICAM (*Mobic, ✦Mobicox*)** ▶L ♀C (D in 3rd trimester) ▶? $
  ADULT - RA/OA: 7.5 mg PO daily. Max dose 15 mg/d.
  PEDS - JRA, ≥2 yo: 0.125 mg/kg PO daily to max of 7.5 mg.
  FORMS - Generic/Trade: Tabs 7.5, 15 mg. Trade only: Suspension 7.5 mg/5 mL (1.5 mg/mL).
  NOTES - Shake susp gently before using. This is not a selective COX-2 inhibitor.

**NABUMETONE (*Relafen*)** ▶L ♀C (D in 3rd trimester) ▶- $$$
  ADULT - RA/OA: Initial: two 500 mg tabs (1000 mg) PO daily. May increase to 1500–2000 mg PO daily or divided bid. Dosages >2000 mg/d have not been studied.
  PEDS - Not approved in children.
  FORMS - Generic only: Tabs 500 & 750 mg.

**NAPROXEN (*Naprosyn, Aleve, Anaprox, EC-Naprosyn, Naprelan*)** ▶L ♀B (D in 3rd trimester) ▶+ $$$
  WARNING - Multiple strengths; see FORMS & write specific product on Rx.
  ADULT - RA/OA, ankylosing spondylitis, pain, dysmenorrhea, acute tendinitis & bursitis, fever: 250–500 mg PO bid. Delayed release: 375–500 mg PO bid (do not crush or chew). Controlled release: 750–1000 mg PO daily. Acute gout: 750 mg PO × 1, then 250 mg PO q8h until the attack subsides. Controlled release: 1000–1500 mg PO × 1, then 1000 mg PO daily until the attack subsides.
  PEDS - JRA: 10–20 mg/kg/d PO divided bid. Max dose 1250 mg/24h. Pain >2 yo: 5–7 mg/kg/dose PO q8–12h.
  UNAPPROVED ADULT - Acute migraine: 750 mg PO × 1, then 250–500 mg PO prn. Migraine prophylaxis, menstrual migraine: 500 mg PO bid beginning 1 d prior to onset of menses and ending on last d of period.
  FORMS - OTC Generic/Trade (Aleve): Tab immediate-release 200 mg. OTC Trade only (Aleve): Capsules & Gelcaps immediate-release 200 mg. Rx Generic/

Trade: Tabs immediate-release (Naprosyn) 250, 375, 500 mg, (Anaprox) 275 mg, 550 mg. Tabs delayed-release enteric coated (EC-Naprosyn) 375, 500 mg. Tabs, controlled-release (Naprelan) 375, 500 mg. Suspension (Naprosyn) 125 mg/5 mL.
  NOTES - All dosing is based on naproxen content; 500 mg naproxen = 550 mg naproxen sodium.

**OXAPROZIN (*Daypro*)** ▶L ♀C (D in 3rd trimester) ▶- $$$
  ADULT - RA/OA: 1200 mg PO daily. Max dose 1800 mg/d or 26 mg/kg/d, whichever is lower.
  PEDS - Not approved in children.
  FORMS - Generic/Trade: Tabs 600 mg, trade scored.

**PIROXICAM (*Feldene, Fexicam*)** ▶L ♀B (D in 3rd trimester) ▶+ $$$
  ADULT - RA/OA: 20 mg PO daily or divided bid.
  PEDS - Not approved in children.
  UNAPPROVED ADULT - Primary dysmenorrhea: 20–40 mg PO daily × 3 d.
  FORMS - Generic/Trade: Caps 10 & 20 mg.

**SULINDAC (*Clinoril*)** ▶L ♀B (D in 3rd trimester) ▶- $$$
  ADULT - RA/OA, ankylosing spondylitis: 150 mg PO bid. Bursitis, tendinitis, acute gout: 200 mg PO bid, decrease after response. Max dose: 400 mg/d.
  PEDS - Not approved in children.
  UNAPPROVED PEDS - JRA: 4 mg/kg/d PO divided bid.
  FORMS - Generic/Trade: Tabs 200 mg. Generic only: Tabs 150 mg.
  NOTES - Sulindac-associated pancreatitis & a potentially fatal hypersensitivity syndrome have occurred.

**TIAPROFENIC ACID (✦*Surgam, Surgam SR*)** ▶K ♀C (D in 3rd trimester) ▶- $$
  ADULT - Canada only. RA or OA: 600 mg PO daily of sustained release, or 300 mg PO bid of regular release. Some OA patients may be maintained on 300 mg/d.
  PEDS - Not approved in children.
  FORMS - Generic/Trade: Tab 300 mg. Trade only: Cap, sustained-release 300 mg. Generic only: Tab 200 mg.
  NOTES - Caution in renal insufficiency. Cystitis has been reported more frequently than with other NSAIDs.

**TOLMETIN (*Tolectin*)** ▶L ♀C (D in 3rd trimester) ▶+ $$$$
  ADULT - RA/OA: 400 mg PO tid to start. Range 600–1800 mg/d PO divided tid.
  PEDS - JRA ≥2 yo: 20 mg/kg/d PO divided tid-qid to start. Range 15–30 mg/kg/d divided tid-qid. Max dose 2g/24h.
  UNAPPROVED PEDS - Pain ≥2 yo: 5–7 mg/kg/dose PO q6–8h. Max dose 2 g/24 h.
  FORMS - Generic/Trade: Tabs 200 (trade scored) & 600 mg. Cap 400 mg.
  NOTES - Rare anaphylaxis.

## ANALGESICS: OPIOID EQUIVALENCY—OVERVIEW*

### Analgesics: Opioid Equivalency—Approximate Equianalgesic

| | IV/SC/IM | PO | | IV/SC/IM | PO |
|---|---|---|---|---|---|
| **Opioid Agonists** | | | | | |
| morphine | 10 mg q3–4h | †30 mg q3–4h; 60 mg q3–4h | oxycodone | not available | 30 mg q3–4h |
| codeine | 75 mg q3–4h | 130 mg q3–4h | oxymorphone | 1 mg q3–4h | n.a. |
| fentanyl | 0.1 mg q1h | n.a. | **Opioid Agonist–Antagonist and Partial Agonist** | | |
| hydromorphone | 1.5 mg q3–4h | 7.5 mg q3–4h | buprenorphine | 0.3–0.4 mg q6–8h | n.a. |
| hydrocodone | not available | 30 mg q3–4h | butorphanol | 2 mg q3–4h | n.a. |
| levorphanol | 2 mg q6–8h | 4 mg q6–8h | nalbuphine | 10 mg q3–4h | n.a. |
| meperidine§ | 100 mg q3h | 300 mg q2–3h | pentazocine | 60 mg q3–4h | 150 mg q3–4h |

†30 mg with around the clock dosing, and 60 mg with a single dose or short-term dosing (ie, the opioid-naïve).
§Doses should be limited to <600 mg/24 h and total duration of use <48 h; not for chronic pain.

### Analgesics: Opioid Equivalency—Recommended starting dose - Adults >50 kg

| | IV/SC/IM | PO | | IV/SC/IM | PO |
|---|---|---|---|---|---|
| **Opioid Agonists** | | | | | |
| morphine | 10 mg q3–4h | 30 mg q3–4h | oxycodone | n.a. | 10 mg q3–4h |
| codeine | 60 mg q2h | 60 mg q3–4h | oxymorphone | 1 mg q3–4h | n.a. |
| fentanyl | 0.1 mg q1h | n.a. | **Opioid Agonist–Antagonist and Partial Agonist** | | |
| hydromorphone | 1.5 mg q3–4h | 6 mg q3–4h | buprenorphine | 0.4 mg q6–8h | n.a. |
| hydrocodone | not available | 10 mg q3–4h | butorphanol | 2 mg q3–4h | n.a. |
| levorphanol | 2 mg q6–8h | 4 mg q6–8h | nalbuphine | 10 mg q3–4h | n.a. |
| meperidine§ | 100 mg q3h | n.r. | pentazocine | n.r. | 50 mg q4–6h |

§Doses should be limited to <600 mg/24 h and total duration of use <48 h; not for chronic pain.

### Analgesics: Opioid Equivalency—Recommended starting dose—Children/Adults 8 to 50 kg

| | IV/SC/IM | PO | | IV/SC/IM | PO |
|---|---|---|---|---|---|
| **Opioid Agonists** | | | | | |
| morphine | 0.1 mg/kg q3–4h | 0.3 mg/kg q3–4h | oxycodone | n.a. | 0.2 mg/kg q3–4h |
| codeine | n.r. | 1 mg/kg q3–4h | oxymorphone | n.r. | n.r. |
| fentanyl | n.r. | n.a. | **Opioid Agonist–Antagonist and Partial Agonist** | | |
| hydromorphone | 0.015 mg/kg q3–4h | 0.06 mg/kg q3–4h | buprenorphine | 0.004 mg/kg q6–8h | n.a. |
| hydrocodone | not available | 0.2 mg/kg q3–4h | butorphanol | n.r. | n.a. |
| levorphanol | 0.02 mg/kg q6–8h | 0.04 mg/kg q6–8h | nalbuphine | 0.1 mg/kg q3–4h | n.a. |
| meperidine§ | 0.75 mg/kg q2–3h | n.r. | pentazocine | n.r. | n.r. |

§Doses should be limited to <600 mg/24 h and total duration of use <48 h; not for chronic pain.

*Approximate dosing, adapted from 1992 AHCPR guidelines, www.ahcpr.gov. IV doses should be titrated slowly with appropriate monitoring. All PO dosing is with immediate-release preparations. Use lower doses initially in those not currently taking opioids. Individualize all dosing, especially in the elderly, children, and patients with chronic pain, opioid tolerance, or hepatic/renal insufficiency. Many recommend initially using lower than equivalent doses when switching between different opioids. Not available = "n.a." Not recommended = "n.r." Methadone is excluded due to poor consensus on equivalence.

## ANALGESICS: Opioid Agonist–Antagonists

**NOTE:** May cause drowsiness and/or sedation, which may be enhanced by alcohol & other CNS depressants. Opioid agonist-antagonists may result in inadequate pain control and/or withdrawal effects in the opioid-dependent. Reserve IM for when alternative routes are not feasible.

**BUPRENORPHINE** (*Buprenex, Subutex*) ▶L ♀C ▶-
©III $ IV, $$$$$ SL
ADULT - Moderate to severe pain: 0.3–0.6 mg IM or slow IV, q6h prn. Max single dose 0.6 mg. Treatment of opioid dependence: Induction 8 mg SL on d 1, 16 mg SL on d 2. Maintenance: 16 mg SL daily. Can individualize to range of 4–24 mg SL daily.
PEDS - Moderate to severe pain: 2–12 yo: 2–6 mcg/kg/dose IM or slow IV q4–6h. Max single dose 6 mcg/kg.
FORMS - Trade only (Subutex): SL tabs 2, 8 mg
NOTES - May cause bradycardia, hypotension & respiratory depression. Concurrent use with diazepam has resulted in respiratory & cardiovascular collapse. For opioid dependence Subutex is preferred over Suboxone for induction. Suboxone preferred for maintenance. Prescribers must complete training and apply for special DEA number. See www.suboxone.com.

**BUTORPHANOL** (*Stadol, Stadol NS*) ▶L ♀C ▶+ ©IV $$$
WARNING - Approved as a nasal spray in 1991 and has been promoted as a safe treatment for migraine headaches. There have been numerous reports of dependence-addiction & major psychological disturbances. These problems have been documented by the FDA. Stadol NS should be used for patients with infrequent but severe migraine attacks for whom all other common abortive treatments have failed. Experts recommend restriction to ≤2 bottles (30 sprays) per mo in patients who are appropriate candidates for this medication.
ADULT - Pain, including post-operative pain: 0.5–2 mg IV q3–4h prn. 1–4 mg IM q3–4h prn. Obstetric pain during labor: 1–2 mg IV/IM at full term in early labor, repeat after 4h. Last resort for migraine pain: 1 mg nasal spray (1 spray in one nostril). If no pain relief in 60–90 min, may give a 2nd spray in the other nostril. Additional doses q3–4h prn.
PEDS - Not approved in children.
FORMS - Generic only: Nasal spray 1 mg/spray, 2.5 mL bottle (14–15 doses/bottle).
NOTES - May increase cardiac workload.

**NALBUPHINE** (*Nubain*) ▶LK ♀? ▶? $
ADULT - Moderate to severe pain: 10–20 mg SC/IM/IV q3–6h prn. Max dose 160 mg/d.
PEDS - Not approved in children.

**PENTAZOCINE** (*Talwin NX*) ▶LK ♀C ▶? ©IV $$$
WARNING - The oral form (Talwin NX) may cause fatal reactions if injected.
ADULT - Moderate to severe pain: Talwin: 30 mg IM/IV q3–4h prn, max dose 360 mg/d. Talwin NX: 1 tab PO q3–4h, max 12 tabs/d.
PEDS - Not approved in children.
FORMS - Generic/Trade: Tab 50 mg with 0.5 mg naloxone, trade scored.
NOTES - Rotate injection sites. Can cause hallucinations, disorientation, and seizures. Concomitant sibutramine may precipitate serotonin syndrome.

## ANALGESICS: Opioid Agonists

**NOTE:** May cause life-threatening respiratory depression. May cause drowsiness and/or sedation, which may be enhanced by alcohol & other CNS depressants. Patients with chronic pain may require more frequent & higher dosing. Opioids commonly create constipation. All opioids are pregnancy class D if used for prolonged periods or in high doses at term.

**CODEINE** ▶LK ♀C ▶- ©II $$
WARNING - Do not use IV in children due to large histamine release and cardiovascular effects. Use in nursing mothers has led to infant death.
ADULT - Mild to moderate pain: 15–60 mg PO/IM/IV/SC q4–6h. Max dose 360 mg in 24 h. Antitussive: 10–20 mg PO q4–6h prn. Max dose 120 mg in 24 h.
PEDS - Mild to moderate pain in ≥1yo: 0.5–1 mg/kg PO/SC/IM q4–6h, max dose 60 mg/dose. Antitussive: 2–5 yo: 2.5–5 mg PO q4–6h prn, max dose: 30 mg/d. 6–12 yo: 5–10 mg PO q4–6h prn, max dose 60 mg/d.
FORMS - Generic only: Tabs 15, 30, & 60 mg. Oral soln: 15 mg/5 mL.

**FENTANYL** (*Duragesic, Actiq, Fentora, Sublimaze, IONSYS*) ▶L ♀C ▶+ ©II $$$$$
WARNING - Duragesic Patches, Actiq, & Fentora are contraindicated in the management of acute or postoperative pain due to potentially life-threatening respiratory depression in opioid non-tolerant patients. Instruct patients and their caregivers that even used patches/lozenges on a stick can be fatal to a child or pet. Dispose via toilet. Actiq & Fentora are not interchangeable. IONSYS: For hospital use only; remove prior to discharge. Can cause life-threatening respiratory depression.
ADULT - Duragesic Patches: Chronic pain: 12.5–100 mcg/h patch q72 h. Titrate dose to the needs of the patient. Some patients require q48 h dosing. May wear more than one patch to achieve the correct analgesic effect. Actiq: Breakthrough cancer pain: 200–1600 mcg sucked over 15 min, if 200 mcg ineffective × 6 units use higher strength. Goal is 4 lozenges on a stick/d in conjunction with long-acting opioid. Buccal tab (Fentora) for breakthrough cancer pain: 100–800 mcg, titrated
**(cont.)**

**FENTANYL** *(cont.)*

to pain relief; may repeat 1x after 30 min during single episode of breakthrough pain. See PI for dose conversion from transmucosal lozenges. Post-operative analgesia: 50–100 mcg IM; repeat in 1–2 h prn. IONSYS: Acute postoperative pain: Specialized dosing.

PEDS - Transdermal (Duragesic): not approved in children <2 yo or in opioid naive. >2 yo: Use adult dosing. Children converting to a 25 mcg patch should be receiving ≥ 45 mg oral morphine equivalents/d. Actiq: not approved <16 yo. IONSYS not approved in children.

UNAPPROVED ADULT - Analgesia/procedural sedation: 50–100 mcg slow IV over 1–2 min; carefully titrate to effect. Analgesia: 50–100 mcg IM q1–2h prn.

UNAPPROVED PEDS - Analgesia: 1–2 mcg/kg/dose IV/IM q30–60 min prn or continuous IV infusion 1–3 mcg/kg/h (not to exceed adult dosing). Procedural sedation: 1 to 3 yo: 2 to 3 mcg/kg/dose; 3 to 12 yo: 1 to 2 mcg/kg/dose; >12 yo: 0.5 to 1 mcg/kg/dose (not to exceed adult dosing); these doses may repeated q30–60 min prn.

FORMS - Generic/Trade: Transdermal patches 12.5, 25, 50, 75, 100 mcg/h. Actiq lozenges on a stick, berry flavored 200, 400, 600, 800, 1,200, 1,600 mcg. Trade only: IONSYS: Iontophoretic transdermal system: 40 mcg fentanyl per activation; max 6 doses per h. Max per system is eighty 40 mcg doses over 24 h. Trade only: (Fentora) buccal tab 100, 200, 300, 400, 600, 800 mcg.

NOTES - Do not use patches for acute pain or in opioid naive patients. Oral transmucosal fentanyl doses of 5 mcg/kg provide effects similar to 0.75–1.25 mcg/kg of fentanyl IM. Lozenges on a stick should be sucked, not chewed. Flush lozenge remnants (without stick) down the toilet. For transdermal systems: apply patch to non-hairy skin. Clip (not shave) hair if you have to apply to hairy area. Fever or external heat sources may increase fentanyl released from patch. Dispose of a used patch by folding with the adhesive side of the patch adhering to itself, then flush it down the toilet immediately upon removal. Do not cut the patch in half. For Duragesic patches and Actiq lozenges on a stick: Titrate dose as high as necessary to relieve cancer pain or other types of non-malignant pain where chronic opioids are necessary. Do not suck, chew or swallow buccal tab. IONSYS: Apply to intact skin on the chest or upper arm. Each dose, activated by the patient, is delivered over a 10-min period. Remove prior to hospital discharge. Do not allow gel to touch mucous membranes. Dispose of using gloves. Keep all forms of fentanyl out of the reach of children or pets. Concomitant use with potent cytochrome P450 3A4 inhibitors such as ritonavir, ketoconazole, itraconazole, troleandomycin, clarithromycin, nelfinavir, and nefazodone may result in an increase in fentanyl plasma concentrations, which could increase or prolong adverse drug effects and may cause potentially fatal respiratory depression.

| **FENTANYL TRANSDERMAL DOSE (Dosing based on ongoing morphine requirement)** | | |
|---|---|---|
| Morphine* (IV/IM) | Morphine* (PO) | Transdermal fentanyl* |
| 8–22 mg/d | 45–134 mg/d | 25 mcg/h |
| 23–37 mg/d | 135–224 mg/d | 50 mcg/h |
| 38–52 mg/d | 225–314 mg/d | 75 mcg/h |
| 53–67 mg/d | 315–404 mg/d | 100 mcg/h |

*For higher morphine doses see product insert for transdermal fentanyl equivalencies.

**HEROIN** ▶LK ♀- ▶? ©I VARIES
ADULT - Drug of abuse
PEDS - Drug of abuse

**HYDROMORPHONE** *(Dilaudid, Dilaudid-5, ✦Hydromorph Contin)* ▶L ♀C ▶? ©II $$
ADULT - Moderate to severe pain: 2–4 mg PO q4–6h. Initial dose (opioid-naive) 0.5–2 mg SC/IM or slow IV q4–6h prn. 3 mg PR q6–8h.
PEDS - Not approved in children.
UNAPPROVED PEDS - Pain ≤12 yo: 0.03–0.08 mg/kg PO q4–6h prn. 0.015 mg/kg/dose IV q4–6h prn. Pain >12 yo: use adult dose.
FORMS - Generic only: Tabs 2, 4 mg. Generic/Trade: Tabs 8 mg (8mg trade scored). Oral solution 5 mg/5 mL. Supp 3 mg.
NOTES - In opioid-naive patients, consider an initial dose of 0.5 mg or less IM/SC/IV. SC/IM/IV doses after initial dose should be individualized. May be given by slow IV injection over 2–5 min. Titrate dose as high as necessary to relieve cancer pain or other types of non-malignant pain where chronic opioids are necessary. 1.5 mg IV = 7.5 mg PO.

**LEVORPHANOL** *(Levo-Dromoran)* ▶L ♀C ▶? ©II $$$$
ADULT - Moderate to severe pain: 2 mg PO q6–8h prn. Increase to 4 mg if necessary.
PEDS - Not approved in children.
FORMS - Generic only: Tabs 2 mg, scored.

**MEPERIDINE** *(Demerol, pethidine)* ▶LK ♀C but + ▶+ ©II $$$
ADULT - Moderate to severe pain: 50–150 mg IM/SC/PO q3–4h prn. OB analgesia: when pains become regular, 50–100 mg IM/SC q1–3h. May also be given slow IV diluted to 10 mg/mL, or by continuous IV infusion diluted to 1 mg/mL.
PEDS - Moderate to severe pain: 1–1.8 mg/kg IM/SC/PO or slow IV (see adult dosing) up to adult dose, q3–4h prn.
FORMS - Generic/Trade: Tabs 50 (trade scored) & 100 mg. Syrup 50 mg/5 mL (trade banana flavored).
NOTES - Avoid in renal insufficiency and in elderly due to risk of metabolite accumulation and increased risk of CNS disturbance and seizures.

**MEPERIDINE** *(cont.)*

Multiple drug interactions including MAOIs & SSRIs. Poor oral absorption/efficacy. 75 mg meperidine IV,IM,SC = 300 mg meperidine PO. Take syrup with ½ glass (4 oz) water. Due to the risk of seizures at high doses, meperidine is not a good choice for treatment of chronic pain. Not recommended in children.

**METHADONE** *(Diskets, Dolophine, Methadose,* ✚*Metadol)* ▶L ♀C ▶? ©II $

WARNING - High doses (mean ~200 mg/d) have been inconclusively associated with arrhythmia (torsade de pointes), particularly in those with pre-existing risk factors. Caution in opioid-naive patients. Elimination half life (8–59 h) far longer than its duration of analgesic action (4–8 h); monitor for respiratory depression & titrate accordingly. Use caution with escalating doses.

ADULT - Severe pain in opioid-tolerant patients: 2.5–10 mg IM/SC/PO q3–4h prn. Opioid dependence: 20–100 mg PO daily.

PEDS - Not approved in children.

UNAPPROVED PEDS - Pain ≤12 yo: 0.7 mg/kg/24h divided q4–6h PO/SC/IM/IV prn. Max 10 mg/dose.

FORMS - Generic/Trade: Tabs 5, 10 mg, Dispersible tabs 40 mg (for opioid dependence only). Oral concentrate (intensol): 10 mg/mL. Generic only: Oral soln 5 & 10 mg/5mL.

NOTES - Titrate dose as high as necessary to relieve cancer pain or other types of non-malignant pain where chronic opioids are necessary. Every 8–12 h dosing may decrease the risk of drug accumulation and overdose. Treatment for opioid dependence >3 wk is maintenance and only permitted in approved treatment programs. Drug interactions leading to decreased methadone levels with enzyme-inducing HIV drugs (eg, efavirenz, nevirapine) and other potent inducers such as rifampin. Monitor for opiate withdrawal symptoms and increase methadone if necessary. Rapid metabolizers may require more frequent daily dosing.

**MORPHINE** *(MS Contin, Kadian, Avinza, Roxanol, Oramorph SR, MSIR, DepoDur,* ✚*Statex, M.O.S., Doloral)* ▶LK ♀C ▶+ ©II $$$$

WARNING - Multiple strengths; see FORMS & write specific product on Rx. Drinking alcohol while taking Avinza or Kadian may result in a rapid release of a potentially fatal dose of morphine.

ADULT - Moderate to severe pain: 10–30 mg PO q4h (immediate-release tabs, or oral soln). Controlled-release (MS Contin, Oramorph SR): 30 mg PO q8–12h. (Kadian): 20 mg PO q12–24h. Extended-release caps (Avinza): 30 mg PO daily. 10 mg q4h IM/SC. 2.5–15 mg/70kg IV over 4–5 min. 10–20 mg PR q4h. Pain with major surgery (DepoDur): 10–15 mg × 1 epidurally at the lumbar level prior to surgery (max dose 20 mg), or 10 mg epidurally after clamping of the umbilical cord with cesarian section.

PEDS - Moderate to severe pain: 0.1–0.2 mg/kg up to 15 mg IM/SC/IV q2–4h.

UNAPPROVED PEDS - Moderate to severe pain: 0.2–0.5 mg/kg/dose PO (immediate release) q4–6h. 0.3–0.6 mg/kg/dose PO q12h (controlled release).

FORMS - Generic/Trade: Tabs, immediate-release 15 & 30 mg. Oral soln: 10 mg/5 mL, 20 mg/5 mL, 20 mg/mL (concentrate). Rectal suppositories 5, 10, 20 & 30 mg. Controlled-release tabs (MS Contin) 15, 30, 60, 100, 200 mg. Trade only: Controlled-release caps (Kadian) 10, 20, 30, 50, 60, 80, 100, 200 mg. , Controlled-release tabs (Oramorph SR) 15, 30, 60, 100 mg. Extended release caps (Avinza) 30, 60, 90, & 120 mg. Generic only: Tabs, immediate-release 10 mg.

NOTES - Titrate dose as high as necessary to relieve cancer pain or other types of non-malignant pain where chronic opioids are necessary. The active metabolites may accumulate in hepatic/renal insufficiency & the elderly leading to increased analgesic & sedative effects. Do not break, chew, or crush MS Contin or Oramorph SR. Kadian & Avinza caps may be opened & sprinkled in applesauce for easier administration, however the pellets should not be crushed or chewed. Doses >1600 mg/d of Avinza contain a potentially nephrotoxic quantity of fumaric acid. Do not mix DepoDur with other medications; do not administer any other medications into epidural space for ≥48 h. Severe opiate overdose with respiratory depression has occurred with intrathecal leakage of DepoDur.

**OXYCODONE** *(Roxicodone, OxyContin, Percolone, OxyIR, OxyFAST,* ✚*Endocodone, Supeudol)* ▶L ♀C ▶- ©II $$$$$

WARNING - Do not Rx Oxycontin tabs on a prn basis. 80 mg tabs for use in opioid-tolerant patients only. Multiple strengths; see FORMS & write specific product on Rx. Do not break, chew, or crush controlled release preparations.

ADULT - Moderate to severe pain: 5 mg PO q4–6h prn. Controlled-release tabs: 10–40 mg PO q12h. (No supporting data for shorter dosing intervals for controlled release tabs.)

PEDS - Not approved in children.

UNAPPROVED PEDS - Pain ≤12 yo: 0.05–0.3 mg/kg/dose q4–6h PO prn to max of 10 mg/dose.

FORMS - Generic/Trade: Immediate-release: Tabs (scored) & caps 5 mg. Tabs 15, 30 mg. Oral soln 5 mg/5 mL. Oral concentrate 20 mg/mL. Generic only: Immediate release tabs 10, 20 mg. Trade only: Controlled-release tabs: 10, 15, 20, 30, 40, 60, 80 mg.

NOTES - Titrate dose as high as necessary to relieve cancer pain or other types of non-malignant pain where chronic opioids are necessary.

**OXYMORPHONE** *(Opana)* ▶L ♀C ▶? ©II $$$$

WARNING - Do not break, chew, dissolve or crush extended release tabs due to a rapid release and absorption of a potentially fatal dose of oxymorphone.

ADULT - Moderate to severe pain: 10–20 mg PO q4–6h (immediate release) or 5 mg q12h

**OXYMORPHONE** (*cont.*)
    (extended release) 1 h before or 2 h after meals.
Titrate q3–7 d until adequate pain relief. 1–1.5 mg
IM/SC q4–6h prn. 0.5 mg IV initial dose in healthy
patients then q4–6h prn, increase dose until pain
adequately controlled.
PEDS - Not approved in children.
FORMS - Trade only: Extended release tabs (Opana
ER) 5, 7.5, 10, 15, 20, 30, 40 mg, Immediate
release tabs (Opana IR) 5, 10 mg.
NOTES - Contraindicated in moderate to severe
hepatic dysfunction. Decrease dose in elderly and
with CrCl <50 mL/min. Avoid alcohol.

**PROPOXYPHENE** (*Darvon-N, Darvon Pulvules*) ▶L ♀C
▶+ ©IV $$
    ADULT - Mild to moderate pain: 65 mg (Darvon)
to 100 mg (Darvon-N) PO q4h prn. Max dose 6
caps/d.
PEDS - Not approved in children.
FORMS - Generic/Trade: Caps 65 mg. Trade only:
Tabs 100 mg (Darvon-N).
NOTES - Caution in renal & hepatic dysfunction. Avoid
in renal insufficiency and in elderly due to risk of
metabolite accumulation, and increased risk of
CNS disturbance, seizures, and QRS prolongation.

---

## ANALGESICS: Opioid Analgesic Combinations

**NOTE:** Refer to individual components for further information. May cause drowsiness and/or sedation, which may
be enhanced by alcohol & other CNS depressants. Opioids, carisoprodol, and butalbital may be habit-forming.
Avoid exceeding 4 g/d of acetaminophen in combination products. Caution people who drink ≥3 alcoholic drinks/d
to limit acetaminophen use to 2.5 g/d due to additive liver toxicity. Opioids commonly cause constipation; con-
current laxatives are recommended. All opioids are pregnancy class D if used for prolonged periods or in high
doses at term.

**ANEXSIA** (hydrocodone + acetaminophen) ▶LK ♀C
▶- ©III $$
    WARNING - Multiple strengths; see FORMS & write
specific product on Rx.
ADULT - Moderate pain: 1 tab PO q4–6h prn.
PEDS - Not approved in children.
FORMS - Generic/Trade: Tabs 5/325, 5/500, 7.5/325,
7.5/650, 10/750 mg hydrocodone/mg acetaminophen, scored.
**CAPITAL WITH CODEINE SUSP** (acetaminophen +
codeine) ▶LK ♀C ▶? ©V $
    ADULT - Moderate pain: 15 mL PO q4h prn.
PEDS - Moderate pain 3–6 yo: 5 mL PO q4–6h prn.
7–12 yo: 10 mL PO q4–6h prn. >12 yo use adult
dose.
FORMS - Generic = oral soln. Trade = susp. Both
codeine 12 mg and acetaminophen 120 mg per 5
mL (trade, fruit punch flavor).
**COMBUNOX** (oxycodone + ibuprofen) ▶L ♀C (D in
3rd trimester) ▶? ©III $$$
    ADULT - Moderate to severe pain: 1 tab PO q6h prn
for ≤7 d. Max dose 4 tabs/24 h.
PEDS - Moderate to severe pain: ≥14 yo: Use adult
dose.
FORMS - Generic/Trade: Tab 5 mg oxycodone/400
mg ibuprofen.
NOTES - For short-term (≤7 d) management of
pain. See NSAIDs-Other subclass warning & indi-
vidual components.
**DARVOCET** (propoxyphene + acetaminophen) ▶L
♀C ▶+ ©IV $$
    WARNING - Multiple strengths; see Forms below &
write specific product on Rx.
ADULT - Moderate pain: 1 tab (100/650 or 100/500)
or 2 tabs (50/325) PO q4h prn.
PEDS - Not approved in children.
FORMS - Generic/Trade: Tabs 50/325 (Darvocet N-50),
100/650 (Darvocet N-100), & 100/500 (Darvocet

A500), mg propoxyphene/mg acetaminophen.
    NOTES - Avoid in renal insufficiency and in elderly
due to risk of metabolite accumulation, and
increased risk of CNS disturbance, seizures, and
QRS prolongation.
**EMPIRIN WITH CODEINE** (aspirin + codeine) (→*292
tab*) ▶LK ♀D ▶- ©III $
    WARNING - Multiple strengths; see FORMS & write
specific product on Rx.
ADULT - Moderate pain: 1–2 tabs PO q4h prn.
PEDS - Not approved in children.
FORMS - Generic only: Tab 325/30 & 325/60 mg
ASA/mg codeine. Empirin brand no longer made.
**FIORICET WITH CODEINE** (acetaminophen +
butalbital + caffeine + codeine) ▶LK ♀C ▶-
©III $$$
    ADULT - Moderate pain: 1–2 caps PO q4h prn, max
dose 6 caps/d.
PEDS - Not approved in children.
FORMS - Generic/Trade: Cap 325 mg acetamino-
phen/50 mg butalbital/40 mg caffeine/30 mg
codeine.
**FIORINAL WITH CODEINE** (aspirin + butalbital + caf-
feine + codeine) (→*Fiorinal C-1/4, Fiorinal C-1/2,
Tecnal C-1/4, Tecnal C-1/2*) ▶LK ♀D ▶- ©III $$$
    ADULT - Moderate pain: 1–2 caps PO q4h prn, max
dose 6 caps/d.
PEDS - Not approved in children.
FORMS - Generic/Trade: Cap 325 mg ASA/50 mg
butalbital/40 mg caffeine/30 mg codeine.
**IBUDONE** (hydrocodone + ibuprofen) ▶LK ♀- ▶?
©III $$$
    ADULT - Moderate pain: 1 tab PO q4–6h prn, max
dose 5 tabs/d.
PEDS - Not approved in children.
FORMS - Generic/Trade: Tab 5/200 mg and 10/200
mg hydrocodone/ibuprofen.
NOTES - See NSAIDs-Other subclass warning.

*LORCET* (hydrocodone + acetaminophen) ▶LK ♀C
▶- ©III $
 WARNING - Multiple strengths; see FORMS & write
 specific product on Rx.
 ADULT - Moderate pain: 1–2 caps (5/500) PO q4–6h
 prn, max dose 8 caps/d. 1 tab PO q4–6h prn
 (7.5/650 & 10/650), max dose 6 tabs/d.
 PEDS - Not approved in children.
 FORMS-Generic/Trade: Caps 5/500 mg, Tabs 7.5/650,
 10/650 mg hydrocodone/acetaminophen.

*LORTAB* (hydrocodone + acetaminophen) ▶LK ♀C
▶- ©III $$
 WARNING - Multiple strengths; see FORMS & write
 specific product on Rx.
 ADULT - Moderate pain: 1–2 tabs 2.5/500 & 5/500
 PO q4–6h prn, max dose 8 tabs/d. 1 tab 7.5/500
 & 10/500 PO q4–6h prn, max dose 5 tabs/d. Elixir
 15 mL PO q4–6h prn, max 6 doses/d.
 PEDS - Not approved in children.
 FORMS - Generic/Trade: Lortab 5/500 (scored),
 Lortab 7.5/500 (trade scored) & Lortab 10/500
 mg hydrocodone/mg acetaminophen. Elixir:
 7.5/500 mg hydrocodone/mg acetaminophen/15
 mL. Trade only: Tabs 2.5/500 mg.

*MAGNACET* (oxycodone + acetaminophen) ▶L ♀C
▶- ©II $$$$
 WARNING - Multiple strengths; see FORMS & write
 specific product on Rx.
 ADULT - Moderate-severe pain: 1–2 tabs PO q6h prn
 (2.5/400). 1 tab PO q6h prn (5/400, 7.5/400, 10/400).
 PEDS - Not approved in children.
 FORMS - Trade only: Tabs 2.5/400, 5/400, 7.5/400,
 10/400 mg oxycodone/acetaminophen.

*MAXIDONE* (hydrocodone + acetaminophen) ▶LK
♀C ▶- ©III $$$
 ADULT - Moderate pain: 1 tab PO q4–6h prn, max
 dose 5 tabs/d.
 PEDS - Not approved in children.
 FORMS - Trade only: Tab 10/750 mg hydrocodone/
 mg acetaminophen.

*MERSYNDOL WITH CODEINE* (acetaminophen +
codeine + doxylamine) ▶LK ♀C ▶? $
 ADULT - Canada only. Headaches, cold symptoms,
 muscle aches, neuralgia: 1–2 tabs PO q4–6h prn.
 Max 12 tabs/24 h.
 PEDS - Not approved in children.
 FORMS - Trade only: OTC tab acetaminophen 325 mg
 + codeine phosphate 8 mg + doxylamine 5 mg.
 NOTES - May be habit-forming. Hepatotoxicity may
 be increased with acetaminophen overdose and
 may be enhanced with concomitant chronic alcohol ingestion.

*NORCO* (hydrocodone + acetaminophen) ▶L ♀C ▶?
©III $$$
 WARNING - Multiple strengths; see FORMS & write
 specific product on Rx.
 ADULT - Moderate to severe pain: 1–2 tabs PO
 q4–6h prn (5/325), max dose 12 tabs/d. 1 tab
 (7.5/325 & 10/325) PO q4–6h prn, max dose 8 &
 6 tabs/d, respectively.
 PEDS - Not approved in children.

 FORMS - Trade only: Tabs 5/325, 7.5/325 & 10/325
 mg hydrocodone/acetaminophen, scored.

*PERCOCET* (oxycodone + acetaminophen) (★*Percocet-
demi, Oxycocet, Endocet*) ▶L ♀C ▶-©II $
 WARNING - Multiple strengths; see FORMS & write
 specific product on Rx.
 ADULT - Moderate-severe pain: 1–2 tabs PO q4–6h
 prn (2.5/325 & 5/325). 1 tab PO q4–6 prn
 (7.5/325, 7.5/500, 10/325 & 10/650).
 PEDS - Not approved in children.
 FORMS - Trade only: Tabs 2.5/325 oxycodone/acet-
 aminophen. Generic/Trade: Tabs 5/325, 7.5/325,
 7.5/500, 10/325, 10/650 mg. Generic only:
 2.5/300, 5/300, 7.5/300, 10/300, 2.5/400, 5/400,
 7.5/400, 10/400, 10/500 mg.

*PERCODAN* (oxycodone + aspirin) (★*Oxycodan,
Endodan*) ▶LK ♀D ▶- ©II $$
 ADULT - Moderate to severe pain: 1 tab PO q6h prn.
 PEDS - Not approved in children.
 FORMS - Generic/Trade: Tab 4.88/325 mg oxycodone/
 ASA (trade scored).

*ROXICET* (oxycodone + acetaminophen) ▶L ♀C ▶-
©II $
 WARNING - Multiple strengths; see FORMS & write
 specific product on Rx.
 ADULT - Moderate to severe pain: 1 tab PO q6h prn.
 Oral soln: 5 mL PO q6h prn.
 PEDS - Not approved in children.
 FORMS - Generic/Trade: Tab 5/325 mg. Cap/Caplet
 5/500 mg. Soln 5/325 per 5 mL, mg oxycodone/
 acetaminophen.

*SOMA COMPOUND WITH CODEINE* (carisoprodol +
aspirin + codeine) ▶L ♀D ▶- ©III $$$
 ADULT - Moderate to severe musculoskeletal pain:
 1–2 tabs PO qid prn.
 PEDS - Not approved in children.
 FORMS - Generic/Trade: Tab 200 mg carisopro-
 dol/325 mg ASA/16 mg codeine.
 NOTES - Refer to individual components. Withdrawal
 with abrupt discontinuation.

*SYNALGOS-DC* (dihydrocodeine + aspirin + caffeine)
▶L ♀C ▶- ©III $
 WARNING - Case reports of prolonged erections
 when taken concomitantly with sildenafil.
 ADULT - Moderate-severe pain: 2 caps PO q4h prn.
 PEDS - Not approved in children.
 FORMS - Trade only: Cap 16 mg dihydroco-
 deine/356.4 mg ASA/30 mg caffeine. "Painpack"
 =12 caps.
 NOTES - Most common use is dental pain. Refer to
 individual components.

*TALACEN* (pentazocine + acetaminophen) ▶L ♀C ▶?
©IV $$$
 ADULT - Moderate pain: 1 tab PO q4h prn.
 PEDS - Not approved in children.
 FORMS - Generic/Trade: Tab 25 mg pentazocine/650
 mg acetaminophen, trade scored.
 NOTES - Serious skin reactions, including erythema
 multiforme & Stevens-Johnson syndrome have
 been reported.

**ANALGESICS—NSAIDs**
- *Salicylic acid derivatives:* aspirin, diflunisal, salsalate, Trilisate.
- *Propionic acids:* flurbiprofen, ibuprofen, ketoprofen, naproxen, oxaprozin.
- *Acetic acids:* diclofenac, etodolac, indomethacin, ketorolac, nabumetone, sulindac, tolmetin.
- *Fenamates:* meclofenamate.
- *Oxicams:* meloxicam, piroxicam.
- *COX-2 inhibitors:* celecoxib.

*If one class fails, consider another.

***TYLENOL WITH CODEINE* (codeine + acetaminophen) (◆*Lenoltec, Emtec, Triatec*) ▶LK ♀C ▶? ©III** (Tabs), V(elixir) $
WARNING - Multiple strengths; see FORMS & write specific product on Rx.
ADULT - Moderate pain: 1–2 tabs PO q4h prn.
PEDS - Moderate pain 3–6 yo: 5 mL PO q4–6h prn. 7–12 yo 10 mL PO q4–6h prn. >12 yo: Use adult dose.
FORMS - Generic only: Tabs Tylenol #2 (15/300). Tylenol with Codeine Elixir 12/120 per 5 mL, mg codeine/mg acetaminophen. Generic/Trade: Tabs Tylenol #3 (30/300), Tylenol #4 (60/300). Canadian forms come with (Lenoltec, Tylenol) or without (Empracet, Emtec) caffeine.
***TYLOX* (oxycodone + acetaminophen) ▶L ♀C ▶- ©II $**
ADULT - Moderate-severe pain: 1 cap PO q6h prn.
PEDS - Not approved in children.
FORMS - Generic/Trade: Cap 5 mg oxycodone/500 mg acetaminophen.
***VICODIN* (hydrocodone + acetaminophen) ▶LK ♀C ▶? ©III $**
WARNING - Multiple strengths; see FORMS & write specific product on Rx.
ADULT - Moderate pain: 5/500 (max dose 8 tabs/d) & 7.5/750 (max dose of 5 tabs/d): 1–2 tabs PO q4–6h prn. 10/660: 1 tab PO q4–6h prn (max of 6 tabs/d).
PEDS - Not approved in children.
FORMS - Generic/Trade: Tabs Vicodin (5/500), Vicodin ES (7.5/750), Vicodin HP (10/660), scored, mg hydrocodone/mg acetaminophen.
***VICOPROFEN* (hydrocodone + ibuprofen) ▶LK ♀- ▶? ©III $$$**

ADULT - Moderate pain: 1 tab PO q4–6h prn, max dose 5 tabs/d.
PEDS - Not approved in children.
FORMS - Generic/Trade: Tab 7.5/200 mg hydrocodone/ibuprofen. Generic only: Tab 2.5/200, 5/200, 10/200 mg.
NOTES - See NSAIDs-Other subclass warning.
***WYGESIC* (propoxyphene + acetaminophen) ▶L ♀C ▶? ©IV $**
ADULT - Moderate pain: 1 tab PO q4h prn.
PEDS - Not approved in children.
FORMS - Generic only: Tab 65 mg propoxyphene/650 mg acetaminophen.
NOTES - Avoid in renal insufficiency and in elderly due to risk of metabolite accumulation, and increased risk of CNS disturbance, seizures, and QRS prolongation.
***XODOL* (hydrocodone + acetaminophen) ▶LK ♀C ▶- ©III $$**
ADULT - Moderate pain: 1 tab PO q4–6 prn, max 6 doses/d.
PEDS - Not approved in children.
FORMS - Trade only: Tabs 5/300, 7.5/300, 10/300 mg hydrocodone/acetaminophen.
***ZYDONE* (hydrocodone + acetaminophen) ▶LK ♀C ▶? ©III $$**
WARNING - Multiple strengths; see FORMS & write specific product on Rx.
ADULT - Moderate pain: 1–2 tabs (5/400) PO q4–6h prn, max dose 8 tabs/d. 1 tab (7.5/400, 10/400) q4–6h prn, max dose 6 tabs/d.
PEDS - Not approved in children.
FORMS - Trade only: Tabs 5/400, 7.5/400, & 10/400 mg hydrocodone/mg acetaminophen.

## ANALGESICS: Opioid Antagonists

**NOTE:** May result in withdrawal in the opioid dependent, including life-threatening withdrawal if administered to neonates born to opioid-dependent mothers. Rare pulmonary edema, cardiovascular instability, hypotension, hypertension, ventricular tachycardia & ventricular fibrillation have been reported in connection with opioid reversal.

**NALOXONE (*Narcan*) ▶LK ♀B ▶? $**
ADULT - Management of opioid overdose: 0.4–2 mg IV. May repeat IV at 2–3 min intervals up to 10 mg. Use IM/SC/ET if IV not available. Intravenous infusion: 2 mg in 500 mL D5W or NS (0.004 mg/mL); titrate according to response. Partial post-operative opioid reversal: 0.1–0.2 mg IV at 2–3 min intervals; repeat IM doses may be required at 1–2 h intervals.

PEDS - Management of opioid overdose: 0.01 mg/kg IV. Give a subsequent dose of 0.1 mg/kg if there is inadequate response. Use IM/SC/ET if IV not available. Partial post-operative opioid reversal: 0.005–0.01 mg IV at 2–3 min intervals.
NOTES - Watch patients for re-emergence of opioid effects.

## ANALGESICS: Other

**ACETAMINOPHEN** (*Tylenol, Panadol, Tempra, parac-etamol, ✦Abenol, Atasol, Pediatrix*) ▶LK ♀B ▶+ $
ADULT - Analgesic/antipyretic: 325–1000 mg PO q4–6h prn. 650 mg PR q4–6h prn. Max dose 4 g/d. OA: extended-release: 2 caplets PO q8h around the clock. Max dose 6 caplets/d.
PEDS - Analgesic/antipyretic: 10–15 mg/kg q4–6h PO/PR prn. Max 5 doses/d.
UNAPPROVED ADULT - OA: 1,000 mg PO qid.
FORMS - OTC: Tabs 325, 500, 650 mg. Chewable Tabs 80 mg. Oral disintegrating Tabs 80, 160 mg. Caps/Gelcaps/Caplet 500 mg. Extended-release caplets 650 mg. Liquid 160 mg/5 mL & 500 mg/15 mL. Infant drops 80 mg/0.8 mL. Suppositories 80, 120, 325, & 650 mg.
NOTES - Risk of hepatotoxicity with chronic use, especially in alcoholics. Caution in those who drink ≥3 drinks/d. Rectal administration may produce lower/less reliable plasma levels.

***CANNIBIS SATIVA L. EXTRACT*** (*✦Sativex*) ▶LK ♀X ▶- $$$$
ADULT - Canada only. Adjunctive treatment for the symptomatic relief of neuropathic pain in multiple sclerosis: Start: 1 spray q4h (max 4 times daily), and titrated upwards as tolerated. Limited experience with >12 sprays/d.
PEDS - Not approved in children.
FORMS - Trade only: Buccal spray, 27 mg/mL delta-9-tetrahydrocannabinol & 25 mg/mL cannabidiol, delivers 100 microliters per actuation, 5.5 mL vials containing up to 51 actuations per vial.
NOTES - Contraindicated in pregnancy, childbearing potential without birth control, history of psychosis, serious heart disease. Contains ethanol. Use cautiously if history of substance abuse.

**CLONIDINE - EPIDURAL** (*Duraclon*) ▶LK ♀C ▶-$$$$$
WARNING - Not recommended for obstetrical, postpartum or peri-operative pain management due to hypotension and bradycardia. Abrupt discontinuation may result in a rapid BP rise.
ADULT - Severe cancer pain in combination with opioids: Specialized epidural dosing.
PEDS - Severe cancer pain in combination with opioids: Specialized epidural dosing.
NOTES - Bradycardia & hypotension common. May be exacerbated by beta-blockers, certain calcium channel blockers and digoxin.

**HYALURONATE** (*Hyalgan, Supartz, ✦Neovisc, Orthovisc*) ▶KL ♀? ▶? $$$$$
WARNING - Do not inject extra-articularly; avoid the synovial tissues & cap. Do not use disinfectants containing benzalkonium chloride for skin preparation.
ADULT - OA (knee): Hyalgan: 2 mL intra-articular injection q wk × 3–5 wk. Supartz: 2.5 mL intra-articular injection q wk × 5 wk. Orthovisc & Neovisc (Canada): 2 mL intra-articular injection

q wk × 3 wk. Inject a local anesthetic SC prior to injections.
PEDS - Not approved in children.
FORMS - Trade only: Hyalgan, Neovisc, Orthovisc: 2 mL vials & prefilled syringes. Supartz: 2.5 mL prefilled syringes.
NOTES - For those who have failed conservative therapy. Caution in allergy to eggs, avian proteins or feathers (except Neovisc - synthetic). Remove synovial fluid or effusion before each injection. Knee pain & swelling most common side effects.

**HYLAN GF-20** (*Synvisc*) ▶KL ♀? ▶? $$$$$
WARNING - Do not inject extra-articularly; avoid the synovial tissues & cap. Do not use disinfectants containing benzalkonium chloride for skin preparation.
ADULT - OA (knee): 2 mL intra-articular injection q wk × 3 wk.
PEDS - Not approved in children.
FORMS - Trade only: 2.25 mL glass syringe w/2 mL drug; 3/pack.
NOTES - For those who have failed conservative therapy. Caution in allergy to eggs, avian proteins or feathers. Remove synovial fluid or effusion before each injection. Knee pain & swelling most common side effects.

**TRAMADOL** (*Ultram, Ultram ER*) ▶KL ♀C ▶- $$$
ADULT - Moderate to moderately severe pain: 50–100 mg PO q4–6h prn. Max dose 400 mg/d. If >75 yo, use <300 mg/d PO in divided doses. If CrCl <30 mL/min, increase the dosing interval to 12 h. If cirrhosis, decrease dose to 50 mg PO q12h. Chronic pain, extended release: 100–300 mg PO daily. Do not use if CrCl <30 mL/min or with severe hepatic dysfunction.
PEDS - Not approved in children <16 yo.
FORMS - Generic/Trade: Tab, immediate-release 50 mg. Trade only: Extended release tabs 100, 200, 300 mg.
NOTES - Contraindicated in acute intoxication with alcohol, hypnotics, centrally acting analgesics, opioids or psychotropic drugs. Seizures and/or serotonin syndrome may occur with concurrent antidepressants, triptans, linezolid, lithium, St John's wort, or enzyme inducing drugs such as ketoconazole & erythromycin; use with caution & adjust dose. Withdrawal symptoms may occur in patients dependent on opioids or with abrupt discontinuation. Overdose treated with naloxone may increase seizures. Carbamazepine decreases tramadol levels. The most frequent side effects are nausea & constipation. ER tabs cannot be crushed, chewed or split.

***WOMEN'S TYLENOL MENSTRUAL RELIEF*** (acetaminophen + pamabrom) ▶LK ♀B ▶+ $
ADULT - Menstrual cramps: 2 caplets PO q4–6h.
PEDS - >12 yo: use adult dose.

**WOMEN'S TYLENOL MENSTRUAL RELIEF (cont.)**
   FORMS - OTC: Caplet 500 mg acetaminophen/25 mg pamabrom (diuretic).
   NOTES - Hepatotoxicity with chronic use, especially in alcoholics.
**ZICONOTIDE (*Prialt*)** ▶Plasma ♀C ▶? $$$$$
   WARNING - Severe psychiatric and neurologic impairment may occur. Monitor for mood changes, hallucinations, or cognitive changes. Contraindicated if history of psychosis.

   ADULT - Severe intractable chronic pain: Specialized intrathecal dosing.
   PEDS - Not approved in children <16 yo.
   NOTES - Contraindicated in patients with history of psychosis, uncontrolled bleeding, spinal canal obstruction or infection at the infusion site. Does not prevent opioid withdrawal; gradually taper while instituting ziconotide therapy. Monitor CK periodically.

## ANESTHESIA: Anesthetics & Sedatives

**ALFENTANIL (*Alfenta*)** ▶L ♀C ▶? ©II $
   ADULT - IV general anesthesia adjunct; specialized dosing.
   PEDS - Not approved in children.
**DESFLURANE (*Suprane*)** ▶Respiratory ♀B ▶+ Varies
   ADULT - General anesthetic gas; specialized dosing.
   PEDS - Not recommended for induction due to high rate of laryngospasm.
   NOTES - Minimum Alveolar Concentration (MAC) 6.0%. Known trigger of malignant hyperthermia; see mhaus.org.
**DEXMEDETOMIDINE (*Precedex*)** ▶LK ♀C ▶? $$$$
   ADULT - ICU sedation <24 h: Load 1 mcg/kg over 10 min followed by infusion 0.2–0.7 mcg/kg/h titrated to desired sedation endpoint.
   PEDS - Not recommended <18 yo.
   NOTES - Alpha 2 adrenergic agonist with sedative properties. Beware of bradycardia and hypotension. Avoid in advanced heart block.
**ENFLURANE (*Ethrane*)** ▶Respiratory/L ♀B ▶? Varies
   ADULT - Rarely-used general anesthetic gas; specialized dosing.
   PEDS - >5 yo: Rarely-used general anesthetic gas; specialized dosing.
   NOTES - Minimum Alveolar Concentration (MAC) 1.68%. Known trigger of malignant hyperthermia; see mhaus.org.
**ETOMIDATE (*Amidate*)** ▶L ♀C ▶? $
   ADULT - Anesthesia induction/rapid sequence intubation: 0.3 mg/kg IV.
   PEDS - Age ≥10 yo: Adult dosing. Age <10 yo: Not approved.
   UNAPPROVED PEDS - Anesthesia induction/rapid sequence intubation: 0.3 mg/kg IV.
   NOTES - Adrenocortical suppression, but rarely of clinical significance.
**HALOTHANE (*Fluothane*)** ▶Respiratory/L ♀C ▶? Varies
   ADULT - Rarely-used general anesthetic gas; specialized dosing.
   PEDS - Rarely-used general anesthetic gas; specialized dosing.
   NOTES - Minimum Alveolar Concentration (MAC) 0.77%. Known trigger of malignant hyperthermia; see mhaus.org.
**ISOFLURANE (*Forane*)** ▶Respiratory ♀C ▶? Varies
   ADULT - General anesthetic gas; specialized dosing.
   PEDS - General anesthetic gas; specialized dosing.
   NOTES - Minimum Alveolar Concentration (MAC) 1.15%. Known trigger of malignant hyperthermia; see mhaus.org.

**KETAMINE (*Ketalar*)** ▶L ♀? ▶? ©III $
   WARNING - Emergence delirium limits value of ketamine in adults; such reactions are rare in children.
   ADULT - Dissociative sedation: 1–2 mg/kg IV over 1–2 min or 4–5 mg/kg IM.
   PEDS - Dissociative sedation: 1–2 mg/kg IV over 1–2 min or 4–5 mg/kg IM.
   NOTES - Raises BP and intracranial pressure; avoid if coronary artery disease, HTN, head or eye injury. Concurrent atropine minimizes hypersalivation; can be combined in same syringe with ketamine for IM use.
**METHOHEXITAL (*Brevital*)** ▶L ♀B ▶? ©IV $
   ADULT - Anesthesia induction: 1–1.5 mg/kg IV.
   PEDS - Anesthesia induction: 6.6–10 mg/kg IM or 25 mg/kg PR.
   UNAPPROVED PEDS - Sedation for diagnostic imaging: 25 mg/kg PR
**MIDAZOLAM (*Versed*)** ▶LK ♀D ▶- ©IV $
   WARNING - Beware of respiratory depression/apnea. Administer with appropriate monitoring.
   ADULT - Sedation/anxiolysis: 0.07–0.08 mg/kg IM (5 mg in average adult); or 1 mg IV slowly q2–3 min up to 5 mg. Anesthesia induction: 0.3–0.35 mg/kg IV over 20–30 sec.
   PEDS - Sedation/anxiolysis: 0.25–1.0 mg/kg to max of 20 mg PO, or 0.1–0.15 mg/kg IM. IV route (6 mo to 5 yo): Initial dose 0.05–0.1 mg/kg IV, then titrated to max 0.6 mg/kg. IV route (6–12 yo): Initial dose 0.025–0.05 mg/kg IV, then titrated to max 0.4 mg/kg.
   UNAPPROVED PEDS - Sedation/anxiolysis: Intranasal 0.2–0.4 mg/kg. Rectal: 0.25–0.5 mg/kg PR. Higher oral dosing: 0.5–0.75 mg/kg PO, max 20 mg/kg. Status epilepticus: Load 0.15 mg/kg IV followed by infusion 1 mcg/kg/min and titrate dose upward q5 min prn.
   FORMS - Oral liquid 2 mg/mL
   NOTES - Use lower doses in the elderly, chronically ill, and those receiving concurrent CNS depressants.
**NITROUS OXIDE (*Entonox*)** ▶Respiratory ♀- ▶? Varies
   ADULT - General anesthetic gas; specialized dosing.
   PEDS - General anesthetic gas; specialized dosing.
   NOTES - Always maintain ≥20% oxygen administration.
**PENTOBARBITAL (*Nembutal*)** ▶LK ♀D ▶? ©II $$
   ADULT - Rarely used; other drugs preferred. Hypnotic: 150–200 mg IM or 100 mg IV at a rate of 50 mg/min, max dose is 500 mg.

**PENTOBARBITAL** (*cont.*)
PEDS - FDA approved for active seizing, but other agents preferred.
UNAPPROVED PEDS - Procedural sedation: 1–6 mg/kg IV, adjusted in increments of 1–2 mg/kg to desired effect, or 2–6 mg/kg IM, max 100 mg. Do not exceed 50 mg/min.
**PROPOFOL** (*Diprivan*) ▶L ♀B ▶- $$$
WARNING - Beware of respiratory depression/apnea. Administer with appropriate monitoring.
ADULT - Anesthesia (<55 yo): 40 mg IV q10 until induction onset (typical 2–2.5 mg/kg). Follow with maintenance infusion generally 100–200 mcg/kg/min. Lower doses in elderly or for sedation. ICU ventilator sedation: infusion 5–50 mcg/kg/min.
PEDS - Anesthesia (≥3 yo): 2.5–3.5 mg/kg IV over 20–30 sec, followed with infusion 125–300 mcg/kg/min. Not recommended if <3 yo or for prolonged ICU use.
UNAPPROVED ADULT - Deep sedation: 1 mg/kg IV over 20–30 sec. Repeat 0.5 mg/kg IV prn. Intubation adjunct: 2.0 to 2.5 mg/kg IV.
UNAPPROVED PEDS - Deep sedation: 1 mg/kg IV (max 40 mg) over 20–30 sec. Repeat 0.5 mg/kg (max 20 mg) IV prn.

NOTES - Avoid with egg or soy allergies. Prolonged infusions may lead to hypertriglyceridemia. Injection pain can be treated or pre-treated with lidocaine 40–50 mg IV.
**REMIFENTANIL** (*Ultiva*) ▶L ♀C ▶? ©II $$
ADULT - IV general anesthesia adjunct; specialized dosing.
PEDS - IV general anesthesia adjunct; specialized dosing.
**SEVOFLURANE** (*Ultane*, ✦*Sevorane*) ▶Respiratory/L ♀B ▶? Varies
ADULT - General anesthetic gas; specialized dosing.
PEDS - General anesthetic gas; specialized dosing.
NOTES - Minimum Alveolar Concentration (MAC) 2.05%. Known trigger of malignant hyperthermia; see mhaus.org.
**SUFENTANIL** (*Sufenta*) ▶L ♀C ▶? ©II $$
ADULT - IV anesthesia adjunct: specialized dosing.
PEDS - IV anesthesia adjunct: specialized dosing.
**THIOPENTAL** (*Pentothal*) ▶L ♀C ▶? ©III $$
ADULT - Anesthesia induction: 3–5 mg/kg IV.
PEDS - Anesthesia induction: 3–5 mg/kg IV.
UNAPPROVED PEDS - Sedation for diagnostic imaging: 25 mg/kg PR
NOTES - Duration 5 min. Hypotension, histamine release, tissue necrosis with extravasation.

## ANESTHESIA: Local Anesthetics

**ARTICAINE** (*Septocaine, Zorcaine*) ▶LK ♀C ▶? $
ADULT - Dental local anesthesia: 4% injection.
PEDS - Dental local anesthesia and ≥4 yo: 4% injection.
FORMS - 4% (includes epinephrine 1:100,000)
NOTES - Do not exceed 7 mg/kg total dose
**BUPIVACAINE** (*Marcaine, Sensorcaine*) ▶LK ♀C ▶? $
ADULT - Local anesthesia, nerve block: 0.25% injection.
PEDS - Not recommended in children <12 yo.
FORMS - 0.25%, 0.5%, 0.75%, all with or without epinephrine.
NOTES - Onset 5 min, duration 2–4h (longer with epi). Amide group. Max dose 2.5 mg/kg alone, or 3.0 mg/kg with epinephrine.
**CHLOROPROCAINE** (*Nesacaine*) ▶LK ♀C ▶? $
ADULT - Local and regional anesthesia: 1%-3% injection.
PEDS - Local and regional anesthesia if ≥3 yo: 1%-3% injection.
FORMS - 1, 2, 3%.
NOTES - Max local dose: 11 mg/kg
*DUOCAINE* (bupivacaine + lidocaine - local anesthetic) ▶LK ♀C ▶? $
ADULT - Local anesthesia, nerve block for eye surgery.
PEDS - Not recommended in children <12 yo.
FORMS - Vials contain bupivacaine 0.375% + lidocaine 1%.
NOTES - Use standard precautions including max dosing without epi for both bupivacaine and lidocaine.

**LIDOCAINE - LOCAL ANESTHETIC** (*Xylocaine*) ▶LK ♀B ▶? $
ADULT - Local anesthesia: 0.5–1% injection.
PEDS - Local anesthesia: 0.5–1% injection.
FORMS - 0.5,1,1.5,2%. With epi: 0.5,1,1.5,2%.
NOTES - Onset <2 min, duration 30–60 min (longer with epi). Amide group. Potentially toxic dose 3–5 mg/kg without epinephrine, and 5–7 mg/kg with epinephrine. Use "cardiac lidocaine" (ie, IV formulation) for Bier blocks at max dose of 3 mg/kg so that neither epinephrine nor methylparaben are injected IV.
**MEPIVACAINE** (*Carbocaine, Polocaine*) ▶LK ♀C ▶? $
ADULT - Nerve block: 1%–2% injection.
PEDS - Nerve block: 1%–2% injection. Use <2% concentration if <3 yo or <30 pounds.
FORMS - 1,1.5,2,3%.
NOTES - Onset 3–5 min, duration 45–90 min. Amide group. Max local dose 5 to 6 mg/kg.
*ORAQUIX* (prilocaine + lidocaine - local anesthetic) ▶LK ♀B ▶? $$
ADULT - Local anesthetic gel applied to periodontal pockets using blunt-tipped applicator: 4% injection.
PEDS - Not approved in children.
FORMS - Gel 2.5% + 2.5% with applicator.
NOTES - Do not exceed max dose for lidocaine or prilocaine.
**PRILOCAINE** (*Citanest*) ▶LK ♀B ▶? $
ADULT - Nerve block and dental procedures: 4% injection.
PEDS - Nerve block and dental procedures, age >9 mo: 4% injection.

(cont.)

**PRILOCAINE** (cont.)
FORMS - 4%, 4% with epinephrine
NOTES - Contraindicated if <6–9 mo old. If <5 yo, max local dose is 3–4 mg/kg (with or without epinephrine). If ≥5 yo, max local dose is 5 mg/kg without epinephrine and 7 mg/kg with epinephrine.

**PROCAINE** (*Novocain*) ▶Plasma ♀C ▶? $
ADULT - Local & regional anesthesia: 1-2% injection. Spinal anesthesia: 10%.
PEDS - Local & regional anesthesia: 1-2% injection. Spinal anesthesia: 10%.
FORMS - 1, 2, 10%.

**ROPIVACAINE** (*Naropin*) ▶LK ♀B ▶? $
WARNING - Inadvertent intravascular injection may result in arrhythmia or cardiac arrest.
ADULT - Local and regional anesthesia: 0.2%-1% injection.
PEDS - Not approved in children.
FORMS - 0.2, 0.5, 0.75, 1%.

**TETRACAINE** (*Pontocaine*, ✦*amethocain*) ▶Plasma ♀C ▶? $
ADULT - Spinal anesthesia
PEDS - Not approved in children.
FORMS - 0.2, 0.3, 1%.

<hr>

## ANESTHESIA: Neuromuscular Blockers

**NOTE:** Should be administered only by those skilled in airway management and respiratory support.

**ATRACURIUM** (*Tracrium*) ▶Plasma ♀C ▶? $
ADULT - Paralysis: 0.4–0.5 mg/kg IV.
PEDS - Paralysis ≥2 yo: 0.4–0.5 mg/kg IV.
NOTES - Duration 15–30 min. Hoffman degradation.

**CISATRACURIUM** (*Nimbex*) ▶Plasma ♀B ▶? $$
ADULT - Paralysis: 0.15–0.2 mg/kg IV.
PEDS - Paralysis: 0.1 mg/kg IV over 5–10 sec.
NOTES - Duration 30–60 min. Hoffman degradation.

**PANCURONIUM** (*Pavulon*) ▶LK ♀C ▶? $
ADULT - Paralysis: 0.04 to 0.1 mg/kg IV.
PEDS - Paralysis (beyond neonatal age): 0.04 to 0.1 mg/kg IV.
NOTES - Duration 45 min. Decrease dose if renal disease.

**ROCURONIUM** (*Zemuron*) ▶L ♀B ▶? $$
ADULT - Paralysis: 0.6 mg/kg IV. Rapid sequence intubation: 0.6 to 1.2 mg/kg IV. Continuous infusion: 10 to 12 mcg/kg/min; first verify spontaneous recovery from bolus dose.
PEDS - Paralysis (age >3 mo): 0.6 mg/kg IV. Continuous infusion: 12 mcg/kg/min; first verify spontaneous recovery from bolus dose.
NOTES - Duration 30 min. Decrease dose if severe liver disease.

**SUCCINYLCHOLINE** (*Anectine, Quelicin*) ▶Plasma ♀C ▶? $
ADULT - Paralysis: 0.6–1.1 mg/kg IV.

PEDS - Paralysis (≥5 yo): 1 mg/kg IV. Paralysis (<5 yo): 2 mg/kg IV.
NOTES - Avoid in hyperkalemia, myopathies, eye injuries, rhabdomyolysis, subacute burn, and syndromes of denervated or disused musculature (eg, paralysis from spinal cord injury or major stroke). If immediate cardiac arrest and ET tube is in correct place & no tension pneumo evident, strongly consider empiric treatment for hyperkalemia. Succinylcholine can trigger malignant hyperthermia; see www.mhaus.org.

**VECURONIUM** (*Norcuron*) ▶LK ♀C ▶? $
ADULT - Paralysis: 0.08–0.1 mg/kg IV bolus. Continuous infusion: 0.8 to 1.2 mcg/kg/min; first verify spontaneous recovery from bolus dose.
PEDS - Paralysis (age ≥10 yr): 0.08–0.1 mg/kg IV bolus. Continuous infusion: 0.8 to 1.2 mcg/kg/min; first verify spontaneous recovery from bolus dose. Age 1–10 yr: may require a slightly higher initial dose and may also require supplementation slightly more often than older patients. Age 7 wk to 1 yr: moderately more sensitive on a mg/kg dose compared to adults and take 1.5 × longer to recover. Age <7 wk: Safety has not been established.
NOTES - Duration 15–30 min. Decrease dose in severe liver disease.

<hr>

## ANTIMICROBIALS: Aminoglycosides

**NOTE:** See also dermatology and ophthalmology

**AMIKACIN** (*Amikin*) ▶K ♀D ▶? $$$
WARNING - Nephrotoxicity, ototoxicity.
ADULT - Gram negative infections: 15 mg/kg/d up to 1500 mg/d IM/IV divided q8–12h. Peak 20–35 mcg/mL, trough <5 mcg/mL.
PEDS - Gram negative infections: 15 mg/kg/d up to 1500 mg/d IM/IV divided q8–12h. Neonates: 10 mg/kg load, then 7.5 mg/kg IM/IV q12h.
UNAPPROVED ADULT - Once daily dosing: 15 mg/kg IV q24h. TB (2nd-line treatment): 15 mg/kg up to 1 g IM/IV daily. 10 mg/kg up to 750 mg IM/IV daily if >59 yo.

UNAPPROVED PEDS - Severe infections: 15–22.5 mg/kg/d IV divided q8h. Some experts recommend 30 mg/kg/d. Once daily dosing: 15 mg/kg IV q24h. Some experts consider once-daily dosing of aminoglycosides investigational in children. TB (2nd-line treatment): 15–30 mg/kg up to 1 g IM/IV daily.
NOTES - May enhance effects of neuromuscular blockers. Avoid other ototoxic/nephrotoxic drugs. Individualize dose in renal dysfunction, burn patients. Base dose on average of actual and ideal body weight in obesity.

**GENTAMICIN (***Garamycin***)** ▶K ♀D ▶+ $
WARNING - Nephrotoxicity, ototoxicity.
ADULT - Gram negative infections: 3–5 mg/kg/d IM/
IV divided q8h. Peak 5–10 mcg/mL, trough <2
mcg/mL. See table for prophylaxis of bacterial
endocarditis.
PEDS - Gram negative infections: 2–2.5 mg/kg IM/
IV q8h. Infants ≥1 wk old, >2 kg: 2.5 mg/kg IM/
IV q8h. Infants <1 wk old, >2 kg: 2.5 mg/kg IM/
IV q12h. Cystic fibrosis: 9 mg/kg/d IV in divided
doses with target peak of 8–12 mcg/mL.
UNAPPROVED ADULT - Once daily dosing for
gram negative infections: 5–7 mg/kg IV q24h.
Endocarditis: 3 mg/kg/d for synergy with another
agent. Give once daily for viridans streptococci,
2–3 divided doses for staphylococci, 3 divided
doses for enterococci.
UNAPPROVED PEDS - Once daily dosing: 5–7 mg/
kg IV q24h. Age <1 wk and full-term: 4 mg/kg IV
q24h. Some experts consider once-daily dosing of
aminoglycosides investigational in children.
NOTES - May enhance effects of neuromuscular
blockers. Avoid other ototoxic/nephrotoxic drugs.
Individualize dose in renal dysfunction, burn
patients. Base dose on average of actual and
ideal body weight in obesity.

**STREPTOMYCIN** ▶K ♀D ▶+ $$$$$
WARNING - Nephrotoxicity, ototoxicity. Monitor audi-
ometry, renal function, and electrolytes.
ADULT - Combined therapy for TB: 15 mg/kg up to 1
g IM/IV daily. 10 mg/kg up to 750 mg IM/IV daily
if >59 yo.
PEDS - Combined therapy for TB: 20–40 mg/kg up
to 1 g IM daily.
UNAPPROVED ADULT - Same IM dosing can be given
IV. *Streptococcal endocarditis:* 7.5 mg/kg IV/
IM bid. Go to www.americanheart.org for further
info.

NOTES - Contraindicated in pregnancy. Obtain baseline audiogram, vestibular and Romberg testing,
and renal function. Monitor renal function and
vestibular and auditory symptoms monthly. May
enhance effects of neuromuscular blockers. Avoid
other ototoxic/nephrotoxic drugs. Individualize
dose in renal dysfunction.

**TOBRAMYCIN (***Nebcin, TOBI***)** ▶K ♀D ▶? $$
WARNING - Nephrotoxicity, ototoxicity.
ADULT - Gram negative infections: 3–5 mg/kg/d IM/
IV divided q8h. Peak 5–10 mcg/mL, trough <2
mcg/mL. Parenteral for cystic fibrosis: 10 mg/
kg/d IV divided q6h with target peak of 8–12
mcg/mL. Nebulized for cystic fibrosis (TOBI): 300
mg neb bid 28 d on, then 28 d off.
PEDS - Gram negative infections: 2–2.5 mg/kg
IV q8h or 1.5–1.9 mg/kg IV q6h. Premature/
full-term neonates ≤1 wk old: Up to 4 mg/
kg/d divided q12h. Parenteral for cystic fibro-
sis: 10 mg/kg/d IV divided q6h with target peak
of 8–12 mcg/mL. Nebulized for cystic fibrosis
(TOBI) ≥6 yo: 300 mg neb bid 28 d on, then
28 d off.
UNAPPROVED ADULT - Once daily dosing: 5–7 mg/
kg IV q24h.
UNAPPROVED PEDS - Once daily dosing: 5–7 mg/
kg IV q24h. Some experts consider once-daily
dosing of aminoglycosides investigational in
children.
FORMS - Trade only: TOBI 300 mg ampules for
nebulizer.
NOTES - May enhance effects of neuromuscular
blockers. Avoid other ototoxic/nephrotoxic drugs.
Individualize dose in renal dysfunction, burn
patients. Base dose on average of actual and
ideal body weight in obesity. Routine monitoring
of tobramycin levels not required with nebulized
TOBI.

## ANTIMICROBIALS: Antifungal Agents—Azoles

**CLOTRIMAZOLE (***Mycelex, ✦Canesten, Clotrimaderm***)**
▶L ♀C ▶? $$$$
ADULT - Oropharyngeal candidiasis: 1 troche dis-
solved slowly in mouth 5x/d × 14 d. Prevention
of oropharyngeal candidiasis in immunocom-
promised patients: 1 troche dissolved slowly in
mouth tid until end of chemotherapy/high-dose
corticosteroids.
PEDS - Oropharyngeal candidiasis ≥3 yo: Use adult
dose.
FORMS - Generic/Trade: Oral troches 10 mg.

**FLUCONAZOLE (***Diflucan***)** ▶K ♀C ▶+ $$$$
ADULT - Vaginal candidiasis: 150 mg PO sin-
gle dose ($). All other dosing regimens IV/PO.
Oropharyngeal/esophageal candidiasis: 200 mg
first d, then 100 mg daily for ≥14 d for oropharyn-
geal, ≥3 wk & continuing for 2 wk past symptom
resolution for esophageal. Systemic candidiasis:
400 mg daily. Candidal UTI, peritonitis: 50–200

mg daily. Cryptococcal meningitis: 400 mg daily
until 10–12 wk after cerebrospinal fluid is culture
negative (see UNAPPROVED ADULT for first-line
regimen). Suppression of cryptococcal meningi-
tis relapse in AIDS: 200 mg daily until immune
system reconstitution. Prevention of candidia-
sis after bone marrow transplant: 400 mg daily
starting several d before neutropenia and contin-
uing until ANC >1000 cells/mm³ × 7 d.
PEDS - All dosing regimens IV/PO. Oropharyngeal/
esophageal candidiasis: 6 mg/kg first d, then 3
mg/kg daily for ≥14 d for oropharyngeal, ≥3
wk & continuing for 2 wk past symptom resolu-
tion for esophageal. Systemic candidiasis: 6–12
mg/kg daily. Cryptococcal meningitis: 12 mg/
kg on first d, then 6 mg/kg daily until 10–12
wk after cerebrospinal fluid is culture negative.
Suppression of cryptococcal meningitis relapse in
AIDS: 6 mg/kg daily.

**(cont.)**

**FLUCONAZOLE** (cont.)

UNAPPROVED ADULT - Onychomycosis, fingernail (2nd line to itraconazole or terbinafine): 150–300 mg PO q wk × 3–6 mo. Onychomycosis, toenail (2nd line to itraconazole or terbinafine): 150–300 mg PO q wk × 6–12 mo. Recurrent vaginal candidiasis: 150 mg PO every third d × 3 doses, then 100–150 mg PO q wk × 6 mo. Non-neutropenic candidemia: 400–800 mg/d IV/PO or 800 mg/d + amphotericin B 0.7 mg/kg/d IV for first 4–7 d. Treat until 14 d past last + blood culture and signs/symptoms resolved. Neutropenic candidemia: 6–12 mg/kg/d IV/PO until 14 d past last + blood culture, signs/symptoms, and neutropenia resolved. Prevention of candidal infections in high-risk neutropenic pts: 400 mg/d during period of risk for neutropenia. Cryptococcal meningitis: Amphotericin B preferably in combo with flucytosine × ≥2 wk (induction), followed by fluconazole 400 mg PO once daily × 8 wk (consolidation), then chronic suppression with fluconazole 200 mg PO once daily until immune system reconstitution.

UNAPPROVED PEDS - Cryptococcal meningitis: Amphotericin B preferably in combo with flucytosine × 2 wk (induction), followed by fluconazole 5–6 mg/kg IV/PO bid × ≥8 wk (consolidation), then chronic suppression with lower dose of fluconazole.

FORMS - Generic/Trade: Tabs 50, 100, 150, 200 mg. 150 mg tab in single-dose blister pack. Susp 10 & 40 mg/mL (35 mL).

NOTES - Hepatotoxicity. Many drug interactions, including increased levels of cyclosporine, phenytoin, theophylline, and increased INR with warfarin. Do not use with cisapride. May inhibit metabolism of fluvastatin, and possibly simvastatin/lovastatin at higher doses. Dosing in renal dysfunction: Reduce maintenance dose by 50% for CrCl 11–50 mL/min. Hemodialysis: Give recommended dose after each dialysis. Single dose during 1st trimester of pregnancy does not appear to increase risk of congenital birth defects.

**ITRACONAZOLE** (*Sporanox*) ▶L ♀C ▶- $$$$$

WARNING - Inhibition of CYP 3A4 metabolism by itraconazole can lead to dangerously high levels of some drugs. High levels of some can prolong QT interval (see QT drugs table). Contraindicated with cisapride, dofetilide, ergot alkaloids, lovastatin, PO midazolam, pimozide, quinidine, simvastatin, triazolam. Negative inotrope; stop treatment if signs/symptoms of heart failure. Not for onychomycosis if heart failure; use for other indications in heart failure only if benefit exceeds risk.

ADULT - Caps - Take caps with full meal. Onychomycosis, toenails: 200 mg PO daily × 12 wk. Onychomycosis "pulse dosing", fingernails: 200 mg PO bid for 1st wk of mo × 2 mo. Test nail specimen to confirm diagnosis before prescribing. Aspergillosis in patients intolerant/refractory

to amphotericin, blastomycosis, histoplasmosis: 200 mg PO bid or daily. Treat for ≥3 mo. For life-threatening infections, load with 200 mg PO tid × 3 d. Oral soln - Swish & swallow in 10 mL increments on empty stomach. Oropharyngeal candidiasis: 200 mg daily × 1–2 wk. Oropharyngeal candidiasis unresponsive to fluconazole: 100 mg bid. Esophageal candidiasis: 100–200 mg daily × ≥3 wk & continuing for 2 wk past symptom resolution.

PEDS - Not approved in children.

UNAPPROVED ADULT - Caps - Onychomycosis "pulse dosing", toenails: 200 mg PO bid for 1st wk of mo × 3–4 mo. Confirm diagnosis with nail specimen lab testing before prescribing.

UNAPPROVED PEDS - Caps for systemic fungal infections, 3–16 yo: 100 mg PO daily. Oropharyngeal candidiasis: Oral solution 2.5 mg/kg PO bid (max 200–400 mg/d) × 7–14 d. Esophageal candidiasis: Oral solution 2.5 mg/kg PO bid or 5 mg/kg PO once daily for minimum of 14–21 d. Caps usually ineffective for esophageal candidiasis.

FORMS - Generic/Trade: Cap 100 mg. Trade only: Oral soln 10 mg/mL (150 mL).

NOTES - Hepatotoxicity, even during 1st wk of therapy. Monitor LFTs if hepatic history; consider monitoring in all. Decreased absorption of itraconazole with antacids, H2 blockers, proton pump inhibitors, or achlorhydria. Itraconazole levels reduced by carbamazepine, isoniazid, nevirapine, phenobarbital, phenytoin, rifabutin & rifampin, and potentially efavirenz. Itraconazole inhibits cytochrome P450 3A4 metabolism of many drugs. Not more than 200 mg bid of itraconazole with unboosted indinavir. May increase adverse effects with trazodone; consider reducing trazodone dose. May increase QT interval with disopyramide or halofantrine. Caps and oral soln not interchangeable. Oral soln may be preferred in serious infections due to greater absorption. Oral soln may not achieve adequate levels in cystic fibrosis patients; consider alternative if no response. Start therapy for onychomycosis on d 1–2 of menses in women of childbearing potential & advise against pregnancy until 2 mo after therapy ends.

**KETOCONAZOLE** (*Nizoral*) ▶L ♀C ▶? + $$$

WARNING - Hepatotoxicity: inform patients of risk & monitor. Do not use with cisapride, midazolam, pimozide, triazolam.

ADULT - Systemic fungal infections: 200–400 mg PO daily.

PEDS - Systemic fungal infections, ≥2 yo: 3.3–6.6 mg/kg PO daily.

UNAPPROVED ADULT - Tinea versicolor: 400 mg PO single dose or 200 mg PO daily × 7 d. Prevention of recurrent mucocutaneous candidiasis in HIV infection: 200 mg PO daily.

UNAPPROVED PEDS - Prevention of recurrent mucocutaneous candidiasis in HIV infection: 5–10 mg/kg/d PO daily or bid; max 400 mg bid.

**KETOCONAZOLE** *(cont.)*
FORMS - Generic/Trade: Tabs 200 mg.
NOTES - Antacids, H2 blockers, proton pump inhibitors, buffered didanosine, achlorhydria decrease absorption. Ketoconazole levels reduced by isoniazid, rifampin, and potentially efavirenz. Avoid >200 mg/d of ketoconazole with ritonavir or Kaletra. Ketoconazole inhibits cytochrome P450 3A4 metabolism of many drugs. May increase adverse effects with trazodone; consider reducing trazodone dose.

**POSACONAZOLE** *(Noxafil)* ▶Glucuronidation ♀C
▶- $$$$$
ADULT - Prevention of invasive Aspergillus or candida infection: 200 mg (5 mL) PO tid. Take with full meal or liquid nutritional supplement.
PEDS - Prevention of invasive Aspergillus or Candida infection, ≥13 yo: 200 mg (5 mL) PO tid. Take with full meal or liquid nutritional supplement.
UNAPPROVED ADULT - Invasive pulmonary aspergillosis: 200 mg PO qid, then 400 mg PO bid when stable. Treat invasive pulmonary aspergillosis for ≥6–12 wk; treat immunosuppressed patients throughout immunosuppression and until lesions resolved.
FORMS - Trade only: Oral susp 40 mg/mL, 105 mL bottle.
NOTES - Consider alternative or monitor for breakthrough fungal infection if patient cannot take with a full meal or liquid nutritional supplement. Monitor for breakthrough fungal infection if severe vomiting/diarrhea. CYP 3A4 inhibitor. Contraindicated with ergot alkaloids and CYP 3A4 substrates that increase the QT interval, including cisapride, pimozide, halofantrine, and quinidine. Consider dosage reduction of vinca alkaloids, calcium channel blockers, lovastatin, simvastatin. Posaconazole levels reduced by rifabutin, phenytoin, and cimetidine; phenytoin and rifabutin levels increased by posaconazole. Do not coadminister unless benefit exceeds risk. Monitor for rifabutin adverse effects. Reduce cyclosporine dose by 25% and tacrolimus dose by 66% when posaconazole started. Monitor levels of cyclosporine, tacrolimus, sirolimus. Monitor for benzodiazepine adverse effects and consider dosage reduction. Increased LFTs and possible hepatotoxicity.

**VORICONAZOLE** *(Vfend)* ▶L ♀D ▶? $$$$$
ADULT - Dilute IV to ≤5 mg/mL and infuse at ≤3 mg/kg/h over 1–2 h. Invasive aspergillosis, or Scedosporium, Fusarium infections: 6 mg/kg IV q12h × 2 doses, then 4 mg/kg IV q12h. When PO tolerated, give 200 mg PO q12h if >40 kg or 100 mg PO q12h if <40 kg. Treat invasive pulmonary aspergillosis for ≥6–12 wk; treat immunosuppressed patients throughout immunosuppression and until lesions resolved. Candidemia in non-neutropenic patients, deep tissue Candida infections: 6 mg/kg IV q12h × 2 doses, then 3–4 mg/kg IV q12h. Treat for ≥2 wk past symptom resolution or last positive culture, whichever

is longer. When PO tolerated, give 200 mg PO q12h if >40 kg or 100 mg PO q12h if <40 kg. Coadministration with efavirenz: voriconazole 400 mg PO bid & efavirenz 300 mg (use caps) PO once daily. See package insert for dosage adjustments due to poor response/adverse effects. Esophageal candidiasis: 200 mg PO q12h if ≥40 kg; 100 mg PO q12h if <40 kg for ≥2 wk and continuing for >1 wk past symptom resolution. Take tabs/susp 1 h before/after meals.
PEDS - Safety & efficacy not established in children <12 yo. Use adult dose if ≥12 yo.
UNAPPROVED ADULT - Invasive aspergillosis, continuation after IV therapy: 4 mg/kg PO q12h; round dose up to convenient tab size. Treat invasive pulmonary aspergillosis for ≥6–12 wk; treat immunosuppressed patients throughout immunosuppression and until lesions resolved.
UNAPPROVED PEDS - Invasive aspergillosis: 5–7 mg/kg IV every 12 h. Invasive aspergillosis, 12–18 yo: 6 mg/kg IV q12h × 2, then 4 mg/kg IV q12h.
FORMS - Trade only: Tabs 50,200 mg (contains lactose), susp 40 mg/mL (75mL).
NOTES - Anaphylactoid reactions (IV only), severe skin reactions & photosensitivity, hepatotoxicity rarely. Transient visual disturbances common; advise against hazardous tasks (if vision impaired), night driving & strong, direct sunlight. Monitor visual (if treated >28 d), liver, and renal function. Monitor pancreatic function if at risk for acute pancreatitis (recent chemotherapy/bone marrow transplant). Many drug interactions. Substrate & inhibitor of CYP 2C9, 2C19, & 3A4. Do not use with carbamazepine, cisapride, ergot alkaloids, lopinavir-ritonavir (Kaletra), phenobarbital, pimozide, quinidine, rifabutin, rifampin, ritonavir 400 mg bid, sirolimus, or St John's wort. Ritonavir decreases voriconazole levels; avoid together unless benefit exceeds risk. Dosage adjustments with cyclosporine, omeprazole, phenytoin, tacrolimus in package insert. Increased INR with warfarin. Could inhibit metabolism of benzodiazepines, calcium channel blockers, statins, and methadone. When combining voriconazole with oral contraceptives monitor for adverse effects based on increased levels of voriconazole, estrogen, and progestin. Do not infuse IV voriconazole at same time as a blood product/ concentrated electrolytes even if given by separate IV lines. IV voriconazole can be infused at the same time as non-concentrated electrolytes/total parenteral nutrition if given by separate lines; give TPN by different port if multi-lumen catheter is used. Vehicle in IV form may accumulate in renal impairment; oral preferred if CrCl <50 mL/min. Mild/moderate cirrhosis (Child-Pugh class A/B): Same loading dose & reduce maintenance dose by 50%. Oral susp stable for 14 d at room temperature.

## ANTIMICROBIALS: Antifungal Agents—Echinocandins

**ANIDULAFUNGIN (*Eraxis*)** ▶Degraded chemically ♀C ▶? $$$$$
ADULT - Candidemia, other systemic candidal infections: 200 mg IV load on d 1, then 100 mg IV once daily until ≥14 d after last positive culture. *Esophageal candidiasis*: 100 mg IV load on d 1, then 50 mg IV once daily for ≥14 d and continuing for ≥7 d after symptoms resolved. Max infusion rate of 1.1 mg/min.
PEDS - Not approved in children.
NOTES - Max infusion rate of 1.1 mg/min to prevent histamine reactions. Diluent contains dehydrated alcohol.

**CASPOFUNGIN (*Cancidas*)** ▶KL ♀C ▶? $$$$$
ADULT - Infuse IV over 1 h. Aspergillosis, candidemia, empiric therapy in febrile neutropenia: 70 mg loading dose on d 1, then 50 mg once daily. Patients taking rifampin: 70 mg once daily. Consider this dose with other enzyme inducers (such as carbamazepine, dexamethasone, efavirenz, nevirapine, phenytoin) or if inadequate response to lower dose in febrile neutropenia or aspergillosis. Esophageal candidiasis: 50 mg daily. Duration of therapy in invasive aspergillosis is based on severity, treatment response, and resolution of immunosuppression. Treat Candidal infections for ≥14 d after last positive culture. Empiric therapy of febrile neutropenia: Treat until neutropenia resolved. If fungal infection confirmed, treat for ≥14 d and continue treatment for ≥7 d after symptoms and neutropenia resolved.
PEDS - Infuse IV over 1 h. Aspergillosis, candidemia, esophageal candidiasis, empiric therapy in febrile neutropenia, 3 mo-17 yo: 70 mg/m² loading dose on d 1, then 50 mg/m² once daily. Consider increasing daily dose to 70 mg/m² up to max of 70 mg once daily if coadministered with enzyme inducers (such as carbamazepine,

dexamethasone, efavirenz, nevirapine, phenytoin, or rifampin) or if inadequate response to lower dose in febrile neutropenia or aspergillosis. Duration of therapy in invasive aspergillosis is based on severity, treatment response, and resolution of immunosuppression. Treat Candidal infections for ≥14 d after last positive culture. Empiric therapy of febrile neutropenia: Treat until neutropenia resolved. If fungal infection confirmed, treat for ≥14 d and continue treatment for ≥7 d after symptoms and neutropenia resolved. If vial strength is available, in order to improve dosing accuracy, use 50-mg vial (5 mg/mL) for pediatric dose <50 mg and 70-mg vial (7 mg/mL) for pediatric dose >50 mg.
NOTES - Administration with cyclosporine increases caspofungin levels & hepatic transaminases; risk of concomitant use unclear. Caspofungin decreases tacrolimus levels. Dosage adjustment in moderate liver dysfunction (Child-Pugh score 7–9): 35 mg IV daily (after 70 mg loading dose in patients with invasive aspergillosis).

**MICAFUNGIN (*Mycamine*)** ▶L, feces ♀C ▶? $$$$$
ADULT - Esophageal candidiasis: 150 mg IV once daily. Candidemia, acute disseminated candidiasis, Candida peritonitis/abscess: 100 mg IV once daily. Prevention of candidal infections in bone marrow transplant patients: 50 mg IV once daily. Infuse over 1 h. Histamine-mediated reactions possible with more rapid infusion. Flush existing IV lines with normal saline before micafungin infusion.
PEDS - Not approved in children.
UNAPPROVED ADULT - Prophylaxis of invasive aspergillosis: 50 mg IV once daily. Infuse IV over 1 h.
NOTES - Increases levels of sirolimus and nifedipine. Not dialyzed. Protect diluted solution from light. Do not mix with other meds; it may precipitate.

## ANTIMICROBIALS: Antifungal Agents—Polyenes

**AMPHOTERICIN B DEOXYCHOLATE (*Fungizone*)** ▶Tissues ♀B ▶? $$$$
WARNING - Do not use IV route for noninvasive fungal infections (oral thrush, vaginal or esophageal candidiasis) in patients with normal neutrophil counts.
ADULT - Life-threatening systemic fungal infections: Test dose 1 mg slow IV. Wait 2–4 h, and if tolerated start 0.25 mg/kg IV daily. Advance to 0.5–1.5 mg/kg/d depending on fungal type. Max dose 1.5 mg/kg/d. Infuse over 2–6 h. Hydrate with 500 mL NS before and after infusion to decrease risk of nephrotoxicity.
PEDS - No remaining FDA approved indications.
UNAPPROVED ADULT - Alternative regimen, life-threatening systemic fungal infections: 1 mg test dose as part of 1st infusion (don't need separate

IV bag); if tolerated continue infusion, giving target dose of 0.5–1.5 mg/kg on 1st d. Candidemia, non-neutropenic pts: 0.6–1.0 mg/kg IV daily; or 0.7 mg/kg IV daily + fluconazole 800 mg/d for 4–7 d, then fluconazole 800 mg/d. Treat until 14 d past last positive blood culture and signs/symptoms resolved. Candidemia, neutropenic pts: 0.7–1.0 mg/kg IV daily until 14 d past last positive blood culture, signs/symptoms, and neutropenia resolved. *Cryptococcal meningitis* in HIV infection: 0.7–1 mg/kg/d IV preferably in combo with flucytosine 25 mg/kg PO q6h × 2 wk. Follow with fluconazole consolidation, then fluconazole chronic suppression until immune reconstitution. *Candidal cystitis*: Irrigate bladder with 50 mcg/mL soln periodically/continuously × 5–10 d.

**AMPHOTERICIN B DEOXYCHOLATE** *(cont.)*

UNAPPROVED PEDS - Systemic life-threatening fungal infections: Test dose 0.1 mg/kg slow IV. Wait 2–4 h, and if tolerated start 0.25 mg/kg IV once daily. Advance to 0.5–1.5 mg/kg/d depending on fungal type. Max dose 1.5 mg/kg/d. Infuse over 2–6 h. Hydrate with 10–15 mL/kg NS before infusion to decrease risk of nephrotoxicity. Alternative dosing regimen: Give 1 mg test dose as part of first infusion (separate IV bag not needed); if tolerated continue infusion, giving target dose of 0.5 to 1.5 mg/kg on first d. Candidemia, non-neutropenic pts: 0.6–1.0 mg/kg IV daily until 14–21 d past signs/symptoms resolved and negative repeat blood culture. Cryptococcal infection in HIV-infected patients: 0.7–1.5 mg/kg IV once daily preferably in combo with flucytosine depending on site and severity of infection. treatment for ≥2 wk, followed by fluconazole consolidation, and then fluconazole chronic suppression. Severe histoplasmosis: 1 mg/kg IV once daily until stable for ≥2–3 wk (treat × 12–16 wk for meningitis), then consolidation & suppressive therapy.

NOTES - Acute infusion reactions, anaphylaxis, nephrotoxicity, hypokalemia, hypomagnesemia, acidosis, anemia. Monitor renal and hepatic function, CBC, serum electrolytes. Lipid formulations better tolerated, preferred in renal dysfunction.

**AMPHOTERICIN B LIPID FORMULATIONS** *(Amphotec, Abelcet, AmBisome)* ▶? ♀B ▶? $$$$$

ADULT - Lipid formulations used primarily in patients refractory/intolerant to amphotericin deoxycholate. Abelcet: Invasive fungal infections: 5 mg/kg/d IV at 2.5 mg/kg/h. Shake infusion bag every 2 h. AmBisome: Infuse IV over 2 h. Empiric therapy of fungal infections in febrile neutropenia: 3 mg/kg/d. Aspergillus, candidal, cryptococcal infections: 3–5 mg/kg/d. Cryptococcal meningitis in HIV infection: 6 mg/kg/d. Amphotec: Test dose of 10 mL over 15–30 min, observe for 30 min, then 3–4 mg/kg/d IV at 1 mg/kg/h.

PEDS - Lipid formulations used primarily in patients refractory/intolerant to amphotericin deoxycholate. Abelcet: Invasive fungal infections: 5 mg/kg/d IV at 2.5 mg/kg/h. Shake infusion bag every 2 h. AmBisome: Infuse IV over 2 h. Empiric therapy of fungal infections in febrile neutropenia: 3 mg/kg/d. Aspergillus, candidal, cryptococcal infections: 3–5 mg/kg/d. Cryptococcal meningitis in HIV infection: 6 mg/kg/d. Amphotec: Aspergillosis: Test dose of 10 mL over 15–30 min, observe for 30 min, then 3–4 mg/kg/d IV at 1 mg/kg/h.

NOTES - Acute infusion reactions, anaphylaxis, nephrotoxicity, hypokalemia, hypomagnesemia, acidosis. Lipid formulations better tolerated than amphotericin deoxycholate, preferred in renal dysfunction. Monitor renal and hepatic function, CBC, electrolytes.

## ANTIMICROBIALS: Antifungal Agents—Other

**FLUCYTOSINE** *(Ancobon)* ▶K ♀C ▶- $$$$$

WARNING - Extreme caution in renal or bone marrow impairment. Monitor hematologic, hepatic, renal function in all patients.

ADULT - Candidal/cryptococcal infections: 50–150 mg/kg/d PO divided qid. Initial dose for cryptococcal meningitis: 100 mg/kg/d PO divided qid.

PEDS - Not approved in children.

UNAPPROVED PEDS - Candidal/cryptococcal infections: 50–150 mg/kg/d PO divided qid.

FORMS - Trade only: Caps 250, 500 mg.

NOTES - Flucytosine is given with other antifungal agents. Myelosuppression. Reduce nausea by taking caps a few at a time over 15 min. Monitor flucytosine levels. Peak 70–80 mg/L, trough 30–40 mg/L. Reduce dose in renal dysfunction. Avoid in children with severe renal dysfunction.

**GRISEOFULVIN** *(Grifulvin V, ✦Fulvicin)* ▶Skin ♀C ▶? $$$$$

ADULT - Tinea: 500 mg PO daily × 4–6 wk for capitis, 2–4 wk for corporis, 4–8 wk for pedis, 4 mo for fingernails, 6 mo for toenails. Can use 1 g/d for pedis and unguium.

PEDS - Tinea: 11 mg/kg PO daily × 4–6 wk for capitis, 2–4 wk for corporis, 4–8 wk for pedis, 4 mo for fingernails, 6 mo for toenails.

UNAPPROVED PEDS - Tinea capitis: AAP recommends 15–20 mg/kg (max 1 g) PO daily × 4–6 wk, continuing for 2 wk past symptom resolution.

Some infections may require 20–25 mg/kg/d or ultramicrosize griseofulvin 5–10 mg/kg (max 750 mg) PO daily.

FORMS - Generic/Trade: Susp 125 mg/5 mL (120 mL), Trade only: Tabs 500 mg.

NOTES - Do not use in liver failure, porphyria. May cause photosensitivity, lupus-like syndrome/exacerbation of lupus. Decreased INR with warfarin, decreased efficacy of oral contraceptives. Ultramicrosize formulations have greater GI absorption, and are available with different strengths and dosing.

**GRISEOFULVIN ULTRAMICROSIZE** *(Gris-PEG)* ▶Skin ♀C ▶? $$$$

ADULT - Tinea: 375 mg PO daily × 4–6 wk for capitis, 2–4 wk for corporis, 4–8 wk for pedis, 4 mo for fingernails, 6 mo for toenails. Can use 750 mg/d for pedis and unguium. Best absorption when given after meal containing fat.

PEDS - Tinea, >2 yo: 7.3 mg/kg PO daily × 4–6 wk for capitis, 2–4 wk for corporis, 4–8 wk for pedis, 4 mo for fingernails, 6 mo for toenails. Give 82.5–165 mg PO daily for 13.6–22.6 kg. Give 165–330 mg for >22.6 kg. Tinea capitis: AAP recommends 5–10 mg/kg (up to 750 mg) PO daily × 4–6 wk, continuing for 2 wk past symptom resolution. Best absorption when given after meal containing fat.

FORMS - Trade only: Tabs 125, 250 mg.

**(cont.)**

**GRISEOFULVIN ULTRAMICROSIZE** (cont.)

NOTES - Do not use in liver failure, porphyria. May cause photosensitivity, lupus-like syndrome/exacerbation of lupus. Decreased INR with warfarin, decreased efficacy of oral contraceptives. Microsize formulations, which have lower GI absorption, are available with different strengths and dosing.

**NYSTATIN** (*Mycostatin*, ✦*Nilstat, Nyaderm, Candistatin*) ▶Not absorbed ♀B ▶? $$

ADULT - Thrush: 4–6 mL PO swish & swallow qid or suck on 1–2 troches 4–5 × daily.

PEDS - Thrush, infants: 2 mL/dose PO with 1 mL in each cheek qid. Premature and low weight infants: 0.5 mL PO in each cheek qid. Thrush, older children: 4–6 mL PO swish & swallow qid or suck on 1–2 troches 4–5 × daily.

FORMS - Generic only: Susp 100,000 units/mL (60 & 480 mL).

**TERBINAFINE** (*Lamisil*) ▶LK ♀B ▶- $

ADULT - Onychomycosis: 250 mg PO daily × 6 wk for fingernails, × 12 wk for toenails.

PEDS - Tinea capitis, ≥4 yo: Give granules once daily with food × 6 wk: 125 mg if <25 kg, 187.5 mg if 25–35 kg, 250 mg if >35 kg.

UNAPPROVED ADULT - Onychomycosis "pulse dosing": 500 mg PO daily for 1st wk of mo × 2 mo for fingernails, 4 mo for toenails.

UNAPPROVED PEDS - Onychomycosis: 67.5 mg PO daily for <20 kg, 125 mg PO daily for 20–40 kg, 250 mg PO daily for >40 kg × 6 wk for fingernails, × 12 wk for toenails.

FORMS - Generic/Trade: Tabs 250 mg. Trade only: Oral granules 125 & 187.5 mg/packet.

NOTES - Hepatotoxicity; monitor AST & ALT at baseline. Neutropenia. May rarely cause or exacerbate lupus. Do not use in liver disease or CrCl ≤50 mL/min. Test nail specimen to confirm diagnosis before prescribing. Inhibitor of CYP 2D6.

## ANTIMICROBIALS: Antimalarials

**NOTE:** For help treating malaria or getting antimalarials, see www.cdc.gov/malaria or call the CDC "malaria hotline" (770) 488–7788 Monday-Friday 8 am to 4:30 pm EST; after h/weekend (770) 488–7100. Pediatric doses of antimalarials should never exceed adult doses.

**CHLOROQUINE** (*Aralen*) ▶KL ♀C but + ▶+ $

WARNING - Review product labeling for precautions and adverse effects before prescribing.

ADULT - Doses as chloroquine phosphate. Malaria prophylaxis, chloroquine-sensitive areas: 500 mg PO q wk from 1–2 wk before exposure to 4 wk after. Malaria: 1 g PO × 1, then 500 mg PO daily × 3 starting 6 h after 1st dose. Total dose is 2.5 g. Extraintestinal amebiasis: 1 g PO daily × 2, then 500 mg PO daily × 2–3 wk.

PEDS - Doses as chloroquine phosphate. Malaria prophylaxis, chloroquine-sensitive areas: 8.3 mg/kg (up to 500 mg) PO q wk from 1–2 wk before exposure to 4 wk after. Malaria: 16.7 mg/kg PO × 1, then 8.3 mg/kg daily × 3 d starting 6 h after 1st dose. Do not exceed adult dose. Chloroquine phosphate 8.3 mg/kg = chloroquine base 5 mg/kg.

FORMS - Generic only: Tabs 250 mg. Generic/Trade: Tabs 500 mg (500 mg phosphate equivalent to 300 mg base).

NOTES - Retinopathy with chronic/high doses; eye exams required. May cause seizures (caution advised if epilepsy); ototoxicity (caution advised if hearing loss); myopathy (discontinue if muscle weakness develops); bone marrow toxicity (monitor CBC if long-term use); exacerbation of psoriasis; torsades. Concentrates in liver; caution advised if hepatic disease, alcoholism, or hepatotoxic drugs. Antacids reduce absorption; give at least 4 h apart. Chloroquine reduces ampicillin absorption; give at least 2 h apart. May increase cyclosporine levels. As little as 1 g can cause fatal overdose in a child. Fatal malaria reported after chloroquine used as malaria prophylaxis in areas with chloroquine resistance; use only in areas without resistance. Maternal antimalarial prophylaxis doesn't harm breast-fed infant or protect infant from malaria.

**FANSIDAR** (sulfadoxine + pyrimethamine) ▶KL ♀C ▶- $

WARNING - Can cause life-threatening Stevens-Johnson syndrome and toxic epidermal necrolysis. Stop treatment at first sign of rash, bacterial/fungal infection, or change in CBC.

ADULT - CDC does not recommend Fansidar for treatment of malaria.

PEDS - CDC does not recommend Fansidar for treatment of malaria.

FORMS - Trade only: Tabs sulfadoxine 500 mg + pyrimethamine 25 mg.

NOTES - CDC does not recommend Fansidar for treatment of malaria due to drug resistance and adverse effects. Do not use in sulfonamide allergy; megaloblastic anemia due to folate deficiency; or for prolonged period in hepatic/renal failure or blood dyscrasia. Can cause hemolytic anemia in G6PD deficiency. Fansidar resistance is common in many malarious regions. Avoid excessive sun exposure.

**HALOFANTRINE** ▶? ♀? ▶? ?

ADULT - CDC does not recommend for treatment of malaria.

PEDS - CDC does not recommend for treatment of malaria.

FORMS - Not available in the US or Canada.

**MALARONE** (atovaquone + proguanil) ▶Fecal excretion; LK ♀C ▶? $$$$

ADULT - Malaria prophylaxis: 1 adult tab PO daily from 1–2 d before exposure until 7 d after. Malaria treatment: 4 adult tabs PO daily × 3 d.

**MALARONE** (cont.)

Take with food/milk at same time each d. Repeat dose if vomiting within 1 h. CDC recommends for presumptive self-treatment of malaria (same dose as for treatment, but not for patients taking it for prophylaxis).

PEDS - Safety & efficacy established in children ≥11 kg for prevention, ≥5 kg for treatment. Prevention of malaria: Give PO daily from 1–2 d before exposure until 7 d after: 1 ped tab for 11–20 kg; 2 ped tabs for 21–30 kg; 3 ped tabs for 31–40 kg; 1 adult tab for >40 kg. Treatment of malaria: Give PO daily × 3 d: 2 ped tabs for 5–8 kg; 3 ped tabs for 9–10 kg; 1 adult tab for 11–20 kg; 2 adult tabs for 21–30 kg; 3 adult tabs for 31–40 kg; 4 adult tabs for >40 kg. Take with food or milk at same time each d. Repeat dose if vomiting occurs within 1 h after dose.

FORMS - Trade only: Adult tabs atovaquone 250 mg + proguanil 100 mg; pediatric tabs 62.5 mg + 25 mg.

NOTES - Vomiting common with malaria treatment doses (consider antiemetic). Monitor parasitemia. Atovaquone levels may be decreased by tetracycline, metoclopramide (use another antiemetic if possible), and rifampin (avoid). Atovaquone can reduce indinavir trough levels. Proguanil may increase the INR with warfarin. If CrCl <30 mL/min avoid for malaria prophylaxis and use cautiously for treatment.

**MEFLOQUINE** (*Lariam*) ▶L ♀C ▶? $$

ADULT - Malaria prophylaxis, chloroquine-resistant areas: 250 mg PO q wk from 1 wk before exposure to 4 wk after. Malaria treatment: 1250 mg PO single dose. Take on full stomach with at least 8 oz water.

PEDS - Malaria treatment: 20–25 mg/kg PO; can divide into 2 doses given 6–8 h apart to reduce risk of vomiting. Repeat full dose if vomiting <30 min after dose; repeat ½ dose if vomiting <30–60 min after dose. Experience limited in infants <3 mo or <5 kg. Malaria prophylaxis: Give PO once weekly starting 1 wk before exposure to 4 wk after: 5–10 kg, 5 mg/kg (prepared by pharmacist); 10–20 kg, ¼ tab; 20–30 kg, ½ tab; 30–45 kg, ¾ tab. Take on full stomach.

UNAPPROVED ADULT - CDC regimen for malaria: 750 mg PO followed by 500 mg PO 6–12 h later, for total of 1250 mg. Quinine + doxycycline/tetracycline/clindamycin or atovaquone-proguanil preferred over mefloquine because of high rate of neuropsychiatric adverse effects with malaria treatment doses of mefloquine.

UNAPPROVED PEDS - Malaria prophylaxis, chloroquine-resistant areas: CDC recommends these PO doses q wk starting 1 wk before exposure to 4 wk after: ≤15 kg, 5 mg/kg; 15–19 kg, ¼ tab; 20–30 kg, ¼ tab; 31–45 kg, ¾ tab; >45 kg, 1 tab. Malaria treatment, <45 kg: 15 mg/kg PO, then 10 mg/kg PO given 8–12 h after first dose. Take on full stomach with at least 8 oz water.

FORMS - Generic/Trade: Tabs 250 mg.

NOTES - Cardiac conduction disturbances. Do not use with ziprasidone. Do not give until 12 h after the last dose of quinidine, quinine, or chloroquine; may cause ECG changes and seizures. Contraindicated for prophylaxis if depression (active/recent), generalized anxiety disorder, psychosis, schizophrenia, other major psychiatric disorder, or history of seizures. Tell patients to discontinue if psychiatric symptoms occur during prophylaxis. May cause drowsiness (warn about hazardous tasks). Can crush tabs and mix with a little water, milk, or other liquid. Pharmacists can put small doses into caps to mask bitter taste. Decreases valproate levels. Rifampin decreases mefloquine levels. Maternal use of antimalarial prophylaxis doesn't harm or protect breastfed infant from malaria.

**PRIMAQUINE** ▶L ♀- ▶- $$

WARNING - Review product labeling for precautions and adverse effects and document normal G6PD level before prescribing.

ADULT - Prevention of relapse, P vivax/ovale malaria: 30 mg base PO daily × 14 d.

PEDS - Not approved in children.

UNAPPROVED ADULT - Pneumocystis in patients intolerant to trimethoprim/sulfamethoxazole: 30 mg primaquine base (2 tabs) PO daily plus clindamycin 600–900 mg IV q8h or 300–450 mg PO q8h × 21 d. Primary prevention of malaria in special circumstances: 30 mg base PO once daily beginning 1–2 d before exposure until 7 d after (consult with malaria expert; contact CDC at 770-488-7788 for info).

UNAPPROVED PEDS - Prevention of relapse, P vivax/ovale malaria: 0.5 mg/kg up to 30 mg base PO once daily × 14 d. Primary prevention of malaria in special circumstances: 0.5 mg/kg up to 30 mg base PO once daily beginning 1–2 d before exposure until 7 d after (consult with malaria expert; contact CDC at 770-488-7788 for info).

FORMS - Generic only: Tabs 26.3 mg (equiv to 15 mg base).

NOTES - Causes hemolytic anemia in G6PD deficiency, methemoglobinemia in NADH methemoglobin reductase deficiency. Contraindicated in pregnancy and G6PD deficiency; screen for deficiency before prescribing. Stop if dark urine or anemia. Avoid in patients with RA or SLE, recent quinacrine use, or use of other bone marrow suppressants.

**QUININE** (*Qualaquin*) ▶L ♀C ▶+? $

ADULT - Malaria: 648 mg PO tid × 3 d (Africa/South America) or 7 d (Southeast Asia). Also give 7-d course of doxycycline, tetracycline or clindamycin.

PEDS - Not approved in children.

UNAPPROVED ADULT - Nocturnal leg cramps: 260–325 mg PO qhs. FDA believes risks outweigh benefits for this indication.

UNAPPROVED PEDS - Malaria: 25–30 mg/kg/d up to 2 g/d PO divided q8h × 3 d (Africa/South **(cont.)**

**QUININE** (*cont.*)
America) or 7 d (Southeast Asia). Also give doxy-cycline, tetracycline or clindamycin.

FORMS - Trade only: Caps 324 mg. Unapproved qui-nine products removed from US market by Feb 2007 with interstate shipment to cease by June 2007.

NOTES - Thrombocytopenia, thrombotic thrombo-cytopenic purpura, hemolytic uremic syndrome, cinchonism, hemolytic anemia with G6PD defi-ciency, cardiac conduction disturbances, hearing impairment. Contraindicated if prolonged QT interval, optic neuritis, myasthenia gravis, or hypersensitivity to quinine, quinidine, or meflo-quine. Many drug interactions. Do not use with erythromycin, rifampin, neuromuscular block-ers. May increase digoxin levels. May decrease theophylline levels. Monitor INR with warfarin. Antacids decrease quinine absorption. Rule out G6PD deficiency in breastfed at-risk infant before giving quinine to mother.

## ANTIMICROBIALS: Antimycobacterial Agents

**NOTE:** Two or more drugs are needed for the treatment of active mycobacterial infections. See guidelines at http://www.thoracic.org/sections/publications/statements/. See www.aidsinfo.nih.gov and www.cdc.gov/tb/TB_HIV_Drugs/default.htm for use of rifamycins with antiretrovirals. Get baseline LFTs, creatinine, and platelet count before treating TB. Evaluate at least monthly for adverse drug reactions. Routine liver and renal function tests not needed unless baseline dysfunction or increased risk of hepatotoxicity.

**CAPREOMYCIN** (*Capastat*) ▶K ♀C ▶? $$$$$
WARNING - Nephrotoxicity, ototoxicity.

ADULT - TB (2nd-line treatment): CDC and ATS rec-ommend 15 mg/kg up to 1 g IM/IV daily. Max 10 mg/kg up to 750 mg IM/IV if >59 yo. Give deep IM injection or infuse IV over 1 h.

PEDS - Not approved in children.

UNAPPROVED PEDS - TB (2nd-line treatment): ATS, CDC, and AAP recommend 15–30 mg/kg/d up to 1 g IM/IV daily. Give deep IM injection or infuse IV over 1 h.

NOTES - Contraindicated in pregnancy. Get baseline audiogram, vestibular and Romberg tests, renal function, serum electrolytes. Monitor renal func-tion and vestibular/auditory symptoms monthly, serum electrolytes at least monthly. May enhance effects of neuromuscular blockers. Avoid other ototoxic/nephrotoxic drugs. Reduce dose and monitor serum levels in renal dysfunction.

**CLOFAZIMINE** (*Lamprene*) ▶Fecal excretion ♀C ▶?- $
ADULT - Approved for leprosy therapy.

PEDS - Not approved in children.

UNAPPROVED ADULT - Mycobacterium avium com-plex in immunocompetent patients: 100–200 mg PO daily until "tan", then 50 mg PO daily or 100 mg PO three times weekly. Use in combina-tion with other antimycobacterial agents. Not for general use in AIDS patients due to increased mortality.

FORMS - Trade only: Caps 50 mg. Distributed only through investigational new drug application. For leprosy, contact National Hansen's Disease Program (phone 225-578-9861). For non-leprosy indications, contact FDA Division of Special Pathogen and Immunologic Drugs Program (phone 301-796-1600).

NOTES - Abdominal pain common; rare reports of splenic infarction, bowel obstruction, and GI bleeding. Pink to brownish-black skin pigmen-tation that may persist for mo to yr after drug is discontinued. Discoloration of urine, body secretions.

**CYCLOSERINE** (*Seromycin*) ▶KL ♀C ▶- $$$$$
ADULT - TB (2nd-line treatment): Manufacturer rec-ommends 250 mg PO bid × 2 wk, then 500–1000 mg/d PO in divided doses. ATS and CDC recom-mend 10–15 mg/kg/d (up to 1 g/d) PO divided bid. Usual dose is 500–750 mg/d PO divided bid. Toxicity more common with >500 mg/d. Monitoring serum levels (peak of 20–35 mcg/mL) may help determine optimal dose. Give pyridoxine 100–200 mg/d PO to minimize neurotoxicity.

PEDS - Not approved in children.

UNAPPROVED PEDS - TB (2nd-line treatment): ATS and CDC recommend 10–15 mg/kg/d PO up to 1 g/d.

FORMS - Trade only: Caps 250 mg.

NOTES - Dose-related neurotoxicity. Contraindicated in epilepsy, depression, severe anxiety, psycho-sis, severe renal dysfunction, frequent alcohol use (may increase seizure risk). Monitor mental status. Ethionamide, isoniazid may increase neurotoxicity. May cause drowsiness (warn about hazardous tasks). May increase phenytoin levels. Do not use if CrCl <50 mL/min unless patient receives hemodialysis.

**DAPSONE** (*Aczone*) ▶LK ♀C ▶- $
ADULT - Leprosy: 100 mg PO daily with rifampin +/− clofazimine or ethionamide. Acne (Aczone): Apply bid.

PEDS - Leprosy: 1 mg/kg (up to 100 mg) PO daily with other antimycobacterial agents. Acne (12–17 yo, Aczone): Apply bid.

UNAPPROVED ADULT - Pneumocystis prophylaxis: 100 mg PO daily. Pneumocystis treatment: 100 mg PO daily with trimethoprim 5 mg/kg PO tid × 21 d.

UNAPPROVED PEDS - Pneumocystis prophylaxis, age ≥1 mo: 2 mg/kg (up to 100 mg) PO daily or 4 mg/kg (up to 200 mg) PO q wk.

FORMS - Generic only: Tabs 25,100 mg. Trade only (Aczone): gel 5% 30 g.

NOTES - Blood dyscrasias, severe allergic skin reactions, sulfone syndrome, hemolysis in G6PD

**DAPSONE** *(cont.)*
deficiency, hepatotoxicity, neuropathy, photosensitivity, leprosy reactional states. Monitor CBC q wk × 4, then monthly × 6, then twice yearly. Monitor LFTs.

**ETHAMBUTOL** *(Myambutol, ✦Etibi)* ▶LK ♀C but + ▶+ $$$$
ADULT - TB: ATS and CDC recommend 15–20 mg/kg PO daily. Dose with whole tabs: 800 mg PO daily if 40–55 kg, 1200 mg PO daily if 56–75 kg, 1600 mg PO daily if 76–90 kg. Base dose on estimated lean body weight. Max dose regardless of weight is 1600 mg/d.
PEDS - TB: ATS and CDC recommend 15–20 mg/kg up to 1 g PO daily. Use cautiously if visual acuity cannot be monitored. Manufacturer recommends against use in children <13 yo.
UNAPPROVED ADULT - Treatment or prevention of recurrent Mycobacterium avium complex disease in HIV infection: 15–25 mg/kg up to 1600 mg PO daily with clarithromycin/azithromycin +/− rifabutin.
UNAPPROVED PEDS - Treatment or prevention of recurrent Mycobacterium avium complex disease in HIV infection: 15 mg/kg up to 900 mg PO daily with clarithromycin/azithromycin +/− rifabutin.
FORMS - Generic/Trade: Tabs 100, 400 mg.
NOTES - Can cause retrobulbar neuritis. Avoid, if possible, in patients with optic neuritis. Test visual acuity and color discrimination at baseline. Ask about visual disturbances monthly. Monitor visual acuity and color discrimination monthly if dose >15–20 mg/kg, duration >2 mo, or renal dysfunction. Advise patients to report any change in vision immediately; do not use in those who cannot report visual symptoms (eg, children, unconscious). Do not give aluminum hydroxide antacid until >4h after ethambutol dose. Reduce dose in renal impairment.

**ETHIONAMIDE** *(Trecator)* ▶L ♀C but − ▶? $$$$$
ADULT - TB (2nd-line treatment): 15–20 mg/kg/d up to 1 g/d PO divided daily-bid. Usual dose is 500–750 mg/d. To improve GI tolerance, can start with 250 mg/d and increase by 250 mg/d every few d, and give with meals or qhs. Give with pyridoxine.
PEDS - TB (2nd-line treatment): AAP, ATS and CDC recommend 15–20 mg/kg/d up to 1 g/d PO. Dose can be divided daily-tid.
FORMS - Trade only: Tab 250 mg.
NOTES - Hepatotoxicity, hypothyroidism. Contraindicated in severe hepatic dysfunction. Monitor LFTs at baseline; monitor monthly if underlying liver disease. Monitor TSH at baseline and monthly. Increases risk of seizures with cycloserine. Advise patients to avoid excessive alcohol ingestion. Drug malabsorption may be present in AIDS patients with TB. Do not use in pregnancy. Reduce dose in renal dysfunction.

**ISONIAZID** *(INH, ✦Isotamine)* ▶LK ♀C but + ▶+ $
WARNING - Hepatotoxicity. Obtain baseline LFTs. Monitor LFTs monthly in high-risk patients (HIV,

signs/history of liver disease, abnormal LFTs at baseline, pregnancy/postpartum, alcoholism/regular alcohol use, some patients >35 yo). Tell all patients to stop isoniazid and call at once if hepatotoxicity symptoms. Discontinue if AST >3 × upper limit of normal with hepatotoxicity symptoms or AST >5 × upper limit of normal without hepatotoxicity symptoms.
ADULT - TB treatment: 5 mg/kg up to 300 mg PO daily or 15 mg/kg up to 900 mg twice weekly. Latent TB: 300 mg PO daily.
PEDS - TB treatment: 10–15 mg/kg up to 300 mg PO daily. Latent TB: 10 mg/kg up to 300 mg PO daily.
UNAPPROVED ADULT - American Thoracic Society regimen, latent tuberculosis: 5 mg/kg up to 300 mg PO daily × 9 mo (6 mo OK if HIV-negative, but less effective than 9 mo).
UNAPPROVED PEDS - American Thoracic Society regimen for latent tuberculosis: 10–20 mg/kg up to 300 mg PO daily for 9 mo.
FORMS - Generic only: Tabs 100,300 mg, syrup 50 mg/5 mL.
NOTES - To reduce risk of peripheral neuropathy, give pyridoxine 25 mg PO daily if alcoholism, diabetes, HIV, uremia, malnutrition, seizure disorder, pregnant/breastfeeding woman, breast-fed infant of INH-treated mother. Many drug interactions.

**KANAMYCIN** *(Kantrex)* ▶K ♀D ▶+ $$$$$
WARNING - Nephrotoxicity, ototoxicity.
ADULT - TB (2nd-line treatment): 15 mg/kg up to 1 g IM/IV daily. 10 mg/kg up to 750 mg IM/IV daily if >59 yo.
PEDS - TB (2nd-line treatment): AAP, ATS and CDC recommend 15–30 mg/kg up to 1 g IM/IV daily.
NOTES - Monitor renal and vestibular function, and audiogram. Avoid other ototoxic/nephrotoxic drugs. Individualize dose in renal dysfunction. May enhance effects of neuromuscular blockers.

**PARA-AMINOSALICYLIC ACID** *(Paser, aminosalicylic acid, PAS, ✦Nemasol Sodium)* ▶K ♀C ▶? $$$$$
ADULT - TB (2nd-line treatment): 4 g granules (1 packet) PO tid. ATS and CDC recommend 8–12 g/d divided bid-tid. Take with acidic food or drink (applesauce, yogurt, fruit juice). Do not chew granules.
PEDS - Not approved in children.
UNAPPROVED PEDS - TB (2nd-line treatment): AAP and ATS recommend 200–300 mg/kg/d up to 10 g/d PO divided bid-qid. Take with acidic food or drink (applesauce, yogurt, fruit juice). Do not chew granules.
FORMS - Trade only: Granules, delayed-release 4 g packets.
NOTES - Hepatotoxicity, hypothyroidism, vitamin B12 deficiency. Monitor LFTs at baseline. Monitor thyroid function at baseline and every 3 mo. Decreases absorption of digoxin, vitamin B12. Increases phenytoin levels. Levels decreased by diphenhydramine; do not use together. Contraindicated in severe renal dysfunction. Do
**(cont.)**

**PARA-AMINOSALICYLIC ACID** *(cont.)*

not use granules if packet is swollen or granules are dark brown or purple. Store packets in refrigerator or freezer. Acid-resistant granule coating protects against conversion to hepatotoxic metabolite in gastric fluid. Granule coating lasts ≥2 h in acidic food/drink (pH <5). Coating may be seen in stool.

**PYRAZINAMIDE** *(PZA, ◆Tebrazid)* ▶LK ♀C ▶? $$$$
WARNING - The ATS and CDC recommend against general use of 2 mo regimen of rifampin + pyrazinamide for latent TB due to reports of fatal hepatotoxicity.
ADULT - TB: ATS and CDC recommend 20–25 mg/kg PO daily. Dose with whole tabs: 1000 mg PO daily if 40–55 kg, 1500 mg daily if 56–75 kg, 2000 mg if 76–90 kg. Base dose on estimated lean body weight. Max dose regardless of weight is 2000 mg PO daily.
PEDS - TB: 15–30 mg/kg up to 2000 mg PO daily.
FORMS - Generic only: Tabs 500 mg.
NOTES - Hepatotoxicity, hyperuricemia (avoid in acute gout). Obtain LFTs at baseline. Monitor periodically in high-risk patients (HIV infection, alcoholism, pregnancy, signs/history of liver disease, abnormal LFTs at baseline). Discontinue if AST >3 × upper limit of normal with hepatotoxicity symptoms or AST >5 × upper limit of normal without hepatotoxicity symptoms. The ATS and CDC recommend against general use of 2 mo regimen of rifampin + pyrazinamide for latent TB due to reports of fatal hepatotoxicity. Consider reduced dose in renal dysfunction.

**RIFABUTIN** *(Mycobutin)* ▶L ♀B ▶? $$$$$
ADULT - Prevention of disseminated Mycobacterium avium complex disease in AIDS: 300 mg PO daily or 150 mg PO bid. Reduce to 150 mg once daily or 300 mg 3 times/wk with fosamprenavir, indinavir, or nelfinavir (without ritonavir). Increase indinavir to 1000 mg q8h if not ritonavir-boosted. Increase nelfinavir to 1250 mg q12h. Reduce rifabutin to 150 mg every other d or three times/wk if regimen includes ritonavir at any dose. Monitor CBC at least weekly with fosamprenavir.
PEDS - Not approved in children.
UNAPPROVED ADULT - TB or Mycobacterium avium complex disease treatment in AIDS: 300 mg PO daily. Reduce to 150 mg once daily or 300 mg 3 times/wk with fosamprenavir, indinavir, nelfinavir. Increase indinavir to 1000 mg q8h if not ritonavir-boosted. Increase nelfinavir to 1250 mg q12h. Reduce rifabutin to 150 mg every other d or three times/wk if regimen includes ritonavir at any dose. Monitor CBC at least weekly with fosamprenavir.
UNAPPROVED PEDS - Mycobacterium avium complex disease. Prophylaxis: ≥6 yo, 300 mg PO daily. <6 yo, 5 mg/kg (up to 300 mg) PO daily. Treatment: 10–20 mg/kg (max 300 mg/d) PO once daily. TB: 10–20 mg/kg (up to 300 mg) PO once daily.
FORMS - Trade only: Caps 150 mg.

NOTES - Uveitis (with high doses or if metabolism inhibited by other drugs), hepatotoxicity, thrombocytopenia, neutropenia. Obtain CBC and LFTs at baseline. Monitor periodically in high-risk patients (HIV infection, alcoholism, pregnancy, signs/history of liver disease, abnormal LFTs at baseline). Do not use alone in patients with active TB. May induce liver metabolism of other drugs including oral contraceptives, protease inhibitors, and azole antifungals. Substrate of CYP 3A4; fluconazole, clarithromycin, and protease inhibitors increase rifabutin levels. Urine, body secretion, soft contact lenses may turn orange-brown. Consider dosage reduction for hepatic dysfunction.

**RIFAMATE** *(isoniazid + rifampin)* ▶LK ♀C but + ▶+ $$$$
WARNING - Hepatotoxicity.
ADULT - Tuberculosis: 2 caps PO daily on empty stomach.
PEDS - Not approved in children.
FORMS - Generic/Trade: Caps isoniazid 150 mg + rifampin 300 mg.
NOTES - See components. Monitor LFTs at baseline and periodically during therapy.

**RIFAMPIN** *(Rimactane, Rifadin, ◆Rofact)* ▶L ♀C but + ▶+ $$$
WARNING - The ATS and CDC recommend against general use of 2 mo regimen of rifampin + pyrazinamide for latent TB due to reports of fatal hepatotoxicity.
ADULT - Tuberculosis: 10 mg/kg up to 600 mg PO/IV daily. Neisseria meningitidis carriers: 600 mg PO bid × 2 d. Take oral doses on empty stomach. IV and PO doses are the same. Neisseria meningitidis carriers: 600 mg PO bid × 2 d. Take on empty stomach. IV & PO doses are the same.
PEDS - Tuberculosis: 10–20 mg/kg up to 600 mg PO/IV daily. Neisseria meningitidis carriers: ≥1 mo, 10 mg/kg up to 600 mg PO bid × 2 d. <1 mo, 5 mg/kg PO bid × 2 d. Take on empty stomach. IV and PO doses are the same. Neisseria meningitidis carriers: age ≥1 mo, 10 mg/kg up to 600 mg PO bid × 2 d. Age <1 mo, 5 mg/kg PO bid × 2 d. Take on empty stomach.
UNAPPROVED ADULT - Prophylaxis of H influenza type b infection: 20 mg/kg up to 600 mg PO daily × 4 d. Leprosy: 600 mg PO q mo with dapsone. American Thoracic Society regimen for latent TB: 10 mg/kg up to 600 mg PO daily × 4 mo. Staphylococcal prosthetic valve endocarditis: 300 mg PO q8 h in combination with gentamicin plus nafcillin, oxacillin, or vancomycin. Take on empty stomach.
UNAPPROVED PEDS - Prophylaxis of H influenza type b infection: ≥1 mo, 20 mg/kg up to 600 mg PO daily × 4 d. <1 mo, 10 mg/kg PO daily × 4 d. Prophylaxis of invasive meningococcal disease: ≥1 mo, 10 mg/kg up to 600 mg PO bid × 2 d. <1 mo, 5 mg/kg PO bid × 2 d. American Thoracic Society regimen for latent tuberculosis:

**RIFAMPIN** *(cont.)*
10–20 mg/kg up to 600 mg PO daily × 4 mo. Take on empty stomach.

FORMS - Generic/Trade: Caps 150,300 mg. Pharmacists can make oral susp.

NOTES - Hepatotoxicity, thrombocytopenia. When treating TB, obtain baseline CBC, LFTs. Monitor periodically in high-risk patients (HIV infection, alcoholism, pregnancy, signs/history of liver disease, abnormal LFTs at baseline). Discontinue if AST >3 × upper limit of normal with hepatotoxicity symptoms or AST >5 × upper limit of normal without hepatotoxicity symptoms. The ATS and CDC recommend against general use of 2 mo regimen of rifampin + pyrazinamide for latent TB due to reports of fatal hepatotoxicity. Induces hepatic metabolism of many drugs; check other sources for dosage adjustments before prescribing. If used with rifampin, consider increasing efavirenz to 800 mg qhs if weight ≥60 kg. Do not use rifampin with standard protease inhibitor regimens. Decreased efficacy of oral contraceptives; use non-hormonal method. Decreased INR with warfarin; monitor daily or as needed. Adjust dose for hepatic impairment. Colors urine, body secretions, soft contact lenses red-orange. IV rifampin is stable for 4h after dilution in dextrose 5%.

**RIFAPENTINE** *(Priftin)* ▶Esterases, fecal ♀C ▶? $$$$
ADULT - TB: 600 mg PO twice weekly × 2 mo, then once weekly × 4 mo. ATS and CDC recommend use only for continuation therapy in selected HIV-negative patients.

PEDS - Not approved in children <12 yo.

FORMS - Trade only: Tabs 150 mg.

NOTES - Hepatotoxicity, thrombocytopenia, exacerbation of porphyria. Obtain CBC and LFTs at baseline. Monitor LFTs periodically in high-risk patients (HIV infection, alcoholism, pregnancy, signs/history of liver disease, abnormal LFTs at baseline). Do not use in porphyria. Urine, body secretions, contact lenses, and dentures may turn red-orange. May induce liver metabolism of other drugs including oral contraceptives. Avoid with protease inhibitors or NNRTIs.

**RIFATER** (isoniazid + rifampin + pyrazinamide) ▶LK ♀C ▶? $$$$$
WARNING - Hepatotoxicity.

ADULT - TB, initial 2 mo of treatment: 6 tabs PO daily if ≥55 kg, 5 tabs daily if 45–54 kg, 4 tabs daily if ≤44 kg. Additional pyrazinamide tabs required to provide adequate dose in patient >90 kg. Take on empty stomach. Can finish treatment with Rifamate.

PEDS - Ratio of formulation may not be appropriate for children <15 yo.

FORMS - Trade only: Tab Isoniazid 50 mg + rifampin 120 mg + pyrazinamide 300 mg.

NOTES - See components. Monitor LFTs at baseline and during therapy. Do not use in patients with renal dysfunction.

## ANTIMICROBIALS: Antiparasitics

**ALBENDAZOLE** *(Albenza)* ▶L ♀C ▶? $$$
ADULT - Hydatid disease, neurocysticercosis: ≥60 kg - 400 mg PO bid. <60 kg - 15 mg/kg/d (up to 800 mg/d) PO divided bid. Treatment duration varies. Take with food.

PEDS - Hydatid disease, neurocysticercosis: ≥60 kg - 400 mg PO bid. <60 kg: 15 mg/kg/d (up to 800 mg/d) PO divided bid. Treatment duration varies. Take with food.

UNAPPROVED ADULT - Hookworm, whipworm, pinworm, roundworm: 400 mg PO single dose. Repeat in 2 wk for pinworm. Cutaneous larva migrans: 200 mg PO bid × 3 d. Giardia: 400 mg PO daily × 5 d.

UNAPPROVED PEDS - Roundworm, hookworm, pinworm, whipworm: 400 mg PO single dose. Repeat in 2 wk for pinworm. Cutaneous larva migrans: 200 mg PO bid × 3 d. Giardia: 400 mg PO daily × 5 d.

FORMS - Trade only: Tabs 200 mg.

NOTES - Associated with bone marrow suppression (especially if liver disease), increased LFTs (common), and acute liver failure (rare). Monitor CBC and LFTs before starting and then q2 wk; discontinue drug if significant changes. Consider corticosteroids & anticonvulsants in neurocysticercosis. Get negative pregnancy test before treatment & warn against getting pregnant until a mo after treatment. Treat close contacts for pinworms. Can crush/chew tabs and swallow with water.

**ATOVAQUONE** *(Mepron)* ▶Fecal ♀C ▶? $$$$$
ADULT - Pneumocystis in patients intolerant to trimethoprim/sulfamethoxazole: Treatment 750 mg PO bid × 21 d. Prevention 1500 mg PO daily. Take with meals.

PEDS - Pneumocystis in patients intolerant to trimethoprim/sulfamethoxazole, 13–16 yo: Treatment, 750 mg PO bid × 21 d. Prevention, 1500 mg PO daily. Take with meals. Efficacy & safety not established for <13 yo.

UNAPPROVED PEDS - Prevention of recurrent Pneumocystis in HIV infection: 1–3 mo, 30 mg/kg PO daily. 4–24 mo, 45 mg/kg PO daily. >24 mo, 30 mg/kg PO daily. Take with meals.

FORMS - Trade only: Susp 750 mg/5 mL (210 mL), foil pouch 750 mg/5 mL (5 & 10 mL).

NOTES - Efficacy of atovaquone may be decreased by lopinavir/ritonavir (Kaletra), rifampin (consider using alternative), rifabutin, rifapentine, and ritonavir.

**IODOQUINOL** *(Yodoxin, diiodohydroxyquin, ✦Diodoquin)* ▶Not absorbed ♀? ▶? $$
ADULT - Intestinal amebiasis: 650 mg PO tid after meals × 20 d.

PEDS - Intestinal amebiasis: 40 mg/kg/d PO divided tid × 20 d. Do not exceed adult dose.

**(cont.)**

**IODOQUINOL** (*cont.*)
FORMS - Generic/Trade: Tabs 650 mg. Trade only: Tabs 210 mg.
NOTES - Optic neuritis/atrophy, peripheral neuropathy with prolonged high doses. Interference with some thyroid function tests for up to 6 mo after treatment.

**IVERMECTIN** (*Stromectol*) ▶L ♀C ▶+ $$
ADULT - Strongyloidiasis: 200 mcg/kg PO single dose. Onchocerciasis: 150 mcg/kg PO q3–12 mo. Take on empty stomach with water.
PEDS - For children ≥15 kg. Strongyloidiasis: 200 mcg/kg PO single dose. Onchocerciasis: 150 mcg/kg PO single dose q 3–12 mo. Take on empty stomach with water.
UNAPPROVED ADULT - Scabies: 200 mcg/kg PO repeated in 2 wk. Pubic lice: 250 mcg/kg PO repeated in 2 wk. Cutaneous larva migrans: 150–200 mcg/kg PO single dose. Take on empty stomach with water.
UNAPPROVED PEDS - Scabies: 200 mcg/kg PO single dose. Cutaneous larva migrans: 150–200 mcg/kg PO single dose. Take on empty stomach with water. Safety and efficacy not established in children <15 kg.
FORMS - Trade only: Tab 3 mg.
NOTES - Mazzotti & ophthalmic reactions with treatment for onchocerciasis. May need repeat/ monthly treatment for strongyloidiasis in immunocompromised/HIV-infected patients.

**MEBENDAZOLE** (*Vermox*) ▶L ♀C ▶? $$
ADULT - Pinworm: 100 mg PO × 1; repeat in 2 wk. Roundworm, whipworm, hookworm: 100 mg PO bid × 3 d.
PEDS - Pinworm: 100 mg PO × 1; repeat dose in 2 wk. Roundworm, whipworm, hookworm: 100 mg PO bid × 3 d.
UNAPPROVED ADULT - Roundworm, whipworm, hookworm: 500 mg PO single dose.
UNAPPROVED PEDS - Roundworm, whipworm, hookworm: 500 mg PO single dose.
FORMS - Generic only: Chew tab 100 mg.
NOTES - Treat close contacts for pinworms.

**NITAZOXANIDE** (*Alinia*) ▶L ♀B ▶? $$$$
ADULT - Cryptosporidial or Giardial diarrhea: 500 mg PO bid with food × 3 d.
PEDS - Cryptosporidial or Giardial diarrhea: 100 mg bid for 1–3 yo, 200 mg bid for 4–11 yo, 500 mg bid for ≥12 yo. Give PO with food × 3 d. Use susp for <12 yo.
UNAPPROVED ADULT - C difficile colitis: 500 mg PO bid × 10 d.
FORMS - Trade only: Oral susp 100 mg/5 mL 60 mL bottle, tab 500 mg.
NOTES - Contains 1.5 g sucrose/5 mL. Turns urine bright yellow. Store at room temperature for up to 7 d.

**PAROMOMYCIN** ▶Not absorbed ♀C ▶- $$$$
ADULT - Intestinal amebiasis: 25–35 mg/kg/d PO divided tid with/after meals × 5–10 d.
PEDS - Intestinal amebiasis: 25–35 mg/kg/d PO divided tid with/after meals × 5–10 d.

UNAPPROVED ADULT - Giardiasis: 500 mg PO tid × 7 d.
UNAPPROVED PEDS - Giardiasis: 25–35 mg/kg/d PO divided tid with/after meals × 7 d.
FORMS - Generic only: Caps 250 mg.
NOTES - Nephrotoxicity possible with systemic absorption in inflammatory bowel disease. Not effective for extra-intestinal amebiasis.

**PENTAMIDINE** (*Pentam, NebuPent*) ▶K ♀C ▶- $$$
ADULT - Pneumocystis treatment: 4 mg/kg IM/ IV daily × 21 d. IV infused over 60–90 min. NebuPent for Pneumocystis prevention: 300 mg nebulized q 4 wk.
PEDS - Pneumocystis treatment: 4 mg/kg IM/IV daily × 21 d. NebuPent not approved in children.
UNAPPROVED PEDS - Pneumocystis prevention, ≥5 yo: 300 mg NebuPent nebulized q 4 wk.
FORMS - Trade only: Aerosol 300 mg.
NOTES - Contraindicated with ziprasidone. Fatalities due to severe hypotension, hypoglycemia, cardiac arrhythmias with IM/IV. Have patient lie down, check BP, and keep resuscitation equipment handy during IM/IV injection. May cause torsades, hyperglycemia, neutropenia, nephrotoxicity, pancreatitis, and hypocalcemia. Monitor BUN, serum creatinine, blood glucose, CBC, LFTs, serum calcium, and ECG. Bronchospasm with inhalation (consider bronchodilator). Reduce IM/IV dose in renal dysfunction.

**PRAZIQUANTEL** (*Biltricide*) ▶LK ♀B ▶- $$$
ADULT - Schistosomiasis: 20 mg/kg PO q4–6h × 3 doses. Liver flukes: 25 mg/kg PO q4–6h × 3 doses.
PEDS - Schistosomiasis: 20 mg/kg PO q4–6h × 3 doses. Liver flukes: 25 mg/kg PO q4–6h × 3 doses.
UNAPPROVED ADULT - Neurocysticercosis: 50 mg/ kg/d PO divided tid × 15 d. Fish, dog, beef, pork intestinal tapeworms: 10 mg/kg PO single dose.
UNAPPROVED PEDS - Neurocysticercosis: 50–100 mg/kg/d PO divided tid × 15 d. Fish, dog, beef, pork intestinal tapeworms: 10 mg/kg PO single dose.
FORMS - Trade only: Tabs 600 mg.
NOTES - Contraindicated in ocular cysticercosis. May cause drowsiness; do not drive or operate machinery for 48 h. Phenytoin, carbamazepine, rifampin (avoid using together), and dexamethasone may lower praziquantel levels enough to cause treatment failure. Take with liquids during a meal. Do not chew tabs. Manufacturer advises against breast feeding until 72 h after treatment.

**PYRANTEL** (*Antiminth, Pin-X, Pinworm, ✦Combantrin*) ▶Not absorbed ♀- ▶? $
ADULT - Pinworm, roundworm: 11 mg/kg up to 1 g PO single dose. Repeat in 2 wk for pinworm.
PEDS - Pinworm, roundworm: 11 mg/kg up to 1 g PO single dose. Repeat in 2 wk for pinworm.
UNAPPROVED ADULT - Hookworm: 11 mg/kg up to 1 g PO daily × 3 d.
UNAPPROVED PEDS - Hookworm: 11 mg/kg up to 1 g PO daily × 3 d.

**PYRANTEL** (*cont.*)
FORMS - OTC Trade only (Pin-X): Susp 144 mg/mL (equivalent to 50 mg/mL of pyrantel base) 30, 60 mL. Tab 720.5 mg (equivalent to 250mg of pyrantel base). OTC Generic only: Cap 180 mg (equivalent to 62.5 mg of pyrantel base).
NOTES - Purging not necessary. Treat close contacts for pinworms.

**PYRIMETHAMINE** (*Daraprim*) ▶L ♀C ▶+ $$
ADULT - Toxoplasmosis, immunocompetent patients: 50–75 mg PO daily × 1–3 wk, then reduce dose by 50% for 4–5 more wk. Give with leucovorin (10–15 mg daily) and sulfadiazine. Reduce initial dose in seizure disorders.
PEDS - Toxoplasmosis: 1 mg/kg/d PO divided bid × 2–4 d, then reduce by 50% × 1 mo. Give with sulfadiazine & leucovorin. Reduce initial dose in seizure disorders.
UNAPPROVED ADULT - CNS toxoplasmosis in AIDS. Acute therapy: 200 mg PO × 1, then 50 mg (<60 kg) to 75 mg (≥60 kg) PO once daily + sulfadiazine 1000 mg (<60 kg) to 1500 mg (≥60 kg) PO q6h + leucovorin 10–20 mg PO once daily (can increase to ≥50 mg/d). Treat for ≥6 wk. Secondary prevention: 25–50 mg PO once daily + sulfadiazine 500–1000 mg PO qid +.leucovorin 10–25 mg PO once daily. Reduce initial dose in seizure disorders.
UNAPPROVED PEDS - Congenital toxoplasmosis: 2 mg/kg PO once daily × 2 d, then 1 mg/kg once daily × 2–6 mo, then 1 mg/kg three times weekly + sulfadiazine 50 mg/kg PO bid. Give leucovorin 10 mg PO/IM with each dose of pyrimethamine. Treat × 1 yr. Acquired toxoplasmosis: 2 mg/kg (up to 50 mg) PO once daily × 3 d, then 1 mg/kg (up to 25 mg) PO once daily + sulfadiazine 25–50 mg/kg PO (up to 1–1.5 g/dose) PO qid. Give leucovorin 10–25 mg/d PO. Treat ≥6 wk followed by chronic suppressive therapy.

FORMS - Trade only: Tabs 25 mg.
NOTES - Hemolytic anemia in G6PD deficiency, dose-related folate deficiency, hypersensitivity. Monitor CBC.

**THIABENDAZOLE** (*Mintezol*) ▶LK ♀C ▶? $
ADULT - Helminths: 22 mg/kg/dose up to 1500 mg PO bid. Treat × 2 d for strongyloidiasis, cutaneous larva migrans. Take after meals.
PEDS - Helminths: 22 mg/kg/dose up to 1500 mg PO bid. Treat × 2 d for strongyloidiasis, cutaneous larva migrans. Limited use in children <13.5 kg. Take after meals.
FORMS - Trade only: Chew tab 500 mg, susp 500 mg/5 mL (120 mL).
NOTES - May cause drowsiness.

**TINIDAZOLE** (*Tindamax*) ▶KL ♀C ▶?- $
ADULT - Trichomoniasis or giardiasis: 2 g PO single dose. Amebiasis: 2 g PO daily × 3 d. Bacterial vaginosis: 2 g PO once daily × 2 d or 1 g PO once daily × 5 d. Take with food.
PEDS - Giardiasis, >3 yo: 50 mg/kg (up to 2 g) PO single dose. Amebiasis, >3 yo: 50 mg/kg (up to 2 g) PO daily × 3 d. Take with food.
UNAPPROVED ADULT - Recurrent/persistent urethritis: 2 g PO single dose.
FORMS - Trade only: Tabs 250,500 mg. Pharmacists can compound oral susp.
NOTES - Give iodoquinol/paromomycin after treatment for amebic dysentery or liver abscess. Disulfiram reaction; avoid alcohol until ≥3 d after treatment. Can minimize infant exposure by withholding breastfeeding for 3 d after maternal single dose. May increase levels of cyclosporine, fluorouracil, lithium, phenytoin, tacrolimus. May increase INR with warfarin. Do not give at same time as cholestyramine. CYP 450 3A4 substrate. For patients undergoing hemodialysis: Give supplemental ½ dose after dialysis session.

## ANTIMICROBIALS: Antiviral Agents—Anti-Cytomegalovirus

**CIDOFOVIR** (*Vistide*) ▶K ♀C ▶- $$$$$
WARNING - Severe nephrotoxicity. Granulocytopenia - monitor neutrophil counts.
ADULT - CMV retinitis: 5 mg/kg IV q wk × 2 wk, then 5 mg/kg every other wk. Give probenecid 2 g PO 3h before and 1 g 2h and 8h after infusion. Give normal saline with each infusion.
PEDS - Not approved in children.
NOTES - Fanconi-like syndrome. Stop nephrotoxic drugs ≥1 wk before cidofovir. Get serum creatinine, urine protein before each dose. See package insert for dosage adjustments based on renal function. Do not use if creatinine >1.5 mg/dl, CrCl ≤55 mL/min, or urine protein ≥100 mg/dl (≥2+). Hold/decrease zidovudine dose by 50% on d cidofovir is given. Tell women not to get pregnant until 1 mo after and men to use barrier contraceptive until 3 mo after cidofovir. Ocular hypotony - monitor intraocular pressure.

**FOSCARNET** (*Foscavir*) ▶K ♀C ▶? $$$$$
WARNING - Nephrotoxicity; seizures due to mineral/electrolyte imbalance.
ADULT - Hydrate before infusion. CMV retinitis: 60 mg/kg IV (over 1 h) q8h or 90 mg/kg IV (over 1.5–2 h) q12h × 2–3 wk, then 90–120 mg/kg IV daily over 2h. Acyclovir-resistant HSV infection: 40 mg/kg IV (over 1 h) q8–12h × 2–3 wk or until healed.
PEDS - Not approved in children. Deposits into teeth & bone of young animals.
UNAPPROVED PEDS - Hydrate before infusion. CMV retinitis: 60 mg/kg IV (over 1 h) q8h or 90 mg/kg IV (over 1.5–2 h) q12h × 2–3 wk, then 90–120 mg/kg IV daily over 2h. Acyclovir-resistant HSV infection: 40 mg/kg IV (over 1 h) q8h × 2–3 wk or until healed. Acyclovir-resistant varicella zoster infection: 40 mg/kg IV q8h × 7–10 d.
NOTES - Granulocytopenia, anemia, vein irritation, penile ulcers. Decreased ionized serum calcium, especially with IV pentamidine. Must use IV pump
**(cont.)**

**FOSCARNET** (*cont.*)

to avoid rapid administration. Monitor renal function, serum calcium, magnesium, phosphate, potassium. Reduce dose in renal impairment. Stop foscarnet if CrCl decreases to <0.4 mL/min/kg.

**GANCICLOVIR** (*DHPG*) ▶K ♀C ▶- $$$$$
WARNING - Neutropenia, anemia, thrombocytopenia. Do not use if ANC <500/mm³ or platelets <25,000/mm³.
ADULT - CMV retinitis. Induction: 5 mg/kg IV q12h × 14–21 d. Maintenance: 6 mg/kg IV daily × 5 d/wk; 5 mg/kg IV daily; 1000 mg PO tid; or 500 mg PO 6 times/d (q3h while awake) with food. Prevention of CMV disease in advanced AIDS: 1000 mg PO tid with food. Prevention of CMV disease after organ transplant: 5 mg/kg IV q12h × 7–14 d, then 6 mg/kg IV daily × 5 d/wk or 1000 mg PO tid with food. Give IV infusion over 1 h.
PEDS - Safety and efficacy not established in children; potential carcinogenic or reproductive adverse effects.
UNAPPROVED PEDS - CMV retinitis in immunocompromised patient: Induction 5 mg/kg IV q12h × 14–21 d. Maintenance 5 mg/kg IV daily or 6 mg/kg IV daily × 5 d/wk. Symptomatic congenital CMV infection: 6 mg/kg IV q12 h × 6 wk.
FORMS - Generic only: Caps 250, 500 mg.
NOTES - Neutropenia (worsened by zidovudine), phlebitis/pain at infusion site, increased seizure risk with imipenem. Monitor CBC, creatinine. Reduce dose if CrCl <70 mL/min. Adequate hydration required. Potential teratogen. Tell women not to get pregnant during & men to use

barrier contraceptive until ≥3 mo after treatment. Potential carcinogen. Follow guidelines for handling/disposal of cytotoxic agents.

**VALGANCICLOVIR** (*Valcyte*) ▶K ♀C ▶- $$$$$
WARNING - Myelosuppression may occur at any time. Monitor CBC frequently. Do not use if ANC <500/mm³, platelets <25,000/mm³, hemoglobin <8 g/dL.
ADULT - CMV retinitis: 900 mg PO bid × 21 d, then 900 mg PO daily. Prevention of CMV disease in high-risk kidney, kidney-pancreas, and heart transplant patients: 900 mg PO daily from within 10 d after transplant until 100 d post-transplant. Give with food. Valganciclovir tabs and ganciclovir caps not interchangeable on mg per mg basis.
PEDS - Safety and efficacy not established in children; potential carcinogenic or reproductive adverse effects.
FORMS - Trade only: Tabs 450 mg.
NOTES - Contraindicated in ganciclovir allergy. Greater bioavailability than oral ganciclovir. Potential teratogen. Tell women not to get pregnant during and men to use barrier contraceptive until ≥3 mo after treatment. CNS toxicity; warn against hazardous tasks. May increase serum creatinine; monitor renal function. Reduce dose if CrCl <60 mL/min. Use ganciclovir instead in hemodialysis patients. Potential drug interactions with didanosine, mycophenolate. Potential carcinogen. Avoid direct contact with broken/crushed tabs; do not intentionally break/crush tabs. Follow guidelines for handling/disposal of cytotoxic agents.

## ANTIMICROBIALS: Antiviral Agents—Anti-Herpetic

**ACYCLOVIR** (*Zovirax*) ▶K ♀B ▶+ $
ADULT - Genital herpes: 200 mg PO q4h (5x/d) × 10 d for first episode, × 5 d for recurrent episodes. Chronic suppression: 400 mg PO bid. Zoster: 800 mg PO q4h (5x/d) × 7–10 d. Chickenpox: 800 mg PO qid × 5 d. IV: 5–10 mg/kg IV q8h, each dose over 1 h. Zoster in immunocompromised patients: 10 mg/kg IV q8h × 7 d. Herpes simplex encephalitis: 10 mg/kg IV q8h × 10 d. Mucosal/cutaneous herpes simplex in immunocompromised patients: 5 mg/kg IV q8h × 7 d.
PEDS - Safety and efficacy of PO acyclovir not established in children <2 yo. Chickenpox: 20 mg/kg PO qid × 5 d. Use adult dose if >40 kg. AAP does not recommend routine treatment of chickenpox with acyclovir. Consider use if >12 yo, chronic cutaneous or pulmonary disease, chronic salicylate use, or short, intermittent or inhaled corticosteroid. Possibly also for secondary case-patients in same household as infected children. IV: 250–500 mg/m² q8h, each dose over 1h. Zoster in immunocompromised patients <12 yo: 20 mg/kg IV q8h × 7 d. Herpes simplex encephalitis: 20 mg/kg IV q8h × 10 d for 3 mo-12 yo, adult dose for ≥12 yo. Neonatal herpes simplex (birth to 3

mo): 10 mg/kg IV q8 h × 10 d; CDC regimen is 20 mg/kg IV q8h × 21 d for disseminated/CNS disease, × 14 d for skin/mucous membranes. Mucosal/cutaneous herpes simplex in immunocompromised patients: 10 mg/kg IV q8h × 7 d for <12 yo, adult dose for ≥12 yo. Treat ASAP after symptom onset.
UNAPPROVED ADULT - Genital herpes: 400 mg PO tid × 7–10 d for first episode, × 5 d for recurrent episodes, × 5–10 d for recurrent episodes in HIV+ patients. Alternative regimens for recurrent episodes in HIV negative patients: 800 mg PO bid × 5 d or 800 mg PO tid × 2 d. Chronic suppression of genital herpes in HIV+ patients: 400–800 mg PO bid-tid. Orolabial herpes (controversial indication): 400 mg PO 5x/d.
UNAPPROVED PEDS - Primary herpes gingivostomatitis: 15 mg/kg PO 5x/d × 7 d. First-episode genital herpes: 80 mg/kg/d PO divided tid (max 1.2 g/d) × 7–10 d. Use dose in unapproved adult for adolescents. Zoster (mild) in mild immunosuppression: 20 mg/kg (max 800 mg/dose) PO qid × 7–10 d. Treat ASAP after symptom onset.
FORMS - Generic/Trade: Caps 200 mg, tabs 400,800 mg. Susp 200 mg/5 mL.

**ACYCLOVIR** *(cont.)*
NOTES - Maintain adequate hydration. Severe drowsiness with acyclovir plus zidovudine. Reduce dose in renal dysfunction and in elderly. Base IV dose on ideal body weight in obese adults.
**FAMCICLOVIR** *(Famvir)* ▶K ♀B ▶? $$
ADULT - Recurrent genital herpes: 1000 mg PO bid × 2 doses. Chronic suppression of genital herpes: 250 mg PO bid. Recurrent herpes labialis: 1500 mg PO single dose. Recurrent orolabial/genital herpes in HIV patients: 500 mg PO bid × 7 d. Zoster: 500 mg PO tid × 7 d. Treat ASAP after symptom onset.
PEDS - Not approved in children.
UNAPPROVED ADULT - First-episode genital herpes: 250 mg PO tid × 7–10 d. Chronic suppression of genital herpes in HIV+ patients: 500 mg PO bid. Chickenpox in young adults: 500 mg PO tid × 5 d. Bell's palsy: 750 mg PO tid plus prednisone 1 mg/kg PO daily × 7 d. Treat ASAP after symptom onset.
UNAPPROVED PEDS - Chickenpox in adolescents: 500 mg PO tid × 5 d. First-episode genital herpes in adolescents: Use dose in unapproved adult.
FORMS - Generic/Trade: Tabs 125, 250, 500 mg.
NOTES - Reduce dose for CrCl <60 mL/min.
**VALACYCLOVIR** *(Valtrex)* ▶K ♀B ▶+ $$$$$
ADULT - First-episode genital herpes: 1 g PO bid × 10 d. Recurrent genital herpes: 500 mg PO bid × 3 d. Chronic suppression of genital herpes in immunocompetent patients: 1 g PO daily.

Can use 500 mg PO daily if ≤9 recurrences/yr; transmission of genital herpes reduced with use of this regimen by source partner, in conjunction with safer sex practices. Chronic suppression of genital herpes in HIV-infected patients: 500 mg PO bid. Herpes labialis: 2 g PO q12h × 2 doses. Zoster: 1 g PO tid × 7 d. Treat ASAP after symptom onset.
PEDS - Herpes labialis, ≥12 yo: 2 g PO q12h × 2 doses. Treat ASAP after symptom onset.
UNAPPROVED ADULT - Recurrent genital herpes: 1 g PO daily × 5 d. Recurrent genital herpes in HIV+ patients: 1 g PO bid × 5–10 d. Bell's palsy: 1 g PO bid plus prednisone 1 mg/kg PO daily × 7 d. Orolabial herpes in immunocompromised patients, including HIV infection: 1 g PO tid × 7 d. Chickenpox in young adults: 1 g PO tid × 5 d. Treat ASAP after symptom onset.
UNAPPROVED PEDS - Chickenpox in adolescents: 1 g PO tid × 5 d. Treat ASAP after symptom onset. First-episode genital herpes in adolescents: Use adult dose.
FORMS - Generic/Trade: Tabs 500,1000 mg.
NOTES - Maintain adequate hydration. CNS and renal adverse effects more common if elderly or renal impairment; avoid inappropriately high doses in these patients. Thrombotic thrombocytopenic purpura/hemolytic uremic syndrome at dose of 8 g/d. Reduce dose for CrCl <50 mL/min. Metabolized to acyclovir.

## ANTIMICROBIALS: Antiviral Agents—Anti-HIV—CCR5 Antagonists

**NOTE:** AIDS treatment guidelines available online at www.aidsinfo.nih.gov. Consider monitoring LFTs in patients receiving highly active anti-retroviral therapy (HAART).

**MARAVIROC** *(Selzentry)* ▶LK ♀B ▶- $$$$$
WARNING - Hepatotoxicity with allergic features. Consider discontinuation if signs/symptoms of hepatitis, or increased LFTs with rash or other systemic symptoms. Caution with baseline liver dysfunction or coinfection with hepatitis B/C.
ADULT - Combination therapy for HIV infection, treatment-experienced patients: 150 mg PO bid with strong CYP 3A4 inhibitors (delavirdine, most protease inhibitors, ketoconazole, itraconazole, clarithromycin); 300 mg PO bid with drugs that are not strong CYP 3A4 inducers/inhibitors (NRTIs, tipranavir-ritonavir, nevirapine, enfuvirtide); 600 mg PO bid with strong CYP 3A4 inducers

(efavirenz, rifampin, carbamazepine, phenobarbital, phenytoin). Tropism test before treatment; not for dual/mixed or CXCR4-tropic HIV infection.
PEDS - Not recommended for <16 yo based on lack of data.
FORMS - Trade only: Tabs 150, 300 mg.
NOTES - Caution for patients with liver dysfunction or coinfection with hepatitis B/C. May increase risk of myocardial ischemia or MI. Theoretical risk of infection/malignancy due to effects on immune system. Metabolized by CYP 3A4; do not use with St John's wort. Coadministration of CYP 3A4 inhibitor in patients with CrCl <50 mL/min may increase maraviroc levels and risk of adverse drug reactions.

## ANTIMICROBIALS: Antiviral Agents–Anti-HIV—Combinations

**NOTE:** AIDS treatment guidelines available online at www.aidsinfo.nih.gov. Consider monitoring LFTs in patients receiving highly active anti-retroviral therapy (HAART). WARNING: Nucleoside reverse transcriptase inhibitors can cause lactic acidosis and hepatic steatosis. Fatalities reported in pregnant women receiving didanosine + stavudine.

*ATRIPLA* **(efavirenz + emtricitabine + tenofovir)** ▶KL ♀D ▶- $$$$$
WARNING - Emtricitabine and tenofovir: Potentially fatal lactic acidosis and hepatosteatosis; severe

acute exacerbation of hepatitis B after discontinuation in patients coinfected with HIV and hepatitis B; not indicated for treatment of hepatitis B.

*(cont.)*

**ATRIPLA** (cont.)
ADULT - Combination therapy for HIV infection: 1 tab PO once daily on empty stomach, preferably at bedtime. Atripla can be used alone or in combo with other anti-retrovirals that are not already in the tab.
PEDS - Safety and efficacy not established.
UNAPPROVED PEDS - Combination therapy for HIV infection, adolescents ≥40 kg: 1 tab PO once daily on empty stomach, preferably at bedtime. Atripla can be used alone or in combo with other anti-retrovirals.
FORMS - Trade only: Tabs efavirenz 600 mg + emtricitabine 200 mg + tenofovir 300 mg.
NOTES - See components. Do not give Atripla with lamivudine. Not for CrCl ≤50 mL/min. Efavirenz induces cytochrome P450 3A4, causing many drug interactions.

**COMBIVIR** (lamivudine + zidovudine) ▶LK ♀C ▶- $$$$$
WARNING - Zidovudine: bone marrow suppression, myopathy. Lamivudine: Severe acute exacerbation of hepatitis B can occur after discontinuation of lamivudine in patients coinfected with HIV + hepatitis B. Monitor closely for ≥2 mo after discontinuing lamivudine in such patients; consider treating hepatitis B.
ADULT - Combination therapy for HIV infection: 1 tab PO bid.
PEDS - Combination therapy for HIV infection, ≥12 yo: 1 tab PO bid.
FORMS - Trade only: Tabs lamivudine 150 mg + zidovudine 300 mg.
NOTES - See components. Monitor CBC. Not for weight <50 kg, CrCl ≤50 mL/min, hepatic dysfunction, or if dosage adjustment required.

**EPZICOM** (abacavir + lamivudine) ▶LK ♀C ▶- $$$$$
WARNING - Abacavir: Potentially fatal hypersensitivity reactions. Abacavir and lamivudine: Lactic acidosis and hepatosteatosis. Lamivudine: Exacerbation of hepatitis B after discontinuation in patients co-infected with HIV and hepatitis B.
ADULT - Combination therapy for HIV infection: 1 tab PO daily.
PEDS - Safety and efficacy not established in children.
FORMS - Trade only: Tabs abacavir 600 mg + lamivudine 300 mg.
NOTES - See components. Contraindicated in patients with previous hypersensitivity reaction to abacavir due to risk of fatal rechallenge reaction. Not for patients with CrCl ≤50 mL/min, hepatic dysfunction, or if dosage adjustment required.

**TRIZIVIR** (abacavir + lamivudine + zidovudine) ▶LK ♀C ▶- $$$$$
WARNING - Abacavir: Life-threatening hypersensitivity (see abacavir entry for details). Never restart after a reaction. Zidovudine: Bone marrow suppression, myopathy.
ADULT - HIV infection, alone (not a preferred regimen) or in combo with other agents: 1 tab PO bid.
PEDS - HIV infection in adolescents ≥40 kg, alone (not a preferred regimen) or in combo with other agents: 1 tab PO bid.
FORMS - Trade only: Tabs abacavir 300 mg + lamivudine 150 mg + zidovudine 300 mg.
NOTES - See components. Monitor CBC. Not for weight <40 kg, CrCl ≤50 mL/min or if dosage adjustment required.

**TRUVADA** (emtricitabine + tenofovir) ▶K ♀B ▶- $$$$$
WARNING - Emtricitabine and tenofovir: Potentially fatal lactic acidosis and hepatosteatosis; severe acute exacerbation of hepatitis B after discontinuation in patients coinfected with HIV and hepatitis B.
ADULT - Combination therapy for HIV infection: 1 tab PO daily.
PEDS - Safety and efficacy not established in children.
UNAPPROVED ADULT - Antiviral-resistant chronic hepatitis B in HIV-coinfected patients: 1 tab PO daily.
FORMS - Trade only: Tabs emtricitabine 200 mg + tenofovir 300 mg.
NOTES - See components. Do not use in a triple nucleoside regimen. Not for patients with CrCl ≤30 mL/min or hemodialysis; hepatic dysfunction; or if dosage adjustment required. Increase dosing interval to q48h if CrCl 30–49 mL/min. Coadminister didanosine and Truvada cautiously; monitor for didanosine adverse effects, and discontinue didanosine if they occur. Reduce didanosine dose to 250 mg in adults >60 kg; dosage adjustment of didanosine unclear if <60 kg. Give Videx EC + Truvada on empty stomach or with light meal. Give buffered didanosine + Truvada on empty stomach. Atazanavir and lopinavir/ritonavir increase tenofovir levels; monitor and discontinue Truvada if tenofovir adverse effects. Tenofovir decreases atazanavir levels. If atazanavir is used with Truvada, use 300 mg atazanavir + 100 mg ritonavir. Do not use Truvada with lamivudine.

---

## ANTIMICROBIALS: Antiviral Agents—Anti-HIV—Fusion Inhibitors

**NOTE:** AIDS treatment guidelines available online at www.aidsinfo.nih.gov. Consider monitoring LFTs in patients receiving highly active anti-retroviral therapy (HAART).

**ENFUVIRTIDE** (*Fuzeon, T-20*) ▶Serum ♀B ▶- $$$$$
WARNING - Not for monotherapy.
ADULT - Combination therapy for HIV infection: 90 mg SC bid. Give each injection at new site in
upper arm, anterior thigh, or abdomen, avoiding areas with current injection site reaction.
PEDS - Combination therapy for HIV infection, 6–16 yo: 2 mg/kg up to 90 mg SC bid. Give each

**ENFUVIRTIDE** *(cont.)*
injection at new site in upper arm, anterior thigh, or abdomen, avoiding areas with current injection site reaction.

FORMS - 30-d kit with vials, diluent, syringes, alcohol wipes. Single-dose vials contain 108 mg to provide 90 mg enfuvirtide.

NOTES - Increased risk of bacterial pneumonia; monitor for signs and symptoms of pneumonia. Biojector 2000 can cause persistent nerve pain if used near large nerves, bruising, hematomas. Anticoagulants, hemophilia, or other coagulation disorder may increase risk of post-injection bleeding. Reconstitute with 1.1 mL sterile water for injection. This provides 1.2 mL of solution, of which only 1 mL (90 mg) is injected. Allow vial to stand until powder dissolves completely (up to 45 min). Do not shake. Second daily dose can be reconstituted ahead of time if stored in refrigerator in original vial and used within 24 h. Return to room temp before injecting. Discard unused solution. Patient education on administration available at 1-877-438-9366 or www.fuzeon.com.

## ANTIMICROBIALS: Antiviral Agents—Anti-HIV—Integrase Strand Transfer Inhibitor

**NOTE:** AIDS treatment guidelines available online at www.aidsinfo.nih.gov. Consider monitoring LFTs in patients receiving highly active anti-retroviral therapy (HAART).

**RALTEGRAVIR** *(Isentress)* ▶Glucuronidation ♀C ▶- $$$$$
WARNING - Not for monotherapy.
ADULT - Combination therapy for treatment-resistant HIV infection: 400 mg PO bid.
PEDS - Safety & efficacy not established in children.

FORMS - Trade only: Tabs 400 mg.
NOTES - Rifampin may reduce raltegravir levels; monitor for reduced efficacy. Myopathy and rhabdomyolysis reported; caution advised for coadministration with drugs that cause myopathy.

## ANTIMICROBIALS: Antiviral Agents—Anti-HIV—Non-Nucleoside Reverse Transcriptase Inhibitors

**NOTE:** Many serious drug interactions - always check before prescribing! See www.aidsinfo.nih.gov and www.cdc.gov/tb/TB_HIV_Drugs/default.htm for AIDS treatment guidelines and the use of rifamycins with NNRTIs. Consider monitoring LFTs in patients receiving highly active anti-retroviral therapy (HAART).

**DELAVIRDINE** *(Rescriptor, DLV)* ▶L ♀C ▶- $$$$$
WARNING - Not for monotherapy.
ADULT - Combination therapy for HIV infection: 400 mg PO tid.
PEDS - Combination therapy for HIV infection, ≥16 yo: 400 mg PO tid. Safety and efficacy not established in younger children.
UNAPPROVED PEDS - Combination therapy for HIV, adolescents <16 yo: 400 mg PO tid.
FORMS - Trade only: Tabs 100, 200 mg.
NOTES - Rash common in 1st first mo of therapy. Can cause Stevens-Johnson syndrome. Many drug interactions. Inhibits cytochrome P450 3A4 & 2C9. Do not use with alprazolam, carbamazepine, cisapride, ergot alkaloids, lovastatin, phenytoin, phenobarbital, pimozide, chronic use of H2 blocker or proton pump inhibitor, rifabutin, rifampin, rifapentine, simvastatin, St John's wort, triazolam. Midazolam contraindicated in labeling; but can use single dose IV cautiously with monitoring for procedural sedation. Monitor LFTs when delavirdine used with saquinavir. May increase fluticasone levels; find alternatives for long-term use. May need to decrease methadone or trazodone dose. See package insert for clarithromycin dosage reduction if CrCl <60 mL/min. Monitor levels of antiarrhythmics, immunosuppressants. Not more than a single 25 mg dose of sildenafil in 48 h. Not more than a single 2.5 mg dose of vardenafil in 24 h. Tadalafil initial dose is 5 mg; not more than 10 mg single dose in 72 h. Monitor INR with warfarin. Take at least 1 h before/after buffered didanosine or antacids. Can dissolve 100 mg tabs in water. Take with acidic drink if achlorhydria.

**EFAVIRENZ** *(Sustiva, EFV)* ▶L ♀D ▶- $$$$$
WARNING - Not for monotherapy.
ADULT - Combination therapy for HIV infection: 600 mg PO qhs. Coadministration with voriconazole: Use voriconazole maintenance dose of 400 mg PO bid & reduce efavirenz to 300 mg (use caps) PO once daily. Avoid with high-fat meal. Take on empty stomach, preferably at bedtime.
PEDS - Consider antihistamine rash prophylaxis before starting. Combination therapy for HIV infection, ≥3 yo: 10–15 kg: 200 mg PO qhs. 15–20 kg: 250 mg qhs. 20 to <25 kg: 300 mg qhs. 25 to <32.5 kg: 350 mg qhs. 32.5 to <40 kg: 400 mg qhs. ≥40 kg: 600 mg qhs. Do not give with high-fat meal.
FORMS - Trade only: Caps 50, 100, 200 mg; tabs 600 mg.
NOTES - Psychiatric/CNS reactions (warn about hazardous tasks), rash (consider antihistamines and/or corticosteroids; stop treatment if severe), increased cholesterol (monitor). To avoid "hangover", give 1st dose at 6–8 pm & start drug over weekend. False-positive with Microgenics cannabinoid screening test. Monitor LFTs if given with ritonavir, hepatotoxic drugs, or to patients with hepatitis B/C. Induces cytochrome P450 3A4. Many drug interactions including decreased levels of anticonvulsants, atorvastatin, diltiazem, itraconazole, methadone, pravastatin, simvastatin, and probably ketoconazole. Do not give with

**(cont.)**

**EFAVIRENZ** (cont.)

cisapride, pimozide, triazolam, ergot alkaloids, or St John's wort. Midazolam contraindicated in labeling; but can use single dose IV cautiously with monitoring for procedural sedation. If used with rifampin, consider increasing efavirenz to 800 mg qhs if weight ≥60 kg. High risk of rash when taken with clarithromycin; consider alternative antimicrobial. Potentially teratogenic; get negative pregnancy test before use by women of child-bearing potential and recommend barrier contraceptive.

**ETRAVIRINE** (*Intelence*) ▶L ♀B ▶- $$$$$
WARNING - Not for monotherapy.
ADULT - Combination therapy for treatment-resistant HIV infection: 200 mg PO bid after meals.
PEDS - Safety and efficacy not established in children.
FORMS - Trade only: Tabs 100 mg.
NOTES - Severe skin reactions, Stevens-Johnson syndrome, hypersensitivity. Induces CYP 3A4 and inhibits CYP 2C9 and 2C19; substrate of CYP 2C9, 2C19, and 3A4. Do not give with efavirenz, nevirapine, ritonavir 600 mg bid; ritonavir-boosted tipranavir/fosamprenavir/atazanavir; St John's wort, rifampin, rifapentine, carbamazepine, phenobarbital, phenytoin. Do not give rifabutin if ritonavir is used; give rifabutin 300 mg once daily with unboosted etravirine. Monitor INR with warfarin. Consider monitoring antiarrhythmic blood levels. Can disperse tabs in water and take immediately if swallowing difficulty.

**NEVIRAPINE** (*Viramune, NVP*) ▶LK ♀C ▶- $$$$$
WARNING - Life-threatening skin reactions, hypersensitivity, and hepatotoxicity. Monitor clinical and lab status intensively during first 18 wk of therapy (risk of rash and/or hepatotoxicity greatest during first 6 wk of therapy) and frequently thereafter. Consider LFTs at baseline, before and 2 wk after dose increase, and at least once monthly. Rapidly progressive liver failure can occur after only a few wk of therapy. Stop nevirapine and never rechallenge if clinical hepatitis, severe rash, or rash with constitutional symptoms/increased LFTs. Obtain LFTs if rash occurs. Risk of hepatotoxicity with rash high in women or high CD4 count (women with CD4 count >250 especially high risk, including pregnant women). Do not use if CD4 count >250 in women or >400 in men unless benefit clearly outweighs risk. Elevated LFTs or hepatitis B/C infection at baseline increases risk of hepatotoxicity. Hepatotoxicity not reported after single doses of nevirapine or in children. Not for monotherapy.
ADULT - Combination therapy for HIV infection: 200 mg PO daily × 14 d, then 200 mg PO bid. Dose titration reduces risk of rash. If rash develops, do not increase dose until it resolves. If stopped for >7 d, restart with initial dose.
PEDS - Combination therapy for HIV infection, age ≥15 d: 150 mg/m² PO once daily × 14 d, then 150 mg/m² bid (max dose 200 mg bid). Dose titration reduces risk of rash. If rash develops, do not increase dose until it resolves. If stopped for >7 d, restart with initial dose. Per HIV guidelines, children ≤8 yo may require up to 200 mg/m² PO bid up to max of 200 mg bid.
UNAPPROVED ADULT - Combination therapy for HIV infection: 200 mg PO daily × 14 d, then 400 mg PO daily. Prevention of maternal-fetal HIV transmission, maternal dosing: 200 mg PO single dose at onset of labor.
UNAPPROVED PEDS - Prevention of maternal-fetal HIV transmission, neonatal dosing: 2 mg/kg PO single dose within 3 d of birth.
FORMS - Trade only: Tabs 200 mg, susp 50 mg/5 mL (240 mL).
NOTES - Cytochrome P450 3A inducer. May require increased methadone dose. Do not give with ketoconazole, hormonal contraceptives, St John's wort. Granulocytopenia more common in children receiving zidovudine and nevirapine.

## ANTIMICROBIALS: Antiviral Agents—Anti-HIV—Nucleoside/Nucleotide Reverse Transcriptase Inhibitors

**NOTE:** See www.aidsinfo.nih.gov and www.cdc.gov/tb/TB_HIV_Drugs/default.htm for AIDS treatment guidelines and use of rifamycins with NRTIs. Consider monitoring LFTs with highly active anti-retroviral therapy (HAART). Can cause lactic acidosis and hepatic steatosis. Fatalities reported in pregnant women receiving didanosine + stavudine.

**ABACAVIR** (*Ziagen, ABC*) ▶L ♀C ▶- $$$$$
WARNING - Potentially fatal hypersensitivity (look for fever, rash, GI symptoms, cough, dyspnea, pharyngitis, or other respiratory symptoms). Stop at once & never rechallenge after suspected reaction. Fatal reactions can recur within h of rechallenge in patients with previously unrecognized reaction. HLA-B*5701 predisposes to hypersensitivity; screen before starting abacavir and avoid if positive test. Label HLA-B*5701 patients as abacavir-allergic in medical record.
ADULT - Combination therapy for HIV infection: 300 mg PO bid or 600 mg PO daily. Severe hypersensitivity may be more common with once-daily dose.
PEDS - Combination therapy for HIV, 3 mo - 16 yo: 8 mg/kg up to 300 mg PO bid. Use adult dose for >16 yo.
FORMS - Trade only: Tabs 300 mg, oral soln 20 mg/mL (240 mL).
NOTES - Dosage reduction for mild hepatic dysfunction (Child-Pugh score 5–6): 200 mg (10 mL of oral soln) PO bid. As of Feb 2008, FDA is investigating possible increased risk of myocardial infarction with abacavir.

**DIDANOSINE** (*Videx, Videx EC, ddI*) ▶LK ♀B ▶- $$$$$
WARNING - Potentially fatal pancreatitis; avoid use with other drugs that can cause pancreatitis. Avoid didanosine + stavudine in pregnancy due to reports of fatal lactic acidosis with pancreatitis or hepatic steatosis.
ADULT - Combination therapy for HIV infection: Buffered powder: 250 mg PO bid for ≥60 kg, 167 mg PO bid for <60 kg. Videx EC: 400 mg PO daily for ≥60 kg, 250 mg PO daily for <60 kg. All formulations usually taken on empty stomach. Dosage reduction of Videx EC with tenofovir: 250 mg if ≥60 kg, 200 mg if <60 kg. Dosage reduction unclear with tenofovir if CrCl <60 mL/min. Give tenofovir + Videx EC on empty stomach or with light meal; give tenofovir + buffered didanosine on empty stomach.
PEDS - Combination therapy for HIV infection: 100 mg/m² PO bid for age 2 wk-8 mo. 120 mg/m² PO bid for age >8 mo. Give on empty stomach. Videx EC not approved for children.
FORMS - Generic/Trade: Pediatric powder for oral solution 10 mg/mL (buffered with antacid), delayed-release caps 200, 250, 400 mg. Trade only: (Videx EC) delayed-release caps 125 mg, chewable tabs 25, 50, 100, 150, 200 mg.
NOTES - As of Feb 2008, FDA is investigating possible increased risk of myocardial infarction with didanosine. Peripheral neuropathy (use cautiously with other neurotoxic drugs), retinal changes, optic neuritis, retinal depigmentation in children, hyperuricemia. Risk of lactic acidosis, pancreatitis, and peripheral neuropathy increased by concomitant stavudine. Diarrhea with buffered powder. See package insert for reduced dose if CrCl <60 mL/min. Do not use with allopurinol. Give some medications at least 1 h (delavirdine, indinavir), 2 h (atazanavir, ciprofloxacin, levofloxacin, norfloxacin, ofloxacin, itraconazole, ketoconazole, ritonavir, dapsone, tetracyclines), or 4 h (moxifloxacin, gatifloxacin) before buffered didanosine. Contraindicated with ribavirin due to risk of didanosine toxicity.

**EMTRICITABINE** (*Emtriva, FTC*) ▶K ♀B ▶- $$$$$
WARNING - Severe acute exacerbation of hepatitis B can occur after discontinuation in patients coinfected with HIV + hepatitis B. Monitor closely for ≥2 mo; consider treating hepatitis B.
ADULT - Combination therapy for HIV infection: 200 mg cap PO daily. Oral soln: 240 mg (24 mL) PO daily.
PEDS - Combination therapy for HIV, ≥3 mo: 6 mg/kg up to 240 mg (24 mL) of oral soln PO once daily. Can give 200 mg cap PO once daily if >33 kg.
UNAPPROVED PEDS - Combination therapy for HIV infection. Oral soln: 3 mg/kg PO once daily for ≤3 mo, 6 mg/kg up to 240 mg for 3 mo-17 yo. Caps, >33 kg: 200 mg PO once daily.
FORMS - Trade only: Caps 200 mg, oral soln 10 mg/mL (170 mL).

NOTES - Lactic acidosis/hepatic steatosis. Exacerbation of hepatitis B after discontinuation in adults with renal dysfunction. Dosage reduction in adults with renal dysfunction. Caps: 200 mg PO q48h if CrCl 30-49 mL/min; 200 mg PO q72h if CrCl 15-29 mL/min; 200 mg PO q96h if CrCl <15 mL/min or hemodialysis. Oral soln: 120 mg q24h if CrCl 30-49 mL/min; 80 mg q24h if CrCl 15-29 mL/min, 60 mg q24h if CrCl <15 mL/min or hemodialysis. Refrigerate oral soln if possible; stable for 3 mo stored at room temp.

**LAMIVUDINE** (*Epivir, Epivir-HBV, 3TC, ◆Heptovir*) ▶K ♀C ▶- $$$$$
WARNING - Lower dose of lamivudine in Epivir-HBV can cause HIV resistance - test for HIV before prescribing Epivir-HBV. Severe acute exacerbation of hepatitis B can occur after discontinuation of lamivudine in patients coinfected with HIV + hepatitis B. Monitor closely for ≥2 mo after discontinuing lamivudine in such patients; consider treating hepatitis B.
ADULT - Epivir for combination therapy for HIV infection: 300 mg PO daily or 150 mg PO bid. Epivir-HBV for chronic hepatitis B: 100 mg PO daily. Co-infection with HIV and hepatitis B requires higher dose of lamivudine for HIV infection.
PEDS - Epivir for HIV infection: 3 mo-16 yo, 4 mg/kg (up to 150 mg) PO bid. Epivir tabs: 75 mg (½ tab) PO bid for 14-21 kg; 75 mg (½ tab) PO q am and 150 mg (1 tab) PO q pm for >21 to <30 kg; 150 mg (1 tab) PO bid for ≥30 kg. Epivir-HBV for chronic hepatitis B, 2-17 yo: 3 mg/kg up to 100 mg PO daily. Co-infection with HIV and hepatitis B requires higher dose of lamivudine for HIV infection.
UNAPPROVED PEDS - Epivir for combination therapy for HIV infection. Adolescents ≥50 kg: 300 mg PO daily. Infants, <30 d old: 2 mg/kg PO bid.
FORMS - Trade only: Epivir, 3TC: Tabs 150 (scored), 300 mg, oral soln 10 mg/mL. Epivir-HBV, Heptovir: Tabs 100 mg, oral soln 5 mg/mL.
NOTES - Lamivudine-resistant hepatitis B reported. Epivir: Pancreatitis in children. Monitor for hepatic decompensation (potentially fatal), neutropenia, and anemia if also receiving interferon for hepatitis C. If hepatic decompensation occurs, consider discontinuing lamivudine, and reducing or discontinuing interferon, and/or ribavirin. Dosage reduction for CrCl <50 mL/min in package insert.

**STAVUDINE** (*Zerit, d4T*) ▶LK ♀C ▶- $$$$$
WARNING - Warn patients to report early signs of lactic acidosis (eg, abdominal pain, N/V, fatigue, dyspnea, weakness). Symptoms can mimic Guillain-Barre syndrome. Stop stavudine if weakness or lactic acidosis. Potentially fatal pancreatitis & hepatotoxicity with didanosine + stavudine +/- hydroxyurea. Avoid this combo in pregnancy.
ADULT - Combination therapy for HIV infection: 40 mg PO q12h; 30 mg PO q12h if <60 kg. Hold
**(cont.)**

**STAVUDINE** *(cont.)*

for peripheral neuropathy. If symptoms resolve completely, can restart at 20 mg PO q12h or 15 mg PO q12h if <60 kg. If symptoms recur, consider stopping permanently.

PEDS - Combination therapy for HIV infection: <30 kg and ≥2 wk old: 1 mg/kg PO bid. 30–59.9 kg: 30 mg bid. ≥60 kg: 40 mg bid.

FORMS - Trade only: Caps 15, 20, 30, 40 mg, oral soln 1 mg/mL (200 mL).

NOTES - Peripheral neuropathy, lactic acidosis, pancreatitis; risk of these adverse reactions increased by concomitant didanosine. Do not use with zidovudine. Dosage reduction for CrCl <50 mL/min in package insert. Oral soln stable in refrigerator for 30 d.

**TENOFOVIR** *(Viread, TDF)* ▶K ♀B ▶- $$$$$

WARNING - Stop tenofovir if hepatomegaly or steatosis occur, even if LFTs normal. Severe acute exacerbation of hepatitis B can occur after discontinuation of tenofovir in patients coinfected with HIV + hepatitis B. Monitor closely for ≥2 mo after discontinuing tenofovir in such patients; consider treating hepatitis B.

ADULT - Combination therapy for HIV infection: 300 mg PO daily with a meal. High rate of virologic failure with tenofovir + didanosine + lamivudine; avoid this regimen.

PEDS - Not approved in children. Decreased bone mineral density reported. Insufficient data to recommend as initial HIV therapy in children.

UNAPPROVED ADULT - Coinfection with HIV + hepatitis B: 300 mg PO daily with a meal.

FORMS - Trade only: Tab 300 mg.

NOTES - Decreased bone mineral density; consider bone monitoring if history of pathologic fracture or high risk of osteopenia. Consider calcium + vitamin D supplement. Tenofovir increases didanosine levels and possibly serious didanosine adverse effects (eg pancreatitis, lactic acidosis, hyperlactatemia, neuropathy). Reduce Videx EC to 250 mg in patients ≥60 kg or 200 mg if <60 kg. Dosage adjustment of Videx EC unclear if CrCl <60 mL/min. Give tenofovir + Videx EC on empty stomach or with light meal; give tenofovir + buffered didanosine on empty stomach. If atazanavir is used with tenofovir, use 300 mg atazanavir + 100 mg ritonavir. Atazanavir and lopinavir/ritonavir increase tenofovir levels; monitor and discontinue tenofovir if adverse effects. Tenofovir can cause renal impairment including acute renal failure & Fanconi syndrome. Avoid tenofovir if current/recent nephrotoxic drug use. Drugs that reduce renal function or undergo renal elimination (eg, acyclovir, adefovir, ganciclovir) may increase tenofovir levels. Monitor creatinine & phosphate if risk/history of renal insufficiency or nephrotoxic drug. Dosage reduction if CrCl <50 mL/min: 300 mg q48h if CrCl 30–49 mL/min; 300 mg twice weekly if CrCl 10–29 mL/min, 300 mg once weekly for dialysis patients (given after dialysis).

**ZIDOVUDINE** *(Retrovir, AZT, ZDV)* ▶LK ♀C ▶- $$$$$

WARNING - Bone marrow suppression, myopathy.

ADULT - Combination therapy for HIV infection: 600 mg/d PO divided bid or tid. IV dosing: 1 mg/kg IV over 1 h 5–6 ×/d. Prevention of maternal-fetal HIV transmission, maternal dosing (>14 wk of pregnancy): 200 mg PO tid or 300 mg PO bid until start of labor. During labor, 2 mg/kg IV over 1 h, then 1 mg/kg/h until delivery.

PEDS - Combination therapy for HIV infection. 6 wk -12 yo: 160 mg/m² up to 200 mg PO q8h. Adolescents: Use adult dose. Prevention of maternal-fetal HIV transmission, infant dosing: 2 mg/kg PO q6h from within 12 h of birth until 6 wk old. Can also give infants 1.5 mg/kg IV over 30 min q6h.

UNAPPROVED PEDS - Combination therapy for HIV infection, 6 wk - 12 yo: 180–240 mg/m² PO q12h.

FORMS - Generic/Trade: Cap 100 mg, tab 300 mg, syrup 50 mg/5 mL (240 mL).

NOTES - Do not use with stavudine. Hematologic toxicity; monitor CBC. Increased bone marrow suppression with ganciclovir or valganciclovir. Granulocytopenia more common in children receiving zidovudine and nevirapine. Monitor for hepatic decompensation, neutropenia, and anemia if also receiving interferon regimen for hepatitis C. If hepatic decompensation occurs, consider discontinuing zidovudine, interferon, and/or ribavirin. See package insert for dosage adjustments based on renal function or hematologic toxicity.

---

## ANTIMICROBIALS: Antiviral Agents—Anti-HIV—Protease Inhibitors

**NOTE:** Many serious drug interactions - always check before prescribing! Protease inhibitors inhibit CYP 3A4. Contraindicated with most antiarrhythmics, cisapride, ergot alkaloids, lovastatin, pimozide, simvastatin, St. John's wort, triazolam; caution with atorvastatin. Midazolam contraindicated in labeling; but can use single dose IV cautiously with monitoring for procedural sedation. See www.aidsinfo.nih.gov and www.cdc.gov/tb/TB_HIV_Drugs/default.htm for use of rifamycins with protease inhibitors. Do not use rifampin with standard protease inhibitor regimens. Monitor INR with warfarin. Avoid inhaled/nasal fluticasone with ritonavir if possible; increased fluticasone levels can cause Cushing's syndrome/adrenal suppression. Other protease inhibitors may increase fluticasone levels; find alternatives for long-term use. Trazodone levels and adverse effects increased by ritonavir and possibly other protease inhibitors; may need to reduce trazodone dose. Not more than a single 25 mg dose of sildenafil in 48 h with protease inhibitors. Vardenafil initial dose is 2.5 mg; not more than a single 2.5 mg dose in 72 h. Sildenafil preferred over vardenafil with unboosted indinavir. Tadalafil initial dose is 5 mg; not more (**cont.**)

than 10 mg single dose in 72 h. Adverse effects include spontaneous bleeding in hemophiliacs, hyperglycemia, hyperlipidemia, immune reconstitution syndrome, and fat redistribution. Coinfection with hepatitis C or other liver disease increases the risk of hepatotoxicity with protease inhibitors; monitor LFTs at least twice in 1st mo of therapy, then every 3 mo.

**ATAZANAVIR (*Reyataz, ATV*) ▶L ♀B ▶- $$$$$**

ADULT - Combination therapy for HIV infection. Therapy-naive patients: 400 mg PO daily. With efavirenz or tenofovir, therapy-naive patients: Atazanavir 300 mg + ritonavir 100 mg all PO daily with food. Therapy-experienced patients: Atazanavir 300 mg PO daily + ritonavir 100 mg PO daily. Give atazanavir with food; give 2 h before or 1 h after buffered didanosine.

PEDS - Combination therapy for HIV infection. Therapy-naïve, ritonavir-intolerant, ≥13 yo and ≥39 kg: 400 mg PO once daily with food. Therapy-naïve, ≥6 yo: Give atazanavir/ritonavir 150/80 mg for 15–<25 kg; 200/100 mg for 25–<32 kg; 250/100 mg for 32–<39 kg; 300/100 mg for ≥39 kg. Therapy-experienced, ≥6 yo: Give atazanavir/ritonavir 200/100 mg for 25–<32 kg; 250/100 mg for 32–<39 kg; 300/100 mg for ≥39 kg. Max dose for atazanavir/ritonavir of 300/100 mg. Do not use in infants; may cause kernicterus.

FORMS - Trade only: Caps 100, 150, 200, 300 mg.

NOTES - Does not appear to increase cholesterol or triglycerides. Asymptomatic increases in indirect bilirubin due to inhibition of UDP-glucuronosyl transferase (UGT); may cause jaundice/scleral icterus. Do not use with indinavir; both may increase bilirubin. Do not use with rifampin. Reduce rifabutin to 150 mg every other d or 300 mg 3 times/wk. Consider other etiology for associated increases in transaminases. May inhibit UGT1A1 metabolism of irinotecan. Can prolong PR interval; rare cases of 2nd degree AV block reported; caution advised for patients with AV block or on drugs that prolong PR interval. Monitor ECG with calcium channel blockers; consider reducing diltiazem dose by 50%. Reduce clarithromycin dose by 50%; consider alternative therapy for indications other than *Mycobacterium avium* complex. Give atazanavir with food. Acid required for absorption; acid-suppressing drugs can cause treatment failure. Proton pump inhibitors: In treatment-naïve patients do not exceed dose equivalent of omeprazole 20 mg; give PPI 12 h before atazanavir 300 mg + ritonavir 100 mg. Do not use PPIs with unboosted atazanavir or in treatment-experienced patients. H2 blockers: Give atazanavir 300 mg + ritonavir 100 mg simultaneously with and/or ≥10 h after H2 blocker, with max dose equivalent of famotidine 40 mg bid for treatment naïve patients and 20 mg bid for treatment experienced patients. For treatment-experienced patients receiving tenofovir and H2 blocker, give atazanavir 400 mg + ritonavir 100 mg once daily with food. Give atazanavir 2 h before or 1 h after antacids or buffered

didanosine. Give atazanavir and EC didanosine at different times. Inhibits cytochrome P450 1A2, 2C9, and 3A4. Use lowest possible dose of atorvastatin/rosuvastatin or consider pravastatin/fluvastatin. Monitor levels of antiarrhythmics, immunosuppressants, tricyclic antidepressants. Increases levels of ethinyl estradiol and norethindrone; use lowest dose of both in oral contraceptives. In mild to moderate hepatic impairment (Child-Pugh class B), consider dosage reduction to 300 mg PO daily with food. Do not use in Child-Pugh Class C. Dosage adjustment, hemodialysis for end-stage renal disease: atazanavir 300 mg + ritonavir 100 mg if treatment-naïve; do not use atazanavir if treatment-experienced.

**DARUNAVIR (*Prezista*) ▶L ♀B ▶- $$$$$**

ADULT - Combination therapy for HIV infection in therapy-experienced patients: 600 mg PO bid boosted by ritonavir 100 mg PO bid with food. Darunavir should always be boosted with ritonavir.

PEDS - Not approved in children.

FORMS - Trade only: Tab 300, 600 mg.

NOTES - Cross-sensitivity with sulfonamides possible; caution if allergy. Hepatotoxicity; monitor AST/ALT more frequently (especially during first few mo of therapy) if patient already has chronic hepatitis, cirrhosis, or elevated transaminase levels. CYP 3A4 inhibitor and substrate. Do not give with lopinavir/ritonavir, saquinavir, or rifampin. Monitor levels of antiarrhythmics. Clarithromycin dosage reduction if CrCl <60 mL/min (see clarithromycin entry for details). Not >200 mg/d ketoconazole or itraconazole. Ritonavir decreases voriconazole levels; do not use darunavir/ritonavir unless benefit exceeds risk. Reduce rifabutin to 150 mg PO every other d. May decrease oral contraceptive efficacy; consider additional or alternative method. Give didanosine 1 h before/2 h after darunavir/ritonavir. Increases pravastatin levels up to 5-fold; use lowest possible dose of pravastatin, rosuvastatin, or atorvastatin or consider using fluvastatin.

**FOSAMPRENAVIR (*Lexiva, 908, ✦Telzir*) ▶L ♀C ▶- $$$$$**

ADULT - Combination therapy for HIV infection. Therapy-naive patients: 1400 mg PO bid (without ritonavir). OR fosamprenavir 1400 mg + ritonavir 200 mg both PO daily. OR 700 mg fosamprenavir + 100 mg ritonavir both PO bid OR 1400 mg + ritonavir 100 mg both PO daily. Protease inhibitor-experienced patients: 700 mg fosamprenavir + 100 mg ritonavir both PO bid. Do not use once-daily regimen. If once-daily ritonavir-boosted regimen given with efavirenz, increase ritonavir to 300 mg/d; no increase of ritonavir dose needed for bid regimen with efavirenz. Can

**(cont.)**

**FOSAMPRENAVIR** (cont.)

give nevirapine with fosamprenavir only if bid ritonavir-boosted regimen used. No meal restrictions for tabs; advise adults to take susp with food. Re-dose if vomiting occurs within 30 min of giving oral susp.

PEDS - Combination therapy for HIV infection. Do not use once-daily dosing of fosamprenavir in children. Therapy-naïve, 2–5 yo: 30 mg/kg susp PO bid (max 1400 mg bid). Therapy naïve, ≥6 yo: 30 mg/kg susp PO bid (max 1400 mg bid) OR 18 mg/kg susp PO bid + ritonavir 3 mg/kg PO bid (max fosamprenavir 700 mg + ritonavir 100 mg PO bid). Can use fosamprenavir 2 tabs bid if ≥47 kg. Protease inhibitor-experienced, ≥6 yo: 18 mg/kg susp PO bid + ritonavir 3 mg/kg PO bid (max fosamprenavir 700 mg + ritonavir 100 mg PO bid). For fosamprenavir + ritonavir, can use fosamprenavir tabs if ≥39 kg and ritonavir caps if >33 kg. Do not use in infants; may cause kernicterus. Advise children to take susp with food. Take tabs without regard to meals. Re-dose if vomiting occurs within 30 min of giving oral susp.

FORMS - Trade only: Tabs 700 mg, susp 50 mg/mL.

NOTES - Life-threatening skin reactions possible (reported with amprenavir). Cross-sensitivity with sulfonamides possible; use caution in sulfonamide-allergic patients. Hypertriglyceridemia; monitor lipids. Fosamprenavir is inhibitor & substrate of cytochrome P450 3A4. Do not use fosamprenavir + ritonavir with flecainide or propafenone. Do not use fosamprenavir with delavirdine, lovastatin, rifampin, or simvastatin. Use lowest possible dose of atorvastatin or rosuvastatin with monitoring for myopathy or consider fluvastatin/pravastatin. Monitor CBC at least weekly if taking rifabutin. Monitor levels of antiarrhythmics, immunosuppressants, tricyclic antidepressants. May need to increase dose of methadone. Monitor INR with warfarin. Not >200 mg/d ketoconazole/itraconazole with fosamprenavir + ritonavir; may need to reduce antifungal dose if >400 mg/d itraconazole/ketoconazole with unboosted fosamprenavir. Not >2.5 mg vardenafil q24h with unboosted fosamprenavir or q72h for fosamprenavir + ritonavir. Do not use hormonal contraceptives. More adverse reactions when fosamprenavir given with Kaletra; appropriate dose for combination therapy unclear. Mild to moderate hepatic dysfunction (Child-Pugh score 5–8): 700 mg PO bid for unboosted fosamprenavir; no data for ritonavir-boosted regimen. Refrigeration not required, but may improve taste of oral susp.

**INDINAVIR** (Crixivan, IDV) ▶LK ♀C ▶- $$$$$

ADULT - Combination therapy for HIV infection: 800 mg PO q8h between meals with water (at least 48 oz/d).

PEDS - Not approved in children. Do not use in infants; may cause kernicterus.

UNAPPROVED ADULT - Combination therapy for HIV infection: 800 mg PO bid with ritonavir 100–200

mg PO bid. Or 400 mg bid with ritonavir 400 mg bid. 600 mg PO bid with Kaletra 400/100 mg PO bid. Can be given without regard to meals when given with ritonavir.

UNAPPROVED PEDS - Combination therapy for HIV infection, adolescents: 800 mg PO q8h between meals with water (at least 48 oz/d). Children: 350–500 mg/m²/dose (max of 800 mg/dose) PO q8h.

FORMS - Trade only: Caps 100, 200, 333, 400 mg.

NOTES - Nephrolithiasis (especially in children), hemolytic anemia, indirect hyperbilirubinemia, possible hepatitis, interstitial nephritis with asymptomatic pyuria. Do not use with atazanavir; both may increase bilirubin. Inhibits cytochrome P450 3A4. Avoid using with carbamazepine if possible. Give indinavir and buffered didanosine 1 h apart on empty stomach. Reduce indinavir dose to 600 mg PO q8h when given with ketoconazole, itraconazole 200 mg bid, or delavirdine 400 mg tid. Increase indinavir dose to 1000 mg PO q8h when given with efavirenz, nevirapine. Do not use with rifampin. Give rifabutin 150 mg once daily with indinavir 1000 mg q8h. With ritonavir-boosted indinavir, reduce rifabutin to 150 mg every other d without increasing indinavir dose. For mild to moderate hepatic cirrhosis, give 600 mg PO q8h. Indinavir not recommended in pregnancy because of dramatic reduction in blood levels.

**LOPINAVIR-RITONAVIR** (Kaletra, LPV/r) ▶L ♀C ▶- $$$$$

ADULT - Combination therapy for HIV infection: Give tabs without regard to meals; give oral soln with food. Therapy-naive patients: 2 tabs (400/100 mg) PO bid or 4 tabs (800/200 mg) once daily. 5 mL PO bid or 10 mL once daily of oral soln. Increase oral soln to 6.5 mL PO bid (not once daily) with efavirenz, nevirapine, fosamprenavir, or nelfinavir (dosage increase not needed with tabs). Therapy-experienced patients: No once-daily regimen. 2 tabs (400/100 mg) PO bid or 5 mL oral soln bid. Increase oral soln to 6.5 mL PO bid with efavirenz, nevirapine, fosamprenavir, or nelfinavir. Consider 3 tabs (600/150 mg) bid with efavirenz, nevirapine, fosamprenavir without ritonavir, or nelfinavir if reduced lopinavir susceptibility suspected. Do not use once-daily dosing in pregnant women.

PEDS - Combination therapy for HIV infection without concomitant efavirenz, nevirapine, fosamprenavir, or nelfinavir. Oral soln, 14 d-6 mo: lopinavir 16 mg/kg or 300 mg/m² PO bid. Oral soln, 6 mo-18 yo: lopinavir 230 mg/m² PO bid OR 12 mg/kg PO bid for 7–<15 kg, 10 mg/kg PO bid for ≥15 kg-<40 kg. Tabs (100 mg/25 mg), 6 mo–18 yo: 2 tabs PO bid for 15–25 kg, 3 tabs PO bid for >25–35 kg, 4 tabs PO bid for >35 kg. Concomitant therapy with efavirenz, nevirapine, fosamprenavir, or nelfinavir, 6 mo-18 yo: lopinavir 300 mg/m² PO bid OR 13 mg/kg PO bid for 7–<15 kg (use oral soln only), 11 mg/kg PO

**LOPINAVIR-RITONAVIR (cont.)**
bid for ≥15–<45 kg (use oral soln or tabs); use adult dose for >45 kg. Give tabs without regard to meals; give oral soln with food. Beware of medication errors with highly concentrated Kaletra oral soln; fatal overdose reported in infant given excessive volume of Kaletra oral soln.

UNAPPROVED ADULT - Combination therapy for HIV infection during rifampin-based therapy for TB: 4 tabs (800/200 mg) PO bid OR 2 tabs (400/100 mg) + ritonavir 300 mg both PO bid. Monitor for hepatotoxicity.

FORMS - Trade only: Caps 133.3/33.3 mg; tabs 200/50 mg, 100/25 mg; oral soln 80/20 mg/mL (160 mL).

NOTES - Medication errors can occur if Keppra (levetiracetam) confused with Kaletra. May cause pancreatitis. Ritonavir (inhibits cytochrome P450 3A4 & 2D6) included in formulation to inhibit metabolism and boost levels of lopinavir. Increases tenofovir levels; monitor for adverse drug reaction. Many other drug interactions including decreased efficacy of oral contraceptives. Ritonavir decreases voriconazole levels; do not give with voriconazole unless benefit exceeds risk. Reduce rifabutin to 150 mg every other d or 3 times/wk. May require higher methadone dose. Avoid inhaled/nasal fluticasone if possible; concomitant use may cause Cushing's syndrome and adrenal suppression. Ritonavir increases trazodone levels and adverse effects; consider reducing trazodone dose. Clarithromycin dosage reduction if CrCl <60 mL/min (see clarithromycin entry for details). Give buffered didanosine 1 h before/2 h after Kaletra oral soln. Kaletra tabs can be given at same time as didanosine without food. Do not give Kaletra with tipranavir 500 mg + ritonavir 200 mg both bid. Monitor INR with warfarin. Do not use once-daily dosing in pregnant women. Oral soln contains alcohol. Use oral soln within 2 mo if patient stores at room temperature. Tabs do not require refrigeration. Do not crush, cut, or chew tabs.

**NELFINAVIR (Viracept, NFV)** ▶L ♀B ▶- $$$$$
ADULT - Combination therapy for HIV infection: 750 mg PO tid or 1250 mg PO bid with meals. Absorption improved when meal contains ≥500 calories with 11–28 g of fat.

PEDS - Combination therapy for HIV infection, ≥2 yo: 45–55 mg/kg PO bid or 25–35 mg/kg PO tid to max of 2500 mg/d. Take with meals. Use powder or 250 mg tabs which can be crushed and mixed with water or other liquids. Do not mix with acidic foods/juice; will taste bitter.

UNAPPROVED PEDS - Combination therapy for HIV infection: Up to 45 mg/kg/dose PO tid with meals. Absorption improved when meal contains ≥500 calories with 11–28 g of fat.

FORMS - Trade only: Tab 250, 625 mg, oral powder 50 mg/g (114 g).

NOTES - Diarrhea common. Inhibits cytochrome P450 3A4. Use lowest possible dose of atorvastatin/ rosuvastatin or consider pravastatin/fluvastatin. Decreases efficacy of oral contraceptives. May require higher methadone dose. Do not use with proton pump inhibitors, rifampin. Give rifabutin 150 mg once daily with nelfinavir 1250 mg bid. Give nelfinavir 2 h before/1 h after buffered didanosine. Oral powder stable for 6 h after mixing if refrigerated. No dosage adjustment for mild hepatic impairment (Child-Pugh Class A); not recommended for more severe hepatic failure (Child-Pugh B/C). Concern about trace amounts of ethyl methanesulfonate (a carcinogen) resolved and restrictions on nelfinavir use in pregnant women and children removed in May 2008.

**RITONAVIR (Norvir, RTV)** ▶L ♀B ▶- $$$$$
WARNING - Contraindicated with many drugs due to risk of drug interactions.
ADULT - Full-dose regimen (600 mg PO bid) poorly tolerated. Lower doses of 100 mg PO daily to 400 mg PO bid used to boost levels of other protease inhibitors. Best tolerated regimen with saquinavir may be ritonavir 400 mg + saquinavir 400 mg both bid. Saquinavir 1000 mg + ritonavir 100 mg both bid also used.

PEDS - Combination therapy for HIV infection, ≥1 mo old: 250 mg/m² PO q12h, increasing by 50 mg/m²/dose every 2–3 d to 400 mg/m² PO q12h. Max dose 600 mg PO bid. Give with meals.

UNAPPROVED ADULT - Combination therapy for HIV infection: 100–200 mg PO bid with indinavir 800 mg PO bid OR ritonavir 400 mg + indinavir 400 mg both bid.

UNAPPROVED PEDS - Used at lower than labeled doses to boost levels of other protease inhibitors.

FORMS - Trade only: Cap 100 mg, oral soln 80 mg/ mL (240 mL).

NOTES - N/V, pancreatitis, alterations in AST, ALT, GGT, CPK, uric acid. Inhibits hepatic cytochrome P450 3A & 2D6. Contraindicated with alfuzosin. Ritonavir decreases voriconazole levels. Do not use ritonavir 400 mg bid with voriconazole; use ritonavir 100 mg bid with voriconazole only if benefit exceeds risk. Not >200 mg/d of ketoconazole with ritonavir. Reduce rifabutin to 150 mg every other d or 3 times/wk with ritonavir alone or ritonavir-boosted protease inhibitors. Can give ritonavir/saquinavir 400/400 mg bid with rifampin; monitor for hepatotoxicity. Not more than a single dose of vardenafil 2.5 mg or tadalafil 10 mg in 72 h with ritonavir. Decreases efficacy of combined oral or patch contraceptives; consider alternative. Increases methadone dosage requirements. May cause serotonin syndrome with fluoxetine. Increases trazodone levels and adverse effects; consider reducing trazodone dose. Clarithromycin dosage reduction if CrCl <60 mL/min (see clarithromycin entry for details). Avoid inhaled/ nasal fluticasone if possible; concomitant use may cause Cushing's syndrome and adrenal suppression. Give ritonavir 2.5h before/after buffered didanosine. Monitor digoxin; may increase levels.

(cont.)

**RITONAVIR** *(cont.)*

Caps and oral soln contain alcohol. Do not refrigerate oral soln. Try to refrigerate caps, but stable for 30 d at <77 degrees F.

**SAQUINAVIR** *(Invirase, SQV)* ▶L ♀B ▶? $$$$$

ADULT - Combination therapy for HIV infection. Regimen must contain ritonavir. Saquinavir 1000 mg + ritonavir 100 mg both PO bid taken within 2 h after meals. Saquinavir 1000 mg + lopinavir-ritonavir (Kaletra) 400/100 mg both PO bid. If serious toxicity occurs, do not reduce Invirase dose; efficacy unclear for lower doses.

PEDS - Combination therapy for HIV, ≥16 yo: Use adult dose.

UNAPPROVED ADULT - Combination therapy for HIV infection during rifampin-based TB therapy: Saquinavir 400 mg + ritonavir 400 mg both PO bid. Monitor for hepatotoxicity.

FORMS - Trade only: Invirase (hard gel) caps 200 mg, tabs 500 mg.

NOTES - Do not use saquinavir with garlic supplements or tipranavir/ritonavir. Delavirdine, omeprazole, or ketoconazole increase saquinavir levels. Monitor LFTs if given with delavirdine. Reduce rifabutin to 150 mg every other d or 3 times/wk. Monitor for increased digoxin levels. May reduce methadone levels. Clarithromycin dosage reduction if CrCl <60 mL/min (see clarithromycin entry for details).

**TIPRANAVIR** *(Aptivus)* ▶Feces ♀C ▶- $$$$$

WARNING - Potentially fatal hepatotoxicity. Monitor clinical status and LFTs frequently. Risk increased by coinfection with hepatitis B/C. Contraindicated in moderate to severe (Child Pugh B/C) hepatic failure. Intracranial hemorrhage can occur with tipranavir + ritonavir; caution if at risk of bleeding from trauma, surgery, other medical conditions, or receiving antiplatelet agents or anticoagulants.

ADULT - HIV infection, boosted by ritonavir in treatment-experienced patients with strains resistant to multiple protease inhibitors: 500 mg + ritonavir 200 mg PO bid with food.

PEDS - HIV infection, boosted by ritonavir in treatment-experienced patients ≥2 yo with strains resistant to multiple protease inhibitors: 14 mg/kg with 6 mg/kg ritonavir (375 mg/m$^2$ with ritonavir 150 mg/m$^2$) PO bid to max of 500 mg with ritonavir 200 mg bid. Dosage reduction for toxicity in patients infected with virus that is not resistant to multiple protease inhibitors: 12 mg/kg with 5 mg/kg ritonavir (290 mg/m$^2$ with 115 mg/m$^2$ ritonavir) bid.

FORMS - Trade only: Caps 250 mg. Oral soln 100 mg/mL (95 mL in unit-ofuse amber glass bottle).

NOTES - Contains sulfonamide moiety; potential for cross-sensitivity unknown. Al/Mg antacids may decrease absorption of tipranavir; separate doses. Ritonavir-boosted tipranavir inhibits CYP 3A4 and 2D6. Contraindicated with CYP 3A4 substrates that can cause life-threatening toxicity at high concentrations. Monitor levels of immunosuppressants, tricyclic antidepressants. May need higher methadone dose. Ritonavir decreases voriconazole levels; do not give together unless benefit exceeds risk. Do not use tipranavir/ritonavir with Kaletra, saquinavir, or rifampin. Decreases ethinyl estradiol levels; consider non-hormonal contraception. Reduce rifabutin to 150 mg PO every other d. Clarithromycin dosage reduction if CrCl <60 mL/min (see clarithromycin entry for details). Caps contain alcohol. Refrigerate bottle of caps before opening. Use caps and oral soln within 60 d of opening container. Oral soln contains 116 IU/mL of vitamin E; advise patients not to take supplemental vitamin E other than a multivitamin.

## ANTIMICROBIALS: Antiviral Agents—Anti-Influenza

**NOTE:** Whenever possible, immunization is the preferred method of prophylaxis. Consider chemoprophylaxis in high-risk patients vaccinated after influenza activity has begun, care-givers for high-risk patients, patients with immunodeficiency (including HIV infection), and those who request it. Provide chemoprophylaxis to all residents during institutional outbreaks of influenza, continuing for ≥2 wk or until 1 wk after end of outbreak. Avoid anti-influenza antivirals from 48 h before until 2 wk after a dose of live influenza vaccine unless medically necessary. Patients with suspected influenza may have primary/concomitant bacterial pneumonia; antibiotics may be indicated.

**AMANTADINE** *(Symmetrel, ✦Endantadine)* ▶K ♀C ▶? $$

WARNING - The CDC recommends against amantadine/rimantadine for treatment/prevention of influenza A in the US due to high levels of resistance.

ADULT - Influenza A: 100 mg PO bid. ≥65 yo: 100 mg PO daily. Parkinsonism: 100 mg PO bid. Max 400 mg/d divided tid-qid. Drug-induced extrapyramidal disorders: 100 mg PO bid. Max 300 mg/d divided tid-qid.

PEDS - Safety and efficacy not established in infants <1 yo. Influenza A, treatment or prophylaxis, ≥10

yo: 100 mg PO bid. 1–9 yo and any child <40 kg: 5 mg/kg/d up to 150 mg/d PO divided bid.

FORMS - Generic only: Cap 100 mg. Generic/Trade: Tab 100 mg, syrup 50 mg/5 mL (480 mL).

NOTES - CNS toxicity, suicide attempts, neuroleptic malignant syndrome with dosage reduction/withdrawal, anticholinergic effects, orthostatic hypotension. Do not stop abruptly in Parkinson's disease. Dosage reduction in adults with renal dysfunction: 200 mg PO 1st d, then 100 mg PO daily for CrCl 30–50 mL/min. 200 mg PO 1st d, then 100 mg PO qod for CrCl 15–29 mL/min. 200 mg PO q wk for CrCl <15 mL/min or hemodialysis.

**OSELTAMIVIR (*Tamiflu*)** ▶LK ♀C ▶? $$$
ADULT - Influenza A/B, treatment: 75 mg PO bid × 5 d starting within 2 d of symptom onset. Prophylaxis: 75 mg PO daily. Start within 2 d of exposure and continue for ≥7 d. Take with food to improve tolerability.
PEDS - Influenza A/B, ≥1 yo: Each dose is 30 mg if ≤15 kg, 45 mg if 16–23 kg, 60 mg if 24–40 kg, 75 mg if >40 kg or ≥13 yo. For treatment, give twice daily × 5 d starting within 2 d of symptoms onset. For prophylaxis, give once daily × 10 d starting within 2 d of exposure. Take with food to improve tolerability. Suspension comes with graduated syringe calibrated to 30, 45, and 60 mg; use 30 mg plus 45 mg to measure 75 mg dose.
FORMS - Trade only: Caps 30, 45, 75 mg, susp 12 mg/mL (25 mL).
NOTES - Not for infants <1 yo; immature blood brain barrier could lead to high oseltamivir levels in CNS. Increased INR with warfarin. Post-marketing reports (mostly from Japan) of self-injury and delirium, primarily among children and adolescents; monitor for abnormal behavior. Dosage adjustment for CrCl 10–30 mL/min: 75 mg PO daily × 5 d for treatment, 75 mg PO qod for prophylaxis. Susp stable for 10 d at room temperature.

**RIMANTADINE (*Flumadine*)** ▶LK ♀C ▶- $$
WARNING - The CDC recommends against amantadine/rimantadine for treatment/prevention

of influenza A in the US due to high levels of resistance.
ADULT - Prophylaxis/treatment of influenza A: 100 mg PO bid. Start treatment ≤48 h of symptom onset and continue × 7 d. Reduce to 100 mg/d if side effects in patients ≥65 yo, severe hepatic dysfunction, CrCl ≤10 mL/min, elderly nursing home patient.
PEDS - Prophylaxis of influenza A, ≥10 yo: 100 mg PO bid. 1–9 yo or any child <40 kg: 5 mg/kg/d up to 150 mg/d PO divided daily or bid.
FORMS - Generic/Trade: Tabs 100 mg. Trade only: Syrup 50 mg/5 mL (240 mL).

**ZANAMIVIR (*Relenza*)** ▶K ♀C ▶? $$$
ADULT - Influenza A/B, treatment: 2 puffs bid × 5 d. Take 2 doses on d 1 at least 2 h apart. Start within 2 d of symptom onset. Influenza A/B, prevention: 2 puffs once daily × 10 d.
PEDS - Influenza A/B, treatment, ≥7 yo: 2 puffs bid × 5 d. Take 2 doses on d 1 at least 2 h apart. Start within 2 d of symptom onset. Influenza A/B, prevention, ≥5 yo: 2 puffs once daily × 10 d.
FORMS - Trade only: Rotadisk inhaler 5 mg/puff (20 puffs).
NOTES - May cause bronchospasm & worsen pulmonary function in asthma or COPD; avoid if underlying airways disease. Stop if bronchospasm/decline in respiratory function. Show patient how to use inhaler.

## ANTIMICROBIALS: Antiviral Agents—Other

**ADEFOVIR (*Hepsera*)** ▶K ♀C ▶- $$$$$
WARNING - Nephrotoxic; monitor renal function. HIV resistance in untreated HIV infection; test for HIV before prescribing. Lactic acidosis with hepatic steatosis. Severe acute exacerbation of hepatitis B can occur after discontinuation of adefovir in patients with HIV + hepatitis B coinfection. Monitor closely for ≥2 mo after discontinuing adefovir in such patients; consider retreating hepatitis B.
ADULT - Chronic hepatitis B: 10 mg PO daily.
PEDS - Chronic hepatitis B, ≥12 yo: 10 mg PO daily.
FORMS - Trade only: Tabs 10 mg.
NOTES - Monitor renal function. See package insert for dosage reduction if CrCl <50 mL/min. Other nephrotoxic drugs may increase risk of nephrotoxicity. Use adefovir plus lamivudine instead of adefovir alone in patients with lamivudine-resistant hepatitis B. Adefovir resistance can cause viral load rebound. Consider change in therapy if persistant serum hepatitis B DNA >1000 copies/mL.

**ENTECAVIR (*Baraclude*)** ▶K ♀C ▶- $$$$$
WARNING - Nucleoside analogues can cause lactic acidosis with hepatic steatosis. Severe acute exacerbation of hepatitis B can occur after discontinuation. Monitor closely for ≥2 mo after discontinuation. Patients coinfected with HIV + hepatitis B should not receive entecavir for

hepatitis B unless they also receive HAART for HIV; failure to treat HIV in such patients could lead to HIV resistance to NRTIs.
ADULT - Chronic hepatitis B: 0.5 mg PO once daily if treatment naive; 1 mg if lamivudine-resistant or history of viremia despite lamivudine treatment. Give on empty stomach (2 h after last meal and 2 h before next meal).
PEDS - Chronic hepatitis B, ≥16 yo: 0.5 mg PO once daily if treatment naive; 1 mg if lamivudine-resistant or history of viremia despite lamivudine treatment.
FORMS - Trade only: Tabs 0.5, 1 mg, solution 0.05 mg/mL (210 mL).
NOTES - Entecavir treatment of co-infected patients not receiving HIV treatment may increase the risk of lamivudine/emtricitabine resistance. Do not mix oral solution with water or other liquid. Reduce dose if CrCl <50 mL/min or dialysis. Give dose after dialysis sessions.

**INTERFERON ALFA-2B (*Intron A*)** ▶K ♀C ▶? + $$$$$
WARNING - May cause or worsen serious neuropsychiatric, autoimmune, ischemic, & infectious diseases. Frequent clinical & lab monitoring required. Stop interferon if signs/symptoms of these conditions are persistently severe or worsen.
ADULT - Chronic hepatitis B: 5 million units/d or 10 million units 3 times/wk SC/IM × 16 wk if HBeAg +, × 48 wk if HBeAg. Chronic hepatitis **(cont.)**

**INTERFERON ALFA-2B** *(cont.)*

C: 3 million units SC/IM 3 times/wk × 16 wk. Continue for 18–24 mo if ALT normalized. Other indications: condylomata acuminata, AIDS-related Kaposi's sarcoma, hairy-cell leukemia, melanoma, follicular lymphoma.

PEDS - Chronic hepatitis C, ≥3 yo: Interferon alfa-2b 3 million units/m² SC 3 times/wk and PO ribavirin according to weight. Ribavirin: 200 mg bid for 25–36 kg; 200 mg q am and 400 mg q pm for 37–49 kg; 400 mg bid for 50–61 kg. Use adult dose for >61 kg. If ribavirin contraindicated use interferon 3–5 million units/m² (max 3 million units/dose) SC/IM three times/wk. Chronic hepatitis B, ≥1 yo: 3 million units/m² three times/wk for first wk, then 6 million units/m² three times/wk (max 10 million units/dose) SC three times/wk.

UNAPPROVED ADULT - Prevention of chronic hepatitis C in acute hepatitis C: 5 million units SC daily × 4 wk then 5 million units SC 3 times/wk × 20 wk. Superficial bladder tumors. Chronic myelogenous leukemia. Cutaneous T-cell lymphoma. Essential thrombocythemia. Non-Hodgkin's lymphoma. Chronic granulocytic leukemia.

FORMS - Trade only: Powder/soln for injection 10, 18, 50 million units/vial. Soln for injection 18, 25 million units/multidose vial. Multidose injection pens 3, 5,10 million units/0.2mL (1.5 mL), 6 doses/pen.

NOTES - Monitor for depression, suicidal behavior (esp. in adolescents), other severe neuropsychiatric effects. Thyroid abnormalities, hepatotoxicity, flu-like symptoms, pulmonary & cardiovascular reactions, retinal damage, neutropenia, thrombocytopenia, hypertriglyceridemia (consider monitoring). Increases theophylline levels. Monitor CBC, TSH, LFTs, electrolytes. Dosage adjustments for hematologic toxicity in package insert.

**INTERFERON ALFACON-1** *(Infergen)* ▶Plasma ♀C ▶? $$$$$

WARNING - May cause or worsen serious neuropsychiatric, autoimmune, ischemic, & infectious diseases. Frequent clinical & lab monitoring required. Stop interferon if signs/symptoms of these conditions are persistently severe or worsen.

ADULT - Chronic hepatitis C: 9 mcg SC 3 times/wk × 24 wk. Increase to 15 mcg SC 3 times/wk × 24 wk if relapse/no response. Reduce to 7.5 mcg SC 3 times/wk if intolerable adverse effects.

PEDS - Not approved in children.

FORMS - Trade only: Vials injectable soln 30 mcg/mL (0.3 mL, 0.5 mL).

NOTES - Monitor for depression, suicidal behavior, other severe neuropsychiatric effects. Thyroid dysfunction, cardiovascular reactions, retinal damage, flu-like symptoms, thrombocytopenia, neutropenia, exacerbation of autoimmune disorders, hypertriglyceridemia (consider monitoring). Monitor CBC, thyroid function. Refrigerate injectable soln.

**INTERFERON ALFA-N3** *(Alferon N)* ▶K ♀C ▶- $$$$$

WARNING - Flu-like syndrome, myalgias, alopecia. Contraindicated in egg protein allergy.

ADULT - Doses vary by indication. Condylomata acuminata, intralesional.

PEDS - Not approved in children.

**PALIVIZUMAB** *(Synagis)* ▶L ♀C ▶? $$$$$

PEDS - Prevention of respiratory syncytial virus pulmonary disease in high-risk patients: 15 mg/kg IM q mo during RSV season with first injection before season starts (November to April in northern hemisphere). Consider for children <2 yo treated for chronic lung disease in last 6 mo or with hemodynamically significant congenital heart disease; infants born <28 wk gestation who are now <12 mo; infants born 29–32 wk gestation who are now <6 mo. Give a dose ASAP after cardiopulmonary bypass (due to decreased palivizumab levels) even if <1 mo after last dose.

NOTES - Preservative-free - use within 6 h of reconstitution. Not more than 1 mL per injection site.

**PEGINTERFERON ALFA-2A** *(Pegasys)* ▶LK ♀C ▶- $$$$$

WARNING - May cause or worsen serious neuropsychiatric, autoimmune, ischemic, & infectious diseases. Frequent clinical & lab monitoring recommended. Discontinue if signs/symptoms of these conditions are persistently severe or worsen.

ADULT - Chronic hepatitis C not previously treated with alfa interferon: 180 mcg SC in abdomen or thigh once weekly for 48 wk +/− PO ribavirin 800–1200 mg/d. Ribavirin dose and duration depends on genotype and body weight (see PO ribavirin entry). Chronic hepatitis C in patients coinfected with HIV: 180 mcg SC once weekly plus ribavirin 800 mg/d PO for 48 wk regardless of genotype. Hepatitis B: 180 mcg SC in abdomen or thigh once weekly for 48 wk.

PEDS - Not approved in children.

FORMS - Trade only: 180 mcg/1 mL solution in single-use vial, 180 mcg/0.5 mL prefilled syringe.

NOTES - Contraindicated in autoimmune hepatitis; hepatic decompensation in cirrhotic patients (Child-Pugh score >6 if HCV only; score ≥6 if HIV co-infected). Monitor for depression, suicidal behavior, relapse of drug addiction, other severe neuropsychiatric effects. Interferons can cause thrombocytopenia, neutropenia, thyroid dysfunction, hyperglycemia, hypoglycemia, cardiovascular events, colitis, pancreatitis, hypersensitivity, flu-like symptoms, pulmonary & ophthalmologic disorders. Risk of severe neutropenia/thrombocytopenia greater in HIV infected patients. Monitor CBC, blood chemistry. Interferons increase risk of hepatic decompensation in hep C/HIV coinfected patients receiving HAART with NRTI. Monitor LFTs and clinical status; discontinue peginterferon if Child-Pugh score ≥6. Exacerbation of hepatitis during treatment of hepatitis B: Monitor LFTs more often and consider dosage reduction if ALT flares. Discontinue treatment if ALT increase is progressive despite dosage reduction or if flares

**PEGINTERFERON** (*cont.*)

accompanied by hepatic decompensation or bilirubin increase. Cytochrome P450 1A2 inhibitor; may increase theophylline levels (monitor). May increase methadone levels. Use cautiously if CrCl <50 mL/min. Dosage adjustments for adverse effects, hepatic dysfunction, or hemodialysis in package insert. Store in refrigerator.

**PEGINTERFERON ALFA-2B** (*PEG-Intron*) ▶K? ♀C ▶- $$$$$

WARNING - May cause or worsen serious neuropsychiatric, autoimmune, ischemic, & infectious diseases. Frequent clinical & lab monitoring recommended. Discontinue if signs/symptoms of these conditions are persistently severe or worsen.

ADULT - Chronic hepatitis C not previously treated with alfa interferon. Give SC once weekly for 1 yr. Dose and vial strength based on weight.

Monotherapy: 1 mcg/kg/wk. ≤45 kg: 40 mcg (0.4 mL, 50 mcg/0.5 mL vial). 46–56 kg: 50 mcg (0.5 mL, 50 mcg/0.5 mL vial). 57–72 kg: 64 mcg (0.4 mL, 80 mcg/0.5 mL vial). 73–88 kg: 80 mcg (0.5 mL, 80 mcg/0.5 mL vial). 89–106 kg: 96 mcg (0.4 mL, 120 mcg/0.5 mL vial). 107–136 kg: 120 mcg (0.5 mL, 120 mcg/0.5 mL vial). 137–160 kg: 150 mcg (0.5 mL, 150 mcg/0.5 mL vial).

In combo with oral ribavirin (see Rebetol entry): 1.5 mcg/kg/wk. <40 kg: 50 mcg (0.5 mL, 50 mcg/0.5 mL vial). 40–50 kg: 64 mcg (0.4 mL, 80 mcg/0.5 mL vial). 51–60 kg: 80 mcg (0.5 mL, 80 mcg/0.5 mL vial). 61–75 kg: 96 mcg (0.4 mL, 120 mcg/0.5 mL vial). 76–85 kg: 120 mcg (0.5 mL, 120 mcg/0.5 mL vial). >95 kg: 150 mcg (0.5 mL, 150 mcg/0.5 mL vial).

Give at bedtime or with antipyretic to minimize flu-like symptoms. Consider stopping if HCV RNA is not below level of detection after 24 wk of therapy.

PEDS - Not approved in children.

FORMS - Trade only: 50, 80, 120, 150 mcg/0.5 mL single-use vials with diluent, 2 syringes, and alcohol swabs. Disposable single-dose Redipen 50, 80, 120, 150 mcg.

NOTES - Monitor for depression, suicidal behavior, other severe neuropsychiatric effects. Thrombocytopenia, neutropenia, thyroid dysfunction, hyperglycemia, cardiovascular events, colitis, pancreatitis, hypersensitivity, flu-like symptoms, pulmonary damage. Use cautiously if CrCl <50 mL/min. Monitor CBC, blood chemistry. May increase methadone levels. Dosage adjustments for adverse effects in package insert. Peginterferon should be used immediately after reconstitution, but can be refrigerated for up to 24 h.

**RIBAVIRIN - INHALED** (*Virazole*) ▶Lung ♀X ▶- $$$$$

WARNING - Beware of sudden pulmonary deterioration with ribavirin. Drug precipitation may cause ventilator dysfunction.

PEDS - Severe respiratory syncytial virus infection: Aerosol 12–18 h/d × 3–7 d.

NOTES - Minimize exposure to health care workers, especially pregnant women.

**RIBAVIRIN-ORAL**(*Rebetol,Copegus,Ribasphere*)▶Cellular, K ♀X ▶- $$$$$

WARNING - Teratogen with extremely long half-life; contraindicated if pregnancy possible in patient/partner. Female patients and female partners of male patients must avoid pregnancy by using 2 forms of birth control during and for 6 mo after stopping ribavirin. Obtain pregnancy test at baseline and monthly. Hemolytic anemia that may worsen cardiac disease. Assess for underlying heart disease before treatment with ribavirin. Do not use in significant/unstable heart disease. Baseline ECG if pre-existing cardiac dysfunction.

ADULT - Chronic hepatitis C. Rebetol in combo with interferon alfa-2b (Intron A): 600 mg PO bid if >75 kg; 400 mg q am and 600 mg q pm if ≤75 kg. Take without regard to meals, but consistently the same. Rebetol in combo with peginterferon alfa 2b (PEG-Intron): 400 mg PO bid with food. Copegus in combo with peginterferon alfa 2a (Pegasys): For genotype 1 or 4, treat × 48 wk with 1200 mg/d if >75 kg; 1000 mg/d if <75 kg. For genotype 2 or 3, treat × 24 wk with 800 mg/d PO. For patients coinfected with HIV: 800 mg/d PO for 48 wk regardless of genotype. Take bid with food. See package inserts for dosage reductions if Hb declines.

PEDS - Rebetol in combo with interferon alfa-2b: For patients ≤25 kg or who cannot swallow caps: 15 mg/kg/d of soln PO divided bid. Caps: 200 mg PO bid for 25–36 kg; 200 mg qam and 400 mg q pm for 37–49 kg; 400 mg bid for 50–61 kg. Use adult dose for >61 kg. Take without regard to meals, but consistently the same.

UNAPPROVED PEDS - Combination therapy with interferon alfa for chronic hepatitis C. 200 mg bid for 25–36 kg; 200 mg qam and 400 mg q pm for 37–49 kg; 400 mg bid for 50–61 kg. Use adult dosing for >61 kg.

FORMS - Generic/Trade: Caps 200 mg, Tabs 200, 500 mg. Generic only: Tabs 400, 600 mg. Trade only (Rebetol): Oral soln 40 mg/mL (100mL).

NOTES - Contraindicated in hemoglobinopathies; autoimmune hepatitis; hepatic decompensation in cirrhotic patients (Child-Pugh score >6 if HCV only; score ≥6 if HIV co-infected). Get CBC at baseline, wk 2 & 4, and prn. Risk of anemia increased if >50 yo or if renal dysfunction. Do not use if CrCl <50 mL/min. Decreased INR with warfarin; monitor INR weekly for 4 wk after ribavirin started/stopped. May increase risk of lactic acidosis with nucleoside reverse transcriptase inhibitors. Avoid didanosine, stavudine, zidovudine.

**TELBIVUDINE** (*Tyzeka*) ▶K ♀B ▶- $$$$$

WARNING - Nucleoside analogues can cause lactic acidosis with hepatic steatosis. Severe acute exacerbation of hepatitis B can occur after discontinuation. Monitor closely for ≥2 mo after discontinuation.

ADULT - Chronic hepatitis B: 600 mg PO once daily.

PEDS - Not approved in children.

**(cont.)**

**TELBIVUDINE** *(cont.)*
FORMS - Trade only: Tabs 600 mg.
NOTES - No dosage adjustment needed for hepatic dysfunction. Renal dysfunction: 600 mg PO q48h

for CrCl 30–49 mL/min; q72h for CrCl <30 mL/min but not hemodialysis; q96h for ESRD. Give dose after hemodialysis session.

## OVERVIEW OF BACTERIAL PATHOGENS (Selected)

### By bacterial class

Gram Positive Aerobic Cocci *Staph epidermidis* (coagulase negative), *Staph aureus* (coagulase positive), Streptococci: *S pneumoniae* (pneumococcus), *S pyogenes* (Group A), *S agalactiae* (Group B), enterococcus
Gram Positive Aerobic/Facultatively Anaerobic Bacilli *Bacillus, Corynebacterium diphtheriae, Erysipelothrix rhusiopathiae, Listeria monocytogenes,* Nocardia
Gram Negative Aerobic Diplococci *Moraxella catarrhalis, Neisseria gonorrhoeae, Neisseria meningitidis*
Gram Negative Aerobic Coccobacilli *Haemophilus ducreyi, Haemophilus influenzae*
Gram Negative Aerobic Bacilli *Acinetobacter,* Bartonella species, *Bordetella pertussis,* Brucella, *Burkholderia cepacia, Campylobacter, Francisella tularensis, Helicobacter pylori, Legionella pneumophila, Pseudomonas aeruginosa, Stenotrophomonas maltophilia, Vibrio cholerae, Yersinia*
Gram Negative Facultatively Anaerobic Bacilli *Aeromonas hydrophila, Eikenella corrodens, Pasteurella multocida,* Enterobacteriaceae: *E coli, Citrobacter, Salmonella, Shigella, Klebsiella, Enterobacter, Hafnia, Serratia, Proteus, Providencia*
Anaerobes *Actinomyces, Bacteroides fragilis, Clostridium botulinum, Clostridium difficile, Clostridium perfringens, Clostridium tetani, Fusobacterium, Lactobacillus, Peptostreptococcus*
Defective Cell Wall Bacteria *Chlamydia pneumoniae, Chlamydia psittaci, Chlamydia trachomatis, Coxiella burnetii, Myocoplasma pneumoniae, Rickettsia prowazekii, Rickettsia rickettsii, Rickettsia typhi, Ureaplasma urealyticum*
Spirochetes *Borrelia burgdorferi, Leptospira, Treponema pallidum*

### By bacterial name

*M avium complex, M kansasii, M leprae, M tuberculosis*
*Acinetobacter*     Gram Negative Aerobic Bacilli
*Actinomyces*     Anaerobes
*Aeromonas hydrophila*     Gram Negative Facultatively Anaerobic Bacilli
*Bacillus*     Gram Positive Aerobic/Facultatively Anaerobic Bacilli
*Bacteroides fragilis*     Anaerobes
*Bartonella species*     Gram Negative Aerobic Bacilli
*Bordetella pertussis*     Gram Negative Aerobic Bacilli
*Borrelia burgdorferi*     Spirochetes
*Brucella*     Gram Negative Aerobic Bacilli
*Burkholderia cepacia*     Gram Negative Aerobic Bacilli
*Campylobacter*     Gram Negative Aerobic Bacilli
*Chlamydia pneumoniae*     Defective Cell Wall Bacteria
*Chlamydia psittaci*     Defective Cell Wall Bacteria
*Chlamydia trachomatis*     Defective Cell Wall Bacteria
*Citrobacter*     Gram Negative Facultatively Anaerobic Bacilli
*Clostridium botulinum*     Anaerobes
*Clostridium difficile*     Anaerobes
*Clostridium perfringens*     Anaerobes
*Clostridium tetani*     Anaerobes
*Corynebacterium diphtheriae*     Gram Positive Aerobic/Facultatively Anaerobic Bacilli
*Coxiella burnetii*     Defective Cell Wall Bacteria
*E coli*     Gram Negative Facultatively Anaerobic Bacilli
*Eikenella corrodens*     Gram Negative Facultatively Anaerobic Bacilli
*Enterobacter*     Gram Negative Facultatively Anaerobic Bacilli
*Enterobacteriaceae*     Gram Negative Facultatively Anaerobic Bacilli
*Enterococcus*     Gram Positive Aerobic Cocci

(cont.)

## OVERVIEW OF BACTERIAL PATHOGENS (Selected) (cont.)

### By bacterial name, (cont.)

*Erysipelothrix rhusiopathiae*   Gram Positive Aerobic/Facultatively Anaerobic Bacilli
*Francisella tularensis*   Gram Negative Aerobic Bacilli
*Fusobacterium*   Anaerobes
*Haemophilus ducreyi*   Gram Negative Aerobic Coccobacilli
*Haemophilus influenzae*   Gram Negative Aerobic Coccobacilli
*Hafnia*   Gram Negative Facultatively Anaerobic Bacilli
*Helicobacter pylori*   Gram Negative Aerobic Bacilli
*Klebsiella*   Gram Negative Facultatively Anaerobic Bacilli
*Lactobacillus*   Anaerobes
*Legionella pneumophila*   Gram Negative Aerobic Bacilli
*Leptospira*   Spirochetes
*Listeria monocytogenes*   Gram Positive Aerobic/Facultatively Anaerobic Bacilli
*M avium complex*   Mycobacteria
*M kansasii*   Mycobacteria
*M leprae*   Mycobacteria
*M tuberculosis*   Mycobacteria
*Moraxella catarrhalis*   Gram Negative Aerobic Diplococci
*Myocoplasma pneumoniae*   Defective Cell Wall Bacteria
*Neisseria gonorrhoeae*   Gram Negative Aerobic Diplococci
*Neisseria meningitidis*   Gram Negative Aerobic Diplococci
*Nocardia*   Gram Positive Aerobic/Facultatively Anaerobic Bacilli
*Pasteurella multocida*   Gram Negative Facultatively Anaerobic Bacilli
*Peptostreptococcus*   Anaerobes
*Pneumococcus*   Gram Positive Aerobic Cocci
*Proteus*   Gram Negative Facultatively Anaerobic Bacilli
*Providencia*   Gram Negative Facultatively Anaerobic Bacilli
*Pseudomonas aeruginosa*   Gram Negative Aerobic Bacilli
*Rickettsia prowazekii*   Defective Cell Wall Bacteria
*Rickettsia rickettsii*   Defective Cell Wall Bacteria
*Rickettsia typhi*   Defective Cell Wall Bacteria
*Salmonella*   Gram Negative Facultatively Anaerobic Bacilli
*Serratia*   Gram Negative Facultatively Anaerobic Bacilli
*Shigella*   Gram Negative Facultatively Anaerobic Bacilli
*Staph aureus (coagulase positive)*   Gram Positive Aerobic Cocci
*Staph epidermidis (coagulase negative)*   Gram Positive Aerobic Cocci
*Stenotrophomonas maltophilia*   Gram Negative Aerobic Bacilli
*Strep agalactiae (Group B)*   Gram Positive Aerobic Cocci
*Strep pneumoniae*   Gram Positive Aerobic Cocci
*Strep pyogenes (Group A)*   Gram Positive Aerobic Cocci
*Streptococci*   Gram Positive Aerobic Cocci
*Treponema pallidum*   Spirochetes
*Ureaplasma urealyticum*   Defective Cell Wall Bacteria
*Vibrio cholerae*   Gram Negative Aerobic Bacilli
*Yersinia*   Gram Negative Aerobic Bacilli

## ANTIMICROBIALS: Carbapenems

**NOTE:** Carbapenems can dramatically reduce valproic acid levels; monitor frequently or switch antibiotic or anticonvulsant.

**DORIPENEM (*Doribax*)** ▶K ♀B ▶? $$$$$
ADULT - 500 mg IV q8h × 5–14 d for complicated intra-abdominal infection, ×10–14 d for complicated UTI or pyelonephritis. Renal dysfunction:

250 mg q8h for CrCl >30 to <50 mL/min; 250 mg q12h for CrCl >10 to <30 mL/min.
PEDS - Not approved in children.

(cont.)

**DORIPENEM** (*cont.*)

NOTES - Possible cross-sensitivity with other beta-lactams; C. difficile associated diarrhea; superinfection.

**ERTAPENEM** (*Invanz*) ▶K ♀B ▶? $$$$$

ADULT - Community-acquired pneumonia, diabetic foot, complicated intra-abdominal, skin, urinary tract, acute pelvic infections: 1g IM/IV over 30 min q24h × ≤14 d for IV, × ≤7 d for IM. Prophylaxis, elective colorectal surgery: 1 g IV 1 h before incision.

PEDS - Community-acquired pneumonia, complicated intra-abdominal, skin, urinary tract, acute pelvic infections (3 mo-12 yo): 15 mg/kg IV/IM q12h (max 1 g/d). Use adult dose for ≥13 yo. Infuse IV over 30 min. Can give IV for ≤14 d, IM for ≤7 d.

NOTES - Possible cross-sensitivity with other beta-lactams; C. difficile associated diarrhea; superinfection; seizures (especially if renal dysfunction or CNS disorder). Not active against Pseudomonas and Acinetobacter species. IM diluted with lidocaine; contraindicated if allergic to amide-type local anesthetics. For adults with renal dysfunction: 500 mg q24h for CrCl ≤30 mL/min or hemodialysis. Give 150 mg supplemental dose if daily dose given within 6 h before hemodialysis session. Do not dilute in dextrose.

**IMIPENEM-CILASTATIN** (*Primaxin*) ▶K ♀C ▶? $$$$$

ADULT - Pneumonia, sepsis, endocarditis, polymicrobic, intra-abdominal, gynecologic, bone & joint, skin infections. Normal renal function, ≥70 kg - Mild infection: 250–500 mg IV q6h. Moderate infection: 500 mg IV q6–8h or 1 g IV q8h. Severe infection: 500 mg IV q6h to 1 g IV q6–8h. Complicated UTI: 500 mg IV q6h. See product labeling for doses in adults <70 kg. Can give up to 1.5 g/d IM for mild/moderate infections.

PEDS - Pneumonia, sepsis, endocarditis, polymicrobic, intra-abdominal, bone & joint, skin infections. Age >3 mo: 15–25 mg/kg IV q6h. 1–3 mo: 25 mg/kg IV q6h. 1–4 wk old: 25 mg/kg IV q8h. <1 wk old: 25 mg/kg IV q12h. Not for children with CNS infections, or <30 kg with renal dysfunction.

UNAPPROVED ADULT - Malignant otitis externa, empiric therapy for neutropenic fever: 500 mg IV q6h.

NOTES - Possible cross-sensitivity with other beta-lactams; C. difficile associated diarrhea; superinfection, seizures (especially if given with ganciclovir, elderly with renal dysfunction, or cerebrovascular or seizure disorder). See product labeling for dose if CrCl <70 mL/min. Not for CrCl <5 mL/min unless dialysis started within 48 h.

**MEROPENEM** (*Merrem IV*) ▶K ♀B ▶? $$$$$

ADULT - Intra-abdominal infections: 1 g IV q8h. Complicated skin infections: 500 mg IV q8h.

PEDS - Meningitis: 40 mg/kg IV q8h for age ≥3 mo; 2 g IV q8h if >50 kg. Intra-abdominal infection: 20 mg/kg IV q8h for age ≥3 mo; 1 g IV q8h for weight >50 kg. Complicated skin infections: 10 mg/kg IV q8h for age ≥3 mo; 500 mg IV q8h for weight >50 kg.

UNAPPROVED ADULT - Meningitis: 40 mg/kg (max 2 g) IV q 8h. Hospital-acquired pneumonia, complicated UTI, malignant otitis externa: 1 g IV q8h.

UNAPPROVED PEDS - Infant >2 kg: 20 mg/kg IV q12h for ≤1 wk old, q8h for 1–4 wk old.

NOTES - Possible cross-sensitivity with other beta-lactams; C. difficile associated diarrhea; superinfection; seizures; thrombocytopenia in renal dysfunction. For adults with renal dysfunction: Give normal dose q12h for CrCl 26–50 mL/min, 50% of normal dose q12h for CrCl 10–25 mL/min, 50% of normal dose q24h for CrCl <10 mL/min.

---

## ANTIMICROBIALS: Cephalosporins—1st Generation

**NOTE:** Cephalosporins are 2nd-line to penicillin for group A strep pharyngitis, can be cross-sensitive with penicillin, and can cause C. difficile associated diarrhea.

**CEFADROXIL** (*Duricef*) ▶K ♀B ▶+ $$$

ADULT - Simple UTI: 1–2 g/d PO divided once daily-bid. Other UTIs: 1 g PO bid. Skin infections: 1 g/d PO divided once daily-bid. Group A strep pharyngitis: 1 g/d PO divided once daily-bid × 10 d. See table for prophylaxis of bacterial endocarditis.

PEDS - UTIs, skin infections: 30 mg/kg/d PO divided bid. Group A streptococcal pharyngitis/tonsillitis, impetigo: 30 mg/kg/d PO divided once daily-bid. Treat pharyngitis for 10 d.

FORMS - Generic/Trade: Tabs 1 g, caps 500 mg, susp 125, 250, & 500 mg/5 mL.

NOTES - Renal dysfunction in adults: 1 g load, then 500 mg PO q12h for CrCl 25–50 mL/min, 500 mg PO q24h for CrCl 10–25 mL/min, 500 mg PO q36h for CrCl <10 mL/min.

**CEFAZOLIN** (*Ancef*) ▶K ♀B ▶+ $$

ADULT - Pneumonia, sepsis, endocarditis, skin, bone & joint, genital infections. Mild infections due to gram-positive cocci: 250–500 mg IM/IV q8h. Moderate/severe infections: 0.5–1 g IM/IV q6–8h. Life-threatening infections: 1–1.5 g IV q6h. Simple UTI: 1 g IM/IV q12h. Pneumococcal pneumonia: 500 mg IM/IV q12h. Surgical prophylaxis: 1 g IM/IV 30–60 min preop, additional 0.5–1 g during surgery >2h, and 0.5–1 g q6–8h × 24h postop. See table for prophylaxis of bacterial endocarditis.

PEDS - Pneumonia, sepsis, endocarditis, skin, bone & joint infections. Mild/moderate infections, age ≥1 mo: 25–50 mg/kg/d IM/IV divided q6–8h. Severe infections, age ≥1 mo: 100 mg/kg/d IV

**CEFAZOLIN** (*cont.*)
divided q6–8h. See table for prophylaxis of bacterial endocarditis.
NOTES - Renal dysfunction in adults: Usual 1st dose, then usual dose q8h for CrCl 35–54 mL/min, 50% of usual dose q12h for CrCl 11–34 mL/min, 50% of usual dose q18–24h for CrCl <10 mL/min. Renal dysfunction in children: Usual 1st dose, then 60% of usual dose q12h for CrCl 40–70 mL/min, 25% of usual dose q12h for 20–40 mL/min, 10% of usual dose q24h for CrCl 5–20 mL/min.

**CEPHALEXIN** (*Keflex, Panixine DisperDose*) ▶K ♀B ▶? $$$
ADULT - Pneumonia, bone, GU infections. Usual dose: 250–500 mg PO qid. Max: 4 g/d. Group A strep pharyngitis, skin infections, simple UTI: 500 mg PO bid. Treat pharyngitis × 10 d. See table for prophylaxis of bacterial endocarditis.
PEDS - Pneumonia, GU, bone, skin infections, group A strep pharyngitis. Usual dose: 25–50 mg/kg/d PO in divided doses. Max dose: 100 mg/kg/d. Can give bid for strep pharyngitis in children >1 yo, skin infections. Group A strep pharyngitis, skin infections, simple UTI in patients >15 yo: 500 mg PO bid. Treat pharyngitis × 10 d. Not for otitis media, sinusitis.
FORMS - Generic/Trade: Caps 250, 500 mg. Generic only: Tabs 250, 500 mg, susp 125 & 250 mg/5 mL. Panixine DisperDose 125, 250 mg scored tabs for oral susp. Trade only: Caps 333, 750 mg.
NOTES - Mix Panixine tab with 2 tsp water and drink mixture, then rinse container with a little water and drink that. Do not chew or swallow tab whole. Use only for doses that can be delivered by half or whole tabs.

## ANTIMICROBIALS: Cephalosporins—2nd Generation

**NOTE:** Cephalosporins are 2nd-line to penicillin for group A strep pharyngitis, can be cross-sensitive with penicillin, and can cause C. difficile associated diarrhea.

**CEFACLOR** (*Ceclor, Raniclor*) ▶K ♀B ▶? $$$$
ADULT - Otitis media, pneumonia, group A strep pharyngitis, UTI, skin infections: 250–500 mg PO tid. Extended release tabs: Acute exacerbation of chronic bronchitis, secondary bacterial infection of acute bronchitis: 500 mg PO bid with food. Group A streptococcal pharyngitis, skin infections: 375 mg PO bid with food. Treat pharyngitis × 10 d.
PEDS - Pneumonia, group A streptococcal pharyngitis, UTI, skin infections: 20–40 mg/kg/d up to 1 g/d PO divided bid for pharyngitis, tid for other infections. Treat pharyngitis × 10d. Otitis media: 40 mg/kg/d PO divided bid.
FORMS - Generic only: Caps 250, 500 mg, susp & chew tabs 125, 187, 250, 375 mg per 5 mL or tab, extended release tabs 375, 500 mg.

**CEFOTETAN** ▶K/BILE ♀B ▶? ?
ADULT - Usual dose: 1–2 g IM/IV q12h. UTI: 0.5–2 g IM/IV q12h or 1–2 g IM/IV q24h. Pneumonia, gynecologic, intra-abdominal, bone & joint infections: 1–3 g IM/IV q12h. Skin infections: 1–2 g IM/IV q12h or 2 g IV q24h. Surgical prophylaxis: 1–2 g IV 30–60 min preop. Give after cord clamp for C-section.
PEDS - Not approved in children.
UNAPPROVED PEDS - Usual dose: 40–80 mg/kg/d IV divided q12h.
NOTES - Hemolytic anemia (higher risk than other cephalosporins), clotting impairment rarely. Disulfiram-like reaction with alcohol. Dosing reduction in adults with renal dysfunction: Usual dose q24h for CrCl 10–30 mL/min, usual dose q48h for CrCl <10 mL/min.

**CEFOXITIN** (*Mefoxin*) ▶K ♀B ▶+ $$$$$
ADULT - Pneumonia, UTI, sepsis, intra-abdominal, gynecologic, skin, bone & joint infections: Uncomplicated, 1 g IV q6–8h. Moderate to severe, 1 g IV q4h or 2 g IV q6–8h. Infections requiring high doses, 2 g IV q4h or 3 g IV q6h.

Uncontaminated gastrointestinal surgery, vaginal/abdominal hysterectomy: 2 g IV 30–60 min preop, then 2 g IV q6h × 24h. C-section: 2 g IV after cord clamped or 2 g IV q4h × 3 doses with 1st dose given after cord clamped.
PEDS - Pneumonia, UTI, sepsis, intra-abdominal, skin, bone & joint infections, age ≥3 mo: 80–160 mg/kg/d IV divided into 4–6 doses, not to exceed 12 g/d. Mild-moderate infections: 80–100 mg/kg/d IV divided into 3–4 doses. Surgical prophylaxis: 30–40 mg/kg IV 30–60 min preop and for not more than 24h postop.
NOTES - Eosinophilia & increased AST with high doses in children. Dosing reduction in adults with renal dysfunction: Load with 1–2 g IV; then 1–2 g IV q8–12h for CrCl 30–50 mL/min, 1–2 g IV q12–24h for CrCl 10–29 mL/min, 0.5–1 g IV q12–24h for CrCl 5–9 mL/min, 0.5 g IV q24–48h for CrCl <5 mL/min. Give 1–2 g loading dose after each hemodialysis.

**CEFPROZIL** (*Cefzil*) ▶K ♀B ▶+ $$$$
ADULT - Group A strep pharyngitis: 500 mg PO daily × 10 d. Sinusitis: 250–500 mg PO bid. Acute exacerbation of chronic/secondary infection of acute bronchitis: 500 mg PO bid. Skin infections: 250–500 mg PO bid or 500 mg PO once daily.
PEDS - Otitis media: 15 mg/kg/dose PO bid. Group A strep pharyngitis: 7.5 mg/kg/dose PO bid × 10 d. Sinusitis: 7.5–15 mg/kg/dose PO bid. Skin infections: 20 mg/kg PO daily. Use adult dose for ≥13 yo.
FORMS - Generic/Trade: Tabs 250,500 mg, susp 125 & 250 mg/5 mL.
NOTES - Give 50% of usual dose at usual interval for CrCl <30 mL/min.

**CEFUROXIME** (*Zinacef, Ceftin*) ▶K ♀B ▶? $$$
ADULT - IM/IV cefuroxime. Uncomplicated pneumonia, simple UTI, skin infections, disseminated gonorrhea: 750 mg IM/IV q8h. Bone & joint, or severe/complicated infections: 1.5 g IV q8h. Sepsis: 1.5

**(cont.)**

**CEFUROXIME** (*cont.*)

g IV q6h to 3 g IV q8h. Gonorrhea: 1.5 g IM single dose split into 2 injections, given with probenecid 1 g PO. Surgical prophylaxis: 1.5 g IV 30–60 min preop, then 750 mg IM/IV q8h for prolonged procedures. Open heart surgery: 1.5 g IV q12h × 4 with 1st dose at induction of anesthesia. Cefuroxime axetil tabs. Group A strep pharyngitis, acute sinusitis: 250 mg PO bid × 10 d. Acute exacerbation of chronic/secondary infection of acute bronchitis, skin infections: 250–500 mg PO bid. Lyme disease: 500 mg PO bid × 14 d for early disease, × 28 d for Lyme arthritis. Simple UTI: 125–250 mg PO bid. Gonorrhea: 1 g PO single dose.

PEDS - IM/IV cefuroxime. Most infections: 50–100 mg/kg/d IM/IV divided q6–8h. Bone & joint infections: 150 mg/kg/d IM/IV divided q8h not to exceed max adult dose. Cefuroxime axetil tabs: Group A strep pharyngitis: 125 mg PO bid × 10 d. Otitis media, sinusitis: 250 mg PO bid × 10 d. Cefuroxime axetil oral susp. Group A strep pharyngitis: 20 mg/kg/d (up to 500 mg/d) PO divided bid × 10 d. Otitis media, sinusitis, impetigo: 30 mg/kg/d (up to 1 g/d) PO divided bid × 10 d. Use adult dose for ≥13 yo.

UNAPPROVED PEDS - Lyme disease: 30 mg/kg/d PO divided bid (max 500 mg/dose) × 14 d for early disease, × 28 d for Lyme arthritis. Community-acquired pneumonia: 150 mg/kg/d IV divided q8h.

FORMS - Generic/Trade: Tabs 125, 250, 500 mg, Susp 125 & 250 mg/5 mL.

NOTES - AAP recommends 5–7 d of therapy for older (≥6 yo) children with non-severe otitis media, and 10 d for younger children and those with severe disease. Dosage adjustment for renal dysfunction in adults: 750 mg IM/IV q12h for CrCl 10–20 mL/min, 750 mg IM/IV q24h for CrCl <10 mL/min. Give supplemental dose after hemodialysis. Tabs & susp not bioequivalent on mg/mg basis. Do not crush tabs.

## ANTIMICROBIALS: Cephalosporins—3rd Generation

**NOTE:** Cephalosporins are 2nd-line to penicillin for group A strep pharyngitis, can be cross-sensitive with penicillin, and can cause C. difficile associated diarrhea.

**CEFDINIR** (*Omnicef*) ▶K ♀B ▶? $$$$

ADULT - Community-acquired pneumonia, skin infections: 300 mg PO bid × 10 d. Sinusitis: 600 mg PO once daily or 300 mg PO bid × 10 d. Group A strep pharyngitis, acute exacerbation of chronic bronchitis: 600 mg PO once daily × 10 d or 300 mg PO bid × 5–10 d.

PEDS - Group A strep pharyngitis, otitis media: 14 mg/kg/d PO divided bid × 5–10 d or once daily × 10 d. Sinusitis: 14 mg/kg/d PO divided once daily-bid × 10 d. Skin infections: 14 mg/kg/d PO divided bid × 10 d. Use adult dose for ≥13 yo.

FORMS - Generic/Trade: Cap 300 mg. Susp 125 & 250 mg/5 mL.

NOTES - AAP recommends 5–7 d of therapy for older (≥6 yo) children with non-severe otitis media, and 10 d for younger children and those with severe disease. Give iron, multivitamins with iron, or antacids ≥2 h before/after cefdinir. Complexation of cefdinir with iron may turn stools red. Dosage reduction for renal dysfunction: 300 mg PO daily for adults with CrCl <30 mL/min. 7 mg/kg/d PO once daily up to 300 mg/d for children with CrCl <30 mL/min. Hemodialysis: 300 mg or 7 mg/kg PO after hemodialysis, then 300 mg or 7 mg/kg PO q48h.

**CEFDITOREN** (*Spectracef*) ▶K ♀B ▶? $$$$

ADULT - Skin infections, group A strep pharyngitis: 200 mg PO bid × 10 d. Give 400 mg bid × 10 d for acute exacerbation of chronic bronchitis, × 14 d for community-acquired pneumonia. Take with food.

PEDS - Not approved for children <12 yo. Skin infections, group A strep pharyngitis, adolescents ≥12 yo: 200 mg PO bid with food × 10 d.

FORMS - Trade only: Tabs 200 mg.

NOTES - Contraindicated if milk protein allergy or carnitine deficiency. Not for long-term use due to potential risk of carnitine deficiency. Do not take with drugs that reduce gastric acid (antacids, H2 blockers, etc). Dosage adjustment for renal dysfunction: Max 200 mg bid if CrCl 30–49 mL/min; max 200 mg once daily if CrCl <30 mL/min.

**CEFIXIME** (*Suprax*) ▶K/Bile ♀B ▶? $$

ADULT - Simple UTI, pharyngitis, acute bacterial bronchitis, acute exacerbation of chronic bronchitis: 400 mg PO once daily. Gonorrhea: 400 mg PO single dose.

PEDS - Otitis media: 8 mg/kg/d susp PO divided once daily-bid. Pharyngitis: 8 mg/kg/d PO divided once daily-bid × 10 d. Use adult dose for >50 kg or ≥13 yo.

UNAPPROVED ADULT - Disseminated gonorrhea, CDC regimen: 500 mg PO bid of susp or 400 mg PO bid of tabs.

UNAPPROVED PEDS - Febrile UTI (3–24 mo): 16 mg/kg PO on first d, then 8 mg/kg PO daily to complete 14 d. Gonorrhea: 8 mg/kg (max 400 mg) PO single dose for <45 kg, 400 mg PO single dose for ≥45 kg.

FORMS - Trade only: Susp 100 & 200 mg/5 mL, Tab 400 mg.

NOTES - Cross-sensitivity with penicillins possible, C. difficile associated diarrhea. Poor activity against S aureus. Increased INR with warfarin. May increase carbamazepine levels. Susp stable at room temp or refrigerated × 14 d. Dosing in renal dysfunction: 75% of usual dose at usual interval for CrCl 21–60 mL/min or hemodialysis. 50% of usual dose at usual interval for CrCl <20 mL/min or continuous peritoneal dialysis.

## SEXUALLY TRANSMITTED DISEASES & VAGINITIS

*Overview:* Treat sexual partners for all except herpes, candida, and bacterial vaginosis. Reference www.cdc. gov/STD/treatment/

*Bacterial vaginosis:* 1) metronidazole 5 g of 0.75% gel intravaginally daily × 5 d OR 500 mg PO bid × 7 d. 2) clindamycin 5 g of 2% cream intravaginally qhs × 7 d. In pregnancy: 1) metronidazole 500 mg PO bid × 7 d OR 250 mg PO tid × 7 d. 2) clindamycin 300 mg PO bid × 7 d.

*Candidal vaginitis:* 1) intravaginal clotrimazole, miconazole, terconazole, nystatin, tioconazole, or butoconazole. 2) fluconazole 150 mg PO single dose.

*Chancroid:* Single dose of: 1) azithromycin 1 g PO or 2) ceftriaxone 250 mg IM.

*Chlamydia:* First line either azithromycin 1 g PO single dose or doxycycline 100 mg PO bid × 7 d. Second line fluoroquinolones or erythromycin. In pregnancy: 1) azithromycin 1 g PO single dose. 2) amoxicillin 500 mg PO tid × 7 d. Repeat nucleic acid amplification test 3 wk after treatment.

*Epididymitis:* 1) ceftriaxone 250 mg IM single dose + doxycycline 100 mg PO bid × 10 d. 2) ofloxacin 300 mg PO bid or levofloxacin 500 mg PO daily × 10 d if enteric organisms suspected, or cephalosporin/ doxycycline allergic.

*Gonorrhea:* Single dose of: 1) ceftriaxone 125 mg IM 2) cefixime 400 mg PO 3) ciprofloxacin 500 mg PO 4) ofloxacin 400 mg PO or 5) levofloxacin 250 mg PO. Treat chlamydia empirically. Cephalosporin desensitization advised for cephalosporin-allergic patients who cannot take fluoroquinolones (eg, pregnant women). Consider azithromycin 2 g PO single dose for uncomplicated gonorrhea, but no efficacy/safety data for this regimen in pregnant women. Due to high resistance rates, quinolones not recommended if infection acquired in Hawaii or California, recent foreign travel by patient/partner, or in men who have sex with men. See health department or www.cdc.gov/std/gisp for current resistance info.

*Gonorrhea, disseminated:* Initially treat with ceftriaxone 1 g IM/IV q24h until 24–48 h after improvement. Second-line alternatives: 1) ciprofloxacin 400 mg IV q12h. 2) ofloxacin 400 mg IV q12h. 3) levofloxacin 250 mg IV qd. 4) cefotaxime 1 g IV q8h. 5) ceftizoxime 1 g IV q8h. Complete 1 wk of treatment with: 1) cefixime 400 mg PO bid. 2) ciprofloxacin 500 mg PO bid. 3) ofloxacin 400 mg PO bid. 4) levofloxacin 500 mg PO daily. Cephalosporin desensitization advised for cephalosporin-allergic patients who cannot take fluoroquinolones (eg, pregnant women). Due to high resistance rates, quinolones not recommended if infection acquired in Hawaii or California, recent foreign travel by patient/partner, or in men who have sex with men. See health department or www.cdc.gov/std/gisp for current resistance info.

*Gonorrhea, meningitis:* ceftriaxone 1–2 g IV q12h for 10–14 d.

*Gonorrhea, endocarditis:* ceftriaxone 1–2 g IV q12h for at least 4 wk.

*Granuloma inguinale:* doxycycline 100 mg PO bid × ≥3 wk and until lesions completely healed. Alternative azithromycin 1 g PO once weekly × 3 wk.

*Herpes simplex (genital, first episode):* 1) acyclovir 400 mg PO tid × 7–10 d. 2) famciclovir 250 PO tid × 7–10 d. 3) valacyclovir 1 g PO bid × 7–10 d.

*Herpes simplex (genital, recurrent):* 1) acyclovir 400 mg PO tid × 5 d. 2) acyclovir 800 mg PO tid × 2 d or bid × 5 d. 3) famciclovir 125 mg PO bid × 5 d. 4) famciclovir 1000 mg PO bid × 1 d. 5) valacyclovir 500 mg PO bid × 3 d. 6) valacyclovir 1 g PO daily × 5 d.

*Herpes simplex (suppressive therapy):* 1) acyclovir 400mg PO bid. 2) famciclovir 250 mg PO bid. 3) valacyclovir 500–1000 mg PO daily.

*Herpes simplex (genital, recurrent in HIV infection):* 1) Acyclovir 400 mg PO tid × 5–10 d. 2) famciclovir 500 mg PO bid × 5–10 d. 3) Valacyclovir 1 g PO bid × 5–10 d.

*Herpes simplex (suppressive therapy in HIV infection):* 1) Acyclovir 400–800 mg PO bid-tid. 2) Famciclovir 500 mg PO bid. 3) Valacyclovir 500 mg PO bid.

*Herpes simplex (prevention of transmission in immunocompetent patients with ≤9 recurrences/yr):* Valacyclovir 500 mg PO daily by source partner, in conjunction with safer sex practices.

*Lymphogranuloma venereum:* 1) doxycycline 100 mg PO bid × 21 d. Alternative: erythromycin base 500 mg PO qid × 21 d.

*Pelvic inflammatory disease (PID), inpatient regimens:* 1) cefoxitin 2 g IV q6h + doxycycline 100 mg IV/PO q12h. 2) clindamycin 900 mg IV q8h + gentamicin 2 mg/kg IM/IV loading dose, then 1.5 mg/kg IM/IV q8h (See gentamicin entry for alternative daily dosing). Can switch to PO therapy within 24 h of improvement.

*Pelvic inflammatory disease (PID), outpatient treatment:* 1) ceftriaxone 250 mg IM single dose + doxycycline 100 mg PO bid +/− metronidazole 500 mg PO bid × 14 d. 2) ofloxacin 400 mg PO bid/levofloxacin 500 mg PO daily +/− metronidazole 500 mg PO bid × 14 d. Due to high resistance rates, quinolones not recommended if infection acquired in Hawaii or California, recent foreign travel by patient/partner, or in men who have sex with men. See health department or www.cdc.gov/std/gisp for current resistance info.

*Proctitis, proctocolitis, enteritis:* ceftriaxone 125 mg IM single dose + doxycycline 100 mg PO bid x7d.

*Sexual assault prophylaxis:* ceftriaxone 125 mg IM single dose + metronidazole 2 g PO single dose + azithromycin 1 g PO single dose/doxycycline 100 mg PO bid × 7 d. Consider giving antiemetic.

(cont.)

*Syphilis (primary and secondary)*: 1) benzathine penicillin 2.4 million units IM single dose; 2) doxycycline 100 mg PO bid × 2 weeks if penicillin allergic.

*Syphilis (early latent, ie, duration <1 y)*: 1) benzathine penicillin 2.4 million units IM single dose; 2) doxycycline 100 mg PO bid × 2 weeks if penicillin allergic.

*Syphilis (late latent or unknown duration)*: 1) benzathine penicillin 2.4 million units IM q week × 3 doses; 2) doxycycline 100 mg PO bid × 4 weeks if penicillin allergic.

*Syphilis (tertiary)*: 1) benzathine penicillin 2.4 million units IM q week × 3 doses; 2) doxycycline 100 mg PO bid × 4 weeks if penicillin allergic.

*Syphilis (neuro)*: 1) penicillin G 18–24 million units/d continuous IV infusion or 3–4 million units IV q4h × 10–14 d; 2) procaine penicillin 2.4 million units IM daily + probenecid 500 mg PO qid, both × 10–14 d.

*Syphilis in pregnancy*: Treat only with penicillin regimen for stage of syphilis as noted above. Use penicillin desensitization protocol if penicillin-allergic.

*Trichomonal vaginitis*: metronidazole 2 g PO single dose (can use in pregnancy) or tinidazole 2 g PO single dose.

*Urethritis, cervicitis*: Test for chlamydia and gonorrhea with nucleic acid amplification test. Treat based on test results or treat presumptively if high-risk of infection (chlamydia: age ≤25 y, new/multiple sex partners, or unprotected sex; gonorrhea: population prevalence >5%), esp. if nucleic acid amplification test unavailable or patient unlikely to return for follow-up.

*Urethritis (persistent/recurrent)*: 1) metronidazole/tinidazole 2 g PO single dose + azithromycin 2 g PO single dose (if not used in first episode).

**CEFOPERAZONE (*Cefobid*)** ▶Bile/K ♀B ▶? $$$$$
ADULT - Peritonitis, sepsis, respiratory, intra-abdominal, skin infections, endometritis, pelvic inflammatory disease & other gynecologic infections: Usual dose 2–4 g/d IV divided q12h. Infections with less sensitive organisms/severe infections: 6–12 g/d IV divided q6–12h. Use q6h for Pseudomonas infections. 1–2 g doses can be given IM.
PEDS - Not approved in children.
UNAPPROVED PEDS - Mild to moderate infections, age ≥1 mo: 100–150 mg/kg/d IM/IV divided q8–12h.
NOTES - Possible clotting impairment. Disulfiram-like reaction with alcohol. Not for meningitis.

**CEFOTAXIME (*Claforan*)** ▶KL ♀B ▶+ $$$$$
ADULT - Pneumonia, sepsis, GU & gynecologic, skin, intra-abdominal, bone & joint infections: Uncomplicated, 1 g IM/IV q12h. Moderate/severe, 1–2 g IM/IV q8h. Infections usually requiring high doses, 2 g IV q6–8h. Life-threatening, 2 g IV q4h. Meningitis: 2g IV q4–6h. Gonorrhea: 0.5–1 g IM single dose.
PEDS - Neonates, ≤1 wk old: 50 mg/kg/dose IV q12h. 1–4 wk old: 50 mg/kg/dose IV q8h. Labeled dose for pneumonia, sepsis, GU, skin, intra-abdominal, bone/joint, CNS infections, 1 mo-12 yo: 50–180 mg/kg/d IM/IV divided q4–6h. AAP recommendations: 225–300 mg/kg/d IV divided q6–8h for S pneumoniae meningitis. Mild to moderate infections: 75–100 mg/kg/d IV/IM divided q6–8h. Severe infections: 150–200 mg/kg/d IV/IM divided q6–8h.
UNAPPROVED ADULT - Disseminated gonorrhea, CDC regimen: 1 g IV q8h.
NOTES - Bolus injection through central venous catheter can cause arrhythmias. Decrease dose by 50% for CrCl <20 mL/min.

**CEFPODOXIME (*Vantin*)** ▶K ♀B ▶? $$$$
ADULT - Acute exacerbation of chronic bronchitis, acute sinusitis: 200 mg PO bid × 10 d. Community-acquired pneumonia: 200 mg PO bid × 14 d. Group A strep pharyngitis: 100 mg PO bid × 5–10 d. Skin infections: 400 mg PO bid × 7–14 d. Simple UTI: 100 mg PO bid × 7 d. Gonorrhea: 200 mg PO single dose. Give tabs with food.
PEDS - 5 mg/kg PO bid × 5 d for otitis media, × 5–10 d for group A strep pharyngitis, × 10 d for sinusitis. Use adult dose for ≥12 yo.
FORMS - Generic/Trade: Tabs 100, 200 mg. Susp 50 & 100 mg/5 mL.
NOTES - AAP recommends 5–7 d of therapy for older (≥6 yo) children with non-severe otitis media, and 10 d for younger children and those with severe disease. Do not give antacids within 2 h before/after cefpodoxime. Dosing in renal dysfunction: Increase dosing interval to q24h for CrCl <30 mL/min. Give 3 times/wk after dialysis session for hemodialysis patients. Susp stable for 14 d refrigerated.

**CEFTAZIDIME (*Ceptaz, Fortaz, Tazicef*)** ▶K ♀B ▶+ $$$$$
ADULT - Simple UTI: 250 mg IM/IV q12h. Complicated UTI: 500 mg IM/IV q8–12h. Uncomplicated pneumonia, mild skin infections: 500 mg – 1 g IM/IV q8h. Serious gynecologic, intra-abdominal, bone & joint, life-threatening infections, meningitis, empiric therapy of neutropenic fever: 2 g IV q8h. Pseudomonas lung infections in cystic fibrosis: 30–50 mg/kg IV q8h to max of 6 g/d.
PEDS - Use sodium formulations in children (Fortaz, Tazicef). UTIs, pneumonia, skin, intra-abdominal, bone & joint infections, 1 mo-12 yo: 100–150 mg/kg/d IV divided q8h to max of 6 g/d. Meningitis,

**CEFTAZIDIME** (cont.)
1 mo–12 yo: 150 mg/kg/d IV divided q8h to max of 6 g/d. Infants up to 4 wk old: 30 mg/kg IV q12h. Use adult dose & formulations if ≥12 yo.
UNAPPROVED ADULT - *P aeruginosa* osteomyelitis of the foot from nail puncture: 2 g IV q8h.
UNAPPROVED PEDS - AAP dosing for infants >2 kg: 50 mg/kg IV q8–12h for <1 wk old, q8h for ≥1 wk old.
NOTES - High levels in renal dysfunction can cause CNS toxicity. Dosing in adults with renal dysfunction: 1 g IV q12h for CrCl 31–50 mL/min; 1 g q24h for CrCl 16–30 mL/min; load with 1 g, then 500 mg q24h for CrCl 6–15 mL/min; load with 1 g, then 500 mg q48h for CrCl <5 mL/min. 1 g IV load in hemodialysis patients, then 1 g IV after hemodialysis sessions.

**CEFTIBUTEN** (*Cedax*) ▶K ♀B ▶? $$$$$
ADULT - Group A strep pharyngitis, acute exacerbation of chronic bronchitis, otitis media not due to S pneumoniae: 400 mg PO once daily × 10 d.
PEDS - Group A strep pharyngitis, otitis media not due to S pneumoniae, age >6 mo: 9 mg/kg up to 400 mg PO once daily. Give susp on empty stomach.
FORMS - Trade only: Cap 400 mg, susp 90 mg/5 mL.
NOTES - Poor activity against *S aureus* and *S pneumoniae*. Dosing in adults with renal dysfunction: 200 mg PO once daily for CrCl 30–49 mL/min, 100 mg PO daily for CrCl 5–29 mL/min. Dosing in children with renal dysfunction: 4.5 mg/kg PO once daily for CrCl 30–49 mL/min, 2.25 mg/kg PO daily for CrCl 5–29 mL/min. Hemodialysis: adults 400 mg PO and children 9 mg/kg PO after each dialysis session. Susp stable for 14 d refrigerated.

**CEFTIZOXIME** (*Cefizox*) ▶K ♀B ▶? $$$$$
ADULT - Simple UTI: 500 mg IM/IV q12h. Pneumonia, sepsis, intra-abdominal, skin, bone & joint infections: 1–2 g IM/IV q8–12h. Pelvic inflammatory disease: 2 g IV q8h. Life-threatening infections: 3–4 g IV q8h. Gonorrhea: 1 g IM single dose. Split 2 g IM dose into 2 injections.
PEDS - Pneumonia, sepsis, intra-abdominal, skin, bone & joint infections, age ≥6 mo: 50 mg/kg/dose IV q6–8h. Up to 200 mg/kg/d for serious infections, not to exceed max adult dose.
UNAPPROVED PEDS - Gonorrhea, CDC regimens: 500 mg IM single dose for uncomplicated; 1 g IV q8h for disseminated infection.
NOTES - Can cause transient rise in eosinophils, ALT, AST, CPK in children. Not for meningitis. Dosing in adults with renal dysfunction: For less severe infection load with 500 mg - 1 g IM/IV, then 500

mg q8h for CrCl 50–79 mL/min, 250–500 mg q12h for CrCl 5–49 mL/min, 500 mg q48h or 250 mg q24h for hemodialysis. For life-threatening infection, give loading dose, then 750 mg - 1.5 g IV q8h for CrCl 50–79 mL/min, 500 mg - 1 g q12h for CrCl 5–49 mL/min, 500 mg - 1 g q48h or 500 mg q24h for hemodialysis. For hemodialysis patients, give dose at end of dialysis.

**CEFTRIAXONE** (*Rocephin*) ▶K/Bile ♀B ▶+ $$$
WARNING - Fatal lung/kidney precipitation of ceftriaxone with calcium has been reported in neonates. Do not mix with calcium-containing products (eg Ringers/Hartmann's soln or TPN containing calcium) and do not administer in the same or different infusion lines or sites in any patient within 48 h of each other.
ADULT - Pneumonia, UTI, pelvic inflammatory disease (hospitalized), sepsis, meningitis, skin, bone & joint, intra-abdominal infections: Usual dose 1–2 g IM/IV q24h (max 4 g/d divided q12h). Gonorrhea: single dose 125 mg IM (250 mg if ambulatory treatment of PID).
PEDS - Meningitis: 100 mg/kg/d (max 4 g/d) IV divided q12–24h. Skin, pneumonia, other serious infections: 50–75 mg/kg/d (max 2 g/d) IM/IV divided q12–24h. Otitis media: 50 mg/kg (max 1 g) IM single dose.
UNAPPROVED ADULT - Lyme disease carditis, meningitis: 2 g IV daily × 14 d. Chancroid: 250 mg IM single dose. Disseminated gonorrhea: 1 g IM/IV q24h. Prophylaxis, invasive meningococcal disease: 250 mg IM single dose.
UNAPPROVED PEDS - Refractory otitis media (no response after 3 d of antibiotics): 50 mg/kg IM q24h × 3 doses. Lyme disease carditis, meningitis: 50–75 mg/kg IM/IV daily (max 2 g/d) × 14 d. Prophylaxis, invasive meningococcal disease: Single IM dose of 125 mg for ≤15 yo, 250 mg for >15 yo. Gonorrhea: 125 mg IM single dose; use adult regimens in STD table if ≥45 kg. Gonococcal bacteremia/arthritis: 50 mg/kg (max 1 g if ≤45 kg) IM/IV daily × 7 d. Gonococcal ophthalmia neonatorum/gonorrhea prophylaxis in newborn: 25–50 mg/kg up to 125 mg IM/IV single dose at birth. Disseminated gonorrhea, infants: 25–50 mg/kg/d IM/IV daily × 7 d. Typhoid fever: 50–75 mg/kg IM/IV daily × 14 d.
NOTES - Can cause prolonged prothrombin time (due to vitamin K deficiency), biliary sludging/symptoms of gallbladder disease. Do not give to neonates with hyperbilirubinemia. Dilute in 1% lidocaine for IM use. Do not exceed 2 g/d in patients with both hepatic & renal dysfunction.

---

## CEPHALOSPORINS—GENERAL ANTIMICROBIAL SPECTRUM

1st **generation**: gram positive (including *Staph aureus*); basic gram negative coverage
2nd **generation**: diminished *Staph aureus*, improved gram negative coverage compared to 1st generation; some with anaerobic coverage
3rd **generation**: further diminished *Staph aureus*, further improved gram negative coverage compared to 1st & 2nd generation; some with Pseudomonal coverage and diminished gram positive coverage
4th **generation**: same as 3rd generation plus coverage against *Pseudomonas*

## ANTIMICROBIALS: Cephalosporins—4th Generation

**NOTE:** Cross-sensitivity with penicillins possible. May cause C. difficile associated diarrhea.

**CEFEPIME (*Maxipime*)** ▶K ♀B ▶? $$$$$
ADULT - Mild, moderate UTI: 0.5–1 g IM/IV q12h. Severe UTI, skin, complicated intra-abdominal infections: 2 g IV q12h. Pneumonia: 1–2 g IV q12h. Empiric therapy of febrile neutropenia: 2 g IV q8h.
PEDS - UTI, skin infections, pneumonia, ≤40 kg: 50 mg/kg IV q12h. Empiric therapy for febrile neutropenia, ≤40 kg: 50 mg/kg IV q8h. Do not exceed adult dose.

UNAPPROVED ADULT - *P aeruginosa* osteomyelitis of the foot from nail puncture: 2 g IV q12h. Meningitis: 2 g IV q8h.
UNAPPROVED PEDS - Meningitis, cystic fibrosis, other serious infections: 50 mg/kg IV q8h (max 6 g/d).
NOTES - In Nov 2007, an FDA-initiated a safety review based on a meta analysis reported higher mortality with cefepime than with other beta lactams, especially in the neutropenic. High levels in renal dysfunction can cause CNS toxicity; dosing for CrCl <60 mL/min in package insert.

## ANTIMICROBIALS: Macrolides

**AZITHROMYCIN (*Zithromax, Zmax*)** ▶L ♀B ▶? $$
ADULT - Community-acquired pneumonia, inpatient: 500 mg IV over 1 h daily × ≥2 d, then 500 mg PO daily × 7–10 d total. Pelvic inflammatory disease: 500 mg IV daily × 1–2 d, then 250 mg PO daily to complete 7 d. Oral for acute exacerbation of chronic bronchitis, community-acquired pneumonia, group A streptococcal pharyngitis (sec-line to penicillin), skin infections: 500 mg PO on 1st d, then 250 mg PO daily to complete 5 d. Acute sinusitis, alternative for acute exacerbation of chronic bronchitis: 500 mg PO daily × 3 d. Chlamydia, chancroid: 1 g PO single dose. Gonorrhea: 2 g PO single dose. Observe patient for ≥30 min for poor GI tolerability. Prevention of disseminated Mycobacterium avium complex disease: 1200 mg PO q wk. Zmax for acute sinusitis, community-acquired pneumonia: 2 g PO single dose taken on empty stomach.
PEDS - Oral for otitis media, community-acquired pneumonia: 10 mg/kg up to 500 mg PO on 1st d, then 5 mg/kg up to 250 mg PO daily to complete 5 d. Acute sinusitis: 10 mg/kg PO daily × 3 d. Short regimens for otitis media: 30 mg/kg PO single dose or 10 mg/kg PO daily × 3 d. Group A streptococcal pharyngitis (sec-line to penicillin): 12 mg/kg up to 500 mg PO daily × 5 d. Take susp on empty stomach.
UNAPPROVED ADULT - See table for prophylaxis of bacterial endocarditis. Nongonococcal urethritis: 1 g PO single dose. See STD table for recurrent/persistent urethritis. Chlamydia in pregnancy: 1 g PO single dose. Campylobacter gastroenteritis: 500 mg PO daily × 3 d. Traveler's diarrhea: 500 mg PO on 1st d, then 250 mg PO daily to complete 5 d; or 1 g PO single dose. Mycobacterium avium complex disease treatment in AIDS: 500 mg PO daily (use ≥2 drugs for active infection). Pertussis treatment/post-exposure prophylaxis: 500 mg PO on 1st d, then 250 mg PO daily to complete 5 d. Early primary/latent syphilis: 2 g PO single dose (CDC recommends only for penicillin-allergic non-pregnant patients; azithromycin treatment failures reported in US).

UNAPPROVED PEDS - Prevention of disseminated Mycobacterium avium complex disease: 20 mg/kg PO q wk not to exceed adult dose. Mycobacterium avium complex disease treatment: 5 mg/kg PO daily (use ≥2 drugs for active infection). Cystic fibrosis & colonized with P aeruginosa (≥6 yo): 250 mg (<40 kg) or 500 mg (≥40 kg) PO three times weekly × 24 wk. Chlamydia trachomatis (≥8 yo, or <8 yo & ≥45 kg): 1 g PO single dose. Pertussis prophylaxis: Infants <6 mo, 10 mg/kg PO once daily × 5 d. Age ≥6 mo; 10 mg/kg (max 500 mg) PO single dose on d 1, then 5 mg/kg (max 250 mg) PO once daily on d 2–5. See table for bacterial endocarditis prophylaxis. Traveler's diarrhea: 5–10 mg/kg PO single dose. Cholera: 20 mg/kg up to 1 g PO single dose.
FORMS - Generic/Trade: Tab 250, 500, 600 mg, Susp 100 & 200/5 mL. Trade only: Packet 1000 mg. Z-Pak: #6, 250 mg tab. Tri-Pak: #3, 500 mg tab. Zmax extended release oral susp: 2 g in 60 mL single dose bottle.
NOTES - Severe allergic/skin reactions rarely, IV site reactions, hearing loss with prolonged use. Potential for QT interval prolongation and torsades cannot be excluded in patients at risk for prolonged cardiac repolarization. Does not inhibit cytochrome P450 enzymes. Do not take at the same time as Al/Mg antacids (except Zmax which can be taken with antacids). Contraindicated with pimozide. Single dose and 3-d regimens cause more vomiting than 5-d regimen for otitis media. Mechanism of action in cystic fibrosis is unknown; macrolides may inhibit P aeruginosa virulence factors or reduce inflammation. Zmax: Store at room temperature and use within 12 h of reconstitution. Additional treatment required for vomiting within 5 min of dose; consider for vomiting within 1 h of dose; unnecessary for vomiting >1 h after dose.

**CLARITHROMYCIN (*Biaxin, Biaxin XL*)** ▶KL ♀C ▶? $$$
ADULT - Group A streptococcal pharyngitis (sec-line to penicillin): 250 mg PO bid × 10 d. Acute sinusitis: 500 mg PO bid × 14 d. Acute exacerbation

**CLARITHROMYCIN** (*cont.*)
of chronic bronchitis (*S pneumoniae/M catarrhalis*), community-acquired pneumonia, skin infections: 250 mg PO bid × 7–14 d. Acute exacerbation of chronic bronchitis (H influenzae): 500 mg PO bid × 7–14 d. H pylori: See table in GI section. Mycobacterium avium complex disease prevention/treatment: 500 mg PO bid. Two or more drugs are needed for the treatment of active mycobacterial infections. Biaxin XL: Acute sinusitis: 1000 mg PO daily × 14 d. Acute exacerbation of chronic bronchitis, community-acquired pneumonia: 1000 mg PO daily × 7 d. Take Biaxin XL with food.
PEDS - Group A streptococcal pharyngitis (sec-line to penicillin), community-acquired pneumonia, sinusitis, otitis media, skin infections: 7.5 mg/kg PO bid × 10 d. *Mycobacterium avium* complex prevention/treatment: 7.5 mg/kg up to 500 mg PO bid. Two or more drugs are needed for the treatment of active mycobacterial infections.
UNAPPROVED ADULT - See table for prophylaxis of bacterial endocarditis. Pertussis treatment/post-exposure prophylaxis: 500 mg PO bid × 7 d. Community-acquired pneumonia: 500 mg PO bid.
UNAPPROVED PEDS - See table for prophylaxis of bacterial endocarditis. Pertussis treatment/post-exposure prophylaxis (≥1 mo): 7.5 mg/kg up to 500 mg PO bid × 7 d.
FORMS - Generic/Trade: Tab 250, 500 mg. Extended release tab 500 mg. Susp 125 & 250 mg/5 mL. Trade only: Biaxin XL-Pak: #14, 500 mg tabs. Generic only: Extended release tab 1000 mg.
NOTES - Rare arrhythmias in patients with prolonged QT. Cytochrome P450 3A4 & 1A2 inhibitor. Contraindicated with cisapride, pimozide. Many drug interactions including increased levels of carbamazepine, cyclosporine, digoxin, disopyramide, lovastatin, rifabutin, simvastatin (avoid), tacrolimus, theophylline. Toxicity with ergotamine, dihydroergotamine, or colchicine (esp. if elderly or renal dysfunction). Monitor INR with warfarin. Clarithromycin levels decreased by efavirenz (avoid concomitant use) and nevirapine enough to impair efficacy in Mycobacterium avium complex disease. AAP recommends 5–7 d of therapy for older (≥6 yo) children with non-severe otitis media, and 10 d for younger children and those with severe disease. Dosage reduction for renal insufficiency in patients taking ritonavir, lopinavir/ritonavir (Kaletra), or ritonavir-boosted tipranavir or darunavir: Decrease by 50% for CrCl 30–60 mL/min, decrease by 75% for CrCl <30 mL/min. Reduce clarithromycin dose by 50% if given with atazanavir; consider alternative for indications other than Mycobacterium avium complex. Do not refrigerate susp.

**ERYTHROMYCIN BASE** (*Eryc, E-mycin, Ery-Tab, ✦Erybid, Erythromid, P.C.E.*) ▶L ♀B ▶+ $
ADULT - Respiratory, skin infections: 250–500 mg PO qid or 333 mg PO tid. Pertussis, treatment/

post-exposure prophylaxis: 500 mg PO q6h × 14 d. S aureus skin infections: 250 mg PO q6h or 500 mg PO q12h. Secondary prevention of rheumatic fever: 250 mg PO bid. Chlamydia in pregnancy, nongonococcal urethritis: 500 mg PO qid × 7 d. Alternative for chlamydia in pregnancy if high dose not tolerated: 250 mg PO qid × 14 d. Erythrasma: 250 mg PO tid × 21 d. Legionnaires' disease: 2 g/d PO in divided doses × 14–21 d.
PEDS - Usual dose: 30–50 mg/kg/d PO divided qid × 10 d. Can double dose for severe infections. Pertussis: 40–50 mg/kg/d PO divided qid × 14 d (azithromycin preferred for infants <1 mo due to risk of hypertrophic pyloric stenosis with erytho). Chlamydia, newborn - <45 kg: 50 mg/kg/d PO divided qid × 14 d.
UNAPPROVED ADULT - Chancroid: 500 mg PO tid × 7 d. Campylobacter gastroenteritis: 500 mg PO bid × 5 d.
FORMS - Generic/Trade: Tab 250, 333, 500 mg, delayed-release cap 250.
NOTES - Rare arrhythmias in patients with prolonged QT. Incidence of sudden death may be increased when erythromycin is combined with potent CYP 3A4 inhibitors. May aggravate myasthenia gravis. Hypertrophic pyloric stenosis in infants primarily ≤2 wk of age. Cytochrome P450 3A4 & 1A2 inhibitor. Many drug interactions including increased levels of carbamazepine, cyclosporine, digoxin, disopyramide, tacrolimus, theophylline, some benzodiazepines and statins (avoid simvastatin). Monitor INR with warfarin. Contraindicated with cisapride, pimozide.

**ERYTHROMYCIN ESTOLATE** ▶L ♀B ▶+ $$
WARNING - Hepatotoxicity, primarily in adults.
ADULT - Other erythromycin forms preferred in adults.
PEDS - Usual dose: 30–50 mg/kg/d PO divided bid-qid. Can double for severe infections. Group A streptococcal pharyngitis: 20–40 mg/kg/d (up to 1 g/d) PO divided bid to qid × 10d. Secondary prevention of rheumatic fever: 250 mg PO bid. Pertussis: 40–50 mg/kg/d PO divided qid × 14 d.
FORMS - Generic: Susp 125 & 250 mg/5 mL.
NOTES - Contraindicated in liver disease. Rare arrhythmias in patients with prolonged QT. Incidence of sudden death may be increased when erythromycin is combined with potent CYP 3A4 inhibitors. May aggravate myasthenia gravis. Hypertrophic pyloric stenosis in infants primarily ≤2 wk of age. Cytochrome 450 3A4 & 1A2 inhibitor. Many drug interactions including increased levels of carbamazepine, cyclosporine, digoxin, disopyramide, tacrolimus, theophylline, some benzodiazepines and statins. Monitor INR with warfarin. Contraindicated with cisapride, pimozide.

**ERYTHROMYCIN ETHYL SUCCINATE** (*EES, Eryped*) ▶L ♀B ▶+ $
ADULT - Usual dose: 400 mg PO qid. Nongonococcal urethritis: 800 mg PO qid × 7 d. Chlamydia in

**ERYTHROMYCIN ETHYL SUCCINATE** *(cont.)*
pregnancy: 800 mg PO qid × 7 d or 400 mg PO qid × 14 d if high dose not tolerated. Secondary prevention of rheumatic fever: 400 mg PO bid. Legionnaires' disease: 3.2 g/d PO in divided doses × 14–21 d.

PEDS - Usual dose: 30–50 mg/kg/d PO divided qid. Max dose: 100 mg/kg/d. Group A streptococcal pharyngitis: 40 mg/kg/d (up to 1 g/d) PO divided bid to qid × 10 d. Secondary prevention of rheumatic fever: 400 mg PO bid. Pertussis: 40–50 mg/kg/d up to 2 g/d PO divided qid × 14 d.

FORMS - Generic/Trade: Tab 400 tab, susp 200 & 400 mg/5 mL. Trade only (EryPed): Susp 100 mg/2.5 mL (50 mL).

NOTES - Rare arrhythmias in patients with prolonged QT. Incidence of sudden death may be increased when erythromycin is combined with potent CYP 3A4 inhibitors. May aggravate myasthenia gravis. Hypertrophic pyloric stenosis in infants primarily ≤2 wk of age. Cytochrome P450 3A4 & 1A2 inhibitor. Many drug interactions including increased levels of carbamazepine, cyclosporine, digoxin, disopyramide, tacrolimus, theophylline, some benzodiazepines and statins (avoid simvastatin). Monitor INR with warfarin. Contraindicated with cisapride, pimozide.

**ERYTHROMYCIN LACTOBIONATE** (*→Erythrocin IV*) ▶L ♀B ▶+ $$$$$
ADULT - For severe infections/PO not possible: 15–20 mg/kg/d (max 4g) IV divided q6h. Legionnaires' disease: 4 g/d IV divided q6h.

PEDS - For severe infections/PO not possible: 15–20 mg/kg/d (max 4g) IV divided q6h.

UNAPPROVED PEDS - 20–50 mg/kg/d IV divided q6h.

NOTES - Dilute and give slowly to minimize venous irritation. Reversible hearing loss (increased risk in elderly given ≥4 g/d), allergic reactions, arrhythmias in patients with prolonged QT, exacerbation of myasthenia gravis. Incidence of sudden death may be increased when erythromycin is combined with potent CYP 3A4 inhibitors. Hypertrophic pyloric stenosis in infants primarily ≤2 wk of age. Cytochrome P450 3A4 & 1A2 inhibitor. Many drug interactions including increased levels of carbamazepine, cyclosporine, digoxin, disopyramide, tacrolimus, theophylline, some benzodiazepines and statins (avoid simvastatin). Monitor INR with warfarin. Contraindicated with cisapride, pimozide.

**PEDIAZOLE** (erythromycin ethyl succinate + sulfisoxazole) ▶KL ♀C ▶- $$
PEDS - Otitis media, age >2 mo: 50 mg/kg/d (based on EES dose) PO divided tid-qid.

FORMS - Generic/Trade: Susp, erythromycin ethyl succinate 200 mg + sulfisoxazole 600 mg/5 mL.

NOTES - Sulfisoxazole: Stevens-Johnson syndrome, toxic epidermal necrolysis, hepatotoxicity, blood dyscrasia, hemolysis in G6PD deficiency. Increased INR with warfarin. Erythromycin: Rare arrhythmias in patients with prolonged QT. Incidence of sudden death may be increased when erythromycin is combined with potent CYP 3A4 inhibitors. May aggravate myasthenia gravis. Cytochrome P450 3A4 & 1A2 inhibitor. Many drug interactions including increased levels of carbamazepine, cyclosporine, digoxin, disopyramide, tacrolimus, theophylline, some benzodiazepines and statins. Monitor INR with warfarin. Contraindicated with cisapride, pimozide. AAP recommends 5–7 d of therapy for older (≥6 yo) children with non-severe otitis media, and 10 d for younger children and those with severe disease.

## PENICILLINS—GENERAL ANTIMICROBIAL SPECTRUM

1st **generation**: Most streptococci; oral anaerobic coverage
2nd **generation**: Most streptococci; Staph aureus
3rd **generation**: Most streptococci; basic gram negative coverage
4th **generation**: Pseudomonas

## ANTIMICROBIALS: Penicillins—1st Generation—Natural

**NOTE:** Anaphylaxis occurs rarely with penicillins; cross-sensitivity with cephalosporins is possible.

**BENZATHINE PENICILLIN** (*Bicillin L-A*, *→Megacillin*) ▶K ♀B ▶? $$
ADULT - Group A streptococcal pharyngitis: 1.2 million units IM single dose. Secondary prevention of rheumatic fever: 1.2 million units IM q mo (q 3 wk for high-risk patients) or 600,000 units IM q 2 wk. Primary, secondary, early latent syphilis: 2.4 million units IM single dose. Tertiary, late latent syphilis: 2.4 million units IM q wk × 3 doses.

PEDS - Group A streptococcal pharyngitis (American Heart Assoc regimen): 600,000 units IM for ≤27 kg, 1.2 million units IM for >27 kg. Secondary prevention of rheumatic fever: 1.2 million units IM q mo (q 3 wk for high-risk patients) or 600,000 units IM q 2 wk. Primary, secondary, early latent syphilis: 50,000 units/kg (up to 2.4 million units) IM single dose. Late latent syphilis: 50,000 units/kg (up to 2.4 million units) IM × 3 weekly doses.

UNAPPROVED ADULT - Prophylaxis of diphtheria/treatment of carriers: 1.2 million units IM single dose.

UNAPPROVED PEDS - Prophylaxis of diphtheria/treatment of carriers: 1.2 million units IM single dose for ≥30 kg or ≥6 yo. 600,000 units IM single dose for <30 kg or <6 yo.

**BENZATHINE PENICILLIN** (*cont.*)
FORMS - Trade only: for IM use, 600,000 units/mL; 1, 2, and 4 mL syringes.
NOTES - Do not give IV. Doses last 2–4 wk. Not for neurosyphilis.

**BICILLIN C-R** (procaine penicillin + benzathine penicillin) ▶K ♀B ▶? $$$
ADULT - Scarlet fever, erysipelas, upper-respiratory, skin and soft-tissue infections due to Group A strep: 2.4 million units IM single dose. Pneumococcal infections other than meningitis: 1.2 million units IM q2–3 d until temperature normal × 48 h. Not for treatment of syphilis.
PEDS - Scarlet fever, erysipelas, upper-respiratory, skin & soft-tissue infections due to Group A strep: 2.4 million units IM for >27 kg, 900,000 units–1.2 million units IM for 13.6–27 kg, 600,000 units IM for <13.6 kg. Pneumococcal infections other than meningitis: 600,000 units IM q2–3 d until temperature normal × 48 h. Not for treatment of syphilis.
FORMS - Trade only: for IM use 300/300 thousand units/mL procaine/benzathine penicillin; 1, 2, and 4 mL syringes.
NOTES - Contraindicated if allergic to procaine. Do not give IV. Do not substitute Bicillin CR for Bicillin LA in treatment of syphilis.

**PENICILLIN G** ▶K ♀B ▶? $$$$
ADULT - Penicillin-sensitive pneumococcal pneumonia: 8–12 million units/d IV divided q4–6h. Penicillin-sensitive pneumococcal meningitis: 24 million units/d IV divided q2–4h. Empiric therapy, native valve endocarditis: 20 million units/d IV continuous infusion or divided q4h plus nafcillin/ oxacillin and gentamicin. Neurosyphilis: 18–24 million units/d continuous IV infusion or 3–4 million units IV q4h × 10–14 d. Bioterrorism anthrax: See www.idsociety.org/BT/ToC.htm.
PEDS - Mild to moderate infections: 25,000–50,000 units/kg/d IV divided q6h. Severe infections including pneumococcal and meningococcal meningitis: 250,000–400,000 units/kg/d IV divided q4–6h. Neonates <1 wk, >2 kg: 25,000–50,000 units/kg IV q8h. Neonates ≥1 wk, >2 kg: 25,000–50,000 units/kg IV q6h. Group B streptococcal meningitis: ≤7 d old, 250,000–450,000 units/kg/d IV divided q8h. >7 d old, 450,000–500,000 units/kg/d IV divided q4–6h. Congenital syphilis: 50,000 units/kg/dose IV q12h during first 7 d of life, then q8h thereafter to complete 10 d. Congenital syphilis or neurosyphilis in children >1 mo old: 50,000 units/kg IV q4–6 h × 10 d.
UNAPPROVED ADULT - Prevention of perinatal group B streptococcal disease: Give to mother 5 million units IV at onset of labor/after membrane rupture, then 2.5 million units IV q4h until delivery. Diphtheria: 100,000–150,000 units/kg/d IV divided q6h × 14 d.
UNAPPROVED PEDS - Diphtheria: 100,000–150,000 units/kg/d IV divided q6h × 14 d.
NOTES - Decrease dose by 50% if CrCl <10 mL/min.

**PENICILLIN V** (*Veetids, ◆PVF-K, Nadopen-V*) ▶K ♀B ▶? $
ADULT - Usual dose: 250–500 mg PO qid. AHA dosing for group A streptococcal pharyngitis: 500 mg PO bid or tid × 10 d. Secondary prevention of
**(cont.)**

| SBE PROPHYLAXIS | |
|---|---|
| **For dental, oral, respiratory tract, or esophageal procedures** | |
| Standard regimen | amoxicillin 2 g PO 1 before procedure |
| Unable to take oral meds | ampicillin 2 g IM/IV within 30 min before procedure |
| Allergic to penicillin | clindamycin 600 mg PO; or cephalexin or cefadroxil 2 g PO; or azithromycin or clarithromycin 500 mg PO 1 h before procedure |
| Allergic to penicillin and unable to take oral meds | clindamycin 600 mg IV; or cefazolin 1 g IM/IV within 30 min before procedure |
| Pediatric drug doses | Total pediatric dose should not exceed adult dose. Amoxicillin 50 mg/kg, ampicillin 50 mg/kg, azithromycin 15 mg/kg, cephalexin 50 mg/kg, cefadroxil 50 mg/kg, cefazolin 25 mg/kg, clarithromycin 15 mg/kg, clindamycin 20 mg/kg. |
| **For GU and GI (excluding esophageal) procedures** | |
| High-risk patients | ampicillin 2 g IM/IV plus gentamicin 1.5 mg/kg (max 120 mg) within 30 min of starting procedure; 6 h later ampicillin 1 g IM/IV or amoxicillin 1 g PO. |
| High-risk patients allergic to ampicillin | vancomycin 1 g IV over 1–2h plus gentamicin 1.5 mg/kg IV/IM (max 120 mg) complete within 30 minutes of starting procedure |
| Moderate-risk patients | amoxicillin 2 g PO or ampicillin 2 g IM/IV within 30 min of starting procedure |
| Moderate-risk patients allergic to ampicillin | vancomycin 1 g IV over 1–2 h complete within 30 min of starting procedure |
| Pediatric drug doses | Total pediatric dose should not exceed adult dose. Amoxicillin 50 mg/kg, ampicillin 50 mg/kg, azithromycin 15 mg/kg, cephalexin 50 mg/kg, cefadroxil 50 mg/kg, cefazolin 25 mg/kg, clarithromycin 15 mg/kg, clindamycin 20 mg/kg. |

**PENICILLIN V (cont.)**
rheumatic fever: 250 mg PO bid. Vincent's infection: 250 mg PO q6–8h.
PEDS - Usual dose: 25–50 mg/kg/d PO divided tid or qid. Use adult dose for ≥12 yo. AHA dosing for group A streptococcal pharyngitis: 250 mg PO bid or tid × 10 d. Secondary prevention of rheumatic fever: 250 mg PO bid.
UNAPPROVED PEDS - Prevention of pneumococcal infections in functional/anatomic asplenia: 125 mg PO bid for <3 yo, 250 mg PO bid for ≥3 yo.
FORMS - Generic/Trade: Tabs 250, 500 mg, oral soln 125 & 250 mg/5 mL.
NOTES - Oral soln stable in refrigerator for 14 d.

**PROCAINE PENICILLIN (Wycillin)** ▶K ♀B ▶? $$$$$
ADULT - Pneumococcal & streptococcal infections, Vincent's infection, erysipeloid: 0.6–1.0 million units IM daily. Neurosyphilis: 2.4 million units IM daily plus probenecid 500 mg PO q6h, both × 10–14 d.
PEDS - Pneumococcal & streptococcal infections, Vincent's infection, erysipeloid, <27 kg: 300,000 units IM daily. AAP dose for mild-to-moderate infections, >1 mo: 25,000–50,000 units/kg/d IM divided daily-bid. Congenital syphilis: 50,000 units/kg IM daily × 10 d.
NOTES - Peak 4h, lasts 24h. Contraindicated if procaine allergy; skin test if allergy suspected. Transient CNS reactions with high doses.

## ANTIMICROBIALS: Penicillins—2nd Generation—Penicillinase-Resistant

NOTE: Anaphylaxis occurs rarely with penicillins; cross-sensitivity with cephalosporins is possible.

**CLOXACILLIN** ▶KL ♀B ▶? $$
ADULT - Staph infections: 250–500 mg PO qid on empty stomach. Severe infections: 1–2 g IV/IM q4h. Staph osteomyelitis: 2 g IV/IM q6h. IV/IM not available in US.
PEDS - Staph infections: 50–100 mg/kg/d PO divided q6h on empty stomach. Use adult dose for ≥20 kg.
FORMS - Canada only. Generic only: Caps 250,500 mg, oral soln 125 mg/5 mL.
NOTES - Oral soln stable in refrigerator for 14 d.

**DICLOXACILLIN (Dynapen)** ▶KL ♀B ▶? $$
ADULT - Usual dose: 250–500 mg PO qid. Take on empty stomach.
PEDS - Mild to moderate upper respiratory, skin & soft-tissue infections, age >1 mo: 12.5 mg/kg/d PO divided q6h. Pneumonia, disseminated infections, age >1 mo: 25 mg/kg/d PO divided qid. Follow-up therapy after IV antibiotics for Staph osteomyelitis: 50–100 mg/kg/d PO divided qid. Use adult dose for ≥40 kg. Give on empty stomach.
FORMS - Generic only: Caps 250, 500 mg.
NOTES - Oral susp stable at room temperature for 7d, in refrigerator 14d.

**NAFCILLIN** ▶L ♀B ▶? $$$$$
ADULT - Staph infections, usual dose: 500 mg IM q4–6h or 500–2000 mg IV q4h. Osteomyelitis: 1–2 g IV q4h. Empiric therapy, native valve

endocarditis: 2 g IV q4h plus penicillin/ampicillin and gentamicin.
PEDS - Staph infections, usual dose: Neonates, 10 mg/kg IM q12h. <40 kg, 25 mg/kg IM q12h.
UNAPPROVED PEDS - Mild to moderate infections: 50–100 mg/kg/d IM/IV divided q6h. Severe infections: 100–200 mg/kg/d IM/IV divided q4–6h. Neonates <1 wk, >2 kg: 25 mg/kg IM/IV q6h. Neonates ≥1 wk, >2 kg: 25–35 mg/kg IM/IV q6h.
NOTES - Reversible neutropenia with prolonged use. Decreased INR with warfarin. Decreased cyclosporine levels.

**OXACILLIN (Bactocill)** ▶KL ♀B ▶? $$$$$
ADULT - Staph infections: 250 mg-2g IM/IV q4–6h. Osteomyelitis: 1.5–2 g IV q4h. Empiric therapy, native valve endocarditis: 2 g IV q4h with penicillin/ampicillin and gentamicin.
PEDS - Mild to moderate infections: 100–150 mg/kg/d IM/IV divided q6h. Severe infections: 150–200 mg/kg/d IM/IV divided q4–6h. Use adult dose for ≥40 kg. AAP regimens for newborns >2 kg: <1 wk, 25–50 mg/kg IM/IV q8h. ≥1 wk, 25–50 mg/kg IM/IV q6h.
NOTES - Hepatic dysfunction possible with doses >12 g/d; monitor LFTs. Oral soln stable for 3 d at room temperature, 14 d refrigerated.

## ANTIMICROBIALS: Penicillins—3rd Generation—Aminopenicillins

NOTE: Anaphylaxis occurs rarely with penicillins; cross-sensitivity with cephalosporins is possible.

**AMOXICILLIN (Amoxil, DisperMox, Moxatag, Trimox, ◆Novamoxin)** ▶K ♀B ▶+ $
ADULT - ENT, skin, GU infections: 250–500 mg PO tid or 500–875 mg PO bid. Pneumonia: 500 mg PO tid or 875 mg PO bid. Group A streptococcal pharyngitis/tonsillitis, ≥12 yo: 775 mg ER tab (Moxatag) PO × 10 d. Do not chew/crush Moxatag tabs. H pylori: See table in GI section. See table for prophylaxis of bacterial endocarditis.

PEDS - ENT, skin, GU infections: 20–40 mg/kg/d PO divided tid or 25–45 mg/kg/d PO divided bid. See "unapproved" for AAP acute otitis media dosing. Pneumonia: 40 mg/kg/d PO divided tid or 45 mg/kg/d PO divided bid. Infants <3 mo: 30 mg/kg/d PO divided q12h. Group A streptococcal pharyngitis/tonsillitis, ≥12 yo: 775 mg ER tab (Moxatag) PO × 10 d. Do not chew/crush Moxatag tabs. See table for bacterial endocarditis prophylaxis.

**AMOXICILLIN** (cont.)

UNAPPROVED ADULT - Acute sinusitis with antibiotic use in past mo &/or drug-resistant S pneumoniae rate >30%: 3–3.5 g/d PO. High-dose for community-acquired pneumonia: 1 g PO tid. Lyme disease: 500 mg PO tid × 14 d for early disease, × 28 d for Lyme arthritis. Chlamydia in pregnancy: 500 mg PO tid × 7 d. Bioterrorism anthrax: See www.idsociety.org/BT/ToC.htm.

UNAPPROVED PEDS - Otitis media (AAP high-dose): 80–90 mg/kg/d PO divided bid-tid. Community-acquired pneumonia, 4 mo–4 yo: 80–100 mg/kg/d PO divided tid-qid. Lyme disease: 50 mg/kg/d (up to 1500 mg/d) PO divided tid × 14 d for early disease, × 28 d for Lyme arthritis. Bioterrorism anthrax: See www.idsociety.org/BT/ToC.htm.

FORMS - Generic/Trade: Caps 250, 500 mg, tabs 500, 875 mg, chews 125, 200, 250, 400mg, susp 125 & 250 mg/5 mL, susp 200 & 400 mg/5 mL. Trade only: Infant drops 50 mg/mL (Amoxil). DisperMox 200, 400, 600 mg tabs for oral susp, Moxatag 775 mg extended-release tab.

NOTES - Rash in patients with mononucleosis. AAP recommends 5–7 d of therapy for older (≥6 yo) children with non-severe otitis media, and 10 d for younger children and those with severe disease. Dosing in adults with renal dysfunction: Do not use 875 mg tab for CrCl <30 mL/min. Use 250–500 mg PO bid for CrCl 10–30 mL/min, 250–500 mg PO daily for CrCl <10 mL/min or hemodialysis. Give additional dose both during & at end of dialysis. Oral susp & infant drops stable for 14 d at room temperature or in the refrigerator. Mix DisperMox tab with 2 tsp water and drink mixture, then rinse container with a little water and drink that. Do not chew or swallow tab whole. Use only for doses that can be delivered by whole tabs.

**AMOXICILLIN-CLAVULANATE** (*Augmentin, Augmentin ES-600, Augmentin XR, ✚Clavulin*) ▶K ♀B ▶? $$$$

ADULT - Pneumonia, otitis media, sinusitis, skin infections, UTIs: Usual dose - 500 mg PO bid or 250 mg PO tid. More severe infections: 875 mg PO bid or 500 mg PO tid. Augmentin XR: 2 tabs PO q12h with meals × 10 d for acute sinusitis, × 7–10 d for community-acquired pneumonia.

PEDS - 200,400 chewables & 200,400/5 mL susp for bid administration: Pneumonia, otitis media, sinusitis: 45 mg/kg/d PO divided bid. (See "unapproved" for AAP high-dose for otitis media.) Less severe infections such as skin, UTIs: 25 mg/kg/d PO divided bid. 125,250 chewables & 125,250/5 mL susp for tid administration: Pneumonia, otitis media, sinusitis: 40 mg/kg/d PO divided tid. Less severe infections such as skin, UTIs: 20 mg/kg/d PO divided tid. Age <3 mo: Use 125 mg/5 mL susp and give 30 mg/kg PO q12 h. Use adult dose for ≥40 kg. Augmentin ES-600 susp for ≥3 mo and <40 kg. Recurrent/persistent otitis media with risk factors (antibiotics for otitis media in past 3 mo and either age ≤2 yo or daycare): 90 mg/kg/d PO divided bid with food × 10 d.

UNAPPROVED ADULT - Prevention of infection after dog/cat bite: 875 mg PO bid or 500 mg PO tid × 3–5 d. Treatment of infected dog/cat bite: 875 mg PO bid or 500 mg PO tid, duration of treatment based on response.

UNAPPROVED PEDS - AAP otitis media, sinusitis: Augmentin ES-600 susp 90 mg/kg/d PO divided bid. Group A streptococcal pharyngitis, repeated culture-positive episodes: 45 mg/kg/d PO divided bid × 10 d.

FORMS - Generic/Trade: (amoxicillin + clavulanate) Tabs 250+125, 500+125, 875+125 mg, chewables and susp 200+28.5, 400+57 mg per tab or 5 mL, (ES) susp 600+42.9 mg/5mL. Trade only: Chewables and susp 125+31.25, 250+62.5 mg per tab or 5 mL. Extended-release tabs (Augmentin XR) 1000+62.5 mg.

NOTES - Rash in patients with mononucleosis; diarrhea common (less diarrhea with bid dosing). AAP recommends 5–7 d of therapy for older (≥6 yo) children with non-severe otitis media, and 10 d for younger children and those with severe disease. Do not interchange Augmentin products with different clavulanate content. 250 mg tab contains too much clavulanate for children <40 kg. Suspensions stable in refrigerator for 10 d. See package insert for dosage reduction of Augmentin tabs if CrCl <30 mL/min. Augmentin XR contraindicated if CrCl <30 mL/min.

**AMPICILLIN** (*Principen, ✚Penbritin*) ▶K ♀B ▶? $ PO $$$$$ IV

ADULT - Usual dose: 1–2 g IV q4–6h or 250–500 mg PO qid. Sepsis, meningitis: 150–200 mg/kg/d IV divided q3–4h. Empiric therapy, native valve endocarditis: 12 g/d IV continuous infusion or divided q4h plus nafcillin/oxacillin and gentamicin. See table for prophylaxis of bacterial endocarditis. Take oral ampicillin on an empty stomach.

PEDS - AAP recommendations: Mild to moderate infections: 100–150 mg/kg/d IM/IV divided q6h or 50–100 mg/kg/d PO divided qid. Severe infections: 200–400 mg/kg/d IM/IV divided q6h. Infants >2 kg: 25–50 mg/kg IV q8h if <1 wk old and q6h if ≥1 wk old. Use adult doses for ≥40 kg. Give oral ampicillin on an empty stomach. Group B streptococcal meningitis: ≤1 wk old, 200–300 mg/kg/d IV divided q8h. ≥1 wk old, 300 mg/kg/d IV divided q4–6h. Give with gentamicin initially. See table for prophylaxis of bacterial endocarditis.

UNAPPROVED ADULT - Prevention of neonatal group B streptococcal disease: Give to mother 2 g IV during labor, then 1–2 g IV q4–6h until delivery.

FORMS - Generic/Trade: Caps 250,500 mg, susp 125 & 250 mg/5 mL.

NOTES - Rash in patients with mononucleosis or taking allopurinol; C. difficile associated diarrhea. Susp stable for 7 d at room temperature, 14 d in the refrigerator. Reduce dosing interval to q12–24h for CrCl <10 mL/min. Give dose after hemodialysis.

**AMPICILLIN-SULBACTAM (*Unasyn*) ▶K ♀B ▶? $$$$$**
ADULT - Skin, intra-abdominal, gynecologic infections: 1.5–3 g IM/IV q6h.
PEDS - Skin infections, ≥1 yo: <40 kg, 300 mg/kg/d IV divided q6h. ≥40 kg: adult dose.
UNAPPROVED ADULT - Community-acquired pneumonia: 1.5–3 g IM/IV q6h with a macrolide or doxycycline.
UNAPPROVED PEDS - AAP regimens. Mild to moderate infections: 100–150 mg/kg/d of ampicillin IM/IV divided q6h. Severe infections: 200–400 mg/kg/d of ampicillin IM/IV divided q6h.
NOTES - Rash in patients with mononucleosis or taking allopurinol; C. difficile associated diarrhea. Dosing in renal impairment: Give usual dose q6–8h for adults with CrCl ≥30 mL/min, q12h for CrCl 15–29 mL/min, q24 h for CrCl 5–14 mL/min.

**PIVAMPICILLIN (*Pondocillin*) ▶K ♀? ▶? $**
ADULT - Canada only. Respiratory tract, ENT, gynecologic, urinary tract infections: Usual dose is 500 mg PO bid; 1000 mg PO bid for severe infections. Treat pharyngitis × 10 d.
PEDS - Canada only. Not recommended for severe infections. Avoid in infants <3 mo. Susp, 3–12 mo: 40–60 mg/kg/d PO divided bid. Susp, ≤10 yo: 25–35 mg/kg/d up to 525 mg PO bid. 5 mL PO bid for 1–3 yo, 7.5 mL PO bid for 4–6 yo, 10 mL PO bid for 7–10 yo. Treat pharyngitis × 10 d.
FORMS - Trade only: Tabs 500 mg (377 mg ampicillin), # 20, oral susp 35 mg/mL (26 mg ampicillin), 100,150, 200 mL bottles.
NOTES - Long-term therapy or repeated courses may increase carnitine excretion; avoid with valproate or in carnitine deficiency. Avoid with lymphocytic leukemia or infectious mononucleosis due to high risk of rash; allopurinol can also increase risk of rash. C. difficile associated diarrhea. Susp stable for 7 d at room temperature, 14 d in the refrigerator. Reduce dose in severe renal dysfunction.

## ANTIMICROBIALS: Penicillins—4th Generation—Extended Spectrum

**NOTE:** Anaphylaxis occurs rarely with penicillins; cross-sensitivity with cephalosporins is possible.

**PIPERACILLIN ▶K/BILE ♀B ▶? $$$$$**
ADULT - Simple UTI, community-acquired pneumonia: 6–8 g/d IM/IV divided q6–12h. Complicated UTI: 8–16 g/d IV divided q6–8h. Serious infections: 12–18 g/d IV divided q4–6h. Max dose: 24 g/d.
PEDS - Safety and efficacy not established in children <12 yo. Use adult dose for ≥12 yo.
UNAPPROVED ADULT - Empiric therapy of neutropenic fever: 3 g IV q4h or 4 g IV q6h with an aminoglycoside.
UNAPPROVED PEDS - Mild to moderate infections: 100–150 mg/kg/d IV divided q6h. Severe infections: 200–300 mg/kg/d IV divided q4–6h.
NOTES - Hypokalemia; bleeding & coagulation abnormalities possible especially with renal impairment. May prolong neuromuscular blockade with non-depolarizing muscle relaxants. May reduce renal excretion of methotrexate; monitor methotrexate levels and toxicity. Adult dosing with renal dysfunction: Serious infections: 4 g IV q8h for CrCl 20–40 mL/min, 4 g IV q12h for CrCl <20 mL/min. Complicated UTI: 3 g IV q8h for CrCl 20–40 mL/min, 3 g IV q12h for CrCl <20 mL/min. Simple UTI: 3 g IV q12h for CrCl <20 mL/min.

**PIPERACILLIN-TAZOBACTAM (*Zosyn*, ✚*Tazocin*) ▶K ♀B ▶? $$$$$**
ADULT - Appendicitis, peritonitis, skin infections, postpartum endometritis, pelvic inflammatory disease, moderate community-acquired pneumonia: 3.375 g IV q6h. Nosocomial pneumonia: 4.5 g IV q6h (with aminoglycoside initially and if P. aeruginosa is cultured).
PEDS - Appendicitis/peritonitis: 100 mg/kg of piperacillin IV q8h for ≥9 mo old; 80 mg/kg q8h for 2–9 mo old; use adult dose if >40 kg.
UNAPPROVED ADULT - Serious infections: 4.5 g IV q6h.
UNAPPROVED PEDS - 300–400 mg/kg/d piperacillin IV divided q6–8h for >6 mo old; 150–300 mg/kg/d IV divided q6–8h for <6 mo old.
NOTES - Hypokalemia; bleeding & coagulation abnormalities possible especially with renal impairment. May prolong neuromuscular blockade with non-depolarizing muscle relaxants. False-positive result possible with Bio-Rad Laboratories Platelia Aspergillus EIA test. May reduce renal excretion of methotrexate; monitor methotrexate levels and toxicity. Dosing in renal impairment: 2.25 g IV q6h for CrCl 20–40 mL/min, 2.25 g IV q8h for CrCl <20 mL/min. Hemodialysis: Max dose of 2.25 g IV q8h plus 0.75 g after each dialysis.

**TICARCILLIN (*Ticar*) ▶K ♀B ▶+ $$$$$**
ADULT - Sepsis, pneumonia, skin & soft tissue, intra-abdominal, female GU infections: 3 g IV q4h or 4 g IV q6h. Simple UTI: 1 g IM/IV q6h. Complicated UTI: 3 g IV q6h.
PEDS - Sepsis, pneumonia, skin & soft tissue, intra-abdominal infections, <40 kg: 200–300 mg/kg/d IV divided q4–6h. Simple UTI, <40 kg: 50–100 mg/kg/d IM/IV divided q6–8h. Complicated UTI, <40 kg: 150–200 mg/kg/d IV divided q4–6h. Use adult dose for ≥40 kg. Severe infections, neonates ≥2 kg: <1 wk, 75 mg/kg IV q8h. >1 wk, 100 mg/kg IV q8h or 75 mg/kg IV q6h.
NOTES - Hypokalemia; bleeding & coagulation abnormalities possible especially with renal impairment. Not more than 2 g/IM injection site. Up to 6.5 mEq sodium/g ticarcillin. Adult dosing with renal dysfunction: 3 g IV load, then 2 g IV q4h for CrCl 30–60 mL/min, 2 g IV q8h for CrCl 10–30 mL/min, 2 g IV q12h or 1 g IM q6h for CrCl

## QUINOLONES- GENERAL ANTIMICROBIAL SPECTRUM

1st **generation**: gram negative (excluding *Pseudomonas*), urinary tract only, no atypicals
2nd **generation**: gram negative (including *Pseudomonas*); *Staph aureus* but not *Pneumococcus*; some atypicals
3rd **generation**: gram negative (including *Pseudomonas*); gram positive (including *Staph aureus* and pneumococcus); expanded atypical coverage
4th **generation**: same as 3rd generation plus enhanced coverage of *pneumococcus*, decreased activity vs. *Pseudomonas*.

**TICARCILLIN** (*cont.*)
<10 mL/min. Liver dysfunction and CrCl <10 mL/min: 2 g IV q24h or 1 g IM q12h. Peritoneal dialysis: 3 g IV q12h. Hemodialysis: 2 g IV q12h and 3 g IV after each dialysis session.

**TICARCILLIN-CLAVULANATE** (*Timentin*) ▶K ♀B ▶? $$$$$
ADULT - Systemic infections or UTIs: 3.1 g IV q4–6h. Gynecologic infections: Moderate, 200 mg/kg/d IV divided q6h. Severe, 300 mg/kg/d IV divided q4h. Adults <60 kg: 200–300 mg/kg/d (based on ticarcillin content) IV divided q4–6h. Use q4h dosing interval for Pseudomonas infections.
PEDS - Mild to moderate infections: ≥60 kg, 3.1 g IV q6h. Age ≥3 mo and <60 kg, 200 mg/kg/d (based on ticarcillin content) IV divided q6h.

Severe infections: ≥60 kg, 3.1 g IV q4h. Age ≥3 mo and <60 kg, 300 mg/kg/d (based on ticarcillin content) IV divided q4h.
NOTES - Timentin 3.1 g = 3 g ticarcillin + 0.1 g clavulanate. Hypokalemia; bleeding & coagulation abnormalities possible especially in patients with renal impairment. 4.75 mEq sodium/g Timentin. IV dosing in adults with renal dysfunction: Load with 3.1 g, then 2 g q4h for CrCl 30–60 mL/min, 2 g q8h for CrCl 10–30 mL/min, 2 g q12h for CrCl <10 mL/min, 2 g q24h for CrCl <10 mL/min and liver dysfunction. Peritoneal dialysis: 3.1 g q12h. Hemodialysis: 3.1 g load, then 2 g q12h and 3.1 g after each dialysis.

## ANTIMICROBIALS: Quinolones—1st Generation

**NOTE:** Important quinolone drug interactions with warfarin, antacids, iron, zinc, magnesium, sucralfate, cimetidine, caffeine, cyclosporine, hydantoins, theophylline, etc.

**NALIDIXIC ACID** (*NegGram*) ▶KL ♀C ▶? $$$$
ADULT - UTI: 1 g PO qid for 1–2 wk, may reduce to 2 g/d thereafter.
PEDS - UTI, age ≥3 mo: 55 mg/kg/d PO divided qid, may reduce to 33 mg/kg/d thereafter. Use cautiously in children; arthropathy observed in animal studies. Stop therapy if arthralgia develops.

FORMS - Trade only: Tabs 0.25, 0.5, 1 g.
NOTES - CNS toxicity; photosensitivity; hemolytic anemia in G6PD deficiency. Contraindicated if seizure history. Monitor CBC and LFTs if used for >2 wk. Do not use with alkylating agents such as melphalan. Give at least 2 h before or after Al/Mg antacids, iron, sucralfate, calcium, zinc, buffered didanosine.

## ANTIMICROBIALS: Quinolones—2nd Generation

**NOTE:** As of April 2007, the CDC no longer recommends fluoroquinolones for gonorrhea because of high resistance rates. Fluoroquinolones can cause tendon rupture (rare; risk increased by corticosteroids, age >60, or organ transplant), phototoxicity (risk varies among agents), C difficile associated diarrhea (risk may vary among agents), QT interval prolongation (risk varies among agents; see QT drugs table), exacerbation of myasthenia gravis, CNS toxicity, peripheral neuropathy (rare), and hypersensitivity. Important quinolone drug interactions with antacids, iron, zinc, magnesium, sucralfate, buffered didanosine, cimetidine, caffeine, cyclosporine, phenytoin, anticoagulants, theophylline, etc.

**CIPROFLOXACIN** (*Cipro, Cipro XR, ProQuin XR*) ▶LK ♀C but teratogenicity unlikely ▶?+ $
WARNING - Tendon rupture (rare; risk increased by corticosteroids, age >60, or organ transplant). Advise patients to stop fluoroquinolone, rest affected area, and seek medical advice for tendon swelling, pain, or inflammation.
ADULT - UTI: 250–500 mg PO bid or 200–400 mg IV q12h. Simple UTI: 250 mg PO bid × 3 d or Cipro XR/Proquin XR 500 mg PO daily × 3 d. Give Proquin XR with main meal of d, preferably dinner. Cipro XR for complicated UTI, uncomplicated pyelonephritis: 1000 mg PO daily × 7–14 d.

Pneumonia, skin, bone/joint infections: 400 mg IV q8–12h or 500–750 mg PO bid. Treat bone/joint infections × 4–6 wk. Acute sinusitis: 500 mg PO bid × 10 d. Chronic bacterial prostatitis: 500 mg PO bid × 28 d. Infectious diarrhea: 500 mg PO bid × 5–7 d. Typhoid fever: 500 mg PO bid × 10 d. Nosocomial pneumonia: 400 mg IV q8h. Complicated intra-abdominal infection (with metronidazole): 400 mg IV q12 h, then 500 mg PO bid. Empiric therapy of febrile neutropenia: 400 mg IV q8h with piperacillin. Bioterrorism anthrax. Inhalation or severe cutaneous anthrax treatment: 400 mg IV q12h with ≥1 other drug

(cont.)

**CIPROFLOXACIN** *(cont.)*
initially, then monotherapy with 500 mg PO bid to complete 60 d. Monotherapy for post-exposure prophylaxis or treatment of less severe cutaneous anthrax: 500 mg PO bid × 60 d. See www.idsociety.org/BT/ToC.htm for more info.

PEDS - Safety and efficacy not established for most indications in children; arthropathy in juvenile animals. Still limited data, but case series of treated children show no evidence of arthropathy other than transient large-joint arthralgias. Musculoskeletal adverse events reported with ciprofloxacin treatment of complicated UTI in peds patients were mild to moderate in severity and resolved within 1 mo after treatment. Complicated UTI, pyelonephritis, 1–17 yo: 6–10 mg/kg IV q8h, then 10–20 mg/kg PO q12h. Max dose is 400 mg IV or 750 mg PO even for peds patients >51 kg. Bioterrorism anthrax. Treatment of inhalation anthrax, severe cutaneous anthrax, or cutaneous anthrax in any case <2 yo: 10–15 mg/kg IV q12h with ≥1 other drug initially, then monotherapy with 10–15 mg/kg up to 500 mg PO bid to complete 60 d. Monotherapy for post-exposure prophylaxis or less severe cutaneous anthrax treatment: 10–15 mg/kg up to 500 mg PO bid × 60 d. See www.idsociety.org/BT/ToC.htm for more info.

UNAPPROVED ADULT - Acute uncomplicated pyelonephritis: 500 mg PO bid × 7 d. Chancroid: 500 mg PO bid × 3 d. Prophylaxis, high-risk GU surgery: 500 mg PO or 400 mg IV. Prophylaxis, invasive meningococcal disease: 500 mg PO single dose. Traveler's diarrhea (treatment preferred over prophylaxis): Treatment - 500 mg PO bid × 1–3 d or 750 mg PO single dose. Prophylaxis - 500 mg PO daily × ≤3 wk. Infectious diarrhea: 500 mg PO bid × 1–3 d for shigella, × 5–7 d for non-typhi salmonella (usually not treated). Malignant otitis externa: 400 mg IV or 750 mg PO q12h. TB (2nd-line treatment): 750–1500 mg/d IV/PO.

UNAPPROVED PEDS - Acute pulmonary exacerbation of cystic fibrosis: 10 mg/kg/dose IV q8h × 7 d, then 20 mg/kg/dose PO q12h to complete 10–21 d of treatment. TB (2nd-line treatment): 10–15 mg/kg PO bid (max: 1.5 g/d). Cholera, 2–15 yo: 20 mg/kg up to 750 mg PO single dose.

FORMS - Generic/Trade: Tabs 100, 250, 500, 750 mg. Extended release tabs 500, 1000 mg. Trade only (ProQuin XR) Extended release tabs 500mg, blister pack 500 mg (#3 tabs).

NOTES - Crystalluria if alkaline urine. Ciprofloxacin inhibits cytochrome P450 1A2, an enzyme that metabolizes caffeine, clozapine, tacrine, theophylline, and warfarin. Give ciprofloxacin immediate-release or Cipro XR 2 h before or 6 h after antacids, iron, sucralfate, calcium, zinc, buffered didanosine, or other highly buffered drugs (Proquin XR is 2h before or 4 h after these multivalent cations). Can give with meals containing dairy products, but not with yogurt, milk, or calcium-fortified fruit juice alone. Do not give Cipro XR within 2h of calcium doses >800 mg. Watch for hypoglycemia with glyburide. Do not give oral susp in feeding tube. Cipro XR, Proquin XR, and immediate-release tabs are not interchangeable. Do not split, crush, or chew Cipro XR or Proquin XR. In patients with complicated UTI or acute pyelonephritis and CrCl <30 mL/min, reduce dose of Cipro XR to 500 mg daily. Dosing of immediate-release ciprofloxacin in adults with renal dysfunction: 250–500 mg PO q12h for CrCl 30–50 mL/min; 250–500 mg PO q18h for 200–400 mg IV q18–24h for CrCl 5–29 mL/min; 250–500 mg PO q24h given after dialysis session for hemodialysis/peritoneal dialysis.

**LOMEFLOXACIN** *(Maxaquin)* ▶LK ♀C ▶? $$$
WARNING - Tendon rupture (rare; risk increased by corticosteroids, age >60, or organ transplant). Advise patients to stop fluoroquinolone, rest affected area, and seek medical advice for tendon swelling, pain, or inflammation.

ADULT - Acute exacerbation of chronic bronchitis not due to *S pneumoniae*, simple UTI due to *K pneumoniae*, P mirabilis, S saprophyticus: 400 mg PO daily × 10 d. Simple E coli UTI: 400 mg PO daily × 3 d. Complicated UTI: 400 mg PO daily × 14 d. Take in the evening to decrease risk of phototoxicity.

PEDS - Safety and efficacy not established in children; arthropathy in juvenile animals.

FORMS - Trade only: Tabs 400 mg.

NOTES - High risk of phototoxicity. Avoid sunlight during and for several d after treatment. Give Al/Mg antacids, sucralfate 4 h before or 2 h after lomefloxacin. Dosing in renal dysfunction: 400 mg PO load, then 200 mg PO daily for CrCl 11–39 mL/min or hemodialysis.

**NORFLOXACIN** *(Noroxin)* ▶LK ♀C ▶? $$$
WARNING - Tendon rupture (rare; risk increased by corticosteroids, age >60, or organ transplant). Advise patients to stop fluoroquinolone, rest affected area, and seek medical advice for tendon swelling, pain, or inflammation.

ADULT - Simple UTI due to *E coli*, K pneumoniae, P mirabilis: 400 mg PO bid × 3 d. UTI due to other organisms: 400 mg PO bid × 7–10 d. Complicated UTI: 400 mg PO bid × 10–21 d. Acute/chronic prostatitis: 400 mg PO bid × 28 d. Take on an empty stomach.

PEDS - Safety and efficacy not established in children; arthropathy in juvenile animals.

UNAPPROVED ADULT - Traveler's diarrhea (treatment preferred over prophylaxis): Treatment - 400 mg PO bid × 1–3 d. Prophylaxis - 400 mg PO daily for up to 3 wk. Infectious diarrhea: 400 mg PO bid × 5–7 d for non-typhi salmonella (usually not treated), × 1–3 d for shigella. Take on an empty stomach.

FORMS - Trade only: Tabs 400 mg.

NOTES - Crystalluria with high doses. Maintain adequate hydration. Norfloxacin inhibits cytochrome P450 1A2, an enzyme that metabolizes caffeine, clozapine, ropinirole, tacrine, theophylline,

**NORFLOXACIN** (*cont.*)

tizanidine, and warfarin. Increased INR with warfarin. Do not take with dairy products. Give antacids, zinc, iron, sucralfate, multivitamins, or buffered didanosine 2 h before/after norfloxacin. Dosing for CrCl <30 mL/min: 400 mg PO daily.

**OFLOXACIN** (*Floxin*) ▶LK ♀C ▶?+ $$$

WARNING - Tendon rupture (rare; risk increased by corticosteroids, age >60, or organ transplant). Advise patients to stop fluoroquinolone, rest affected area, and seek medical advice for tendon swelling, pain, or inflammation.

ADULT - Acute exacerbation of chronic bronchitis, community-acquired pneumonia, skin infections: 400 mg PO bid × 10 d. Simple UTI due to E coli, K pneumoniae: 200 mg PO bid × 3 d. Simple UTI due to other organisms: 200 mg PO bid × 7 d. Complicated UTI: 200 mg PO bid × 10 d. Chronic bacterial prostatitis: 300 mg PO bid × 6 wk.

PEDS - Safety and efficacy not established in children; arthropathy in juvenile animals.

UNAPPROVED ADULT - Epididymitis: 300 mg PO bid × 10 d. Traveler's diarrhea, treatment: 300 mg PO bid × 1–3 d. Infectious diarrhea: 300 mg PO bid × 1–3 d for shigella, 5–7 d for non-typhi salmonella (usually not treated). TB (2nd-line treatment): 600–800 mg PO daily.

FORMS - Generic/Trade: Tabs 200, 300, 400 mg.

NOTES - May prolong QT interval; avoid using in proarrhythmic conditions or with drugs that prolong QT interval, including Class 1A and Class III antiarrhythmics. Give antacids, iron, sucralfate, multivitamins containing zinc, buffered didanosine 2h before or after ofloxacin. May decrease metabolism of theophylline, increase INR with warfarin. Monitor glucose with antidiabetic agents. Can cause false positive on opiate urine screening immunoassay; may need confirmation test. Dosing in renal dysfunction: Usual dose given q24h for CrCl 20–50 mL/min, 50% of usual dose q24h for CrCl <20 mL/min.

## ANTIMICROBIALS: Quinolones—3rd Generation

NOTE: As of April 2007, the CDC no longer recommends fluoroquinolones for gonorrhea because of high resistance rates. Can cause tendon rupture (rare; risk increased by corticosteroids, age >60, or organ transplant), C. difficile associated diarrhea (risk may vary among agents), phototoxicity (risk varies among agents), CNS toxicity, peripheral neuropathy (rare), hypersensitivity, and QT interval prolongation (risk varies among agents). Avoid using in proarrhythmic conditions or with drugs that prolong QT including Class 1A and Class III antiarrhythmics. Important quinolone drug interactions with antacids, iron, zinc, magnesium, sucralfate, cimetidine, caffeine, cyclosporine, phenytoin, anticoagulants, theophylline, etc.

**LEVOFLOXACIN** (*Levaquin*) ▶KL ♀C ▶? $$$$

WARNING - Tendon rupture (rare; risk increased by corticosteroids, age >60, or organ transplant). Advise patients to stop fluoroquinolone, rest affected area, and seek medical advice for tendon swelling, pain, or inflammation.

ADULT - IV & PO doses are the same. 750 mg once daily × 5 d for community-acquired pneumonia, acute sinusitis, or complicated UTI/acute pyelonephritis; × 7–14 d for nosocomial pneumonia or complicated skin infections. 500 mg once daily × 7 d for acute exacerbation of chronic bronchitis, × 7–10 d for uncomplicated skin infections, × 7–14 d for community-acquired pneumonia, × 10–14 d for acute sinusitis, × 28 d for chronic bacterial prostatitis. 250 mg PO daily × 3 d for simple UTI, × 10 d for complicated UTI or acute pyelonephritis. Post-exposure anthrax prophylaxis: 500 mg PO once daily × 60 d. See www.idsociety.org/BT/ToC.htm for more info. Infuse IV doses over 60 min (250–500 mg) to 90 min (750 mg). Take oral soln on empty stomach.

PEDS - Safety and efficacy not established in children; arthropathy in juvenile animals.

Musculoskeletal disorders (primarily mild arthralgias during treatment) reported in children.

UNAPPROVED ADULT - Legionnaires' disease: 1 g IV/PO on 1st d, then 500 mg IV/PO once daily. Chlamydia, epididymitis: See STD table. TB (2nd-line treatment): 500–1000 mg/d IV/PO. Traveler's diarrhea, treatment: 500 mg PO once daily × 1–3 d. Infectious diarrhea: 500 mg PO once daily × 1–3 d for shigella, × 5–7 d for salmonella.

FORMS - Trade only: Tabs 250, 500, 750 mg, oral soln 25 mg/mL. Leva-Pak: #5, 750 mg tabs.

NOTES - Give Mg/Al antacids, iron, sucralfate, multivitamins containing zinc, buffered didanosine 2 h before/after PO levofloxacin. Increased INR with warfarin. Monitor glucose with antidiabetic agents. Can cause false positive on opiate urine screening immunoassay; may need confirmation test. Dosing in renal dysfunction: For most indications and CrCl <50 mL/min, load with 500 mg, then 250 mg daily for CrCl 20–49 mL/min, 250 mg q48h for CrCl 10–19 mL/min, hemodialysis, peritoneal dialysis. For complicated UTI/pyelonephritis and CrCl 10–19 mL/min, give 250 mg q48h.

## ANTIMICROBIALS: Quinolones—4th Generation

NOTE: As of April 2007, the CDC no longer recommends fluoroquinolones for gonorrhea because of high resistance rates. Can cause tendon rupture (rare; risk increased by corticosteroids, age >60, or organ transplant), C. difficile associated diarrhea (risk may vary among agents), phototoxicity (risk varies among agents), CNS toxicity,

(cont.)

peripheral neuropathy (rare), hypersensitivity, and QT interval prolongation (risk varies among agents; see QT drugs table). Avoid using in proarrhythmic conditions or with drugs that prolong QT interval, including Class 1A and Class III antiarrhythmics. Important quinolone drug interactions with antacids, iron, zinc, magnesium, sucralfate, cimetidine, caffeine, cyclosporine, phenytoin, anticoagulants, theophylline, etc. Monitor INR with warfarin.

**GEMIFLOXACIN (Factive)** ▶Feces, K ♀C ▶- $$$
WARNING - Tendon rupture (rare; risk increased by corticosteroids, age >60, or organ transplant). Advise patients to stop fluoroquinolone, rest affected area, and seek medical advice for tendon swelling, pain, or inflammation.
ADULT - Acute exacerbation of chronic bronchitis: 320 mg PO daily × 5 d. Community-acquired pneumonia: 320 mg PO daily × 5–7 d (x 7 d for multi-drug resistant S pneumoniae).
PEDS - Safety and efficacy not established in children; arthropathy in juvenile animals.
FORMS - Trade only: Tabs 320 mg.
NOTES - Maintain fluid intake to prevent crystalluria. Give 2 h before or 3 h after Al/Mg antacids, iron, multivitamins with zinc, buffered didanosine. Give ≥2 h before sucralfate. May increase INR with warfarin. Discontinue if rash develops. Dosage reduction for CrCl ≤40 mL/min, hemodialysis, or CAPD: 160 mg PO daily.

**MOXIFLOXACIN (Avelox)** ▶LK ♀C ▶- $$$$
WARNING - Tendon rupture (rare; risk increased by corticosteroids, age >60, or organ transplant).
Advise patients to stop fluoroquinolone, rest affected area, and seek medical advice for tendon swelling, pain, or inflammation.
ADULT - 400 mg PO/IV daily × 5 d (chronic bronchitis exacerbation), 5–14 d (complicated intra-abdominal infection; usually given IV initially), 7 d (uncomplicated skin infections), 10 d (acute sinusitis), 7–14 d (community acquired pneumonia, including penicillin-resistant S pneumoniae), 7–21 d (complicated skin infections). IV infused over 60 min.
PEDS - Safety and efficacy not established in children; arthropathy in juvenile animals.
UNAPPROVED ADULT - TB (2nd-line treatment): 400 mg IV/PO daily.
FORMS - Trade only: Tabs 400 mg.
NOTES - Do not exceed recommended IV dose or infusion rate due to QT prolongation risk. Contraindicated with ziprasidone. Give tabs ≥4 h before or 8 h after Mg/Al antacids, iron, multivitamins with zinc, sucralfate, buffered didanosine. Avoid in moderate or severe hepatic insufficiency.

## ANTIMICROBIALS: Sulfonamides

**NOTE:** Sulfonamides can cause Stevens-Johnson syndrome; toxic epidermal necrolysis; hepatotoxicity; blood dyscrasias; hemolysis in G6PD deficiency. Avoid maternal sulfonamides when the breastfed infant is ill, stressed, premature, has hyperbilirubinemia, or has glucose-6-phosphate dehydrogenase deficiency.

**SULFADIAZINE** ▶K ♀C ▶+ $$$$
ADULT - Usual dose: 2–4 g PO initially, then 2–4 g/d divided into 3–6 doses. Secondary prevention of rheumatic fever: 1 g PO daily. Toxoplasmosis treatment: 1–1.5 g PO qid with pyrimethamine and leucovorin.
PEDS - Not for infants <2 mo, except as adjunct to pyrimethamine for congenital toxoplasmosis. Usual dose: Give 75 mg/kg PO initially, then 150 mg/kg/d up to 6 g/d divided into 4–6 doses. Secondary prevention of rheumatic fever, <27 kg: 500 mg PO daily. Use adult dose for >27 kg.
UNAPPROVED ADULT - CNS toxoplasmosis in AIDS. Acute therapy: Pyrimethamine 200 mg PO × 1, then 50 mg (<60 kg) to 75 mg (≥60 kg) PO once daily + sulfadiazine 1000 mg (<60 kg) to 1500 mg (≥60 kg) PO q6h + leucovorin 10–20 mg PO once daily (can increase to ≥50 mg). Secondary prevention: Pyrimethamine 25–50 mg PO once daily + sulfadiazine 500–1000 mg PO qid + leucovorin 10–25 mg PO once daily.
UNAPPROVED PEDS - Not for infants <2 mo, except as adjunct to pyrimethamine for congenital toxoplasmosis. AAP regimen for toxoplasmosis: 100–200 mg/kg/d PO with pyrimethamine and leucovorin (duration varies). Secondary prevention after CNS toxoplasmosis in HIV infection:
85–120 mg/kg/d PO divided in 2–4 doses with pyrimethamine and leucovorin.
FORMS - Generic only: Tab 500 mg.
NOTES - Not effective for streptococcal pharyngitis. Maintain fluid intake to prevent crystalluria & stone formation. Reduce dose in renal insufficiency. May increase INR with warfarin. May increase levels of methotrexate, phenytoin.

**SULFISOXAZOLE (Gantrisin Pediatric)** ▶KL ♀C ▶+ $
PEDS - Usual dose: 75 mg/kg PO load, then 150 mg/kg/d PO divided q4–6h (max 6 g/d). Not for infants <2 mo, except as adjunct to pyrimethamine for congenital toxoplasmosis.
UNAPPROVED PEDS - Prophylaxis for recurrent otitis media: 50 mg/kg PO qhs.
FORMS - Trade only: susp 500 mg/5 mL. Generic only: Tabs 500 mg.
NOTES - May increase levels of methotrexate, phenytoin. Significantly increased INR with warfarin; avoid concomitant use if possible. Reduce dose in renal failure. Maintain fluid intake to prevent crystalluria/stone formation.

**TRIMETHOPRIM-SULFAMETHOXAZOLE (Bactrim, Septra, Sulfatrim, cotrimoxazole)** ▶K ♀C ▶+ $
ADULT - UTI, shigellosis, acute exacerbation of chronic bronchitis: 1 tab PO bid, double strength (DS, 160 TMP/800 SMX). Travelers' diarrhea: 1

**TRIMETHOPRIM-SULFAMETHOXAZOLE** *(cont.)*
DS tab PO bid × 5 d. Pneumocystis treatment: 15–20 mg/kg/d (based on TMP) IV divided q6–8h or PO divided tid × 21 d total. Pneumocystis prophylaxis: 1 DS tab PO daily.
PEDS - UTI, shigellosis, otitis media: 5 mL susp/10 kg (up to 20 mL)/dose PO bid. Pneumocystis treatment: 15–20 mg/kg/d (based on TMP) IV divided q6–8h or 5 mL susp/8 kg/dose PO q6h. Pneumocystis prophylaxis: 150 mg/m²/d (based on TMP) PO divided bid on 3 consecutive d each wk. Do not use in infants <2 mo; may cause kernicterus.
UNAPPROVED ADULT - Bacterial prostatitis: 1 DS tab PO bid × 10–14 d for acute, × 1–3 mo for chronic. Sinusitis: 1 DS tab PO bid × 10 d. Burkholderia cepacia pulmonary infection in cystic fibrosis: 5 mg/kg (based on TMP) IV q6h. Pneumocystis prophylaxis: 1 SS tab PO daily. Primary prevention of toxoplasmosis in AIDS: 1 DS PO daily. Pertussis: 1 DS tab PO bid × 14 d (sec-line to macrolides). High-dose for community-acquired MRSA skin infections: 2 DS tabs PO bid-tid × 7–10 d.

UNAPPROVED PEDS - Head lice unresponsive to usual therapy: 10 mg/kg/d (based on TMP) PO divided bid × 10 d in combo with standard doses of permethrin 1%. Pertussis: 8 mg/kg/d (based on TMP) PO divided bid × 14 d (sec-line to macrolides).
FORMS - Generic/Trade: Tabs 80 mg TMP/400 mg SMX (single strength), 160 mg TMP/800 mg SMX (double strength; DS), susp 40 mg TMP/200 mg SMX per 5 mL. 20 mL susp = 2 SS tabs = 1 DS tab.
NOTES - Not effective for streptococcal pharyngitis. No activity against penicillin-nonsusceptible pneumococci. Bone marrow depression with high IV doses. Significantly increased INR with warfarin; avoid concomitant use if possible. Increases levels of methotrexate, phenytoin. Rifampin reduces TMP/SMX levels. AAP recommends 5–7 d of therapy for older (≥6 yo) children with non-severe otitis media, and 10 d for younger children and those with severe disease. Dosing in renal dysfunction: Use 50% of usual dose for CrCl 15–30 mL/min. Don't use for CrCl <15 mL/min.

## ANTIMICROBIALS: Tetracyclines

**NOTE:** Tetracyclines can cause photosensitivity and pseudotumor cerebri (avoid with isotretinoin, which is also linked to pseudotumor cerebri). May decrease efficacy of oral contraceptives. Increased INR with warfarin. May increase risk of ergotism with ergot alkaloids.

**DEMECLOCYCLINE** *(Declomycin)* ▶K, feces ♀D ▶?+ $$$$$
ADULT - Usual dose: 150 mg PO qid or 300 mg PO bid on empty stomach.
PEDS - Avoid in children <8 yo due to teeth staining. Usual dose: 6.6–13.2 mg/kg/d PO divided bid-qid on empty stomach.
UNAPPROVED ADULT - SIADH: 600–1200 mg/d PO given in 3–4 divided doses.
FORMS - Generic/Trade : Tabs 150,300 mg.
NOTES - Diabetes insipidus, high risk of photosensitivity. Caution in renal dysfunction; doxycycline preferred. Absorption impaired by iron, calcium, Al/Mg antacids. Take with fluids (not milk) to decrease esophageal irritation. SIADH onset of action occurs within 5–14 d; do not increase dose more frequently than q3–4 d. Increased INR with warfarin. May decrease oral contraceptive effectiveness.

**DOXYCYCLINE** *(Adoxa, Doryx, Monodox, Oracea, Periostat, Vibramycin, Vibra-Tabs, ✦Doxycin)* ▶LK ♀D ▶?+ $
ADULT - Usual dose: 100 mg PO bid on first d, then 100 mg/d PO daily or divided bid. Severe infections: 100 mg PO bid. Chlamydia, nongonococcal urethritis: 100 mg PO bid × 7 d. Acne vulgaris: Up to 100 mg PO bid. Periostat for periodontitis: 20 mg PO bid 1 h before breakfast and dinner. Oracea for inflammatory rosacea (papules & pustules): 40 mg PO once every morning on empty stomach. Cholera: 300 mg PO single dose. Primary, secondary, early latent syphilis if penicillin-allergic: 100 mg PO bid × 14 d. Late latent or

tertiary syphilis if penicillin allergic: 100 mg PO bid × 4 wk. Not for neurosyphilis. Malaria prophylaxis: 100 mg PO daily starting 1–2d before exposure until 4 wk after. Intravenous: 200 mg on first d in 1–2 infusions, then 100–200 mg/d in 1–2 infusions. Bioterrorism anthrax: 100 mg bid × 60 d. Use IV with ≥1 other drug for initial treatment of inhalation or severe cutaneous anthrax. PO monotherapy for less severe cutaneous anthrax or post-exposure prophylaxis. See www.idsociety.org/BT/ToC.htm for more info.
PEDS - Avoid in children <8 yo due to teeth staining. Usual dose, children ≤45 kg: 4.4 mg/kg/d PO divided bid on first d, then 2.2–4.4 mg/kg/d PO divided daily or bid. Use adult dose for children >45 kg. Malaria prophylaxis: 2 mg/kg/d up to 100 mg PO daily starting 1–2 d before exposure until 4 wk after. Most PO and IV doses are equivalent. Bioterrorism anthrax: 100 mg bid for >8 yo and >45 kg, 2.2 mg/kg bid for >8 yo and ≤45 kg, or ≤8 yo. Treat × 60 d. Use IV with ≥1 other drug for initial treatment of inhalation anthrax, severe cutaneous anthrax, or cutaneous anthrax in any case <2 yo. PO monotherapy for less severe cutaneous anthrax and post-exposure prophylaxis. See www.idsociety.org/BT/ToC.htm for more info.
UNAPPROVED ADULT - See sexually-transmitted diseases table for granuloma inguinale, lymphogranuloma venereum, pelvic inflammatory disease treatment. Lyme disease: 100 mg PO bid × 14 d for early disease, × 28 d for Lyme

**(cont.)**

**DOXYCYCLINE** *(cont.)*

arthritis. Prevention of Lyme disease in highly endemic area, with deer tick attachment ≥48 h: 200 mg PO single dose with food within 72 h of tick bite. Ehrlichiosis: 100 mg IV/PO bid × 7–14 d. Malaria, co-therapy with quinine/quinidine: 100 mg IV/PO bid × 7 d. Lymphatic filariasis: 100 mg PO bid × 8 wk.

UNAPPROVED PEDS - Avoid in children <8 yo due to teeth staining. Lyme disease: 4 mg/kg/d PO divided bid (max 200 mg/d) × 14 d for early disease, × 28 d for Lyme arthritis. Malaria, co-therapy with quinine/quinidine: 2.2 mg/kg IV/PO bid (max 100 mg bid) × 7 d.

FORMS - Generic/Trade: Tabs 75,100 mg, caps 20, 50,100 mg. Susp 25 mg/5 mL (60 mL). Trade only: (Vibramycin) Syrup 50 mg/5 mL (480 mL). Delayed Release (Doryx): Tabs 75,100 mg, Caps 40 mg (Oracea). Generic only: Caps 75,150 mg tabs 50,150 mg.

NOTES - Photosensitivity, pseudotumor cerebri, increased BUN, painful IV infusion. Do not use Oracea for treatment of infections. Do not give antacids or calcium supplements within 2 h of doxycycline. Barbiturates, carbamazepine, rifampin, and phenytoin may decrease doxycycline levels. Preferred over tetracycline in renal dysfunction. Take with fluids to decrease esophageal irritation; can take with food/milk. Can break Doryx tabs and give immediately in a spoonful of applesauce. Do not crush or chew delayed-release pellets in tab. Maternal antimalarial prophylaxis doesn't harm breast-fed infant or protect infant from malaria.

**MINOCYCLINE** *(Minocin, Dynacin, Solodyn, ✚Enca)* ▶LK ♀D ▶? + $$$

ADULT - Usual dose: 200 mg IV/PO 1st dose, then 100 mg q12hr. IV and PO doses are the same. Not more than 400 mg/d IV. Solodyn for inflammatory non-nodular moderate to severe acne: 1 mg/kg PO once daily. Dose is 45 mg for 45–<60 kg, 90 mg for 60–90 kg, 135 mg for 91–136 kg.

PEDS - Avoid in children <8 yo due to teeth staining. Usual dose: 4 mg/kg PO 1st dose, then 2 mg/kg bid. IV and PO doses are the same. Solodyn for inflammatory non-nodular moderate to severe acne, ≥12 yo: 1 mg/kg PO once daily. Dose is 45–<60 kg, 90 mg for 60–90 kg, 135 mg for 91–136 kg.

UNAPPROVED ADULT - Acne vulgaris (traditional dosing before Solodyn): 50 mg PO bid. RA: 100 mg PO bid.

FORMS - Generic/Trade: Caps, tabs 50, 75, 100 mg. Trade only (Solodyn): Extended release tabs 45, 90, 135 mg.

NOTES - Dizziness, hepatotoxicity, lupus. Do not use Solodyn for treatment of infections. Do not give antacids or calcium supplements within 2h of minocycline. May cause drowsiness. Take with fluids (not milk) to decrease esophageal irritation. Use with caution in renal dysfunction; doxycycline preferred.

**OXYTETRACYCLINE** *(Terramycin)* ▶LK ♀D ▶? + $$$

ADULT - Usual dose: 250 mg IM q24h or 300 mg/d divided q8–12h. IM oxytetracycline provides low and erratic blood levels; switch to a PO tetracycline as soon as possible.

PEDS - Avoid in children <8 yo due to teeth staining. Usual dose: 15–25 mg/kg/d up to 250 mg/d IM. May give in divided doses q8–12h. IM oxytetracycline provides low and erratic blood levels; switch to a PO tetracycline as soon as possible.

NOTES - Contains 2% lidocaine and sodium formaldehyde sulfoxylate (avoid in sulfite-sensitive patients). Use with caution in renal dysfunction; doxycycline preferred.

**TETRACYCLINE** *(Sumycin)* ▶LK ♀D ▶? + $

ADULT - Usual dose: 250–500 mg PO qid on empty stomach. H pylori: See table in GI section. Primary, secondary, early latent syphilis if penicillin-allergic: 500 mg PO qid × 14 d. Late latent syphilis if penicillin allergic: 500 mg PO qid × 28 d.

PEDS - Avoid in children <8 yo due to teeth staining. Usual dose: 25–50 mg/kg/d PO divided bid-qid on empty stomach.

UNAPPROVED ADULT - Malaria, co-therapy with quinine: 250 mg PO qid × 7 d.

UNAPPROVED PEDS - Malaria, co-therapy with quinine: 25 mg/kg/d PO divided qid × 7 d.

FORMS - Generic/Trade: Caps 250, 500 mg. Trade only: Tabs 250, 500 mg, susp 125 mg/5 mL.

NOTES - Increased BUN/hepatotoxicity in patients with renal dysfunction. Increased INR with warfarin. Do not give antacids or calcium supplements within 2 h of tetracycline. Use with caution in renal dysfunction; doxycycline preferred. Take with fluids (not milk) to decrease esophageal irritation.

## ANTIMICROBIALS: Other

**AZTREONAM** *(Azactam)* ▶K ♀B ▶ + $$$$$

ADULT - UTI: 500 mg-1 g IM/IV q8–12h. Pneumonia, sepsis, skin, intra-abdominal, gynecologic infections: Moderate, 1–2 g IM/IV q8–12h. Severe or P aeruginosa infections, 2 g IV q6–8h. Use IV route for doses >1 g.

PEDS - Serious gram-negative infections, usual dose: 30 mg/kg IV q6–8h.

UNAPPROVED ADULT - Meningitis: 2 g IV q6–8h.

UNAPPROVED PEDS - P aeruginosa pulmonary infection in cystic fibrosis: 50 mg/kg/dose IV q6–8h.

NOTES - Dosing in adults with renal dysfunction: 1–2 g IV load, then 50% of usual dose for CrCl 10–30 mL/min. 0.5–2 g IV load, then 25% of usual dose for CrCl <10 mL/min. For life-threatening infections, also give 12.5% of initial dose after each hemodialysis.

**CHLORAMPHENICOL** *(Chloromycetin)* ▶LK ♀C ▶ - $$$$$

WARNING - Serious & fatal blood dyscrasias. Dose-dependent bone marrow suppression common.

ADULT - Typhoid fever, rickettsial infections: 50 mg/kg/d IV divided q6h. Up to 75–100 mg/kg/d

**CHLORAMPHENICOL** *(cont.)*

IV for serious infections untreatable with other agents.

PEDS - Severe infections including meningitis: 50–100 mg/kg/d IV divided q6h. AAP recommends 75–100 mg/kg/d for invasive pneumococcal infections only in patients with life-threatening beta-lactam allergy.

NOTES - Monitor CBC every 2 d. Monitor serum levels. Therapeutic peak: 10–20 mcg/mL. Trough: 5–10 mcg/mL. Use cautiously in acute intermittent porphyria/G6PD deficiency. Gray baby syndrome in preemies and newborns. Barbiturates, rifampin decrease chloramphenicol levels. Chloramphenicol increases barbiturate, phenytoin levels and may increase INR with warfarin. Dosing in adults with hepatic dysfunction: 1 g IV load, then 500 mg q6h.

**CLINDAMYCIN** *(Cleocin, +Dalacin C)* ▶L ♀B ▶?+ $$$

WARNING - C. difficile associated diarrhea.

ADULT - Serious anaerobic, streptococcal, Staph infections: 600–900 mg IV q8h or 150–450 mg PO qid. See tables for prophylaxis of bacterial endocarditis and treatment of sexually transmitted diseases (pelvic inflammatory disease).

PEDS - Serious anaerobic, streptococcal, Staph infections: 20–40 mg/kg/d IV divided q6–8h or 8–20 mg/kg/d (as caps) PO divided tid-qid or 8–25 mg/kg/d (as palmitate oral soln) PO divided tid-qid. Do not give <37.5 mg of oral soln PO tid for ≤10 kg. Infants <1 mo: 15–20 mg/kg/d IV divided tid-qid. See table for prophylaxis of bacterial endocarditis.

UNAPPROVED ADULT - Bacterial vaginosis: 300 mg PO bid × 7 d. Oral/dental infection: 300 mg PO qid. Prevention of perinatal group B streptococcal disease: 900 mg IV to mother q8h until delivery. CNS toxoplasmosis, AIDS (with leucovorin, pyrimethamine): Acute treatment 600 mg PO/IV q6h; secondary prevention 300–450 mg PO q6–8h. Group A streptococcal pharyngitis, repeated culture-positive episodes: 600 mg/d PO in 2–4 divided doses × 10 d. Malaria, co-therapy with quinine/quinidine: 10 mg/kg base IV loading dose followed by 5 mg/kg IV q8h or 20 mg/kg/d base PO divided tid to complete 7 d.

UNAPPROVED PEDS - Group A streptococcal pharyngitis, repeated culture-positive episodes: 20–30 mg/kg/d PO divided q8h × 10 d. Otitis media: 30–40 mg/kg/d PO divided tid. Toxoplasmosis, substitute for sulfadiazine in sulfonamide-intolerant children: 5–7.5 mg/kg (up to 600 mg/dose) PO/IV qid + pyrimethamine + leucovorin. Malaria, co-therapy with quinine/quinidine: 10 mg/kg base IV loading dose followed by 5 mg/kg IV q8h or 20 mg/kg/d base PO divided tid to complete 7 d.

FORMS - Generic/Trade: Cap 75, 150, 300 mg. Trade only: Oral soln 75 mg/5 mL.

NOTES - Not for meningitis. Not more than 600 mg/IM injection site. Avoid if lincomycin hypersensitivity.

**COLISTIMETHATE** *(Coly-Mycin M Parenteral)* ▶K ♀C ▶? $$$$$

ADULT - Gram-negative infections, esp. *P aeruginosa:* 2.5–5 mg/kg/d IM/IV divided q6–12h or IV continuous infusion. Inject IV slowly over 3–5 min q12h. For continuous infusion, inject half of daily dose over 3–5 min; give remainder as continuous infusion over 22–23h starting 1–2 h after first injection. Base dose on ideal body weight in obesity.

PEDS - Gram-negative infections, esp. *P aeruginosa:* 2.5–5 mg/kg/d IM/IV divided q6–12h or IV continuous infusion. Inject IV slowly over 3–5 min q12h. For continuous infusion, inject half of daily dose over 3–5 min; give remainder as continuous infusion over 22–23 h starting 1–2 h after first injection. Base dose on ideal body weight in obesity.

UNAPPROVED ADULT - Cystic fibrosis: Use nebulizer solution promptly after it is made. Storage for >24 h increases the formation of polymyxin E1 which may cause pulmonary toxicity.

NOTES - Each vial contains 150 mg colistin activity. May enhance neuromuscular junction blockade by aminoglycosides, neuromuscular blockers. Can cause transient neurologic symptoms that can be relieved by dosage reduction. See package insert for dosage adjustment in adults with renal dysfunction.

**DAPTOMYCIN** *(Cubicin, Cidecin)* ▶K ♀B ▶? $$$$$

ADULT - Complicated skin infections: 4 mg/kg IV once daily × 7–14 d. S aureus bacteremia, including endocarditis: 6 mg/kg IV once daily × ≥2–6 wk. Infuse over 30 min.

PEDS - Not approved in children.

NOTES - May cause myopathy; monitor CK levels weekly. Stop if myopathy symptoms and CK >5 × upper limit of normal, or no symptoms and CK ≥10 × upper limit of normal. Consider withholding statins during daptomycin treatment. May cause neuropathy. Can falsely elevate PT with certain thromboplastin reagents; can minimize effect by drawing PT/INR sample just before daptomycin dose or use another reagent. Not effective for community-acquired pneumonia. Dosage reduction in adults with CrCl <30 mL/min: 4 mg/kg IV q48h. Reconstituted soln stable for up to 12 h at room temp or 48 h in refrigerator (combined time in vial + IV bag).

**DROTRECOGIN** *(Xigris)* ▶Plasma ♀C ▶? $$$$$

ADULT - To reduce mortality in sepsis: 24 mcg/kg/h IV × 96 h. Reduced mortality only in patients with APACHE II score ≥25.

PEDS - Not approved in children, and was ineffective in a clinical trial of severe sepsis in children with a trend toward increased CNS bleeding.

NOTES - Can cause severe bleeding. Contraindicated with conditions and drugs that increase risk of bleeding; see package insert for details. Xigris may not be indicated in patients with single organ dysfunction and recent surgery; these patients do

(cont.)

**DROTRECOGIN** (cont.)

not have high enough risk of mortality to require treatment and Xigris increased mortality. Criteria for use include systemic inflammatory response plus acute organ dysfunction. Stop infusion 2 h before invasive procedure, or if bleeding occurs. May prolong APTT. Complete IV infusion within 12 h of reconstitution. Do not expose IV solution to heat or direct sunlight.

**FOSFOMYCIN** (*Monurol*) ▶K ♀B ▶? $$

ADULT - Simple UTI in women: One 3 g packet PO single dose. Dissolve granules in 1/2 cup of water.

PEDS - Not approved in children <12 yo.

FORMS - Trade only: 3 g packet of granules.

NOTES - Metoclopramide decreases urinary excretion of fosfomycin. No benefit with multiple dosing. Single dose less effective than ciprofloxacin or TMP/SMX; equivalent to nitrofurantoin.

**LINCOMYCIN** (*Lincocin*) ▶LK ♀C ▶- $$$$$

WARNING - *C difficile* associated diarrhea.

ADULT - Serious gram-positive infections: 600 mg IM q12–24h. 600–1000 mg IV q8–12h. Max IV daily dose is 8 g. Dilute to 1 g/100 mL or less, and infuse over at least 1 h. Reserve for patients who are allergic or do not respond to penicillins.

PEDS - Serious gram-positive infections, >1 mo: 10–20 mg/kg/d IV divided q8–12h. Dilute to 1 g/100 mL or less, and infuse over at least 1 h. Reserve for patients who are allergic or do not respond to penicillins.

NOTES - Do not use in patients with clindamycin hypersensitivity. Monitor hepatic and renal function and CBC during prolonged therapy. Do not coadminister with erythromycin due to potential antagonism. May enhance effects of neuromuscular blockers. Reduce dose by 25% to 30% in patients with severe renal dysfunction and consider monitoring levels.

**LINEZOLID** (*Zyvox*, ✦*Zyvoxam*) ▶Oxidation/K ♀C ▶? $$$$$

ADULT - IV & PO doses are the same. Vancomycin-resistant E. faecium infections: 600 mg IV/PO q12h × 14–28 d. Pneumonia, complicated skin infections (including diabetic foot): 600 mg IV/PO q12h × 10–14 d. Uncomplicated skin infections: 400 mg PO q12h × 10–14 d. Infuse over 30–120 min.

PEDS - Pneumonia, complicated skin infections, ≤11 yo: 10 mg/kg IV/PO q8h × 10–14 d. Vancomycin-resistant E. faecium infections, ≤11 yo: 10 mg/kg IV/PO q8h × 14–28 d. Uncomplicated skin infections: 10 mg/kg PO q8h if <5 yo, q12h if 5–11 yo × 10–14 d.

FORMS - Trade only: Tabs 600 mg, susp 100 mg/5 mL.

NOTES - Myelosuppression. Monitor CBC weekly, esp. if >2 wk of therapy, pre-existing myelosuppression, other myelosuppressive drugs, or chronic infection treated with other antibiotics. Consider stopping if myelosuppression occurs or worsens. Peripheral and optic neuropathy,

primarily in those treated for >1 mo. Ophthalmic exam recommended for visual changes at any time; monitor visual function in all treated for ≥3 mo. In a study comparing linezolid with vancomycin, oxacillin, or dicloxacillin for catheter-related bloodstream infections, mortality was increased in linezolid-treated patients infected only with gram-negative bacteria. Inhibits MAO; may interact with adrenergic and serotonergic drugs, high tyramine foods. Limit tyramine to <100 mg/meal. Reduce initial dose of dopamine/epinephrine. Serotonin syndrome reported with concomitant administration of serotonergic drugs (SSRIs). Store susp at room temperature; stable for 21 d. Gently turn bottle over 3–5 times before giving a dose; do not shake.

**METHENAMINE HIPPURATE** (*Hiprex, Urex*) ▶KL ♀C ▶? $$$

ADULT - Long-term suppression of UTI: 1 g PO bid.

PEDS - Long-term suppression of UTI: 0.5–1 g PO bid for 6–12 yo, 1 g PO bid for >12 yo.

FORMS - Generic/Trade: Tabs 1g

NOTES - Not for UTI treatment. Contraindicated if renal or severe hepatic impairment, severe dehydration. Acidify urine if Proteus, Pseudomonas infections. Give 1–2 g vitamin C PO q4h if urine pH >5. Avoid sulfonamides, alkalinizing foods & medications.

**METHENAMINE MANDELATE** (*Mandelamine*) ▶KL ♀C ▶? $$$

ADULT - Long-term suppression of UTI: 1 g PO qid after meals and qhs.

PEDS - Long-term suppression of UTI: 18.4 mg/kg PO qid for <6 yo, 500 mg PO qid for 6–12 yo. Give after meals and qhs.

FORMS - Generic/Trade: Tabs 0.5,1 g.

NOTES - Not for UTI treatment. Contraindicated with renal or severe hepatic impairment, severe dehydration. Acidify urine for Proteus, Pseudomonas infections. If urine pH >5, give 1–2 g vitamin C PO q4h. Avoid sulfonamides, alkalinizing foods/medications.

**METRONIDAZOLE** (*Flagyl*, ✦*Florazole ER, Trikacide, Nidazol*) ▶KL ♀B ▶?- $

ADULT - Trichomoniasis: Treat patient & sex partners with 2 g PO single dose (may be used in pregnancy per CDC), 250 mg PO tid × 7 d, or 375 mg PO bid × 7 d. Flagyl ER for bacterial vaginosis: 750 mg PO daily × 7 d on empty stomach. H pylori: See table in GI section. Anaerobic bacterial infections: Load 1 g or 15 mg/kg IV, then 500 mg or 7.5 mg/kg IV/PO q6–8h, each IV dose over 1h (not to exceed 4 g/d). Prophylaxis, colorectal surgery: 15 mg/kg IV completed 1 h preop, then 7.5 mg/kg IV q6h × 2 doses. Acute amebic dysentery: 750 mg PO tid × 5–10 d. Amebic liver abscess: 500–750 mg PO tid × 5–10 d.

PEDS - Amebiasis: 35–50 mg/kg/d PO (max of 750 mg/dose) divided tid × 10 d.

UNAPPROVED ADULT - Bacterial vaginosis: 500 mg PO bid × 7 d. Bacterial vaginosis in pregnancy:

**METRONIDAZOLE** (cont.)
500 mg PO bid or 250 mg PO tid × 7 d. Trichomoniasis (CDC alternative to single dose): 500 mg PO bid × 7 d. Pelvic inflammatory disease & recurrent/persistent urethritis: see STD table. *Clostridium difficile* diarrhea: 250 mg PO qid or 500 mg PO tid × 10 d. Giardia: 250 mg PO tid × 5–7 d.

UNAPPROVED PEDS - Clostridium difficile diarrhea: 30–50 mg/kg/d PO divided tid or qid × 7–10 d (not to exceed adult dose). Trichomoniasis: 5 mg/kg PO tid (max 2 g/d) × 7 d. Giardia: 15 mg/kg/d PO divided tid × 5–7 d. Anaerobic bacterial infections: 30 mg/kg/d IV/PO divided q6h, each IV dose over 1h (not to exceed 4 g/d).

FORMS - Generic/Trade: Tabs 250,500 mg, ER tabs 750 mg, Caps 375 mg.

NOTES - Peripheral neuropathy (chronic use), seizures. Disulfiram reaction; avoid alcohol until ≥1 d after treatment with tabs, ≥3 d with caps/ Flagyl ER. Do not give within 2 wk of disulfiram. Interacts with barbiturates, lithium, phenytoin. Increased INR with warfarin. Darkens urine. Give iodoquinol/paromomycin after treatment for amebic dysentery or liver abscess. Can minimize infant exposure by withholding breastfeeding for 12–24 h after maternal single dose. Decrease dose in liver dysfunction.

**NITROFURANTOIN** (*Furadantin, Macrodantin, Macrobid*) ▶KL ♀B ▶+? $$
WARNING - Pulmonary fibrosis with prolonged use.
ADULT - Acute uncomplicated cystitis: 50–100 mg PO qid with food/milk × 7 d or × 3 d after sterile urine. Long-term suppressive therapy: 50–100 mg PO qhs. Sustained release Macrobid: 100 mg PO bid with food/milk × 7 d.
PEDS - UTI: 5–7 mg/kg/d PO divided qid × 7 d or × 3 d after sterile urine. Long-term suppressive therapy: Doses as low as 1 mg/kg/d PO divided daily-bid. Give with food/milk. Macrobid, >12 yo: 100 mg PO bid with food/milk × 7 d.
FORMS - Nitrofurantoin macrocrystals (Macrodantin) generic/trade: Caps 25,50,100 mg. Nitrofurantoin macrocrystals/monohydrate (Macrobid) generic/trade: Caps 100 mg. Furadantin: Susp 25 mg/ 5 mL.
NOTES - Contraindicated if CrCl <60 mL/min, pregnancy ≥38 wk, infant <1 mo. Hemolytic anemia in G6PD deficiency (including susceptible infants exposed through breast milk), hepatotoxicity, peripheral neuropathy. May turn urine brown. Do not use for complicated UTI or pyelonephritis.

**RIFAXIMIN** (*Xifaxan*) ▶Feces, no GI absorption ♀C ▶? $$
ADULT - Travelers diarrhea: 200 mg PO tid × 3 d.
PEDS - Not approved in children <12 yo.
FORMS - Trade only: Tab 200 mg.
NOTES - Not effective for diarrhea complicated by fever/blood in stool or caused by pathogens other than E coli. Consider switching to another agent if diarrhea persists for 24–48 h or worsens.

**SYNERCID** (quinupristin + dalfopristin) ▶Bile ♀B ▶? $$$$$
ADULT - Vancomycin-resistant E faecium infections (Not active against E. faecalis): 7.5 mg/kg IV q8h. Complicated staphylococcal/streptococcal skin infections: 7.5 mg/kg IV q12h. Infuse over 1 h.
PEDS - Safety and efficacy not established in children.
UNAPPROVED PEDS - Vancomycin-resistant E faecium infections (Not active against E. faecalis): 7.5 mg/kg IV q8h. Complicated staphylococcal/ streptococcal skin infections: 7.5 mg/kg IV q12h. Infuse over 1 h.
NOTES - Venous irritation (flush with D5W after peripheral infusion; do not use normal saline/ heparin), arthralgias/myalgias, hyperbilirubinemia. Cytochrome P450 3A4 inhibitor. Increases levels of cyclosporine, midazolam, nifedipine, and others.

**TELITHROMYCIN** (*Ketek*) ▶LK ♀C ▶? $$$
WARNING - Contraindicated in myasthenia gravis due to reports of exacerbation, including fatal acute respiratory depression. Warn patients about exacerbation of myasthenia gravis, hepatotoxicity, visual disturbances, and loss of consciousness.
ADULT - Community-acquired pneumonia: 800 mg PO daily × 7–10 d. Indications for acute sinusitis & acute exacerbation of chronic bronchitis removed from labeling in Jan 07 because potential benefit no longer justifies risk of adverse effects.
PEDS - Safety and efficacy not established in children.
FORMS - Trade only: 300,400 mg tabs. Ketek Pak: #10, 400 mg tabs.
NOTES - May prolong QT interval. Avoid in proarrhythmic conditions or with drugs that prolong QT interval. Life-threatening hepatotoxicity. Monitor for signs/symptoms of hepatitis. Contraindicated if history of hepatitis due to any macrolide or telithromycin. Contraindicated in myasthenia gravis. Cytochrome P450 3A4 substrate and inhibitor. Contraindicated with cisapride, pimozide, rifampin, ergot alkaloids. Withhold simvastatin, lovastatin, or atorvastatin during course of telithromycin. Consider monitoring INR with warfarin. Give telithromycin and theophylline at least 1 h apart. Monitor for increased toxicity of digoxin, midazolam, metoprolol. Cytochrome P450 3A4 inducers (ie phenytoin, carbamazepine) could reduce telithromycin levels. Dosage adjustment for CrCl <30 mL/min (including hemodialysis) is 600 mg once daily. On dialysis d, give after hemodialysis session. Dosage adjustment for CrCl <30 mL/min with hepatic dysfunction is 400 mg once daily.

**TIGECYCLINE** (*Tygacil*) ▶Bile, K ♀D ▶?+ $$$$$
ADULT - Complicated skin or intra-abdominal infections: 100 mg IV first dose, then 50 mg IV q12h. Infuse over 30–60 min.

(cont.)

**TIGECYCLINE** (cont.)
PEDS - Not approved in children. Avoid in children <8 yo due to teeth staining.
NOTES - May decrease efficacy of oral contraceptives. Monitor INR with warfarin. Dosage adjustment for severe liver dysfunction (Child Pugh C): 100 mg IV first dose, then 25 mg IV q12h.

**TRIMETHOPRIM** (*Primsol, ✦Proloprim*) ▶K ♀C ▶- $
ADULT - Uncomplicated UTI: 100 mg PO bid or 200 mg PO daily.
PEDS - Safety not established in infants <2 mo; Otitis media, age ≥6 mo (not for M catarrhalis): 10 mg/kg/d PO divided bid × 10 d.
UNAPPROVED ADULT - Prophylaxis of recurrent UTI: 100 mg PO qhs. Pneumocystis treatment: 5 mg/kg PO tid with dapsone 100 mg PO daily × 21 d.
FORMS - Generic only: Tabs 100,200 mg. Primsol: Oral soln 50 mg/5 mL.
NOTES - Contraindicated in megaloblastic anemia due to folate deficiency. Blood dyscrasias. Trimethoprim alone not first-line for otitis media. Inhibits metabolism of phenytoin and procainamide. Dosing in adults with renal dysfunction: 50 mg PO q12h for CrCl 15–30 mL/min. Do not use if CrCl <15 mL/min.

**VANCOMYCIN** (*Vancocin*) ▶K ♀C ▶? $$$$$
ADULT - Severe Staph infections, endocarditis: 1g IV q12h, each dose over 1h or 30 mg/kg/d IV divided q12h. Empiric therapy, native valve endocarditis: 15 mg/kg (max 2 g/d unless levels monitored) IV q12h with gentamicin. Clostridium difficile

diarrhea: 500–2000 mg/d PO divided tid to qid × 7–10 d. IV administration ineffective for this indication. See table for prophylaxis of bacterial endocarditis.
PEDS - Severe Staph infections, endocarditis: 10 mg/kg IV q6h. Infants <1 wk old: 15 mg/kg IV load, then 10 mg/kg q12h. Infants 1 wk - 1 mo: 15 mg/kg IV load, then 10 mg/kg q8h. Clostridium difficile diarrhea: 40–50 mg/kg/d up to 500 mg/d PO divided qid × 7–10 d. IV administration ineffective for this indication.
UNAPPROVED ADULT - Clostridium difficile diarrhea: 125 mg PO qid × 7–10 d.
UNAPPROVED PEDS - AAP dosing for infants: 10–15 mg/kg IV q8–12h for infants <1 wk. 10–15 mg/kg IV q6–8h for infants ≥1 wk. Bacterial meningitis: 60 mg/kg/d IV divided q6h. Nonmeningeal pneumococcal infections: 40–45 mg/kg/d IV divided q6h.
FORMS - Trade only: Caps 125, 250 mg
NOTES - "Red Neck" (or "Red Man") syndrome with rapid IV administration, vein irritation with IV extravasation, reversible neutropenia, ototoxicity or nephrotoxicity rarely. Enhanced effects of neuromuscular blockers. Use caution with other ototoxic/nephrotoxic drugs. Role of levels is controversial, but one approach is peak 30–40 mcg/mL 1.5–2.5 h after 1-h infusion, trough 5–20 mcg/mL. Individualize dose if renal dysfunction. Oral vancomycin poorly absorbed; do not use for extraluminal infections.

## CARDIOVASCULAR: ACE Inhibitors

**NOTE:** See also antihypertensive combinations. Hyperkalemia possible, especially if used concomitantly with other drugs that increase K+ (including K+ containing salt substitutes) and in patients with heart failure, diabetes mellitus, or renal impairment. Monitor closely for hypoglycemia during first mo of treatment when combined with insulin or oral antidiabetic agents. An increase in serum creatinine up to 35% above baseline is acceptable and is not reason to withhold therapy unless hyperkalemia occurs. ACE inhibitors are contraindicated during pregnancy. Contraindicated with a history of angioedema. Consider intestinal angioedema if abdominal pain (with or without N/V). African Americans and smokers may be at higher risk for angioedema. Swelling of tongue, glottis, or larynx may result in airway obstruction, especially with history of airway surgery. Rarely associated with syndrome starting with cholestatic jaundice or hepatitis progressing to fulminant hepatic necrosis and sometimes death. Increases risk of hypotension with volume depleted or hyponatremic patients. African Americans may need higher dose to achieve adequate response. Renoprotection and decreased cardiovascular morbidity/mortality seen with some ACE inhibitors are most likely a class effect. Patients may develop hypoglycemia (rare) when ACE inhibitors are given with insulin or oral antidiabetic medications. Anaphylactoid reactions have been reported when ACE inhibitor patients are dialyzed with high-flux membranes (eg, AN69) or undergoing low-density lipoprotein apheresis with dextran sulfate absorption. Nitritoid reactions (facial flushing, nausea, vomiting, hypotension) have been reported with concomitant gold injections.

**BENAZEPRIL** (*Lotensin*) ▶LK ♀- ▶? $$
ADULT - HTN: Start 10 mg PO daily, usual maintenance dose 20–40 mg PO daily or divided bid, max 80 mg/d, but added effect not apparent above 40 mg/d. Elderly, renal impairment, or concomitant diuretic therapy: Start 5 mg PO daily.
PEDS - HTN: Start 0.2 mg/kg/d (max 10 mg/d) as monotherapy; doses >0.6 mg/kg/d (or >40 mg/d) have not been studied. Do not use if age <6 yr or if glomerular filtration rate <30 mL/min.

UNAPPROVED ADULT - Renoprotective dosing: 10 mg PO daily. Heart failure: Start 5 mg PO daily, usual 5–20 mg/d, max 40 mg/d (in 1–2 doses).
FORMS - Generic/Trade: Tabs, non-scored 5, 10, 20, 40 mg.
NOTES - BID dosing may be required for 24-h BP control.

**CAPTOPRIL** (*Capoten*) ▶LK ♀- ▶+ $
ADULT - HTN: Start 25 mg PO bid-tid, usual maintenance dose 25–150 mg PO bid-tid, max 450 mg/d. Elderly, renal impairment, or concomitant diuretic therapy: Start 6.25–12.5 mg PO bid-tid.

**CAPTOPRIL** (*cont.*)
Heart failure: Start 6.25–12.5 mg PO tid, usual 50–100 mg PO tid, max 450 mg/d. Diabetic nephropathy: 25 mg PO tid.
PEDS - Not approved in children.
UNAPPROVED ADULT - Hypertensive urgency: 12.5–25 mg PO, repeated once or twice if necessary at intervals of ≥30–60 min.
UNAPPROVED PEDS - Neonates: 0.1–0.4 mg/kg/d PO divided q6–8h. Infants: initial dose 0.15–0.3 mg/kg/dose, titrate to effective dose, max dose 6 mg/kg/d divided daily-qid. Children: initial dose 0.3–0.5 mg/kg/dose PO q8h, titrate to effective dose, max dose 6 mg/kg/d (not to exceed 450 mg/d) divided bid-qid.
FORMS - Generic/Trade: Tabs, scored 12.5, 25, 50, 100 mg.
NOTES - A captopril solution or susp (1 mg/mL) can be made by dissolving Tabs in distilled water or flavored syrup. The solution is stable for 7days at room temperature.

**CILAZAPRIL** (*◆Inhibace*) ▶LK ♀- ▶? $
ADULT - Canada only. HTN: Initial dose 2.5 mg PO daily, usual maintenance dose 2.5–5 mg daily, max 10 mg daily. Elderly or concomitant diuretic therapy: initiate 1.25 mg PO daily. Heart failure adjunct: Initially 0.5 mg PO daily, increase to usual maintenance of 1–2.5 mg daily. Renal Impairment with CrCl 10–40 mL/min, initiate 0.5 mg daily, max 2.5mg/d. CrCl <10 mL/min

0.25–0.5 mg once or twice per wk, adjust dose according to BP response.
PEDS - Not approved in children.
FORMS - Generic/Trade: Tabs, scored 1, 2.5, 5 mg.
NOTES - Reduce dose in hepatic/renal impairment

**ENALAPRIL** (*Enalaprilat, Vasotec*) ▶LK ♀- ▶+ $$
ADULT - HTN: Start 5 mg PO daily, usual maintenance dose 10–40 mg PO daily or divided bid, max 40 mg/d. If oral therapy not possible, can use enalaprilat 1.25 mg IV q6h over 5 min, and increase up to 5 mg IV q6h if needed. Renal impairment or concomitant diuretic therapy: Start 2.5 mg PO daily. Heart failure: Start 2.5 mg PO bid, usual 10–20 mg PO bid, max 40 mg/d.
PEDS - Not approved in children.
UNAPPROVED ADULT - Hypertensive crisis: enalaprilat 1.25–5 mg IV q6h. Renoprotective dosing: 10–20 mg PO daily.
UNAPPROVED PEDS - HTN: Start 0.1 mg/kg/d PO daily or divided bid, titrate to effective dose, max dose 0.5 mg/kg/d; 0.005–0.01 mg/kg/dose IV q8–24 h.
FORMS - Generic/Trade: Tabs, scored 2.5, 5 mg, non-scored 10, 20 mg.
NOTES - BID dosing may be required for 24-h BP control. An enalapril oral susp (0.2 mg/mL) can be made by dissolving one 2.5 mg tab in 12.5 mL sterile water, use immediately. Enalaprilat is the active metabolite of enalapril.

**HYPERTENSION THERAPY\***

| Area of Concern | Blood Pressure Target | Preferred Therapy | Comments |
|---|---|---|---|
| General coronary artery disease prevention | <140/90 mm Hg | ACE inhibitor, angiotensin receptor blocker, calcium channel blocker, thiazide, or combination. Start 2 drugs if systolic BP ≥160 or diastolic BP ≥100 | None |
| High coronary artery disease risk | <130/80 mm Hg | ACE inhibitor, angiotensin receptor blocker, calcium channel blocker, thiazide, or combination. Start 2 drugs if systolic BP ≥160 or diastolic BP ≥100 | High coronary artery disease risk is diabetes mellitus, chronic kidney disease, known coronary artery disease or risk equivalent (eg, peripheral artery disease, abdominal aortic aneurysm), 10-year Framingham risk score ≥10% |
| Stable angina, unstable angina, MI | <130/80 mm Hg | Beta–blocker plus either an ACE inhibitor or an angiotensin receptor blocker | May add dihydropyridine calcium channel blocker or thiazide. Use beta–blockers only if hemodynamically stable. If beta-blocker contraindications or intolerable side effects (and no bradycardia or heart failure), may substitute verapamil or diltiazem |
| Left heart failure | <120/80 mm Hg | Beta–blocker plus either an ACE inhibitor or an angiotensin receptor blocker, plus a loop or thiazide diuretic, plus an aldosterone antagonist (if NYHA class III or IV, or if clinical heart failure and LV ejection fraction <40%) | Avoid verapamil, diltiazem, clonidine, alpha-blockers. For blacks with New York Heart Association class III or IV heart failure, consider adding hydralazine/isosorbide dinitrate |

\*All patients should attempt lifestyle modifications: optimize weight, healthy diet, sodium restriction, exercise, smoking cessation alcohol moderation. Adapted from *Circulation* 2007;115:2761–2788.

| ACE INHIBITOR DOSING | Hypertension | | Heart Failure | | |
|---|---|---|---|---|---|
| | Initial | Max/day | Initial | Target | Max |
| benazepril (*Lotensin*) | 10 mg qd* | 80 mg | n.r. | n.r. | n.r. |
| captopril (*Capoten*) | 25 mg bid/tid | 450 mg | 6.25–12.5 mg tid | 50 mg tid | 150 mg tid |
| enalapril (*Vasotec*) | 5 mg qd* | 40 mg | 2.5 mg bid | 10 mg bid | 20 mg bid |
| fosinopril (*Monopril*) | 10 mg qd* | 80 mg | 10 mg qd | 20 mg qd | 40 mg qd |
| lisinopril (*Zestril/ Prinivil*) | 10 mg qd | 80 mg | 5 mg qd | 20 mg qd | 40 mg qd |
| moexipril (*Univasc*) | 7.5 mg qd* | 30 mg | n.r. | n.r. | n.r. |
| perindopril (*Aceon*) | 4 mg qd* | 16 mg | n.r. | n.r. | n.r. |
| quinapril (*Accupril*) | 10–20 mg qd* | 80 mg | 5 mg bid | 10 mg bid | 20 mg bid |
| ramipril (*Altace*) | 2.5 mg qd* | 20 mg | 2.5 mg bid | 5 mg bid | 10 mg bid |
| trandolapril (*Mavik*) | 1–2 mg qd* | 8 mg | 1 mg qd | 4 mg qd | 4 mg qd |

Data taken from prescribing information. *May require bid dosing for 24-h BP control. n.r.=not recommended.

**FOSINOPRIL (*Monopril*)** ▶LK ♀- ▶? $
ADULT - HTN: Start 10 mg PO daily, usual maintenance dose 20–40 mg PO daily or divided bid, max 80 mg/d, but added effect not apparent above 40 mg/d. Elderly, renal impairment, or concomitant diuretic therapy: Start 5 mg PO daily. Heart failure: Start 5–10 mg PO daily, usual 20–40 mg PO daily, max 40 mg/d.
PEDS - HTN: 6–16 yr & weight >50 kg: 5–10 mg PO daily.
UNAPPROVED ADULT - Renoprotective dosing: 10–20 mg PO daily.
FORMS - Generic/Trade: Tabs, scored 10, non-scored 20, 40 mg.
NOTES - Elimination 50% renal, 50% hepatic. Accumulation of drug negligible with impaired renal function.

**LISINOPRIL (*Prinivil, Zestril*)** ▶K ♀- ▶? $
ADULT - HTN: Start 10 mg PO daily, usual maintenance dose 20–40 mg PO daily, max 80 mg/d, but added effect not apparent above 40 mg/d. Renal impairment or concomitant diuretic therapy: Start 2.5–5 mg PO daily. Heart failure, acute MI: Start 2.5–5 mg PO daily, usual 5–20 mg PO daily, max 40 mg/d.
PEDS - HTN ≥6 yo: 0.07 mg/kg PO daily; 5 mg/d max. Not recommended <6 yo or with glomerular filtration rate <30 mL/min/1.73 meters squared.
UNAPPROVED ADULT - Renoprotective dosing: 10–20 mg PO daily.
FORMS - Generic/Trade: Tabs, non-scored (Zestril) 2.5, 5, 10, 20, 30, 40 mg. Tabs, scored (Prinivil) 10, 20, 40 mg.

**MOEXIPRIL (*Univasc*)** ▶LK ♀- ▶? $$
ADULT - HTN: Start 7.5 mg PO daily, usual maintenance dose 7.5–30 mg PO daily or divided bid, max 30 mg/d. Renal impairment or concomitant diuretic therapy: Start 3.75 mg PO daily; max 15 mg/d with renal impairment.
PEDS - Not approved in children.
FORMS - Generic/Trade: Tabs, scored 7.5, 15 mg.
NOTES - BID dosing may be required for 24-h BP control.

**PERINDOPRIL (*Aceon, ✦Coversyl*)** ▶K ♀- ▶? $$$
ADULT - HTN: Start 4 mg PO daily, usual maintenance dose 4–8 mg PO daily or divided bid, max 16 mg/d. Renal impairment or concomitant diuretic therapy: Start 2 mg PO daily or divided bid. Reduction of cardiovascular events in stable coronary artery disease: Start 4 mg PO daily × 2 wk, max 8 mg/d. Elderly (>70 yr): 2 mg PO daily × 1 wk, 4 mg PO daily × 1 wk, max 8 mg/d.
PEDS - Not approved in children.
UNAPPROVED ADULT - Heart failure: Start 2 mg PO daily, max dose 16 mg daily. Recurrent stroke prevention: 4 mg PO daily with indapamide.
FORMS - Trade only: Tabs, scored 2, 4, 8 mg.
NOTES - BID dosing does not provide clinically significant BP lowering compared to once daily dosing.

**QUINAPRIL (*Accupril*)** ▶LK ♀- ▶? $$
ADULT - HTN: Start 10–20 mg PO daily (start 10 mg/d if elderly), usual maintenance dose 20–80 mg PO daily or divided bid, max 80 mg/d, but added effect not apparent above 40 mg/d. Renal impairment or concomitant diuretic therapy: Start 2.5–5 mg PO daily. Heart failure: Start 5 mg PO bid, usual maintenance dose 20–40 mg/d divided bid.
PEDS - Not approved in children.
FORMS - Generic/Trade: Tabs, scored 5, non-scored 10, 20, 40 mg.
NOTES - BID dosing may be required for 24-h BP control.

**RAMIPRIL (*Altace*)** ▶LK ♀- ▶? $$$
ADULT - HTN: Start 2.5 mg PO daily, usual maintenance dose 2.5–20 mg PO daily or divided bid, max 20 mg/d. Renal impairment or concomitant diuretic therapy: Start 1.25 mg PO daily. Heart failure post-MI: Start 2.5 mg PO bid, usual maintenance dose 5 mg PO bid. Reduce risk of MI, stroke, death from cardiovascular causes: Start 2.5 mg PO daily for 1 wk, then 5 mg daily for 3 wk, increase as tolerated to maintenance dose 10 mg daily.
PEDS - Not approved in children.

**RAMIPRIL** (*cont.*)
UNAPPROVED ADULT - Renoprotective dosing: Titrate to 10 mg PO daily.
FORMS - Generic/Trade: Caps 1.25, 2.5, 5, 10 mg. Trade only: Tabs 1.25, 2.5, 5, 10 mg.
NOTES - BID dosing may be required for 24-h BP control. cap contents can be sprinkled on applesauce and eaten or mixed with 120 mL of water or apple juice and swallowed. Mixtures are stable for 24 h at room temperature or 48 h refrigerated. Hypoglycemia may occur with co-administration with insulin or hypoglycemic agents.

**TRANDOLAPRIL** (*Mavik*) ▶LK ♀- ▶? $$
ADULT - HTN: Start 1 mg PO daily in non-black patients or 2 mg PO daily in black patients, usual maintenance dose 2–4 mg PO daily or divided bid, max 8 mg/d, but added effect not apparent above 4 mg/d. Renal impairment or concomitant diuretic therapy: Start 0.5 mg PO daily. Heart failure/post-MI: Start 0.5–1 mg PO daily, titrate to target dose 4 mg PO daily.
PEDS - Not approved in children.
FORMS - Generic/Trade: Tabs, 1, 2, 4 mg.

## CARDIOVASCULAR: Aldosterone Antagonists

**NOTE:** Hyperkalemia possible, especially if used concomitantly with other drugs that increase K+ and in patients with renal impairment.

**EPLERENONE** (*Inspra*) ▶L ♀B ▶? $$$$
ADULT - HTN: Start 50 mg PO daily, increase after 4 wk if needed to max dose 50 mg bid. Start 25 mg daily if concomitant drugs that mildly inhibit CYP 3A4 isoenzyme (eg, erythromycin, verapamil, fluconazole, saquinavir). Improve survival of stable patients with left ventricular systolic dysfunction (EF ≤40%) and heart failure post-MI: Start 25 mg PO daily; titrate to target dose 50 mg PO daily within 4 wk, if tolerated.
PEDS - Not approved in children.
FORMS - Trade only: Tabs non-scored 25, 50 mg
NOTES - Contraindicated in all patients with potassium >5.5 mEq/L; CrCl ≤30 mL/min; strong CYP 3A4 inhibitors (ketoconazole, itraconazole, nefazodone, troleandomycin, clarithromycin, ritonavir, nelfinavir). For treatment of HTN, contraindications include Type 2 DM with microalbuminuria; serum creat >2 mg/dL in males or >1.8 mg/dL in females; CrCl <50 mL/min; concomitant therapy with K+ supplements, K-sparing diuretics. Hyperkalemia more common with concomitant ACE inhibitors/ARBs. Measure serum K+ before initiating, within 1st wk , at 1 mo after starting treatment or dose adjustment, then prn. Monitor lithium levels. Monitor BP if used with NSAIDs.

**SPIRONOLACTONE** (*Aldactone*) ▶LK ♀D ▶+ $
ADULT - Edema (heart failure, cirrhotic ascites, nephrotic syndrome): Start 100 mg PO daily or divided bid, maintain for 5 d, increase as needed to achieve diuretic response, usual dose range 25–200 mg/d. Other diuretics may be needed. HTN: 50–100 mg PO daily or divided bid, generally used in combination with a thiazide diuretic to maintain serum potassium, increase dose as needed based on serum potassium and BP. Diuretic-induced hypokalemia: 25–100 mg PO daily when potassium supplements/sparing regimens inappropriate. Primary hyperaldosteronism, maintenance therapy: 100–400 mg/d PO until surgery or indefinitely if surgery not an option. Cirrhotic ascites: Start 100 mg once daily or in divided doses. Dose may range from 25–200 mg/d.
PEDS - Edema: 3.3 mg/kg PO daily or divided bid.
UNAPPROVED ADULT - Severe heart failure: Start 12.5–25 mg PO daily, usual maintenance dose 25–50 mg daily. Hirsutism: 50–200 mg PO daily, maximal regression of hirsutism in 6 mo. Acne: 50–200 mg PO daily.
UNAPPROVED PEDS - Edema/HTN: 1–3.3 mg/kg/d, PO daily or divided bid, max 200 mg/d.
FORMS - Generic/Trade: Tabs, non-scored 25; scored 50,100 mg.
NOTES - Dosing more frequently than BID not necessary. Hyperkalemia more likely with ≥50 mg/d and with concomitant ACE inhibitors or K+ supplements.

## CARDIOVASCULAR: Angiotensin Receptor Blockers (ARBs)

**NOTE:** See also antihypertensive combinations. An increase in serum creatinine up to 35% above baseline is acceptable and is not reason to withhold therapy unless hyperkalemia occurs. ARB use during pregnancy may cause injury or death to the developing fetus: use reliable form of contraception in women of child bearing age; discontinue as soon as pregnancy is detected. Use with caution in patients with a history of ACE inhibitor-induced angioedema. African Americans may be at higher risk for angioedema. Rare cases of angioedema and rhabdomyolysis have been reported with ARBs. Increased risk of hypotension with volume-depleted, hyponatremic patients, or during anesthesia/major surgery. Coadministration with NSAIDS, including selective COX-2 inhibitors, may further deteriorate renal function (usually reversible) and decrease antihypertensive effects.

**CANDESARTAN** (*Atacand*) ▶K ♀- ▶? $$$
ADULT - HTN: Start 16 mg PO daily, max 32 mg/d. Volume depleted patients: Start 8 mg PO daily. Reduce cardiovascular death and hospitalizations
from heart failure (NYHA II-IV and ejection fraction ≤40%): Start 4 mg PO daily, may double dose q2 wk; max 32 mg/d; has an added effect when used with ACE inhibitor.

(cont.)

**CANDESARTAN** *(cont.)*
PEDS - Not approved in children.
UNAPPROVED ADULT - Reduce heart failure hospitalizations in chronic heart failure & ejection fraction >40%: Start 4 mg PO daily, double dose q 2 wk; target dose 32 mg/d.
FORMS - Trade only: Tabs, non-scored 4, 8, 16, 32 mg.
NOTES - May increase lithium levels. Initiate/titrate cautiously with heart failure; with symptomatic hypotension, may need to reduce dose temporarily and give fluids.

**EPROSARTAN** *(Teveten)* ▶Fecal excretion ♀- ▶? $$$
ADULT - HTN: Start 600 mg PO daily, max 800 mg/d given daily or divided bid.
PEDS - Not approved in children.
FORMS - Trade only: Tabs non-scored 400, 600 mg.

**IRBESARTAN** *(Avapro)* ▶L ♀- ▶? $$$
ADULT - HTN: Start 150 mg PO daily, max 300 mg/d. Volume depleted patients: Start 75 mg PO daily. Type 2 diabetic nephropathy: Start 150 mg PO daily, target dose 300 mg daily.
PEDS - Not approved in children.
FORMS - Trade only: Tabs, non-scored 75, 150, 300 mg.

**LOSARTAN** *(Cozaar)* ▶L ♀- ▶? $$$
ADULT - HTN: Start 50 mg PO daily, max 100 mg/d given daily or divided bid. Volume-depleted patients or history of hepatic impairment: Start 25 mg PO daily. Stroke risk reduction in patients with HTN & left ventricular hypertrophy (does not appear to apply to Blacks): Start 50 mg PO daily. If need more BP reduction add HCTZ 12.5 mg PO daily; then increase losartan to 100 mg PO, then increase HCTZ to 25mg/d. Type 2 diabetic nephropathy: Start 50 mg PO daily, target dose 100 mg daily.
PEDS - HTN: Start 0.7 mg/kg/d (up to 50 mg), doses >1.4 mg/kg/d (or >100 mg) have not been studied. Do not use if age <6 yr or if glomerular filtration rate <30 mL/min.

UNAPPROVED ADULT - Heart failure: Start 12.5 mg PO daily, target dose 50 mg daily. Renoprotective dosing: Start 50 mg PO daily, increase to 100 mg daily as needed for BP control.
FORMS - Trade only: Tabs, non-scored 25, 50, 100 mg.
NOTES - Black patients with HTN & left ventricular hypertrophy may not have the same stroke risk reduction than non-Blacks. Monitor BP control when adding or discontinuing rifampin, fluconazole, or erythromycin.

**OLMESARTAN** *(Benicar)* ▶K ♀- ▶? $$$
ADULT - HTN: Start 20 mg PO daily, max 40 mg/d.
PEDS - Not approved in children.
FORMS - Trade only: Tabs, non-scored 5, 20, 40 mg.

**TELMISARTAN** *(Micardis)* ▶L ♀- ▶? $$$
ADULT - HTN: Start 40 mg PO daily, max 80 mg/d.
PEDS - Not approved in children.
FORMS - Trade only: Tabs, non-scored 20, 40, 80 mg.
NOTES - Swallow tabs whole, do not break or crush. Caution in hepatic insufficiency. May need to monitor digoxin levels when initiating, adjusting dose, or discontinuing.

**VALSARTAN** *(Diovan)* ▶L ♀- ▶? $$$
ADULT - HTN: Start 80-160 mg PO daily, max 320 mg/d. Heart failure: Start 40 mg PO bid, target dose 160 mg bid; there is no evidence of added benefit when used with adequate dose of ACE inhibitor. Reduce mortality/morbidity post-MI with left ventricular systolic dysfunction/failure: Start 20 mg PO daily, increase to 40 mg PO bid within 7 d, target dose 160 mg bid.
PEDS - HTN: Start 1.3 mg/kg/d (up to 40 mg), max 2.7 mg/kg/d (or 160 mg). Do not use if <6 yo.
UNAPPROVED ADULT - Renoprotective dosing: 80-160 mg PO daily.
FORMS - Trade only: Tabs, scored 40 mg, nonscored 80, 160, 320 mg.

## CARDIOVASCULAR: Antiadrenergic Agents

**CLONIDINE** *(Catapres, Catapres-TTS, ✦Dixarit)* ▶LK ♀C ▶? $$
ADULT - HTN: Start 0.1 mg PO bid, usual maintenance dose 0.2-1.2 mg/d divided bid-tid, max 2.4 mg/d. Transdermal (Catapres-TTS): Start 0.1 mg/24 h patch q wk, titrate to desired effect, max effective dose 0.6 mg/24 h (two, 0.3 mg/24 h patches).
PEDS - HTN: Start 5-7 mcg/kg/d PO divided q6-12 h, titrate at 5-7 d intervals to 5-25 mcg/kg/d divided q6h; max 0.9 mg/d. Transdermal therapy not recommended in children.
UNAPPROVED ADULT - HTN urgency: Initially 0.1-0.2 mg PO, followed by 0.1 mg q1h as needed up to a total dose of 0.5-0.7 mg. Menopausal flushing: 0.1-0.4 mg/d PO divided bid-tid; transdermal applied weekly 0.1 mg/d. Tourette's syndrome: 3-5 mcg/kg/d PO divided bid-qid. Opioid withdrawal, adjunct: 0.1-0.3 mg PO tid-qid or 0.1-0.2 mg PO

q4h tapering off over d 4-10. Alcohol withdrawal, adjunct: 0.1-0.2 mg PO q4h prn. Smoking cessation: Start 0.1 mg PO bid, increase 0.1 mg/d at weekly intervals to 0.75 mg/d as tolerated; transdermal (Catapres TTS): 0.1-0.2 mg/24 h patch q wk for 2-3 wk after cessation. ADHD: 5 mcg/kg/d PO × 8 wk. Post-traumatic stress disorder: Start 0.1 mg PO hs, max 0.6 mg/d in divided doses.
UNAPPROVED PEDS - ADHD: Start 0.05 mg PO qhs, titrate based on response over 8 wk to max 0.2 mg/d (<45 kg) or 0.4 mg/d (> 45 kg) in 2-4 divided doses. Tourette's syndrome: 3-5 mcg/kg/d PO divided bid-qid.
FORMS - Generic/Trade: Tabs, non-scored 0.1, 0.2, 0.3 mg. Trade only: transdermal weekly patch 0.1 mg/d (TTS-1), 0.2 mg/d (TTS-2), 0.3 mg/d (TTS-3).
NOTES - Sedation. Bradycardia. Rebound HTN with abrupt discontinuation of tabs, especially at doses ≥0.8 mg/d. Taper therapy over 4-7 d

**CLONIDINE** (*cont.*)
to avoid rebound HTN. Dispose of used patches carefully, keep away from children. Remove patch before MRI to avoid skin burns.

**⋁DOXAZOSIN** (*Cardura, Cardura XL*) ▶L ♀C ▶? $$
WARNING - Not first line agent for HTN. Increased risk of heart failure in patients who used doxazosin compared to diuretic in treating HTN.
ADULT – BPH, immediate release: Start 1 mg PO qhs, titrate by doubling the dose over at least 1–2 wk intervals up to a max of 8 mg PO qhs. Extended release (not approved for HTN): Start 4 mg PO qam with breakfast, titrate dose in 3–4 wk to max dose 8 mg PO qam. HTN: Start 1 mg PO qhs, max 16 mg/d. Avoid use of doxazosin alone to treat combined HTN and BPH.
PEDS - Not approved in children.
UNAPPROVED ADULT - Promote spontaneous passage of ureteral calculi: 4 mg (XL formulation only) PO daily usually combined with an NSAID, antiemetic and opioid of choice.
FORMS - Generic/Trade: Tabs, scored 1, 2, 4, 8 mg. Trade only (Cardura XL): Tabs, extended-release 4, 8 mg.
NOTES - Dizziness, drowsiness, lightheadedness, syncope. Bedtime dosing may minimize side effects. Initial 1 mg dose is used to decrease postural hypotension that may occur after the first few doses. If therapy is interrupted for several d, restart at the 1 mg dose. Monitor BP after first dose, after each dose adjustment, and periodically thereafter. Contraindicated with vardenafil or tadalafil; increases risk of hypotension.

**GUANABENZ** (*Wytensin*) ▶LK ♀C ▶- $$$
WARNING - Sedation, rebound HTN with abrupt discontinuation especially with high doses.
ADULT - HTN: Start 2–4 mg PO bid, max 32 mg bid.
PEDS - Children >12 yr of age: initial dose 0.5–2 mg/d divided bid, usual maintenance dose 4–24 mg/d divided bid.
FORMS - Generic only: Tabs, 4, 8 mg.
NOTES - Sedation. Rebound HTN with abrupt discontinuation, especially at higher doses (32 mg/d). Taper therapy over 4–7 d to avoid rebound HTN.

**GUANFACINE** (*Tenex*) ▶K ♀B ▶? $
ADULT - HTN: Start 1 mg PO qhs, increase to 2–3 mg qhs if needed after 3–4 wk, max 3 mg/d.
PEDS - HTN: ≥12 yr of age, same as adult.
UNAPPROVED PEDS - ADHD: Start 0.5 mg PO daily, titrate by 0.5 mg q3–4 d as tolerated to 0.5 mg PO tid.
FORMS - Generic/Trade: Tabs, non-scored 1, 2 mg.
NOTES - Most of the drug's therapeutic effect is seen at 1 mg/d. Rebound HTN with abrupt discontinuation, but generally BP returns to pretreatment measurements slowly without ill effects. Less sedation and hypotension compared to clonidine.

**METHYLDOPA** (*Aldomet*) ▶LK ♀B ▶+ $
ADULT - HTN: Start 250 mg PO bid-tid, usual maintenance dose 500–3000 mg/d divided bid-qid, max 3000 mg/d. Hypertensive crisis: 250–500 mg IV q6h, max 1gm IV q6h, max 4000 mg/d.

PEDS - HTN: 10 mg/kg/d PO divided bid-qid, titrate dose to a max dose 65 mg/kg/d or 3000 mg/d, whichever is less.
FORMS - Generic only: Tabs, non-scored 125, 250, 500 mg.
NOTES - Not 1st or 2nd line for HTN (other agents preferred) except pregnancy-induced HTN. IV form has a slow onset of effect and other agents preferred for rapid reduction of BP. Hemolytic anemia possible.

**PRAZOSIN** (*Minipress*) ▶L ♀C ▶? $$
WARNING - Not first line agent for hypertension. Increased heart failure risk in patients who used doxazosin compared to diuretic in treating HTN.
ADULT - HTN: Start 1 mg PO bid-tid, usual maintenance dose 20 mg/d divided bid-tid, max 40 mg/d, but doses >20 mg/d usually do not increase efficacy.
PEDS - Not approved in children.
UNAPPROVED ADULT - Post-traumatic stress disorder: Start 1 mg PO hs, increase weekly by 1–2 mg/d to max dose of 20 mg/d. Doses >10 mg/d are divided early evening and hs.
UNAPPROVED PEDS - HTN: Start 0.005 mg/kg PO single dose; increase slowly as needed up to maintenance dose 0.025–0.150 mg/kg/d divided q6 h; max dose 0.4 mg/kg/d.
FORMS - Generic/Trade: Caps 1, 2, 5 mg.
NOTES - To avoid syncope, start with 1 mg qhs, and increase dose gradually. Contraindicated with vardenafil or tadalafil; increases risk of hypotension.

**RESERPINE** (*Serpasil*) ▶LK ♀C ▶- $
ADULT - HTN: Start 0.05–0.1 mg PO daily or 0.1 mg PO qod, max dose 0.25 mg/d.
PEDS - Not approved in children.
FORMS - Generic only: Tabs, scored 0.1, 0.25 mg.
NOTES - Should be used in combination with a diuretic to counteract fluid retention and augment BP control. May cause depression at higher doses, avoid use in patients with depression or active peptic ulcer disease.

**TERAZOSIN** (*Hytrin*) ▶LK ♀C ▶? $$
WARNING - Not first line agent for HTN. Increased risk of heart failure in patients who used related-drug doxazosin compared to diuretic in treating HTN.
ADULT - HTN: Start 1 mg PO qhs, usual effective dose 1–5 mg PO daily or divided bid, max 20 mg/d. BPH: Start 1 mg PO qhs, titrate dose in a stepwise fashion to 2, 5, or 10 mg PO qhs to desired effect. Treatment with 10 mg PO qhs for 4–6 wk may be needed to assess benefit. Max 20 mg/d.
PEDS - Not approved in children.
FORMS - Generic/Trade: Tabs & Caps 1, 2, 5, 10 mg.
NOTES - Dizziness, drowsiness, lightheadedness, syncope. Bedtime dosing may minimize side effects. Initial 1 mg dose is used to decrease **(cont.)**

**TERAZOSIN** *(cont.)*
postural hypotension that may occur after the first few doses. If therapy is interrupted for several d, restart at the 1 mg dose. Monitor BP after first dose, after each dose adjustment, and periodically thereafter. Contraindicated with vardenafil or tadalafil; increases risk of hypotension.

## SELECTED DRUGS THAT MAY PROLONG THE QT INTERVAL

| | | | |
|---|---|---|---|
| alfuzosin | erythromycin*† | nicardipine | sotalol*† |
| amiodarone*† | felbamate | octreotide | sunitinib |
| apomorphine | flecainide* | ofloxacin | tacrolimus |
| arsenic trioxide* | foscarnet | ondansetron | tamoxifen |
| azithromycin* | fosphenytoin | pentamidine*† | telithromycin* |
| chloroquine* | gemifloxacin | phenothiazines‡ | thioridazine |
| chlorpromazine | granisetron | pimozide*† | tizanidine |
| cisapride*† | haloperidol*‡ | polyethylene glycol (PEG-salt solution)§ | tolterodine |
| clarithromycin* | ibutilide*† | procainamide* | vardenafil |
| clozapine | indapamide* | quetiapine‡ | venlafaxine |
| cocaine* | isradipine | quinidine*† | visicol§ |
| dasatinib | levofloxacin* | quinine | voriconazole* |
| disopyramide*† | lithium | ranolazine | vorinostat |
| dofetilide* | mefloquine | risperidone‡ | ziprasidone‡ |
| dolasetron | methadone*† | salmeterol | |
| droperidol* | moexipril/HCTZ | sertraline | |
| epirubicin | moxifloxacin | | |

**NOTE:** This table may not include all drugs that prolong the QT interval or cause torsades. Risk of drug-induced QT prolongation may be increased in women, elderly, hypokalemia, hypomagnesemia, bradycardia, starvation, CHF, & CNS injuries. Hepatorenal dysfunction & drug interactions can increase the concentration of QT interval-prolonging drugs. Coadministration of QT interval-prolonging drugs can have additive effects. Avoid these (and other) drugs in congenital prolonged QT syndrome (www.qtdrugs.org). *Torsades reported in product labeling/case reports. †Increased risk in women. ‡QT prolongation: thioridazine > ziprasidone > risperidone, quetiapine, haloperidol. §May be due to electrolyte imbalance.

## CARDIOVASCULAR: Anti-Dysrhythmics/Cardiac Arrest

**ADENOSINE** *(Adenocard)* ▶Plasma ♀C ▶? $$$
ADULT - PSVT conversion (not A-fib): 6 mg rapid IV & flush, preferably a central line. If no response after 1–2 min then 12 mg. A third dose of 12 mg may be given prn.
PEDS - PSVT conversion <50 kg: initial dose 50–100 mcg/kg IV, give subsequent doses q1–2 min prn by increasing 50–100 mcg/kg each time, up to a max single dose of 300 mcg/kg or 12 mg whichever is less. ≥50 kg: Same as adult.
UNAPPROVED PEDS - PSVT conversion: Initial dose 0.1–0.2 mg/kg IV bolus.
NOTES - Half-life is <10 sec. Give doses by rapid IV push followed by normal saline flush. Need higher dose if on theophylline or caffeine, lower dose if on dipyridamole or carbamazepine. May cause respiratory collapse in patients with asthma, COPD. Use in setting with cardiac resuscitation readily available. Do not confuse with adenosine phosphate used for the symptomatic relief of varicose vein complications.

**AMIODARONE** *(Cordarone, Pacerone)* ▶L ♀D ▶- $$$$
WARNING - Life-threatening pulmonary and hepatoxicity. Proarrhythmic. Contraindicated in cardiogenic shock and with marked sinus bradycardia or 2nd/3rd degree heart block if no pacemaker. For life-threatening ventricular arrhythmias, give loading doses as inpatient.
ADULT - Life-threatening ventricular arrhythmia without cardiac arrest: Load 150 mg IV over 10 min, then 1 mg/min × 6 h, then 0.5 mg/min × 18h. Mix in D5W. Oral loading dose 800–1600 mg PO daily for 1–3 wk, reduce dose to 400–800 mg daily for 1 mo when arrhythmia is controlled or adverse effects are prominent, then reduce to lowest effective dose, usually 200–400 mg daily.
PEDS - Not approved in children.
UNAPPROVED ADULT - Refractory atrial fibrillation: loading dose 600–800 mg PO daily for 7–14 d, then 200–400 mg daily. Maintain sinus rhythm with A-fib: 100–400 mg PO daily. Shock-

**AMIODARONE** (*cont.*)

refractory VF/pulseless VT: 300 mg or 5 mg/kg IV bolus followed by unsynchronized shock, additional 150 mg bolus may be given if serious arrhythmias recur. Stable monomorphic ventricular tachycardia: 150 mg IV over 10 min, repeat q10–15 min prn.

UNAPPROVED PEDS - May cause death or other serious side effects in children (see NOTES); do not use in infants <30 d of age and use only if medically warranted if >30 d of age. Ventricular arrhythmia: IV therapy limited data; 5 mg/kg IV over 30 min; followed by 5 mcg/kg/min infusion; increase infusion as needed up to max 10 mcg/kg/min or 20 mg/kg/d. Give loading dose in 1 mg/kg aliquots with each aliquot given over 5–10 min; do not exceed 30 mg/min.

FORMS - Trade only (Pacerone): Tabs, 100, 300 mg. Generic/Trade: Tabs, scored 200, 400 mg.

NOTES - Consider inpatient rhythm monitoring during initiation of therapy, especially when treating life-threatening arrhythmias. Consult cardiologist before using with other antiarrhythmic agents. Do not use with iodine allergy. Photosensitivity with oral therapy. Hypo or hyperthyroidism possible. Monitor LFTs, TFTs, and PFTs. Prompt ophthalmic examination needed with changes in visual acuity or decreased peripheral vision. Most manufacturers of laser refractive devices contraindicate eye laser surgery when taking amiodarone. Long elimination half-life, approximately 25–50 d. Drug interactions may persist after discontinuance due to long half-life. May increase levels of substrates of p-glycoprotein and drugs metabolized by CYP450 enzymes (CYP1A2, CYP2C9, CYP2D6, CYP3A4). Co-administration of fluoroquinolones, macrolides, loratadine, trazodone, or azoles may prolong QTc. May double or triple phenytoin level. May increase cyclosporine levels. May increase digoxin levels; discontinue digoxin or reduce dose by 50%. May increase INR with warfarin therapy up to 100%; reduce warfarin dose by 33–50%. Increased risk of myopathy when used with simvastatin or lovastatin. Caution with simvastatin >20 mg/d, lovastatin >40 mg/d, or atorvastatin; increases risk of myopathy and rhabdomyolysis. Co-administration with clopidogrel may result in ineffective platelet inhibition. Do not use with grapefruit juice. Use cautiously with beta blockers and calcium channel blockers. Protease inhibitors, cimetidine may increase levels. Give bid if intolerable GI effects occur with once-daily dosing. IV therapy may cause hypotension and bradycardia in adults. Administer IV infusion using a nonevacuated glass bottle and in-line IV filter. Use central line when concentration >2 mg/mL. May cause congenital hypothyroidism and hyperthyroidism if given during pregnancy. Avoid use in children <1 mo of age: IV form contains benzyl alcohol, which may cause gasping syndrome (gasping respirations, hypotension, bradycardia, and cardiovascular collapse). In children 1 mo to 15 yr of age may cause life-threatening hypotension, bradycardia, and AV block. May adversely affect male reproductive tract development in infants & toddlers from plasticizer exposure from IV tubing; use syringes instead of IV tubing to administer doses to infants and toddlers.

**ATROPINE (AtroPen)** ►K ♀C ▶– $

ADULT - Bradyarrhythmia/CPR: 0.5–1.0 mg IV q3–5 min, max 0.04 mg/kg (3 mg). Treatment of muscarinic symptoms of insecticide or nerve agent poisonings: Mild symptoms: 1 injection of 2 mg auto-injector pen, 2 additional injections after 10 min may be given in rapid succession if severe symptoms develop. Severe symptoms: 3 injections of 2 mg pen in rapid succession. Administer injection in mid-lateral thigh. Max 3 injections.

PEDS - CPR: 0.02 mg/kg/dose IV q5 min for 2–3 doses prn (max single dose 0.5 mg); minimum single dose, 0.1 mg; max cumulative dose 1 mg. Treatment of muscarinic symptoms of insecticide or nerve agent poisonings: Follow adult dosing instructions, but if <7 kg use 0.25 mg pen, if 7–18 kg use 0.5 mg pen, if 18–41 kg use 1 mg pen, if >41 kg use 2 mg pen.

UNAPPROVED ADULT - ET administration prior to IV access: 2–2.5 × the recommended IV dose in 10 mL of NS or distilled water.

FORMS - Trade only: Prefilled auto-injector pen: 0.25 mg (yellow), 0.5 mg (blue), 1 mg (dark red), 2 mg (green).

NOTES - Injector should be used by someone who has adequate training in recognizing & treating nerve agent or insecticide intoxication. Seek immediate medical attention after injection(s).

**BICARBONATE** ►K ♀C ▶? $

ADULT - Cardiac arrest: 1 mEq/kg/dose IV initially, followed by repeat doses up to 0.5 mEq/kg at 10 min intervals during continued arrest. Severe acidosis: 2–5 mEq/kg dose IV administered as a 4–8 h infusion. Repeat dosing based on lab values.

PEDS - Cardiac arrest: Neonates or infants <2 yr of age, 1 mEq/kg dose IV slow injection initially, followed by repeat doses up to 1 mEq/kg at 10 min intervals during continued arrest. To avoid intracranial hemorrhage due to hypertonicity, use a 1:1 dilution of 8.4% (1 mEq/mL) sodium bicarbonate and dextrose 5% or use the 4.2% (0.5 mEq/mL) product.

UNAPPROVED ADULT - Prevention of contrast-induced nephropathy: Administer sodium bicarbonate 154 mEq/L soln at 3 mL/kg/h IV × 1h before contrast, followed by infusion of 1 mL/kg/h × 6 h post-procedure. If >110 kg dose based on 110 kg weight.

NOTES - Full correction of bicarbonate deficit should not be attempted during the first 24h. May paradoxically exacerbate intracellular acidosis.

**DIGOXIN (Lanoxin, Lanoxicaps, Digitek)** ▶KL ♀C ▶+ $
ADULT - Systolic heart failure/rate control of chronic A-fib: <70 yr: 0.25 mg PO daily; >70 yr: 0.125 mg PO daily; impaired renal function: 0.0625–0.125 mg PO daily; titrate based on response. Rapid A-fib: Load 0.5 mg IV, then 0.25 mg IV q6h × 2 doses, maintenance 0.125–0.375 mg IV/PO daily; titrate to minimum effective dose. Other agents (ie, beta blockers, diltiazem, verapamil) generally more effective in controlling ventricular rate in A-fib.
PEDS - Arrhythmia: Oral total loading dose with tabs or elixir: premature neonate, 20–30 mcg/kg; full-term neonate, 25–35 mcg/kg; 1–24 mo, 35–60 mcg/kg; 2–5 yr, 30–40 mcg/kg; 5–10 yr, 20–35 mcg/kg; >10 yr, 10–15 mcg/kg. Initially, give half of the total loading dose; other half of loading dose may be given in 6–8h after reassessment. Use 25–35% of oral loading dose in divided doses (bid) for < 10 yr for maintenance dose. Caution - pediatric doses are in mcg, elixir product is labeled in mg/mL.
UNAPPROVED ADULT - Reentrant PSVT (after carotid massage, IV adenosine, IV beta blocker, IV diltiazem): 8–15 mcg/kg IV, give 50% of total dose initially, 25% 4–6 h later, and then the final 25% 4–6 h later.
FORMS - Generic/Trade: Tabs, scored (Lanoxin, Digitek) 0.125, 0.25 mg; elixir 0.05 mg/mL. Trade only: Caps (Lanoxicaps), 0.1, 0.2 mg.
NOTES - Consider patient specific characteristics (weight, CrCl, age, factors likely to alter pharmacokinetic/dynamic profile of digoxin) when dosing; see package insert for alterations based on weight & renal function. Adjust dose based on response and therapeutic serum levels (range from 0.8–2.0 ng/mL). Heart failure may respond at lower levels (≥0.5 ng/mL) while A-fib may need higher. Serum digoxin concentration of 0.5–0.8 ng/mL (compared to higher serum concentrations) is associated with decreased mortality in men with stable heart failure and ejection fraction ≤45%. Toxicity exacerbated by hypokalemia. 100 mcg Lanoxicaps = 125 mcg tabs or elixir. Avoid administering IM due to severe local irritation. Elimination prolonged with renal impairment, monitor levels carefully. Many drug and herb interactions.

**DIGOXIN IMMUNE FAB (Digibind, Digifab)** ▶K ♀C ▶? $$$$$
ADULT - Digoxin toxicity: 2–20 vials IV, one formula is: Number vials = (serum dig level in ng/mL) × (kg)/100.
PEDS - Same as adult.
NOTES - Do not draw serum digoxin concentrations after administering digoxin-immune Fab; levels will be falsely elevated for several d. One vial binds approximately 0.5 mg digoxin.

**DISOPYRAMIDE (Norpace, Norpace CR, ✦Rythmodan, Rythmodan-LA)** ▶KL ♀C ▶+ $$$$
WARNING - Proarrhythmic. Increased mortality in patients with non-life threatening ventricular

arrhythmias and structural heart disease (ie, MI, LV dysfunction).
ADULT - Rarely indicated, consult cardiologist. Ventricular arrhythmia: 400–800 mg PO daily in divided doses (immediate-release, q6h or extended-release, q12h). With cardiomyopathy or possible cardiac decompensation, limit initial dose to 100 mg of immediate-release q6–8h; do not give a loading dose. With liver disease or moderate renal impairment (CrCl>40): 400 mg/d PO in divided doses. Use immediate release form when CrCl ≤40 mg/dL: CrCl 30–40 mg/dL: 100 mg q8h; CrCl 15–30 mg/dL: 100 mg q12h; CrCl <15 mg/dL: 100 mg q24h.
PEDS - Ventricular arrhythmia: Divide dose q6h. <1 yr, 10–30 mg/kg/d; 1–4 yr, 10–20 mg/kg/d; 4–12 yr, 10–15 mg/kg/d; 12–18 yr, 6–15 mg/kg/d.
UNAPPROVED ADULT - Maintain sinus rhythm with A-fib: 400–750 mg/d in divided doses.
FORMS - Generic/Trade: Caps, immediate-release 100, 150 mg; extended-release 150 mg. Trade only: Caps, extended-release 100 mg.
NOTES - Consider inpatient rhythm monitoring during initiation of therapy, especially when treating life-threatening arrhythmias. Anticholinergic side effects (dry mouth, constipation, blurred vision, urinary hesitancy) commonly occur. Reduce dose in patients with CrCl <40 mL/min. Initiate as an outpatient with extreme caution. May start 6–12 h after last dose of quinidine, or 3–6 h after last dose of procainamide. May start extended release form 6 h after last dose of immediate release form.

**DOFETILIDE (Tikosyn)** ▶KL ♀C ▶- $$$$
WARNING - Rarely indicated; available only to hospitals and prescribers who have received appropriate dosing and treatment initiation education. Contraindicated if CrCl is <20 mL/min or QTc interval >440 msec, or >500 msec in patients with ventricular conduction abnormalities. Must be initiated or re-initiated in a facility that can provide CrCl calculation, ECG monitoring, and cardiac resuscitation. Monitor in this setting for ≥3 d. Do not discharge if ≤12 h since electrical or pharmacological conversion to normal sinus rhythm.
ADULT - Conversion of A-fib/flutter: Specialized dosing based on creatinine clearance and QTc interval.
PEDS - Not approved in children.
FORMS - Trade only: Caps, 0.125, 0.25, 0.5 mg.
NOTES - Use with heart rate <50 bpm has not been studied. Serum K+, Mg++ should be within normal range prior to initiating and during therapy. Monitor K+ and Mg++ (low levels increase risk of arrhythmias). Assess CrCl and QTc prior to first dose. Continuously monitor ECG during hospital initiation and adjust dose based on QTc interval. Effects may be increased by known cytochrome P450 3A4 inhibitors and drugs that inhibit renal elimination. Contraindicated with HCTZ (alone

**DOFETILIDE** (*cont.*)

or with triamterene), trimethoprim, verapamil, cimetidine, prochlorperazine, megestrol, and ketoconazole. Using with phenothiazines, cisapride, tricyclic antidepressants, macrolides, fluoroquinolones may increase QTc.

**FLECAINIDE (*Tambocor*)** ▶K ♀C ▶- $$$$

WARNING - Proarrhythmic. Increased mortality in patients with non-life threatening ventricular arrhythmias, structural heart disease (ie, MI, LV dysfunction); not recommended for use with chronic atrial fibrillation.

ADULT - Prevention of paroxysmal atrial fib/flutter or PSVT, with symptoms & no structural heart disease: Start 50 mg PO q12h, may increase by 50 mg bid q4 d, max 300 mg/d. Life-threatening ventricular arrhythmias without structural heart disease: Start 100 mg PO q12h, may increase by 50 mg bid q 4 d, max 400 mg/d. With severe renal impairment (CrCl<35 mL/min): Start 50 mg PO bid.

PEDS - Consult pediatric cardiologist.

UNAPPROVED ADULT - Cardioversion of recent onset atrial fib: 200–300 mg PO single dose. Maintain sinus rhythm with A-fib: 200–300 mg/d in divided doses. Outpatient prn therapy for recurrent atrial fib in highly-select patients ("pill-in-the-pocket"): Single dose PO of 300 mg (if ≥70 kg) or 200 mg (if <70 kg).

FORMS - Generic/Trade: Tabs, non-scored 50, scored 100, 150 mg.

NOTES - Consider inpatient rhythm monitoring during initiation of therapy, especially when treating life-threatening arrhythmias. Do not use with structural heart disease. Use with AV nodal slowing agent (beta blocker, verapamil, diltiazem) to minimize risk of 1:1 atrial flutter. Reduce dose if QRS widening >20% from baseline or if 2nd/3rd degree AV block. Correct hypo/hyperkalemia before giving. Increases digoxin level 13–19%. Consult cardiologist before using with other antiarrhythmic agents. Reduce dose of flecainide 50% when used with amiodarone. Quinidine, cimetidine may increase levels. Use cautiously with disopyramide, verapamil, or impaired hepatic function. Use cautiously with impaired renal function; will take >4 d to reach new steady state level. Target trough level 0.2–1 mcg/mL.

**IBUTILIDE (*Corvert*)** ▶K ♀C ▶? $$$$$

WARNING - Proarrhythmic; only administer by trained personnel with continuous ECG monitoring.

ADULT - Recent onset A-fib/flutter: Patients >60 kg: 1 mg (10 mL) IV over 10 min, may repeat once if no response after 10 additional min. Patients <60 kg: 0.01 mg/kg over 10 min, may repeat if no response after 10 additional min. Useful in combination with DC cardioversion if DC cardioversion alone is unsuccessful.

PEDS - Not approved in children.

NOTES - Serum K+, Mg++ should be within normal range prior to initiating and during therapy. Monitor K+ and Mg++ (low levels increase risk

of arrhythmias). Keep on cardiac monitor ≥4 h. Use with caution, if at all, when QT interval is >500 ms, severe LV dysfunction, or in patients already using class Ia or III antiarrhythmics. Stop infusion when arrhythmia is terminated.

**ISOPROTERENOL (*Isuprel*)** ▶L ♀C ▶? $$$

ADULT - Refractory bradycardia or third degree AV block: 0.02–0.06 mg (1–3 mL of a 1:50,000 dilution) IV bolus or IV infusion (2 mg in 250 mL D5W = 8 mcg/mL) at 5 mcg/min; 5 mcg/min = 37 mL/h. General dose range 2–20 mcg/min.

PEDS - Refractory bradycardia or third degree AV block: Start IV infusion 0.05 mcg/kg/min, increase every 5–10 min by 0.1 mcg/kg/min until desired effect or onset of toxicity, max 2 mcg/kg/min. 10 kg: 0.1 mcg/kg/min = 8 mL/h.

**LIDOCAINE (*Xylocaine, Xylocard*)** ▶LK ♀B ▶? $

ADULT - Ventricular arrhythmia: Load 1 mg/kg IV, then 0.5 mg/kg IV q8–10min as needed to max 3 mg/kg. IV infusion: 4 gm in 500 mL D5W (8 mg/mL) at 1–4 mg/min.

PEDS - Ventricular arrhythmia: Loading dose 1 mg/kg IV/intraosseous slowly; may repeat for 2 doses 10–15 min apart; max 3–5 mg/kg in one h. ET tube: Use 2–2.5 times IV dose. IV infusion: 4 gm in 500 mL D5W (8 mg/mL) at 20–50 mcg/kg/min. 10 kg: 40 mcg/kg/min = 3 mL/h.

UNAPPROVED ADULT - ET administration prior to IV access: 2–2.5 × the recommended IV dose in 10 mL of NS or distilled water. Shock refractory VF/pulseless VT: 1–1.5 mg/kg IV push × 1, then 0.5–0.75 mg/kg IV push q5–10 min as needed to max 3 mg/kg.

NOTES - Reduce infusion in heart failure, liver disease, elderly. Not for routine use after acute MI. Monitor for CNS side effects with prolonged infusions.

**MEXILETINE (*Mexitil*)** ▶L ♀C ▶- $$$

WARNING - Proarrhythmic. Increased mortality in patients with non-life threatening ventricular arrhythmias and structural heart disease (ie, MI, LV dysfunction).

ADULT - Rarely indicated, consult cardiologist. Ventricular arrhythmia: Start 200 mg PO q8h with food or antacid, max dose 1,200 mg/d. Patients responding to q8h dosing may be converted to q12h dosing with careful monitoring, max 450 mg/dose q12h.

PEDS - Not approved in children.

FORMS - Generic only: Caps, 150, 200, 250 mg.

NOTES - Patients may require decreased dose with severe liver disease. CNS side effects may limit dose titration. Monitor level when given with phenytoin, rifampin, phenobarbital, cimetidine, fluvoxamine. May increase theophylline level.

**PROCAINAMIDE (*Pronestyl*)** ▶LK ♀C ▶? $

WARNING - Proarrhythmic. Increased mortality in patients with non-life threatening ventricular arrhythmias and structural heart disease (ie, MI, LV dysfunction). Positive ANA titer, blood dyscrasias, and lupus erythematosus-like syndrome.

(cont.)

**PROCAINAMIDE** (cont.)

ADULT - Ventricular arrhythmia: Load 100 mg IV q10 min or 20 mg/min (150 mL/h) until: 1) QRS widens >50%, 2) dysrhythmia suppressed, 3) hypotension, or 4) total of 17 mg/kg or 1000 mg. Infusion 2g in 250 mL D5W (8 mg/mL) at 2–6 mg/min (15–45 mL/h). If rhythm unresponsive, guide therapy by serum procainamide/NAPA levels.

PEDS - Not approved in children.

UNAPPROVED ADULT - Shock responsive VF/pulseless VT: up to 50 mg/min until: 1) QRS widens >50%, 2) dysrhythmia suppressed, 3) hypotension, or 4) total of 17 mg/kg or 1000 mg. Maintain sinus rhythm with A-fib: 1000–4000 mg/d in divided doses. Restoration of sinus rhythm in atrial fibrillation with Wolf-Parkinson-White syndrome (preexcitation) 100 mg IV q10 min or 20 mg/min. until: 1) QRS widens >50%, 2) dysrhythmia suppressed, 3) hypotension, or 4) total of 17 mg/kg or 1000 mg.

UNAPPROVED PEDS - Arrhythmia: 2–6 mg/kg IV over 5 min, max loading dose 100 mg, repeat loading dose every 5–10 min as needed up to max 15 mg/kg; 20–80 mcg/kg/min IV infusion, max dose 2 g/d. Consult peds cardiologist or intensivist.

**PROPAFENONE (Rythmol, Rythmol SR)** ▶L ♀C ▶? $$$$

WARNING - Proarrhythmic. Increased mortality in patients with non-life threatening ventricular arrhythmias and structural heart disease (ie, MI, LV dysfunction).

ADULT - Prevention of paroxysmal atrial fib/flutter or PSVT, with symptoms & no structural heart disease; or life-threatening ventricular arrhythmias: Start (immediate release) 150 mg PO q8h; may increase after 3–4 d to 225 mg PO q8h; max 900 mg/d. Prolong time to recurrence of symptomatic atrial fib without structural heart disease: 225 mg SR PO q12h, may increase ≥5 d to 325 mg PO q12h, max 425 mg q12h.

PEDS - Not approved in children.

UNAPPROVED ADULT - Cardioversion of recent onset atrial fib: 600 mg PO single dose. Outpatient prn therapy for recurrent atrial fib in highly-select patients ("pill-in-the-pocket"): Single dose PO of 600 mg (if ≥70 kg) or 450 mg (if <70 kg).

FORMS - Generic/Trade: Tabs (immediate release), scored 150, 225, 300 mg. Trade only: SR, caps 225, 325, 425 mg.

NOTES - Consider inpatient rhythm monitoring during initiation of therapy, especially when treating life-threatening arrhythmias. Do not use with structural heart disease or for ventricular rate control during atrial fib. Consider using with AV nodal slowing agent (beta blocker, verapamil, diltiazem) to minimize risk of 1:1 atrial flutter. Reduce dose if QRS widening >20% from baseline or if 2nd/3rd degree AV block. Correct hypo/hyperkalemia and low magnesium before giving. Consult cardiologist before using with other antiarrhythmic agents. May increase digoxin level 35–85%. May increase beta blocker, cyclosporine, desipramine, haloperidol, imipramine, theophylline, venlafaxine levels. Increases warfarin activity; monitor INR. Amiodarone, cimetidine, desipramine, erythromycin, ketoconazole, paroxetine, ritonavir, saquinavir, sertraline may increase level and risk of QT prolongation. Instruct patient to report any changes in OTC, prescription, supplement use and symptoms that may be associated with altered electrolytes (prolonged/excessive diarrhea, sweating, vomiting, thirst, appetite loss). Reduce dose 70–80% with impaired hepatic function. Use cautiously with impaired renal function. Bioavailability of 325 mg SR bid = 150 mg immediate release tid. Poorly metabolized by 10% population; reduce dose & monitor for toxicity.

**QUINIDINE  (◆Biquin Durules)** ▶LK ♀C ▶+ $$$-Gluconate, $-Sulfate

WARNING - Proarrhythmic. Increased mortality in patients with non-life threatening arrhythmias and structural heart disease (ie, MI, LV dysfunction).

ADULT - Arrhythmia: gluconate, extended-release: 324–648 mg PO q8–12h; sulfate, immediate-release: 200–400 mg PO q6–8h; sulfate, extended-release: 300–600 mg PO q8–12h. Consider inpatient rhythm and QT monitoring during initiation of therapy. Life-threatening malaria: Load with 10 mg/kg (max 600 mg) IV over 1–2 h, then 0.02 mg/kg/min for ≥24h. Dose given as quinidine gluconate. When parasitemia <1% and PO meds tolerated, convert to PO quinine to complete 3 d (Africa/South America) or 7 d (Southeast Asia). Also give doxycycline, tetracycline, or clindamycin.

PEDS - Not approved in children.

UNAPPROVED PEDS - Arrhythmia: Test dose (oral sulfate or IM/IV gluconate) 2 mg/kg (max 200 mg). Sulfate: 15–60 mg/kg/d PO divided q6h. Life-threatening malaria: Load with 10 mg/kg IV over 1–2 h, then 0.02 mg/kg/min × ≥24h. Dose given as quinidine gluconate. When parasitemia <1% and PO meds tolerated, convert to PO quinine to complete 3 d (Africa/South America) or 7 d (Southeast Asia). Also give doxycycline, tetracycline, or clindamycin.

FORMS - Generic gluconate: Tabs, extended-release non-scored 324 mg. Generic sulfate: Tabs, scored immediate-release 200, 300 mg, Tabs, extended-release 300 mg.

NOTES - QRS widening, QT interval prolongation (risk increased by hypokalemia, hypomagnesemia, or bradycardia), hypotension, hypoglycemia. Contraindicated with ziprasidone. Monitor EKG and BP. Drug interactions with some antiarrhythmics, digoxin, phenytoin, phenobarbital, rifampin, verapamil. Do not chew, break, or crush extended-release tabs. Do not use with digitalis toxicity, hypotension, AV/bundle branch block, or myasthenia gravis. Quinidine gluconate 267 mg = quinidine sulfate 200 mg.

## LDL CHOLESTEROL GOALS*

### Definitions

| | |
|---|---|
| Risk factors | "Risk factors": Cigarette smoking, HTN (BP ≥140/90 mm Hg or on antihypertensive meds), low HDL (<40 mg/dL), family hx of CHD (1 relative: male <55 yo, female <65 yo), age (male ≥45 yo, female ≥55 yo). |
| Lifestyle changes | "Lifestyle changes" refer to dietary modification, weight reduction, exercise. |
| Equivalent risk | "Equivalent risk" defined as diabetes, other atherosclerotic disease (peripheral artery disease, abdominal aortic aneurysm, symptomatic carotid artery disease), or multiple risk factors such that 10 yr risk >20%. |

| Risk Category | LDL Goal | Lifestyle Changes at LDL | Also Consider Meds at LDL |
|---|---|---|---|
| High risk: CHD or equivalent risk, 10-yr risk >20% | <100 mg/dL; optional <70 with very high risk factors | ≥100 mg/dL | ≥100 mg/dL (<100: consider Rx options) |
| Moderately-high risk: 2+ risk factors, 10-yr risk 10–20% | <130 mg/dL | ≥130 mg/dL | ≥130 mg/dL (100–129: consider Rx options) |
| Moderate risk: 2+ risk factors, 10-yr risk <10% | <130 mg/dL | ≥130 mg/dL | ≥160 mg/dL |
| Lower risk: 0–1 risk factor | <160 mg/dL | ≥160 mg/dL | ≥190 mg/dL (160–189: Rx optional) |

*All 10-yr risks based upon Framingham stratification; calculator available at: http://hin.nhlbi.nih.gov/atpiii/calculator.asp?usertype=prof. CHD=coronary heart disease. LDL=low density lipoprotein. Adapted from NCEP: *JAMA* 2001; 285:2486.

## LIPID REDUCTION BY CLASS/AGENT*

| Drug Class/ Agent | Specific Drugs | Low Density Lipoprotein (LDL) | High Density Lipoprotein (HDL) | Triglycerides |
|---|---|---|---|---|
| Bile acid sequestrants | Cholestyramine (4–16 g), colestipol (5–20 g), colesevelam (2.6–3.8 g) | decrease 15–30% | increase 3–5% | No change or increase |
| Cholesterol absorption inhibitor | Ezetimibe (10 mg). When added to statin therapy, will decrease LDL 25%, increase HDL 3%, decrease TG 14% in addition to statin effects. | decrease 18% | increase 1% | decrease 8% |
| Fibrates | Fenofibrate (145–200 mg), gemfibrozil (600 mg bid) | decrease 5–20% | increase 10–20% | decrease 20–50% |
| Lovastatin + extended release niacin | Advicor (20/1000–40/2000 mg) | decrease 30–42% | increase 20–30% | decrease 32–44% |
| Niacin | Extended release nicotinic acid (Niaspan 1–2 g), immediate release (crystalline) nicotinic acid (1.5–3 g), sustained release nicotinic acid (Slo-Niacin 1–2 g) | decrease 5–25% | increase 15–35% | decrease 20–50% |
| Omega 3 fatty acids | Omacor 4 g | No change or increase | increase 9% | decrease 45% |
| Statins | Atorvastatin (10–80 mg), fluvastatin (20–80 mg), lovastatin (20–80 mg), pravastatin (20–80 mg), rosuvastatin (5–40 mg), simvastatin (20–80 mg) | decrease 18–63% | increase 5–15% | decrease 7–35% |
| Simvastatin + ezetimibe | Vytorin 10/10–10/80 mg | decrease 45–60% | increase 6–10% | decrease 23–31% |

*Adapted from NCEP: *JAMA* 2001; 285:2486 and prescribing information.

**SOTALOL** (*Betapace, Betapace AF, ◆Rylosol*) ▶K ♀B ▶- $$$$
WARNING - Patients should be in a facility for ≥3 d with ECG monitoring, cardiac resuscitation available, and creatinine clearance calculated when initiating or re-initiating Betapace AF. Do not substitute Betapace for Betapace AF.
ADULT - Ventricular arrhythmia (Betapace), symptomatic A-fib/A-flutter (Betapace AF): Start 80

mg PO bid, usual maintenance dose 160–320 mg/d divided bid, max 640 mg/d.
PEDS - Not approved in children.
FORMS - Generic/Trade: Tabs, scored 80,120,160,240 mg, Tabs, scored (Betapace AF) 80,120,160 mg.
NOTES - Proarrhythmic. Caution, higher incidence of torsades de pointes with doses >320 mg/d, in women, or heart failure. Adjust dose if CrCl <60 mL/min.

## CARDIOVASCULAR: Anti-Hyperlipidemic Agents—Bile Acid Sequestrants

**CHOLESTYRAMINE** (*Questran, Questran Light, Prevalite, LoCHOLEST, LoCHOLEST Light*) ▶Not absorbed ♀C ▶+ $$$
ADULT - Elevated LDL cholesterol: Start 4 g PO daily-bid before meals, usual maintenance 12–24 g/d in divided doses bid-qid before meals, max 24 g/d.
PEDS - Not approved in children.
UNAPPROVED ADULT - Cholestasis-associated pruritus: 4–8 g bid-tid. Diarrhea: 4–16 g/d.
UNAPPROVED PEDS - Elevated LDL cholesterol: Start 240 mg/kg/d PO divided bid before meals, usual maintenance 8–16 g/d divided tid.
FORMS - Generic/Trade: Powder for oral susp, 4 g cholestyramine resin/9 g powder (Questran, LoCHOLEST), 4 g cholestyramine resin/5 g powder (Questran Light), 4 g cholestyramine resin/5.5 g powder (Prevalite, LoCHOLEST Light). Each available in bulk powder and single dose packets.
NOTES - Administer other drugs at least 1 h before or 4–6 h after cholestyramine to avoid decreased absorption of the other agent. BID dosing recommended, but may divide up to 6x/d. Mix powder with 60–180 mL of water, milk, fruit juice, or drink. Avoid carbonated liquids for mixing. GI problems common, mainly constipation. May cause elevated triglycerides; do not use when triglycerides >400 mg/dL.
**COLESEVELAM** (*Welchol*) ▶Not absorbed ♀B ▶+ $$$$$
ADULT - Glycemic control or type 2 diabetes or reduce elevated LDL cholesterol: 3 tabs PO bid with meals or 6 tabs once daily with a meal, max dose 6 tabs/d. Same dose when used with statins or other agents.

PEDS - Not approved in children.
FORMS - Trade only: Tabs, non-scored, 625 mg.
NOTES - Take with a full glass of water or other non-carbonated liquid. GI problems common, mainly constipation. May cause elevation of triglycerides. Do not use when triglycerides >500 mg/dL, or with a history of bowel obstruction or triglyceride-induced pancreatitis. Administer other drugs ≥4 h before colesevelam to avoid decreased absorption of the other agent; may decrease levels of glyburide, levothyroxine, oral contraceptives containing ethinyl estradiol and norethindrone, phenytoin, warfarin.
**COLESTIPOL** (*Colestid, Colestid Flavored*) ▶Not absorbed ♀B ▶+ $$$
ADULT - Elevated LDL cholesterol: Tabs: Start 2 g PO daily-bid, max 16 g/d. Granules: Start 5 g PO daily-bid, increase by 5 g increments as tolerated at 1–2 mo intervals, max 30 g/d.
PEDS - Not approved in children.
UNAPPROVED PEDS - 125–250 mg/kg/d PO in divided doses bid-qid, dosing range 10–20 g/d.
FORMS - Generic/Trade: Tab 1 g. Granules for oral susp, 5 g/7.5 g powder.
NOTES - Administer other drugs ≥1 h before or 4–6 h after colestipol to avoid decreased absorption of the other agent. Mix granules in at least 90 mL of water, milk, fruit juice, or drink. Avoid carbonated liquids for mixing. Swallow tabs whole with a full glass of liquid to avoid tab disintegration in the esophagus. GI problems common, mainly constipation. May cause elevated triglycerides; do not use when triglycerides >400 mg/dL.

## CARDIOVASCULAR: Anti-Hyperlipidemic Agents—HMG-CoA Reductase Inhibitors ("Statins") & Combinations

**NOTE:** Hepatotoxicity - monitor LFTs initially, approximately 12 wk after starting/titrating therapy, then annually or more frequently if indicated. May initiate, continue, or increase dose of statin with modest LFT elevation (<3 times upper limit of normal). Repeat LFTs and rule out other causes with isolated, asymptomatic LFT elevation >3 times upper limit of normal. Consider continuing vs. discontinuing statin or reducing statin dose. Patients with chronic liver disease, nonalcoholic fatty liver, or nonalcoholic steatohepatitis may receive statins. Discontinue statin with objective evidence of liver injury; seek cause; consider referral to gastroenterologist or hepatologist. Evaluate muscle symptoms & creatine kinase before starting therapy. Evaluate muscle symptoms 6–12 wk after starting/increasing therapy & at each follow-up visit. Obtain creatine kinase when patient complains of muscle soreness, tenderness, weakness, or pain. Teach patients to report promptly unexplained muscle pain, tenderness, or weakness; rule out common causes; discontinue if myopathy diagnosed or suspected. With tolerable muscle complaints or asymptomatic creatine kinase increase <10 times upper limit of normal, continue statin at same or reduced

(cont.)

dose; use symptoms to guide continuing/discontinuing statin. With intolerable muscle symptoms with/without creatine kinase elevation, discontinue statin; when asymptomatic, may restart same/different statin at same/lower dose. With rhabdomyolysis, discontinue statin, provide IV hydration; weigh risk/benefit of statin therapy when recovered. These factors increase risk of myopathy: advanced age (especially >80, women >men); multisystem disease (eg, chronic renal insufficiency, especially due to diabetes); multiple medications; perioperative periods; alcohol abuse; grapefruit juice (>1 quart/d); specific concomitant medications: fibrates (especially gemfibrozil), nicotinic acid (rare), cyclosporine, erythromycin, clarithromycin, itraconazole, ketoconazole, protease inhibitors, nefazodone, verapamil, amiodarone. Weigh potential risk of combination therapy against potential benefit.

**ADVICOR (lovastatin + niacin) ▶LK ♀X ▶- $$$$**
ADULT - Hyperlipidemia: 1 tab PO qhs with a low-fat snack. Establish dose using extended-release niacin first, or if already on lovastatin substitute combo product with lowest niacin dose.
PEDS - Not approved in children.
FORMS - Trade only: Tabs, non-scored extended release lovastatin/niacin 20/500, 20/750, 20/1000, 40/1000 mg.
NOTES - Do not exceed >40/2000 mg. Do not break, chew, or crush. Swallow whole. Aspirin or NSAID 30 min prior may decrease niacin flushing reaction. Niacin may worsen glucose control, peptic ulcer disease, gout, headaches, and menopausal flushing. Significantly lowers LDL-cholesterol and triglycerides, raises HDL-cholesterol. Do not use with potent inhibitors of cytochrome P450 3A4 enzyme system (clarithromycin, erythromycin, grapefruit juice >1 quart/d, HIV protease inhibitors, itraconazole, ketoconazole, nefazodone, telithromycin); increases risk of myopathy. Do not exceed 20 mg/d of lovastatin component when used with cyclosporine, danazol, fibrates, or niacin ≥1 g/d; do not exceed 40 mg/d of lovastatin component when used with amiodarone or verapamil. With concomitant cyclosporine or danazol, start with 10 mg daily of lovastatin component.

**ATORVASTATIN (Lipitor) ▶L ♀X ▶- $$$**
ADULT - Hyperlipidemia/prevention of cardiovascular events, including Type 2 DM: Start 10 mg PO daily, 40 mg daily for LDL-C reduction >45%, increase at ≥4-wk intervals to a max of 80 mg/d.
PEDS - Hyperlipidemia, ≥10 yr: Same as adult.
UNAPPROVED ADULT - Prevention of cardiovascular events & death post-acute coronary syndrome or with stable CAD, or prevention of stroke/cardiovascular events with recent stroke/TIA & no CHD: 80 mg PO daily.
FORMS - Trade only: Tabs, non-scored 10,20,40, 80 mg.
NOTES - Concomitant administration of azole antifungals, erythromycin, clarithromycin, cyclosporine, combinations of HIV protease inhibitors, nefazodone, fibrates, niacin, grapefruit and grapefruit juice increase the risk of myopathy and possible rhabdomyolysis. Do not exceed 10 mg/d when used with cyclosporine. Use >20 mg/d cautiously when used with clarithromycin or combinations of HIV protease inhibitors; increased risk of myopathy. May increase plasma levels of digoxin. Give either 1 h before or 4 h after colestipol or cholestyramine.

**CADUET (amlodipine + atorvastatin) ▶L ♀X ▶- $$$$**
ADULT - Simultaneous treatment of HTN and hypercholesterolemia: Establish dose using component drugs first. Dosing interval: daily
PEDS - Not approved in children.
FORMS - Trade only: Tabs, 2.5/10, 2.5/20, 2.5/40, 5/10, 5/20, 5/40, 5/80, 10/10, 10/20, 10/40, 10/80 mg.

**FLUVASTATIN (Lescol, Lescol XL) ▶L ♀X ▶- $$$**
ADULT - Hyperlipidemia: Start 20 mg PO qhs for LDL-C reduction of <25%, 40–80 mg qhs for LDL-C reduction of ≥25%, max 80 mg/d, give 80 mg daily (Lescol XL) or 40 mg bid. Prevention of cardiac events post percutaneous coronary intervention: 80 mg of extended release PO daily, max 80 mg daily.
PEDS - Hyperlipidemia: Start 20 mg PO qhs, max 80 mg daily (XL) or divided bid.
FORMS - Trade only: Caps, 20, 40 mg; tab, extended-release, non-scored 80 mg.
NOTES - Not metabolized substantially by the cytochrome P450 isoenzyme 3A4, so less potential for drug interactions. Increased risk of myopathy and rhabdomyolysis when used with a fibric acid agent, niacin, or colchicine. Give either 1 h before or 4 h after colestipol or cholestyramine.

**LOVASTATIN (Mevacor, Altoprev) ▶L ♀X ▶- $**
ADULT - Hyperlipidemia/prevention of cardiovascular events: Start 20 mg PO daily with the evening meal, increase at ≥4 wk intervals to max 80 mg/d (daily or divided bid). Altocor dosed daily with max dose 60 mg/d.
PEDS - Hyperlipidemia, ≥10 yr: Same as adult.
FORMS - Generic/Trade: Tabs, non-scored 20,40 mg. Trade only: Tabs, extended-release (Altoprev) 20,40,60 mg.
NOTES - Do not use with potent inhibitors of cytochrome P450 3A4 enzyme system (clarithromycin, erythromycin, grapefruit juice >1 quart/d, HIV protease inhibitors, itraconazole, ketoconazole, nefazodone, telithromycin); increases risk of myopathy. Do not exceed 20 mg/d when used with cyclosporine, danazol, fibrates, or niacin ≥1 g/d; do not exceed 40 mg/d when used with amiodarone or verapamil. With concomitant cyclosporine or danazol, start with 10 mg daily. Give either 1 h before or 4 h after colestipol or cholestyramine. Measure LFTs prior to starting if history of liver disease or if using ≥40 mg/d.

**PRAVASTATIN (Pravachol) ▶L ♀X ▶- $$$**
ADULT - Hyperlipidemia/prevention of cardiovascular events: Start 40 mg PO daily, increase

(cont.)

**PRAVASTATIN** (*cont.*)
at ≥4-wk intervals to max 80 mg/d. Renal or hepatic impairment: Start 10 mg PO daily.
PEDS - Hyperlipidemia, 8–13 yo: 20 mg PO daily. 14–18 yo: 40 mg PO daily.
FORMS - Generic/Trade: Tabs, non-scored 10, 20, 40, 80 mg. Generic only: Tabs 30 mg.
NOTES - Not metabolized substantially by the cytochrome P450 isoenzyme 3A4, less potential for drug interactions. Increased risk of myopathy and rhabdomyolysis when used with a fibric acid agent. Give either 1 h before or 4 h after colestipol or cholestyramine.

**ROSUVASTATIN** (*Crestor*) ▶L ♀X ▶- $$$$
ADULT - Hyperlipidemia/slow progression of atherosclerosis: Start 10 mg daily, may adjust dose after 2–4 wk. Do not start with 40 mg; use 40 mg only with severe hypercholesterolemia when treatment goal not achieved with 20 mg/d. Consider 20 mg starting dose when LDL-C >190 mg/dL. Severe renal impairment: Start 5 mg PO daily, max 10 mg/d. With predisposing factors for myopathy (renal impairment, advanced age, hypothyroidism): Start 5 mg PO daily. Asians: Start 5 mg PO daily, max 20 mg daily.
PEDS - Canada only: May use with age >8 yr with homozygous familial hypercholesterolemia. Specialist should supervise use.
FORMS - Trade only: Tabs, non-scored 5, 10, 20, 40 mg.
NOTES - Do not exceed 10 mg/d with severe renal impairment, gemfibrozil, or the combination of lopinavir and ritonavir. Do not exceed 5 mg/d with cyclosporine. Give aluminum & magnesium containing antacids >2 h after rosuvastatin. May potentiate effects of warfarin; monitor INR. Proteinuria, with unknown clinical significance, reported with 40 mg/d; consider dose reduction when using 40 mg/d with unexplained persistent proteinuria. May increase levels of ethinyl estradiol & norgestrel. Use cautiously with other drugs that may decrease levels/activity of endogenous steroid hormones (ketoconazole, spironolactone, cimetidine). Asians may have higher blood concentrations & more risk of side effects than Caucasians. Temporarily withhold with acute, serious condition suggestive of myopathy or predisposing to renal failure from rhabdomyolysis (eg, sepsis, hypotension, dehydration, major surgery, trauma, severe metabolic/endocrine/electrolyte disorders, uncontrolled seizures). Give either 1 h before or 4 h after colestipol or cholestyramine.

**SIMCOR** (simvastatin + niacin) ▶LK ♀X ▶- $$$
ADULT - Hyperlipidemia: 1 tab PO qhs with a low-fat snack. If niacin naïve or switching from immediate release niacin, start: 20/500 mg PO q pm. If receiving extended release niacin, do not start with > 40/2000 mg PO q pm. Max 40/2000 mg/d.
PEDS - Not approved in children.
FORMS - Trade only: Tabs, non-scored extended release simvastatin/niacin 20/500, 20/750, 20/1000 mg.
NOTES - Do not exceed >40/2000 mg. Do not break, chew, or crush. Swallow whole. Aspirin or NSAID 30 min prior may decrease niacin flushing reaction. Niacin may worsen glucose control, peptic ulcer disease, gout, headaches, and menopausal flushing. Significantly lowers LDL-cholesterol and triglycerides, raises HDL-cholesterol. Do not use with potent inhibitors of cytochrome P450 3A4 enzyme system (clarithromycin, erythromycin, grapefruit juice >1 quart/d, HIV protease inhibitors, itraconazole, ketoconazole, nefazodone, telithromycin); increases risk of myopathy. Do not use with cyclosporine, danazol, or fibrates. Do not exceed 20 mg/d of simvastatin component when used with amiodarone or verapamil. May increase INR when added to warfarin.

| STATINS* | Minimum Dose for 30–40% LDL Reduction | LDL | LFT Monitoring |
|---|---|---|---|
| | atorvastatin 10 mg | −39% | Baseline, 12 wk, semiannually |
| | fluvastatin 40 mg bid | −36% | Baseline, 8 wk |
| | fluvastatin XL 80 mg | −35% | Baseline, 8 wk |
| | lovastatin 40 mg | −31% | Baseline, 6 & 12 wk, semiannually |
| | pravastatin 40mg | −34% | Baseline, prior to dose increase |
| | rosuvastatin 5 mg | −45% | Baseline, 12 wk, semiannually |
| | simvastatin 20 mg | −38% | Get LFTs prior to & 3 mo after dose increase to 80 mg, then semiannually for first yr |

*Adapted from Circulation 2004;110:227–239. Data taken from prescribing information for primary hypercholesterolemia. LDL= low-density lipoprotein, LFT = liver function tests. Will get ~6% decrease in LDL with every doubling of dose. ACC/AHA/NHLBI schedule for LFT monitoring: baseline, ~12 wk after starting therapy, annually, when clinically indicated. Stop statin therapy if LFTs are >3 times upper limit of normal.

**♂SIMVASTATIN (Zocor)** ▶L ♀X ▶- $$$$
ADULT - Hyperlipidemia: Start 20–40 mg PO q pm.
Reduce cardiovascular mortality/events in high
risk for coronary heart disease event (existing
coronary heart disease, DM, peripheral vascular disease, history of stroke or cerebrovascular disease): 40 mg q pm. Increase prn at ≥4 wk
intervals to max 80 mg/d.
PEDS - Hyperlipidemia, ≥10 yr: Start 10 mg PO q
pm, max 40 mg/d.
FORMS - Generic/Trade: Tabs, non-scored 5, 10, 20,
40, 80 mg. Generic only: Orally disintegrating
tabs 10, 20, 40 ,80 mg.
NOTES - Do not use with potent inhibitors of cytochrome P450 3A4 enzyme system (clarithromycin,
erythromycin, grapefruit juice >1 quart/d, HIV
protease inhibitors, itraconazole, ketoconazole,
nefazodone, telithromycin); increases risk of
myopathy. Do not exceed 10 mg/d when used
with gemfibrozil, cyclosporine, danazol; or 20
mg/d when used with amiodarone or verapamil;
increased risk of myopathy. Use caution with
other fibrates, niacin ≥1 g/d; increases risk
of myopathy. Give either 1 h before or 4 h after
colestipol or cholestyramine.

**VYTORIN (ezetimibe + simvastatin)** ▶L ♀X ▶- $$$$
ADULT - Hyperlipidemia: Start 10/20 mg PO q pm,
max 10/80 mg/d. Start 10/40 if need >55% LDL
reduction.
PEDS - Not approved in children.
FORMS - Trade only: Tabs, non-scored ezetimibe/
simvastatin 10/10, 10/20, 10/40, 10/80 mg.

## CARDIOVASCULAR: Anti-Hyperlipidemic Agents—Other

**BEZAFIBRATE, ◆BEZALIP** ▶K ♀D ▶- $$$
ADULT - Canada only. Hyperlipidemia/hypertrig-
lyceridemia: 200 mg of immediate release PO
bid-tid, or 400 mg of sustained release PO q am
or q evening with or after food. Reduce dose in
renal insufficiency or dialysis. The 400 mg SR tab
should not be used if CrCl <60 mL/min or creat
>1.5 mg/dL.
PEDS - Not approved in children.
FORMS - Trade only: Immediate release tab: 200 mg.
Sustained release tab: 400 mg.
NOTES - Increased risk of myopathy and rhabdomy-
olysis when used with a statin. May increase the
effect of warfarin; reduce oral anticoagulant dose
by ~50%; monitor INR. Do not use in primary bil-
iary cirrhosis. Take either ≥2 h before or ≥4 h
after colestipol or cholestyramine.

**EZETIMIBE (Zetia, ◆Ezetrol)** ▶L ♀C ▶? $$$$
WARNING - May increase cyclosporine levels.
ADULT - Hyperlipidemia: 10 mg PO daily alone or in
combination with statin or fenofibrate.
PEDS - Not approved in children.
FORMS - Trade only: Tabs non-scored 10 mg
NOTES - Take either ≥2 h before or ≥4 h after
colestipol or cholestyramine. Monitor cyclospor-
ine levels (may increase). When used with statin,
monitor LFTs at initiation and then per statin
instructions.

**⌐FENOFIBRATE (TriCor, Antara, Lipofen, Triglide, ◆Lipidil
Micro, Lipidil Supra, Lipidil EZ)** ▶LK ♀C ▶- $$$
ADULT - Hypertriglyceridemia: Tricor tabs: Start
48–145 mg PO daily, max 145 mg/d. Antara:
43–130 mg PO daily; max 130 mg daily. Fenoglide:
40–120 mg PO daily; max 120 mg daily. Lipofen:
50–150 mg PO daily, max 150 mg daily. Lofibra:
54–200 mg PO daily, max 200 mg daily. Triglide:
50–160 mg PO daily, max 160 mg daily. Generic
tabs: 54–160 mg, max 160 mg daily. Generic
caps: 67–200 mg PO daily, max 200 mg daily.
Hypercholesterolemia/mixed dyslipidemia: Tricor
tabs: 145 mg PO daily. Antara: 130 mg PO
daily. Fenoglide: 120 mg daily. Lipofen: 150 mg
daily. Lofibra: 160–200 mg daily, max 200 mg
daily. Triglide: 160 mg daily. Generic tabs: 160
mg daily. Generic caps: 200 mg PO daily. Renal
impairment, elderly: Tricor tabs: Start 48 mg PO
daily; Antara: Start 43 mg PO daily; Fenoglide:
40 mg daily/Lipofen: Start 50 mg daily; Triglide:
Start 50 mg PO daily; generic tabs: Start 40–54
mg PO daily; generic caps 43 mg PO daily.
PEDS - Not approved in children.
FORMS - Generic only: Tabs, non-scored 54, 160
mg. Generic caps, 67, 134, 200 mg. Trade only:
Tricor tabs, non-scored 48,145 mg. Antara caps
43, 130 mg. Fenoglide non-scored tabs 40, 120
mg. Lipofen non-scored tabs 50,100,150 mg.
Lofibra tabs, non-scored 54, 160 mg. Triglide
tabs, non-scored 50, 160 mg. Lofibra caps, 67,
134, 200 mg.
NOTES - All formulations, except Antara, Tricor, and
Triglide, should be taken with food to increase
plasma concentrations. Conversion between
forms: Generic 200 mg cap with food = 145
mg Tricor; Antara 130 mg = 200 mg Lofibra or
generic under low-fat fed conditions; Lipofen 150
mg with food = Tricor 160 mg with food. Monitor
LFTs, dose related hepatotoxicity. Increased risk
of myopathy and rhabdomyolysis when used with
a statin. May increase the effect of warfarin,
monitor INR. Tricor 48 mg and 145 mg replaces
Tricor 54 mg and 160 mg.

**GEMFIBROZIL (Lopid)** ▶LK ♀C ▶? $$$
ADULT - Hypertriglyceridemia/primary prevention
of artery heart disease: 600 mg PO bid 30 min
before meals.
PEDS - Not approved in children.
FORMS - Generic/Trade: Tabs, scored 600 mg.
NOTES - Increased risk of myopathy and rhabdomy-
olysis when used with a statin or with moderate/
severe renal dysfunction. May increase the effect
of warfarin, monitor INR. Increased risk of hypo-
glycemia when used with repaglinide: avoid com-
bination use. Avoid itraconazole with combined
gemfibrozil and repaglinide.

ACE Inhibitor/Diuretic: Accuretic, Capozide, Inhibace Plus, Lotensin HCT, Monopril HCT, Prinzide, Uniretic, Vaseretic, Zestoretic.
ACE Inhibitor/Calcium Channel Blocker: Lexxel, Lotrel, Tarka.
Angiotensin Receptor Blocker/Diuretic: Atacand HCT, Avalide, Benicar HCT, Diovan HCT, Hyzaar, Micardis HCT, Teveten HCT.
Beta-blocker/Diuretic: Corzide, Inderide, Lopressor HCT, Tenoretic, Timolide, Ziac.
Diuretic Combinations: Aldactazide, Dyazide, Maxzide, Maxzide-25, Moduretic, Triazide.
Diuretic/Miscellaneous Antihypertensive: Aldoril, Apresazide, Chlorpres, Minizide, Renese-R, Ser-Ap-Es.
Other: BiDil.

## CARDIOVASCULAR: Antihypertensive Combinations

NOTE: Dosage should first be adjusted by using each drug separately. See component drugs for metabolism, pregnancy, and lactation.

*ACCURETIC* (quinapril + hydrochlorothiazide) ▶See component drugs ♀See component drugs ▶See component drugs $$
ADULT - HTN: Establish dose using component drugs first. Dosing interval: daily.
PEDS - Not approved in children.
FORMS - Generic/Trade: Tabs, 10/12.5, 20/12.5, 20/25 mg.

*ALDACTAZIDE* (spironolactone + hydrochlorothiazide) ▶See component drugs ♀See component drugs ▶See component drugs $$
ADULT - HTN: Establish dose using component drugs first. Dosing interval: daily-bid.
PEDS - Not approved in children.
FORMS - Generic/Trade: Tabs, non-scored 25/25. Trade only: Tabs, scored 50/50 mg.

*ALDORIL* (methyldopa + hydrochlorothiazide) ▶See component drugs ♀See component drugs ▶See component drugs $$
ADULT - HTN: Establish dose using component drugs first. Dosing interval: bid.
PEDS - Not approved in children.
FORMS - Generic only: Tabs, non-scored, 250/15, 250/25, 500/30 mg.

*APRESAZIDE* (hydralazine + hydrochlorothiazide) ▶See component drugs ♀See component drugs ▶See component drugs $$
ADULT - HTN: Establish dose using component drugs first. Dosing interval: bid.
PEDS - Not approved in children.
FORMS - Generic only: Caps 25/25, 50/50 mg.

*ATACAND HCT* (candesartan + hydrochlorothiazide, ✦Atacand Plus) ▶See component drugs ♀See component drugs ▶See component drugs $$$
ADULT - HTN: Establish dose using component drugs first. Dosing interval: daily.
PEDS - Not approved in children.
FORMS - Trade only: Tab, non-scored 16/12.5, 32/12.5, 32/25 mg.

*AVALIDE* (irbesartan + hydrochlorothiazide) ▶See component drugs ♀See component drugs ▶See component drugs $$$
ADULT - HTN: Establish dose using component drugs first. Dosing interval: daily. HTN, initial therapy for patients needing multiple medications: Start 150/12.5 PO daily, may increase after 1–2 wk, max 300/25 daily.

PEDS - Not approved in children.
FORMS - Trade only: Tabs, non-scored 150/12.5, 300/12.5, 300/25 mg.

*AZOR* (amlodipine + olmesartan) ▶See component drugs ♀See component drugs ▶See component drugs $$$
ADULT - HTN: Establish dose using component drugs first. Dosing interval: daily.
PEDS - Not approved in children.
FORMS - Trade only: Tabs, non-scored 5/20, 5/40, 10/20, 10/40 mg.

*BENICAR HCT* (olmesartan + hydrochlorothiazide) ▶See component drugs ♀See component drugs ▶See component drugs $$$
ADULT - HTN: Establish dose using component drugs first. Dosing interval: daily.
PEDS - Not approved in children.
FORMS - Trade only: Tabs, non-scored 20/12.5, 40/12.5, 40/25 mg.

*CAPOZIDE* (captopril + hydrochlorothiazide) ▶See component drugs ♀See component drugs ▶See component drugs $$
ADULT - HTN: Establish dose using component drugs first. Dosing interval: bid-tid.
PEDS - Not approved in children.
FORMS - Generic/Trade: Tabs, scored 25/15, 25/25, 50/15, 50/25 mg.

*CLORPRES* (clonidine + chlorthalidone) ▶See component drugs ♀See component drugs ▶See component drugs $$$$
ADULT - HTN: Establish dose using component drugs first. Dosing interval: bid-tid.
PEDS - Not approved in children.
FORMS - Trade only: Tabs, scored 0.1/15, 0.2/15, 0.3/15 mg.

*CORZIDE* (nadolol + bendroflumethiazide) ▶See component drugs ♀See component drugs ▶See component drugs $$$
ADULT - HTN: Establish dose using component drugs first. Dosing interval: daily.
PEDS - Not approved in children.
FORMS - Generic/Trade: Tabs 40/5, 80/5 mg.

*DIOVAN HCT* (valsartan + hydrochlorothiazide) ▶See component drugs ♀See component drugs ▶See component drugs $$$
ADULT - HTN: Establish dose using component drugs first. Dosing interval: daily.

**DIOVAN HCT** (*cont.*)
PEDS - Not approved in children.
FORMS - Trade only: Tabs, non-scored 80/12.5, 160/12.5, 320/12.5, 160/25, 320/25 mg.

**DYAZIDE (triamterene + hydrochlorothiazide)** ▶See component drugs ♀See component drugs ▶See component drugs $
ADULT - HTN: Establish dose using component drugs first. Dosing interval: daily.
PEDS - Not approved in children.
FORMS - Generic/Trade: Caps, (Dyazide) 37.5/25 mg. Generic only: Caps, 50/25 mg.
NOTES - Dyazide 37.5/25 cap same combination as Maxzide-25 tab.

**EXFORGE (amlodipine + valsartan)** ▶See component drugs ♀See component drugs ▶See component drugs $$$
ADULT - HTN: Establish dose using component drugs first. Dosing interval: daily. HTN, initial therapy for patients needing multiple medications: Start 5/160 PO daily, may increase after 1–2 wk, max 10/320 daily.
PEDS - Not approved in children.
FORMS - Trade only: Tabs, non-scored 5/160, 5/320, 10/160, 10/320 mg.

**HYZAAR (losartan + hydrochlorothiazide)** ▶See component drugs ♀See component drugs ▶See component drugs $$$
ADULT - HTN: Establish dose using component drugs first. Dosing interval: daily. Severe HTN: Start 50/12.5 PO daily, may increase to 100/25 PO daily after 2–4 wk. Stroke risk reduction in HTN & left ventricular hypertrophy (stroke risk reduction may not occur in Blacks): Establish dose using component drugs first. Dosing interval: daily.
PEDS - Not approved in children.
FORMS - Trade only: Tabs, non-scored 50/12.5, 100/12.5, 100/25 mg.

**INDERIDE (propranolol + hydrochlorothiazide)** ▶See component drugs ♀See component drugs ▶See component drugs $$
ADULT - HTN: Establish dose using component drugs first. Dosing interval: daily-bid.
PEDS - Not approved in children.
FORMS - Generic/Trade: Tabs, scored 40/25, 80/25 mg.
NOTES - Do not crush or chew cap contents. Swallow whole.

**INHIBACE PLUS (cilazapril + hydrochlorothiazide)** ▶See component drugs ♀See component drugs ▶See component drugs $$
ADULT - Canada only, HTN: Establish dose using component drugs first. Dosing interval daily.
PEDS - Not approved in children.
FORMS - Generic/Trade: Tabs, scored 5 mg cilazapril + 12.5 mg HCTZ.

**LEXXEL (enalapril + felodipine)** ▶See component drugs ♀See component drugs ▶See component drugs $$
ADULT - HTN: Establish dose using component drugs first. Dosing interval: daily.
PEDS - Not approved in children.
FORMS - Trade only: Tabs, non-scored 5/2.5, 5/5 mg.
NOTES - Do not crush or chew, swallow whole.

**LOPRESSOR HCT (metoprolol + hydrochlorothiazide)** ▶See component drugs ♀See component drugs ▶See component drugs $$$
ADULT - HTN: Establish dose using component drugs first. Dosing interval: daily-bid.
PEDS - Not approved in children.
FORMS - Generic/Trade: Tabs, scored 50/25, 100/25, 100/50 mg.

**LOTENSIN HCT (benazepril + hydrochlorothiazide)** ▶See component drugs ♀See component drugs ▶See component drugs $$
ADULT - HTN: Establish dose using component drugs first. Dosing interval: daily.
PEDS - Not approved in children.
FORMS - Generic/Trade: Tabs, scored 5/6.25, 10/12.5, 20/12.5, 20/25 mg.

**LOTREL (amlodipine + benazepril)** ▶See component drugs ♀See component drugs ▶See component drugs $$$
ADULT - HTN: Establish dose using component drugs first. Dosing interval: daily.
PEDS - Not approved in children.
FORMS - Generic/Trade: Cap, 2.5/10, 5/10, 5/20, 10/20 mg. Trade only: Cap, 5/40, 10/40 mg.

**MAXZIDE (triamterene + hydrochlorothiazide, ✦Triazide)** ▶See component drugs ♀See component drugs ▶See component drugs $
ADULT - HTN: Establish dose using component drugs first. Dosing interval: daily.
PEDS - Not approved in children.
FORMS - Generic/Trade: Tabs, scored (Maxzide-25) 37.5/25 (Maxzide) 75/50 mg.

**MAXZIDE-25 (triamterene + hydrochlorothiazide)** ▶See component drugs ♀See component drugs ▶See component drugs $
ADULT - HTN: Establish dose using component drugs first. Dosing interval: daily.
PEDS - Not approved in children.
FORMS - Generic/Trade: Tabs, scored (Maxzide-25) 37.5/25 mg, (Maxzide) 75/50 mg.

**MICARDIS HCT (telmisartan + hydrochlorothiazide, ✦Micardis Plus)** ▶See component drugs ♀See component drugs ▶See component drugs $$$
ADULT - HTN: Establish dose using component drugs first. Dosing interval: daily.
PEDS - Not approved in children.
FORMS - Trade only: Tabs, non-scored 40/12.5, 80/12.5, 80/25 mg.
NOTES - Swallow tabs whole, do not break or crush. Caution in hepatic insufficiency.

**MINIZIDE (prazosin + polythiazide)** ▶See component drugs ♀See component drugs ▶See component drugs $$$
ADULT - HTN: Establish dose using component drugs first. Dosing interval: bid-tid.
PEDS - Not approved in children.
FORMS - Trade only: Cap, 1/0.5, 2/0.5, 5/0.5 mg.

**MODURETIC (amiloride + hydrochlorothiazide, ✦Moduret)** ▶See component drugs ♀See component drugs ▶See component drugs $
ADULT - HTN: Establish dose using component drugs first. Dosing interval: daily.

(cont.)

**MODURETIC** *(cont.)*
PEDS - Not approved in children.
FORMS - Generic only: Tabs, scored 5/50 mg.
**MONOPRIL HCT (fosinopril + hydrochlorothiazide)**
▶See component drugs ♀See component drugs
▶See component drugs $$
ADULT - HTN: Establish dose using component drugs first. Dosing interval: daily.
PEDS - Not approved in children.
FORMS - Generic/Trade: Tabs, non-scored 10/12.5, scored 20/12.5 mg.
**PRINZIDE (lisinopril + hydrochlorothiazide)** ▶See component drugs ♀See component drugs ▶See component drugs $$
ADULT - HTN: Establish dose using component drugs first. Dosing interval: daily.
PEDS - Not approved in children.
FORMS - Generic/Trade: Tabs, non-scored 10/12.5, 20/12.5, 20/25 mg.
**TARKA (trandolapril + verapamil)** ▶See component drugs ♀See component drugs ▶See component drugs $$$
ADULT - HTN: Establish dose using component drugs first. Dosing interval: daily.
PEDS - Not approved in children.
FORMS - Trade only: Tabs, non-scored 2/180, 1/240, 2/240, 4/240 mg.
NOTES - Contains extended release form of verapamil. 'Do not chew or crush, swallow whole.
**TEKTURNA HCT (aliskiren + hydrochlorothiazide)**
▶See component drugs ♀See component drugs
▶See component drugs $$$
ADULT - HTN: Establish dose using component drugs first. Dosing interval: daily.
PEDS - Not approved in children.
FORMS - Trade only: Tabs, non-scored 150/12.5, 150/25, 300/12.5, 300/25 mg.
**TENORETIC (atenolol + chlorthalidone)** ▶See component drugs ♀See component drugs ▶See component drugs $
ADULT - HTN: Establish dose using component drugs first. Dosing interval: daily.
PEDS - Not approved in children.

FORMS - Generic/Trade: Tabs, scored 50/25, non-scored 100/25 mg.
**TEVETEN HCT (eprosartan + hydrochlorothiazide)**
▶See component drugs ♀See component drugs
▶See component drugs $$$
ADULT - HTN: Establish dose using component drugs first. Dosing interval: daily.
PEDS - Not approved in children.
FORMS - Trade only: Tabs, non-scored 600/12.5, 600/25 mg.
**UNIRETIC (moexipril + hydrochlorothiazide)** ▶See component drugs ♀See component drugs ▶See component drugs $$
ADULT - HTN: Establish dose using component drugs first. Dosing interval: daily-bid.
PEDS - Not approved in children.
FORMS - Generic/Trade: Tabs, scored 7.5/12.5, 15/12.5, 15/25 mg.
**VASERETIC (enalapril + hydrochlorothiazide)** ▶See component drugs ♀See component drugs ▶See component drugs $$
ADULT - HTN: Establish dose using component drugs first. Dosing interval: daily-bid.
PEDS - Not approved in children.
FORMS - Generic/Trade: Tabs, non-scored 5/12.5, 10/25 mg.
**ZESTORETIC (lisinopril + hydrochlorothiazide)** ▶See component drugs ♀See component drugs ▶See component drugs $$
ADULT - HTN: Establish dose using component drugs first. Dosing interval: daily.
PEDS - Not approved in children.
FORMS - Generic/Trade: Tabs, non-scored 10/12.5, 20/12.5, 20/25 mg.
**ZIAC (bisoprolol + hydrochlorothiazide)** ▶See component drugs ♀See component drugs ▶See component drugs $$
ADULT - HTN: Establish dose using component drugs first. Dosing interval: daily.
PEDS - Not approved in children.
FORMS - Generic/Trade: Tabs, non-scored 2.5/6.25, 5/6.25, 10/6.25 mg.

## CARDIOVASCULAR: Antihypertensives—Other

**ALISKIREN (Tekturna)** ▶LK ♀- ▶-? $$$
ADULT - HTN: 150 mg PO daily, max 300 mg/d.
PEDS - Not approved in children.
FORMS - Trade only: Tabs, non-scored 150, 300 mg.
NOTES - Not studied with severe renal impairment (creat ≥1.7 mg/dL for women, ≥2.0 mg/dL for men, and/or estimated GFR <30 mL/min), heart failure, or with max doses of ACEIs. Best absorbed on empty stomach. High fat meals decrease absorption. May decrease effects of furosemide. Monitor potassium and renal function when given with related medications (ie. ACEIs, ARBs). May increase creatine kinase, uric acid levels. Do not use with cyclosporine. Co-administration with potent P-glycoprotein inhibitors (ketoconazaone or avorvastatin) increase aliskiren levels.

**AMBRISENTAN (Letairis)** ▶L ♀X ▶-? $$$$$
WARNING - Hepatotoxicity; monitor LFTs prior to starting therapy & monthly thereafter; discontinue with LFTs > 5x upper limit of normal; LFT elevations and bilirubin >2x upper limit of normal; or signs/symptoms of liver dysfunction. Contraindicated in pregnancy due to birth defects; women of child bearing age must use ≥2 reliable methods of contraception. Women of childbearing age need pregnancy test prior to starting therapy & monthly thereafter.
ADULT - Pulmonary arterial hypertension: Start 5 mg PO daily; if tolerated, may increase to 10 mg/d.
PEDS - Not approved in children.
FORMS - Trade only: Tabs, unscored 5,10 mg.

**AMBRISENTAN** (cont.)
NOTES - Available only through access program by calling 866-664-5327. Monitor hemoglobin at initiation, after 1 mo of therapy, then periodically. Concomitant cyclosporine may increase levels; caution also with strong CYP3A-inhibitors (eg, ketoconazole), CYP2C19-inhibitors (eg, omeprazole), and inducers of P-gp, CYPs, and UGTs.

**DIAZOXIDE** (*Hyperstat, Proglycem*) ▶L ♀C ▶- $$$$$
ADULT - Severe HTN: 1–3 mg/kg (up to 150 mg) IV q5–15 min until BP is controlled. Hypoglycemia: initially 3 mg/kg/d PO divided equally q8h, usual maintenance dose 3–8 mg/kg/d divided equally q8–12 h, max 10–15 mg/kg/d.
PEDS - Severe HTN: same as adult. Hypoglycemia: neonates and infants, initially 10 mg/kg/d divided equally q8h, usual maintenance dose 8–15 mg/kg/d divided equally q8–12h; children, same as adult.
UNAPPROVED ADULT - Preeclampsia/eclampsia: 30 mg IV every few min until control of BP is achieved.
FORMS - Trade only: Susp 50 mg/mL (30 mL).
NOTES - Severe hyperglycemia possible. Monitor for edema and heart failure exacerbation during administration; diuretic therapy may be needed.

**FENOLDOPAM** (*Corlopam*) ▶LK ♀B ▶? $$$
ADULT - Severe HTN: 10 mg in 250 mL D5W (40 mcg/mL), start at 0.1 mcg/kg/min (for 70 kg adult = 11 mL/h), titrate q15 min, usual effective dose 0.1–1.6 mcg/kg/min. Lower initial doses (0.03–0.1 mcg/kg/min) associated with less reflex tachycardia.
PEDS - Reduce BP: Start 0.2 mcg/kg/min, increase by up to 0.3–0.5 mcg/kg/min q 20–30 min. Max infusion 0.8 mcg/kg/min. Administer in hospital by continuous infusion pump; use max 4 h; monitor BP & HR continuously. Refer to package insert for dilution instructions & infusion rates.
UNAPPROVED ADULT - Prevention of contrast nephropathy in those at risk (conflicting evidence of efficacy): Start 0.03 mcg/kg/min infusion 60 min prior to dye. Titrate infusion q15min up to 0.1 mcg/kg/min if BP tolerates. Maintain infusion (with concurrent saline) up to 4–6 h after procedure.
NOTES - Avoid combined use with beta blockers; if must be done, watch for sudden hypotension. Patients at high-risk for contrast nephropathy include age >70, creat >1.5 mg/dL, HTN, DM, heart failure. Use cautiously with glaucoma or increased intraocular HTN. Concurrent acetaminophen may increase fenoldopam levels.

**HYDRALAZINE** (*Apresoline*) ▶LK ♀C ▶+ $
ADULT - HTN: Start 10 mg PO bid-qid for 2–4 d, increase to 25 mg bid-qid, then 50 mg bid-qid if necessary, max 300 mg/d. Hypertensive emergency: 10–50 mg IM or 10–20 mg IV. Use lower doses initially & repeat prn to control BP. Preeclampsia/eclampsia: 5–10 mg IV initially, followed by 5–10 mg IV every 20–30 min as needed to control BP.

PEDS - Not approved in children.
UNAPPROVED ADULT - Heart failure: Start 10–25 mg PO tid, target dose 75 mg tid, max 100 mg tid. Use in combination with isosorbide dinitrate for patients intolerant to ACE inhibitors
UNAPPROVED PEDS - HTN: Start 0.75–1 mg/kg/d PO divided bid-qid, increase slowly over 3–4 wk up to 7.5 mg/kg/d; initial IV dose 1.7–3.5 mg/kg/d divided in 4–6 doses. HTN urgency: 0.1–0.2 mg/kg IM/IV q4–6 h as needed. Max single dose, 25 mg PO and 20 mg IV.
FORMS - Generic only: Tabs, non-scored 10, 25, 50, 100 mg.
NOTES - Headache, nausea, dizziness, tachycardia, peripheral edema, lupus-like syndrome. Usually used in combination with diuretic and beta-blocker to counter side effects.

**MECAMYLAMINE** (*Inversine*) ▶K ♀C ▶- $$$$$
ADULT - Severe HTN: Start 2.5 mg PO bid, increase as needed by 2.5 mg increments no sooner than every 2 d, usual maintenance dose 25 mg/d divided bid-qid.
PEDS - Not approved in children.
FORMS - Trade only: Tabs, scored, 2.5 mg.
NOTES - Orthostatic hypotension, especially during dosage titration. Monitor BP standing and supine. Rebound, severe hypertension with sudden drug withdrawal. Discontinue slowly and use other antihypertensives.

**METYROSINE** (*Demser*) ▶K ♀C ▶? $$$$$
ADULT - Pheochromocytoma: Start 250 mg PO qid, increase by 250–500 mg/d as needed, max dose 4 g/d.
PEDS - Pheochromocytoma >12 yo: Same as adult.
FORMS - Trade only: Caps, 250 mg.

**MINOXIDIL** (*Loniten*) ▶K ♀C ▶+ $$
ADULT - Refractory HTN: Start 2.5–5 mg PO daily, increase at no less than 3 d intervals, usual dose 10–40 mg daily, max 100 mg/d.
PEDS - Not approved in children <12 yo.
UNAPPROVED PEDS - HTN: Start 0.2 mg/kg PO daily, increase every 3 d as needed up to 0.25–1 mg/kg/d daily or divided bid; max 50 mg/d.
FORMS - Generic only: Tabs, scored 2.5, 10 mg.
NOTES - Edema, weight gain, hypertrichosis, may exacerbate heart failure. Usually used in combination with a diuretic and a beta-blocker to counteract side effects .

**NITROPRUSSIDE** (*Nipride, Nitropress*) ▶RBC's ♀C ▶- $
WARNING - May cause significant hypotension. Reconstituted solution must be further diluted before use. Cyanide toxicity may occur, especially with high infusion rates (10 mcg/kg/min), hepatic/renal impairment, and prolonged infusions (>3–7 d). Protect from light.
ADULT - Hypertensive emergency: 50 mg in 250 mL D5W (200 mcg/mL), start at 0.3 mcg/kg/min (for 70 kg adult = 6 mL/h) via IV infusion, titrate slowly, usual range 0.3–10 mcg/kg/min, max 10 mcg/kg/min.
PEDS - Severe HTN: Same as adult.

(cont.)

**NITROPRUSSIDE** (*cont.*)
   NOTES - Discontinue if inadequate response to 10 mcg/kg/min after 10 min. Cyanide toxicity with high doses, hepatic/renal impairment, and prolonged infusions, check thiocyanate levels. Protect IV infusion minibag from light.

**PHENOXYBENZAMINE** (*Dibenzyline*) ▶KL ♀C ▶? $$$$$
   ADULT - Pheochromocytoma: Start 10 mg PO bid, increase slowly qod as needed, usual dose 20–40 mg bid-tid, max 120 mg/d.
   PEDS - Not approved in children.
   UNAPPROVED PEDS - Pheochromocytoma: 0.2 mg/kg/d PO daily, initial dose ≤10 mg, increase slowly qod as needed, usual dose 0.4–1.2 mg/kg/d.
   FORMS - Trade only: Caps, 10 mg.
   NOTES - Patients should be observed after each dosage increase for symptomatic hypotension and other adverse effects. Do not use for essential HTN.

**PHENTOLAMINE** (*Regitine, Rogitine*) ▶Plasma ♀C ▶? $$$
   ADULT - Diagnosis of pheochromocytoma: 5 mg IV/IM. Rapid IV administration is preferred. An immediate, marked decrease in BP should occur, typically, 60 mm Hg SBP and 25 mm Hg DBP decrease in 2 min. HTN during pheochromocytoma surgery: 5 mg IV/IM 1–2h pre-op, 5 mg IV during surgery prn.
   PEDS - Diagnosis of pheochromocytoma: 0.05–0.1 mg/kg IV/IM, up to 5 mg per dose. Rapid IV administration is preferred. An immediate, marked decrease in BP should occur, typically, 60 mm Hg SBP and 25 mm Hg DBP decrease in 2 min. HTN during pheochromocytoma surgery: 0.05–0.1 mg/kg IV/IM 1–2h pre-op, repeat q2–4h prn.
   UNAPPROVED ADULT - IV extravasation of catecholamines: 5–10 mg in 10 mL NS, inject 1–5 mL SC (in divided doses) around extravasation site. Hypertensive crisis: 5–15 mg IV.
   UNAPPROVED PEDS - IV extravasation of catecholamines: neonates, 2.5–5 mg in 10 mL NS, inject 1 mL SC (in divided doses) around extravasation site; children, same as adult.
   NOTES - Weakness, flushing, hypotension; priapism with intracavernous injection. Use within 12h of extravasation. Distributed to hospital pharmacies, at no charge, only for use in life-threatening situations. Call (888) 669–6682 for ordering.

# CARDIOVASCULAR: Antiplatelet Drugs

**ABCIXIMAB** (*ReoPro*) ▶Plasma ♀C ▶? $$$$$
   ADULT - Platelet aggregation inhibition, prevention of acute cardiac ischemic events associated with PTCA: 0.25 mg/kg IV bolus over 1 min via separate infusion line 10–60 min before procedure, then 0.125 mcg/kg/min up to 10 mcg/min infusion for 12h. Unstable angina not responding to standard therapy when percutaneous coronary intervention (PCI) is planned within 24h: 0.25 mg/kg IV bolus over 1 min via separate infusion line, followed by 10 mcg/min IV infusion for 18–24h, concluding 1h after PCI.
   PEDS - Not approved in children.
   NOTES - Thrombocytopenia possible. Discontinue abciximab, heparin, and aspirin if uncontrollable bleeding occurs.

**AGGRENOX** (aspirin + dipyridamole) ▶LK ♀D ▶? $$$$
   ADULT - Prevention of stroke after TIA/stroke: 1 cap PO bid.
   PEDS - Not approved in children.
   FORMS - Trade only: Caps, 25 mg aspirin/200 mg extended-release dipyridamole.
   NOTES - Do not crush or chew Caps. May need supplemental aspirin for prevention of MI.

**CLOPIDOGREL** (*Plavix*) ▶LK ♀B ▶? $$$$
   WARNING - Rarely may cause life-threatening thrombotic thrombocytopenia purpura (TTP), usually during the first 2 wk of therapy.
   ADULT - Reduction of thrombotic events after recent AMI, recent stroke, established peripheral arterial disease: 75 mg PO daily. Acute coronary syndrome, non-ST segment elevation: 300 mg loading dose, then 75 mg PO daily in combination with aspirin PO daily. ST segment elevation MI: Start with/without 300 mg loading dose, then 75 mg PO daily in combination with aspirin, with/without thrombolytics.
   PEDS - Not approved in children.
   UNAPPROVED ADULT - Medical treatment, without stent, of unstable angina/non-ST segment elevation MI: 300–600 mg loading dose, then 75 mg daily in combination with aspirin for ≥1 mo and ideally up to 1 yr. Medical treatment, without stent and with/without thrombolytics, of ST segment elevation MI: 300 mg loading dose, then 75 mg daily in combination with aspirin for ≥14 d and up to 1 yr. Before/when percutaneous coronary intervention performed: 600 mg; consider using 300 mg if patient received thrombolytic within 12–24 h. Post bare metal stent placement: 75 mg daily in combination with aspirin for ≥1 mo and ideally up to 1 yr. Post drug eluting stent placement: 75 mg daily in combination with aspirin ≥1 yr (in patients not at high risk for bleeding). Post percutaneous coronary brachytherapy: 75 mg daily in combination with aspirin indefinitely. Acute coronary syndrome with aspirin allergy or reduction of thrombotic events in high-risk patient after TIA: 75 mg PO daily.
   FORMS - Generic/Trade: Tab, non-scored 75, 300 mg.
   NOTES - Prolongs bleeding time. Discontinue use 7 d before surgery, except in first yr post-coronary stent implantation. Loading dose 300 mg PO >6 h prior to procedure may be used for prevention of cardiac stent occlusion. Contraindicated with active pathologic bleeding (peptic ulcer or intracranial bleed). Concomitant ASA increases bleeding risk. Cardiovascular (but not stroke) patients may receive additional benefit when given with ASA. Should not be used with aspirin for primary prevention of cardiovascular events.

**DIPYRIDAMOLE (*Persantine*)** ▶L ♀B ▶? $$$
ADULT - Prevention of thromboembolic complications of cardiac valve replacement: 75–100 mg PO qid in combination with warfarin.
PEDS - Not approved in children <12 yo.
UNAPPROVED ADULT - Platelet aggregation inhibition: 150–400 mg/d PO divided tid-qid.
FORMS - Generic/Trade: Tabs, non-scored 25, 50, 75 mg.
NOTES - Not effective for angina; may cause chest pain when used in coronary artery disease.

**EPTIFIBATIDE (*Integrilin*)** ▶K ♀B ▶? $$$$$
ADULT - Acute coronary syndrome (unstable angina/non-ST-segment elevation MI): Load 180 mcg/kg IV bolus, then IV infusion 2 mcg/kg/min for up to 72 h. If percutaneous coronary intervention (PCI) occurs during the infusion, continue infusion for 18–24 h after procedure. PCI: Load 180 mcg/kg IV bolus just before procedure, followed by infusion 2 mcg/kg/min and a 2nd 180 mcg/kg IV bolus 10 min after the first bolus. Continue infusion for up to 18–24 h (minimum 12 h) after the procedure. Renal impairment (CrCl <50 mL/min): No change in bolus dose; decrease infusion to 1 mcg/kg/min. Obese patient (>121 kg): Max bolus dose 22.6 mg; max infusion rate 15 mg/h. Renal impairment and obese: Max bolus dose 22.6 mg; max infusion rate 7.5 mg/h.
PEDS - Not approved in children.
NOTES - Discontinue infusion prior to CABG. Thrombocytopenia possible. Concomitant aspirin & heparin/enoxaparin use recommended, unless contraindicated. Contraindicated in dialysis patients.

**TICLOPIDINE (*Ticlid*)** ▶L ♀B ▶? $$$$$
WARNING - May cause life-threatening neutropenia, agranulocytosis, and thrombotic thrombocytopenia purpura (TTP). TTP usually occurs during the first two wk of treatment. Monitor CBC routinely.
ADULT - Due to adverse effects, clopidogrel preferred. Platelet aggregation inhibition/reduction of thrombotic stroke: 250 mg PO bid with food. Prevention of cardiac stent occlusion: 250 mg PO bid in combo with aspirin 325 mg PO daily for up to 30 d post stent implantation.
PEDS - Not approved in children.
UNAPPROVED ADULT - Due to adverse effects, clopidogrel preferred. Prevention of graft occlusion with CABG: 250 mg PO bid.
FORMS - Generic/Trade: Tab, non-scored 250 mg.
NOTES - Check CBC every 2 wk during the first 3 mo of therapy. Neutrophil counts usually return to normal within 1–3 wk following discontinuation. Loading dose 500 mg PO on d 1 may be used for prevention of cardiac stent occlusion.

**TIROFIBAN (*Aggrastat*)** ▶K ♀B ▶? $$$$$
ADULT - Acute coronary syndromes (unstable angina and non-Q wave MI): Start 0.4 mcg/kg/min IV infusion for 30 min, then decrease to 0.1 mcg/kg/min for 48–108 h or until 12–24 h after coronary intervention.
PEDS - Not approved in children.
NOTES - Thrombocytopenia possible. Concomitant aspirin & heparin/enoxaparin use recommended, unless contraindicated. Dose heparin to keep PTT twice normal. Decrease bolus dose and rate of infusion by 50% in patients with CrCl <30 mL/min. Dilute concentrate solution before using.

## CARDIOVASCULAR: Beta Blockers

**NOTE:** See also antihypertensive combinations. Not first-line for HTN unless to treat angina, post-MI, left ventricular dysfunction. Abrupt discontinuation may precipitate angina, myocardial infarction, arrhythmias, or rebound hypertension; discontinue by tapering over 2 wk. Avoid using nonselective beta-blockers and use agents with beta-1 selectivity cautiously in asthma/COPD. Beta-1 selectivity diminishes at high doses. Avoid in decompensated heart failure, sick sinus syndrome, and severe peripheral artery disease. Avoid agents with intrinsic sympathomimetic activity post-AMI. May mask hypoglycemic response. Cross sensitivity between beta blockers can occur. Discontinue beta-blocker several d before discontinuing concomitant clonidine to minimize the risk of rebound hypertension. With pheochromocytoma, give beta blocker only after initiating alpha blocker; using beta blocker alone may increase BP due to the attenuation of beta-mediated vasodilatation in skeletal muscle. Some inhalation anesthetics may increase the cardiodepressant effect of beta-blockers. Concomitant amiodarone, digoxin, or non-dihydropyridine calcium channel blockers may increase risk of bradycardia.

**ACEBUTOLOL (*Sectral*, ✦*Rhotral*)** ▶LK ♀B ▶- $$
ADULT - HTN: Start 400 mg PO daily or 200 mg PO bid, usual maintenance 400–800 mg/d, max 1200 mg/d. Twice daily dosing appears to be more effective than daily dosing.
PEDS - Not approved in children <12.
UNAPPROVED ADULT - Angina: Start 200 mg PO bid, increase as needed up to 800 mg/d.
FORMS - Generic/Trade: Caps, 200, 400 mg.
NOTES - Has mild intrinsic sympathomimetic activity (partial beta agonist activity). Beta1 receptor selective.

**ATENOLOL (*Tenormin*)** ▶K ♀D ▶- $
WARNING - Avoid abrupt cessation in coronary heart disease or HTN.
ADULT - Acute MI: 5 mg IV over 5 min, repeat in 10 min, follow with 50 mg PO 10 min after IV dosing in patients tolerating the total IV dose, increase as tolerated to 100 mg/d given daily or divided bid. HTN: Start 25–50 mg PO daily or divided bid, max 100 mg/d. Renal impairment, elderly: Start 25 mg PO daily, increase as needed. Angina: Start 50 mg PO daily or divided bid, increase as needed to max of 200 mg/d.

(cont.)

**ATENOLOL** *(cont.)*
PEDS - Not approved in children.
UNAPPROVED ADULT - Reduce perioperative cardiac events (death) in high risk patients undergoing noncardiac surgery: Start 5–10 mg IV prior to anesthesia, then 50–100 mg PO daily during hospitalization (max 7 d). Maintain HR between 55–65 bpm. Hold dose for HR <55 bpm and SBP <100 mm Hg. Reentrant PSVT associated w/ST-elevation MI (after carotid massage, IV adenosine): 2.5–5 mg over 2 min to 10 mg max over 10–15 min. Rate control of atrial fibrillation/flutter: Start 25 mg PO daily, titrate to desired heart rate.
UNAPPROVED PEDS - HTN: 1–1.2 mg/kg/dose PO daily, max 2 mg/kg/d.
FORMS - Generic/Trade: Tabs, non-scored 25, 100 mg; scored, 50 mg.
NOTES - Doses >100 mg/d usually do not provide further BP lowering. Beta1 receptor selective. Risk of hypoglycemia to neonates born to mothers using atenolol at parturition or while breastfeeding. May be less effective for HTN than other beta-blockers.

**BETAXOLOL** *(Kerlone)* ▶LK ♀C ▶? $$
ADULT - HTN: Start 5–10 mg PO daily, max 20 mg/d. Renal impairment, elderly: Start 5 mg PO daily, increase as needed.
PEDS - Not approved in children.
FORMS - Generic/Trade: Tabs, scored 10 mg, non-scored 20 mg.
NOTES - Beta1 receptor selective.

**BISOPROLOL** *(Zebeta, ✦Monocor)* ▶LK ♀C ▶? $$
ADULT - HTN: Start 2.5–5 mg PO daily, max 20 mg/d. Renal impairment: Start 2.5 mg PO daily, increase as needed.
PEDS - Not approved in children.
UNAPPROVED ADULT - Compensated heart failure: Start 1.25 mg PO daily, double dose every 2 wk as tolerated to max 10 mg/d. Reduce perioperative cardiac events (death, MI) in high risk patients undergoing noncardiac surgery: Start 5 mg PO daily, at least 1 wk prior to surgery, increase to 10 mg daily to maintain HR <60 bpm, continue for 30 d postop. Hold dose for HR <50 bpm or SBP <100 mm Hg.
FORMS - Generic/Trade: Tabs, scored 5 mg, non-scored 10 mg.
NOTES - Monitor closely for heart failure exacerbation and hypotension when titrating dose. Avoid in decompensated heart failure (ie, NYHA class IV heart failure or pulmonary edema). Stabilize dose of digoxin, diuretics, and ACEI before starting bisoprolol. Beta1 receptor selective.

**CARVEDILOL** *(Coreg, Coreg CR)* ▶L ♀C ▶? $$$$
ADULT - Heart failure: immediate release: Start 3.125 mg PO bid, double dose q2 wk as tolerated up to max of 25 mg bid (if <85 kg) or 50 mg bid (if >85 kg). Heart failure, sustained release: Start 10 mg PO daily, double dose q2 wk as tolerated up to max of 80 mg/d. Reduce cardiovascular risk in post-MI with LV dysfunction, immediate release: Start 3.125–6.25 mg PO bid, double dose

q 3–10 d as tolerated to max of 25 mg bid. LV dysfunction post-MI, sustained release: Start 10–20 mg PO daily, double dose q 3–10 d as tolerated to max of 80 mg/d. HTN, immediate release: Start 6.25 mg PO bid, double dose q7–14 d as tolerated to max 50 mg/d. HTN, sustained release: Start 20 mg PO daily, double dose q7–14 d as tolerated to max 80 mg/d.
PEDS - Not approved in children.
FORMS - Generic/Trade: Tabs, immediate-release non-scored 3.125, 6.25, 12.5, 25 mg. Trade only: Caps, extended-release 10, 20, 40, 80 mg.
NOTES - Avoid in asthma, hepatic impairment, and acute decompensated heart failure (ie, requiring IV inotropes or pulmonary edema). Monitor closely for heart failure exacerbation and hypotension (particularly orthostatic) when titrating dose. Stabilize dose of digoxin, diuretics, and ACEI before starting carvedilol. Reduce the dose with bradycardia (<55 beats/min). May reversibly elevate LFTs. Take with food to decrease orthostatic hypotension. Separate Coreg CR and alcohol (including medications containing alcohol) by at least 2 h. Give Coreg CR in the morning. The contents of Coreg CR may be sprinkled over applesauce and consumed immediately. Dosing conversion from immediate release to sustained release: 3.125 mg bid = 10 mg CR; 6.25 mg bid = 20 mg CR; 12.5 mg bid = 40 mg CR; 25 mg bid = 80 mg CR.

**ESMOLOL** *(Brevibloc)* ▶K ♀C ▶? $
ADULT - SVT/HTN emergency: Mix infusion 5 g in 500 mL (10 mg/mL), load with 500 mcg/kg IV over 1 min (70 kg: 35 mg or 3.5 mL) then IV infusion 50 mcg/kg/min for 4 min (70 kg: 100 mcg/kg/min = 40 mL/h). If optimal response is not attained, repeat IV load and increase IV infusion to 100 mcg/kg/min for 4 min. If necessary, additional boluses (500 mcg/kg/min over 1 min) may be given followed by IV infusion with increased dose by 50 mcg/kg/min for 4 min. Max IV infusion rate 200 mcg/kg/min.
PEDS - Not approved in children.
UNAPPROVED PEDS - Same schedule as adult except loading dose 100–500 mcg/kg IV over 1 min and IV infusion 25–100 mcg/kg/min. IV infusions may be increased by 25–50 mcg/kg/min every 5–10 min. Titrate dose based on patient response.
NOTES - Hypotension. Beta1 receptor selective. Half-life = 9 min.

**LABETALOL** *(Trandate)* ▶LK ♀C ▶+ $$$
ADULT - HTN: Start 100 mg PO bid, usual maintenance dose 200–600 mg bid, max 2400 mg/d. HTN emergency: Start 20 mg slow IV injection, then 40–80 mg IV q10min as needed up to 300 mg total cumulative dose or start 0.5–2 mg/min IV infusion, adjust rate as needed up to total cumulative dose 300 mg.
PEDS - Not approved in children.
UNAPPROVED PEDS - HTN: 4 mg/kg/d PO divided bid, increase as needed up to 40 mg/kg/d. IV:

**LABETALOL** (*cont.*)
Start 0.3–1 mg/kg/dose (max 20 mg) slow IV injection q10 min or 0.4–1 mg/kg/h IV infusion up to 3 mg/kg/h.
FORMS - Generic/Trade: Tabs, scored 100, 200, 300 mg.
NOTES - Hypotension. Contraindicated in asthma/COPD. Alpha1, beta1, and beta2 receptor blocker.

**METOPROLOL** (*Lopressor, Toprol-XL, ✦Betaloc*) ▶L ♀C ▶? $$
WARNING - Avoid abrupt cessation in ischemic heart disease or HTN.
ADULT - Acute MI: 5 mg IV q5–15 min up to 15 mg, then start 50 mg PO q6h for 48h, then 100 mg PO bid as tolerated. If usual IV dose is not tolerated, start 25–50 mg PO q6h. If early IV therapy is contraindicated, patient should be titrated to 100 mg PO bid as soon as possible. HTN (immediate release): Start 100 mg PO daily or in divided doses, increase as needed up to 450 mg/d; may require multiple daily doses to maintain 24 h BP control. HTN (extended release): Start 25–100 mg PO daily, increase as needed q 1 wk up to 400 mg/d. Heart failure: Start 12.5–25 mg (extended-release) PO daily, double dose every 2 wk as tolerated up to max 200 mg/d. Angina: Start 50 mg PO bid (immediate release) or 100 mg PO daily (extended-release), increase as needed up to 400 mg/d.
PEDS - HTN ≥6 yo: Start 1 mg/kg, max 50 mg/daily. Not recommended <6 yo.
UNAPPROVED ADULT - Heart failure: Start 6.25 PO bid, max 75 mg bid. Atrial tachyarrhythmia, except with Wolff-Parkinson-White syndrome: 2.5–5 mg IV q2–5 min as needed to control rapid ventricular response, max 15 mg over 10–15 min. Reentrant PSVT (after carotid massage, IV adenosine): 2.5–5 mg q 2–5 min to 15 mg max over 10–15 min. Reduce perioperative cardiac events (death) in high-risk patients undergoing noncardiac surgery: Start 100 mg (extended release) 2 h prior to anesthesia, then 50–100 mg (extended release) PO daily or 2.5–5 mg IV q6 h during hospitalization (max 7 d). Maintain HR between 55–65 bpm. Hold dose for HR <55 bpm and SBP <100 mm Hg. Rate control of atrial fibrillation/flutter: Start 25 mg PO bid, titrate to desired heart rate.
FORMS - Generic/Trade: Tabs, scored 50, 100 mg, extended-release 25, 50, 100, 200 mg. Generic only: Tabs, scored 25 mg.
NOTES - Monitor closely for heart failure exacerbation and hypotension when titrating dose. Avoid use in patients with decompensated heart failure (ie, NYHA class IV heart failure or pulmonary edema. Stabilize dose of digoxin, diuretics, and ACEI before starting metoprolol. Beta1 receptor selective. Extended-release tabs may be broken in half, but do not chew or crush. Avoid using extended release tabs with verapamil, diltiazem, or peripheral vascular disease. May need lower doses in elderly. Monitor BP with potent CYP 2D6

inhibitors that may increase levels (eg, bupropion, cimetidine, diphenhydramine, fluoxetine, hydroxychloroquine, paroxetine, propafenone, quinidine, thioridazine, ritonavir, terbinafine). Take with food.

**NADOLOL** (*Corgard*) ▶K ♀C ▶- $$
ADULT - HTN: Start 20–40 mg PO daily, usual maintenance dose 40–80 mg/d, max 320 mg/d. Renal impairment: Start 20 mg PO daily, adjust dosage interval based on severity of renal impairment - CrCl 31–50 mL/min, q24–36h; CrCl 10–30 mL/min, q24–48h; CrCl <10 mL/min, q40–60h. Angina: Start 40 mg PO daily, usual maintenance dose 40–80 mg/d, max 240 mg/d.
PEDS - Not approved in children.
UNAPPROVED ADULT - Prevent rebleeding esophageal varices: 40–160 mg/d PO. Titrate dose to reduce heart rate to 25% below baseline. Ventricular arrhythmia: 10–640 mg/d PO.
FORMS - Generic/Trade: Tabs, scored 20, 40, 80, 120, 160 mg.
NOTES - Beta1 and beta2 receptor blocker.

**NEBIVOLOL** (*Bystolic*) ▶L ♀C ▶- $$$
WARNING - Avoid abrupt cessation in coronary heart disease or HTN.
ADULT - HTN: Start 5 mg PO daily, max 40 mg/d. Severe renal impairment (CrCl <30 mL/min), moderate hepatic impairment: Start 2.5 mg PO daily, increase cautiously.
PEDS - Not approved in children.
FORMS - Trade only: Tabs, non-scored 2.5, 5, 10 mg.
NOTES - Do not use with severe liver impairment.

**OXPRENOLOL** (✦ *Trasicor, Slow-Trasicor*) ▶L ♀D ▶- $$
ADULT - Canada only. Mild to moderate HTN, usually in combination with a thiazide-type diuretic: Regular release: Initially 20 mg PO tid, titrate upwards prn to usual maintenance 120–320 mg/d divided bid-tid. Alternatively, may substitute an equivalent daily dose of sustained release product; do not exceed 480 mg/d.
PEDS - Not approved in children.
FORMS - Trade only: Regular release tabs: 40, 80 mg. Sustained release tabs: 80, 160 mg.
NOTES - Caution in bronchospasm, diabetes, or heart failure. Has mild intrinsic sympathomimetic activity (partial beta agonist activity). No dose adjustment in impaired renal function. Empty matrix of sustained release tab may be excreted and found in the feces.

**PENBUTOLOL** (*Levatol*) ▶LK ♀C ▶? $$$$
ADULT - HTN: Start 20 mg PO daily, usual maintenance dose 20–40 mg, max 80 mg/d.
PEDS - Not approved in children.
FORMS - Trade only: Tabs, scored 20 mg.
NOTES - Has mild intrinsic sympathomimetic activity (partial beta agonist activity). Beta1 and beta2 receptor blocker.

**PINDOLOL** (✦ *Visken*) ▶K ♀B ▶? $$$
ADULT - HTN: Start 5 mg PO bid, usual maintenance dose 10–30 mg/d, max 60 mg/d.

(cont.)

**PINDOLOL (cont.)**
PEDS - Not approved in children.
UNAPPROVED ADULT - Angina: 15–40 mg/d PO in divided doses tid-qid.
FORMS - Generic only: Tabs, scored 5, 10 mg.
NOTES - Has intrinsic sympathomimetic activity (partial beta agonist activity). Beta1 and beta2 receptor blocker. Contraindicated with thioridazine.

**PROPRANOLOL (Inderal, Inderal LA, InnoPran XL) ▶L ♀C ▶+ $$**
WARNING - Avoid abrupt cessation in coronary heart disease or HTN.
ADULT - HTN: Start 20–40 mg PO bid, usual maintenance dose 160–480 mg/d, max 640 mg/d; extended-release (Inderal LA): start 60–80 mg PO daily, usual maintenance dose 120–160 mg/d, max 640 mg/d; extended-release (InnoPran XL): start 80 mg qhs (10 PM), max 120 mg qhs. Angina: Start 10–20 mg PO tid/qid, usual maintenance 160–240 mg/d, max 320 mg/d; extended-release (Inderal LA): start 80 mg PO daily, same usual dosage range and max for HTN. Migraine prophylaxis: Start 40 mg PO bid or 80 mg PO daily (extended-release), max 240 mg/d. Supraventricular tachycardia or rapid atrial fibrillation/flutter: 10–30 mg PO tid-qid. MI: 180–240 mg/d PO in divided doses bid-qid. Pheochromocytoma surgery: 60 mg PO in divided doses bid-tid beginning 3 d before surgery, use in combination with an alpha blocking agent. IV: reserved for life-threatening arrhythmia, 1–3 mg IV, repeat dose in 2 min if needed, additional doses should not be given in <4h. Not for use in hypertensive emergency. Essential tremor: Start 40 mg PO bid, titrate prn to 120–320 mg/d.
PEDS - HTN: Start 1 mg/kg/d PO divided bid, usual maintenance dose 2–4 mg/kg/d PO divided bid, max 16 mg/kg/d.

UNAPPROVED ADULT - Prevent rebleeding esophageal varices: 20–180 mg PO bid. Titrate dose to reduce heart rate to 25% below baseline. Control heart rate with A-fib: 80–240 mg/d daily or in divided doses.
UNAPPROVED PEDS - Arrhythmia: 0.01–0.1 mg/kg/dose (max 1 mg/dose) by slow IV push. Manufacturer does not recommend IV propranolol in children.
FORMS - Generic/Trade: Tabs, scored 40, 60, 80. Caps, extended-release 60, 80, 120, 160 mg. Generic only: Solution 20 & 40 mg/5 mL. Tabs, 10, 20 mg. Trade only: (InnoPran XL qhs) 80, 120 mg.
NOTES - Beta1 and beta2 receptor blocker. Do not substitute extended-release product for immediate-release product on mg-for-mg basis. Dosage titration may be necessary with extended-release product when converting from immediate-release Tabs. Extended-release Caps (Inderal LA) may be opened, and the contents sprinkled on food for administration. Cap contents should be swallowed whole without crushing or chewing. Contraindicated with thioridazine. InnoPran XL is a chronotherapeutic product; give at bedtime to blunt early morning surge in BP. Concomitant use of alcohol may increase propranolol levels.

**TIMOLOL (Blocadren) ▶LK ♀C ▶+ $$$**
ADULT - HTN: Start 10 mg PO bid, usual maintenance 20–40 mg/d, max 60 mg/d. MI: 10 mg PO bid, started 1–4 wk post-MI. Migraine headaches: Start 10 mg PO bid, use 20 mg/d daily or divided bid for prophylaxis, increase as needed up to max 60 mg/d. Stop therapy if satisfactory response not obtained after 6–8 wk of max dose.
PEDS - Not approved in children.
UNAPPROVED ADULT - Angina: 15–45 mg/d PO divided tid-qid.
FORMS - Generic only: Tabs, 5, 10, 20 mg.
NOTES - Beta1 and beta2 receptor blocker.

## CARDIOVASCULAR: Calcium Channel Blockers (CCBs)—Dihydropyridines

**NOTE:** See also antihypertensive combinations. Peripheral edema, especially with higher doses. Extended/controlled/sustained-release tabs should be swallowed whole; do not chew or crush. Avoid concomitant grapefruit/grapefruit juice, which may enhance effect. Avoid in decompensated heart failure.

**AMLODIPINE (Norvasc) ▶L ♀C ▶? $$$**
ADULT - HTN: Start 2.5 to 5 mg PO daily, max 10 daily. Coronary artery disease: Start 5 mg PO daily, usual maintenance dose 10 mg PO daily.
PEDS - HTN (6–17 yo): 2.5–5 mg PO daily.
UNAPPROVED PEDS - HTN: Start 0.1–0.2 mg/kg/d PO daily, max 0.3 mg/kg/d.
FORMS - Generic/Trade: Tabs, non-scored 2.5, 5, 10 mg. Generic only: Orally disintegrating tabs 2.5, 5, 10 mg.

**FELODIPINE (Plendil, ◆Renedil) ▶L ♀C ▶? $$**
ADULT - HTN: Start 2.5–5 mg PO daily, usual maintenance dose 5–10 mg/d, max 10 mg/d.
PEDS - Not approved in children.
FORMS - Generic/Trade: Tabs, extended-release, non-scored 2.5, 5, 10 mg.
NOTES - Extended-release tab. May increase tacrolimus concentration; monitor level.

**ISRADIPINE (DynaCirc, DynaCirc CR) ▶L ♀C ▶? $$$$**
ADULT - HTN: Start 2.5 mg PO bid, usual maintenance 5–10 mg/d, max 20 mg/d divided bid (max 10 mg/d in elderly). Controlled-release (DynaCirc CR): Start 5 mg PO daily, usual maintenance dose 5–10 mg/d, max 20 mg/d.
PEDS - Not approved in children.
FORMS - Trade only: Tabs, controlled-release 5, 10 mg. Generic only: Immediate release caps 2.5, 5 mg.

**NICARDIPINE (Cardene, Cardene SR) ▶L ♀C ▶? $$**
ADULT - HTN: sustained-release (Cardene SR), Start 30 mg PO bid, usual maintenance dose 30–60 mg PO bid, max 120 mg/d; immediate-release, Start 20 mg PO tid, usual maintenance dose 20–40 mg PO tid, max 120 mg/d. Hypertensive emergency/short-term management of acute HTN: Begin IV infusion at 5 mg/h, titrate infusion rate by 2.5

**NICARDIPINE** *(cont.)*

mg/h q15min as needed, max 15 mg/h. Angina: immediate-release, Start 20 mg PO tid, usual maintenance dose 20–40 mg tid.

PEDS - Not approved in children.

UNAPPROVED PEDS - HTN: 0.5–3 mcg/kg/min IV infusion.

FORMS - Generic/Trade: Caps, immediate-release 20, 30 mg. Trade only: Caps, sustained-release 30, 45, 60 mg.

NOTES - Hypotension, especially with immediate-release Caps and IV. Decrease dose if hepatically impaired. Use sustained-release Caps for HTN only, not for angina.

**NIFEDIPINE** *(Procardia, Adalat, Procardia XL, Adalat CC, ✦Adalat XL, Adalat PA)* ▶L ♀C ▶+ $$

ADULT - HTN: extended-release, Start 30–60 mg PO daily, max 120 mg/d. Angina: extended-release, Start 30–60 mg PO daily, max 120 mg/d; immediate-release, Start 10 mg PO tid, usual maintenance dose 10–20 mg tid, max 120 mg/d.

PEDS - Not approved in children.

UNAPPROVED ADULT - Preterm labor: loading dose 10 mg PO q20–30 min if contractions persist up to 40 mg within the first h. After contractions are controlled, maintenance dose: 10–20 mg PO q4–6h or 60–160 mg extended release PO daily. Duration of treatment has not been established. Promotes spontaneous passage of

ureteral calculi: extended release, 30 mg PO daily × 10–28 d.

UNAPPROVED PEDS - HTN: 0.25–0.5 mg/kg/dose PO q4–6 h as needed, max 10 mg/dose or 3 mg/kg/d. Doses <0.25 mg/kg may be effective.

FORMS - Generic/Trade: Caps, 10, 20 mg. Tabs, extended-release 30, 60, 90 mg.

NOTES - Immediate-release cap should not be chewed and swallowed or given sublingually; may cause excessive hypotension, stroke. Do not use immediate-release caps for treating HTN, hypertensive emergencies, or ST-elevation MI. Extended-release tabs can be substituted for immediate-release caps at the same dose in patients whose angina is controlled.

**NISOLDIPINE** *(Sular)* ▶L ♀C ▶? $$$

ADULT - HTN: Start 17 mg PO daily, may increase by 8.5 mg weekly, max 34 mg/d. Impaired hepatic function, elderly: Start 8.5 mg PO daily, titrate as needed.

PEDS - Not approved in children.

UNAPPROVED ADULT - Not approved in children.

FORMS - Trade only: Tabs, extended-release 8.5, 17, 25.5, 34 mg. These replace the former 10, 20, 30, 40 mg tabs.

NOTES - Take on an empty stomach. Sular 8.5, 17, 25.5, 34 mg replace 10, 20, 30, 40 mg respectively.

## CARDIOVASCULAR: Calcium Channel Blockers (CCBs)—Other

**NOTE:** See also antihypertensive combinations. Avoid in decompensated heart failure or 2nd/3rd degree heart block.

**DILTIAZEM** *(Cardizem, Cardizem LA, Cardizem CD, Cartia XT, Dilacor XR, Diltiazem CD, Diltzac, Diltia XT, Tiazac, Taztia XT)* ▶L ♀C ▶+ $$

ADULT - Atrial fibrillation/flutter, PSVT: 20 mg (0.25 mg/kg) IV bolus over 2 min. If needed and patient tolerated IV bolus with no hypotension, rebolus 15 min later with 25 mg (0.35 mg/kg). IV infusion: Start 10 mg/h, increase by 5 mg/h (usual range 5–15 mg/h). Once daily, extended-release (Cardizem CD, Cartia XT, Dilacor XR, Diltia XT, Taztia XT, Tiazac); HTN: Start 120–240 mg PO daily, usual maintenance range 240–360 mg/d, max 540 mg/d. Once daily, graded extended-release (Cardizem LA), HTN: Start 180–240 mg, max 540 mg/d. Twice daily, sustained-release (Cardizem SR), HTN: Start 60–120 mg PO bid, max 360 mg/d. Immediate-release, angina: Start 30 mg PO qid, max 360 mg/d divided tid-qid. Extended-release, angina: 120–180 mg PO daily, max 540 mg/d. Once daily, graded extended-release (Cardizem LA), angina: Start 180 mg PO daily, doses >360 mg may provide no additional benefit.

PEDS - Not approved in children. Diltiazem injection should be avoided in neonates due to potential toxicity from benzyl alcohol in the injectable product .

UNAPPROVED ADULT - Control heart rate with A-fib: 120–360 mg/d daily or in divided doses.

UNAPPROVED PEDS - HTN: Start 1.5–2 mg/kg/d PO divided tid-qid, max 3.5 mg/kg/d.

FORMS - Generic/Trade: Tabs, immediate-release, non-scored (Cardizem) 30, scored 60, 90, 120 mg; Caps, extended-release (Cardizem CD, Cartia XT daily) 120, 180, 240, 300, 360 mg, (Diltzac, Taztia XT, Tiazac daily) 120, 180, 240, 300, 360, 420 mg, (Dilacor XR, Diltia XT) 120, 180, 240 mg. Trade only: Tabs, extended-release graded (Cardizem LA daily) 120, 180, 240, 300, 360, 420 mg.

NOTES - Contraindicated in acute MI and pulmonary congestion, hypotension, sick sinus syndrome without pacemaker, second or third degree AV block without pacemaker, Wolff-Parkinson-White syndrome with rapid A-fib/flutter. Contents of extended-release caps may be sprinkled over food. Do not chew or crush cap contents. May accumulate with hepatic impairment; dose based on clinical response. Cardizem LA is a chrono-therapeutic product; give at bedtime to blunt early morning surge in BP. May increase levels of buspirone, quinidine.

**VERAPAMIL** *(Isoptin SR, Calan, Covera-HS, Verelan, Verelan PM, ✦Veramil)* ▶L ♀C ▶+ $$

ADULT - SVT: 5–10 mg (0.075–0.15 mg/kg) IV over 2 min. A 2nd dose of 10 mg IV may be given 15–30 min later if needed. PSVT/rate control with atrial fibrillation: 240–480 mg/d PO divided tid-qid.

**(cont.)**

**VERAPAMIL** (cont.)

Angina: Start 40–80 mg PO tid-qid, max 480 mg/d; sustained-release (Isoptin SR, Calan SR, Verelan), start 120–240 mg PO daily, max 480 mg/d (use bid dosing for doses >240 mg/d with Isoptin SR and Calan SR); extended-release (Covera-HS), start 180 mg PO qhs, max 480 mg/d. HTN: Same as angina, except (Verelan PM) start 100–200 mg PO qhs, max 400 mg/d; (Covera-HS) start 180 mg PO qhs, max 480 mg/d; immediate-release tabs should be avoided in treating HTN.

PEDS - SVT: (1–15 yo) 2–5 mg (0.1–0.3 mg/kg) IV, max dose 5 mg. Repeat dose once in 30 min if needed, max 2nd dose 10 mg. Immediate-release and sustained-release tabs not approved in children.

FORMS - Generic/Trade: Tabs, immediate-release, scored (Calan) 40, 80, 120 mg; Tabs, sustained-release, non-scored (Isoptin SR) 120, scored 180, 240 mg; Caps, sustained-release (Verelan)

120,180, 240, 360 mg; Caps, extended-release (Verelan PM) 100, 200, 300 mg. Trade only: Tabs, extended-release (Covera HS) 180, 240 mg.

NOTES - Contraindicated in severe LV dysfunction, hypotension, sick sinus syndrome, second or third degree AV block without pacemaker, A-fib/flutter conducted via accessory pathway (ie, Wolff-Parkinson-White). Avoid concomitant grapefruit juice (enhances effect). Scored, sustained-release tabs (Calan SR, Isoptin SR) may be broken and each piece swallowed whole, do not chew or crush. Other extended-release tabs (Covera HS) should be swallowed whole. Contents of sustained-release caps may be sprinkled on food (eg, apple sauce). Do not chew or crush cap contents. Coadministration with aspirin may increase bleeding times. Use cautiously with impaired renal/hepatic function. Covera-HS and Verelan PM are chronotherapeutic products; give at bedtime to blunt early morning surge in BP.

## CARDIOVASCULAR: Diuretics—Carbonic Anhydrase Inhibitors

**ACETAZOLAMIDE** (*Diamox, Diamox Sequels*) ▶LK ♀C ▶+ $
ADULT - Glaucoma: 250 mg PO up to qid (immediate release) or 500 mg PO up to bid (sustained release). Max 1g/d. Acute glaucoma: 250 mg IV q4h or 500 mg IV initially with 125–250 mg q4h, followed by oral therapy. Mountain sickness prophylaxis: 125–250 mg PO bid-tid, beginning 1–2 d prior to ascent and continuing ≥5 d at higher altitude. Edema: Rarely used, start 250–375 mg IV/PO qam given intermittently (qod or 2 consecutive d followed by none for 1–2 d) to avoid loss of diuretic effect.
PEDS - Diuretic: 5 mg/kg PO/IV qam.
UNAPPROVED PEDS - Glaucoma: 8–30 mg/kg/d PO, divided tid. Acute glaucoma: 5–10 mg/kg IV every 6h.

FORMS - Generic only: Tabs, 125, 250 mg. Trade only (Sequels): Caps, extended-release 500 mg.
NOTES - A susp (250 mg/5 mL) can be made by crushing and mixing tabs in flavored syrup. The susp is stable for 7 d at room temperature. One tab may be softened in 2 teaspoons of hot water, then add to 2 teaspoons of honey or syrup, and swallowed at once. Tabs and compounded susp may have a bitter taste. Use cautiously in sulfa allergy. Prompt descent is necessary if severe forms of high altitude sickness occur (eg, pulmonary or cerebral edema). Test the drug for tolerance/allergies 1–2 wk before initial dosing prior to ascent.

## CARDIOVASCULAR: Diuretics—Loop

**NOTE:** Give 2nd dose of bid schedule in mid afternoon to avoid nocturia. Rare hypersensitivity in patients allergic to sulfa-containing drugs, except ethacrynic acid.

**BUMETANIDE** (*Bumex, ✦Burinex*) ▶K ♀C ▶? $
ADULT - Edema: 0.5–2 mg PO daily, repeat doses at 4–5 h intervals as needed until desired response is attained, max 10 mg/d; 0.5–1 mg IV/IM, repeat doses at 2–3 h intervals as needed until desired response is attained, max 10 mg/d. Dosing for 3–4 consecutive d followed by no drug for 1–2 d is acceptable. BID dosing may enhance diuretic effect. IV injections should be over 1–2 min. An IV infusion may be used, change bag every 24 h.
PEDS - Not approved in children.
UNAPPROVED PEDS - Edema: 0.015–0.1 mg/kg/dose PO/IV/IM daily or qod.
FORMS - Generic/Trade: Tabs, scored 0.5, 1, 2 mg.
NOTES - 1 mg bumetanide is roughly equivalent to 40 mg oral furosemide. IV administration is preferred when GI absorption is impaired.

**ETHACRYNIC ACID** (*Edecrin*) ▶K ♀B ▶? $$$
ADULT - Edema: 0.5–1 mg/kg IV, max 100 mg/dose; 25 mg PO daily on d one, followed by 50 mg PO bid on d two, followed by 100 mg PO in the morning and 50–100 mg PO in the evening depending on the response to the morning dose, max 400 mg/d.
PEDS - Not approved in children.
UNAPPROVED ADULT - HTN: 25 mg PO daily, max 100 mg/d divided bid-tid.
UNAPPROVED PEDS - Edema: 1 mg/kg IV; 25 mg PO daily, increase slowly by 25 mg increments as needed. Ethacrynic acid should not be administered to infants.
FORMS - Trade only: Tabs, scored 25 mg.
NOTES - Rarely used. Ototoxicity possible. Does not contain a sulfonamide group; may be useful in sulfonamide-allergic patients. Do not administer

**ETHACRYNIC ACID** (*cont.*)

SC or IM due to local irritation. IV ethacrynic acid should be reconstituted to a concentration of 50 mg/mL and given slowly by IV infusion over 20–30 min. May increase lithium levels.

**FUROSEMIDE** (*Lasix*) ▶K ♀C ▶? $

ADULT - Edema: Start 20–80 mg IV/IM/PO, increase dose by 20–40 mg every 6–8h until desired response is achieved, max 600 mg/d. Give maintenance dose daily or divided bid. IV infusion: 0.05 mg/kg/h, titrate rate to desired response. HTN: Start 20–40 mg bid, adjust dose as needed based on BP response. Use lower doses in elderly. Thiazide diuretics generally preferred for HTN.

PEDS - Edema: 0.5–2 mg/kg/dose IV/IM/PO q6–12h, max 6 mg/kg/dose. IV infusion: 0.05 mg/kg/h, titrate rate to achieve desired response.

FORMS - Generic/Trade: Tabs, non-scored 20, scored 40, 80 mg. Generic only: Oral solution 10 mg/mL, 40 mg/5 mL.

NOTES - Loops are diuretic of choice with decreased renal function (CrCl <30 mL/min or creat >2.5 mg/dL). Oral absorption may decrease in acute heart failure exacerbation. Bioequivalence of oral form is 50% of IV dose. Monitor renal function in elderly.

**TORSEMIDE** (*Demadex*) ▶LK ♀B ▶? $

ADULT - Edema: Start 5–20 mg IV/PO daily, double dose as needed to desired response, max 200 mg as a single dose. HTN: Start 5 mg PO daily, increase as needed every 4–6 wk, max 100 mg PO daily or divided bid. Thiazide diuretics generally preferred for HTN.

PEDS - Not approved in children.

FORMS - Generic/Trade: Tabs, scored 5, 10, 20, 100 mg.

NOTES - Loop diuretics are agent of choice for edema with decreased renal function (CrCl <30 mL/min or creat >2.5 mg/dl).

## CARDIOVASCULAR: Diuretics—Potassium Sparing

**NOTE:** See also antihypertensive combinations and aldosterone antagonists. Beware of hyperkalemia. Use cautiously with other agents that may cause hyperkalemia (ie, ACEIs, ARBs).

**AMILORIDE** (*Midamor*) ▶LK ♀B ▶? $$

ADULT - Diuretic-induced hypokalemia: Start 5 mg PO daily, increase prn, max 20 mg/d. Edema/HTN: Start 5 mg PO daily in combination with another diuretic, usually a thiazide for HTN, increase prn, max 20 mg/d. Other diuretics may need to be added when treating edema.

PEDS - Not approved in children.

UNAPPROVED ADULT - Hyperaldosteronism: 10–40 mg PO daily. Do not use combination product (Moduretic) for treatment of hyperaldosteronism.

UNAPPROVED PEDS - Edema: 0.625 mg/kg daily for children weighing 6–20 kg.

FORMS - Generic only: Tabs, non-scored 5 mg.

NOTES - Spironolactone is generally preferred for treating primary hyperaldosteronism.

**TRIAMTERENE** (*Dyrenium*) ▶LK ♀B ▶- $$$

ADULT - Edema (cirrhosis, nephrotic syndrome, heart failure): Start 100 mg PO bid, max 300 mg/d. Most patients can be maintained on 100 mg PO daily or qod after edema is controlled. Other diuretics may be needed.

PEDS - Not approved in children.

UNAPPROVED PEDS - Edema: 4 mg/kg/d divided bid after meals, increase to 6 mg/kg/d if needed, max 300 mg/d.

FORMS - Trade only: Caps 50, 100 mg.

NOTES - Combo product with HCTZ (eg, Dyazide, Maxide) available for HTN.

## CARDIOVASCULAR: Diuretics—Thiazide Type

**NOTE:** See also antihypertensive combinations. Possible hypersensitivity in sulfa allergy. Should be used for most patients with HTN, alone or combined with other anti-hypertensive agents. Thiazides are not recommended for pregnancy-induced HTN. Coadministration with NSAIDS, including selective COX-2 inhibitors, may reduce the antihypertensive, diuretic, and natriuretic effects of thiazides. Thiazide-induced hypokalemia is associated with increased fasting blood glucose and new onset diabetes; target potassium ≥4.0 mg/dL to decrease risk; may use thiazide in combination with oral potassium supplementation, ACE inhibitor, ARB, or potassium-sparing diuretic to maintain K+ level.

**CHLOROTHIAZIDE** (*Diuril*) ▶L ♀C, D if used in pregnancy-induced HTN ▶+ $

ADULT - HTN: Start 125–250 mg PO daily or divided bid, max 1000 mg/d divided bid. Edema: 500–2000 mg PO/IV daily or divided bid. Dosing on alternate d or for 3–4 consecutive d followed by no drug for 1–2 d is acceptable.

PEDS - Edema: Infants: Start 10–20 mg/kg/d PO daily or divided bid, up to 30 mg/kg/d divided bid. Children 6 mo-2 yo: 10–20 mg/kg/d PO daily or divided bid, max 375 mg/d. Children 2–12 yo: start 10–20 mg/kg/d PO daily or divided bid,

up to 1g/d. IV formulation not recommended for infants or children.

FORMS - Trade only: Susp 250 mg/5 mL. Generic only: Tabs, scored 250, 500 mg.

NOTES - Do not administer SC or IM.

**CHLORTHALIDONE** (*Thalitone*) ▶L ♀B, D if used in pregnancy-induced HTN ▶+ $

ADULT - HTN: For generics, start 12.5–25 mg PO daily, usual maintenance dose 12.5–50 mg/d, max 50 mg/d. For Thalitone, start 15 mg PO daily, usual maintenance 30–45 mg/d, max 50 mg/d. Edema: For generics, start 50–100 mg PO daily

**(cont.)**

**CHLORTHALIDONE** (*cont.*)
after breakfast or 100 mg qod or 100 mg 3 times/ wk, usual maintenance dose 150–200 mg/d, max 200 mg/d. For Thalitone, start 30–60 mg PO daily or 60 mg qod, usual maintenance dose 90–120 mg PO daily or qod.
PEDS - Not approved in children.
UNAPPROVED ADULT - Nephrolithiasis: 25–50 mg PO daily.
UNAPPROVED PEDS - Edema: 2 mg/kg PO 3 times weekly.
FORMS - Trade only: Tabs, non-scored (Thalitone) 15 mg. Generic only: Tabs non-scored 25, 50 mg.
NOTES - Thalitone has greater bioavailability than generic forms, do not interchange. Doses greater than 50 mg/d for HTN are usually associated with hypokalemia with little added BP control.
**HYDROCHLOROTHIAZIDE** (*HCTZ, Esidrix, Oretic, Microzide, HydroDiuril*) ▶L ♀B, D if used in pregnancy-induced HTN ▶+ $
ADULT - HTN: Start 12.5–25 mg PO daily, usual maintenance dose 12.5–25 mg/d, max 50 mg/d. Edema: 25–100 mg PO daily or in divided doses or 50–100 mg PO qod or 3–5 d/wk, max 200 mg/d.
PEDS - Edema: 1–2 mg/kg/d PO daily or divided bid, max 37.5 mg/d in infants up to 2 yo, max 100 mg/d in children 2–12 yo.
UNAPPROVED ADULT - Nephrolithiasis: 50–100 mg PO daily.
FORMS - Generic/Trade: Tabs, scored 25, 50 mg; Cap 12.5 mg.
NOTES - Doses as low as 6.25 mg daily may be effective in combination with other antihypertensives. Doses ≥50 mg/d for HTN may cause hypokalemia with little added BP control.

**INDAPAMIDE** (*Lozol, ✦Lozide*) ▶L ♀B, D if used in pregnancy-induced HTN ▶? $
ADULT - HTN: Start 1.25–2.5 mg PO daily, max 5 mg/d. Edema/Heart failure: 2.5–5 mg PO qam.
PEDS - Not approved in children.
FORMS - Generic only: Tabs, non-scored 1.25, 2.5 mg.
**METHYCLOTHIAZIDE** (*Enduron*) ▶L ♀B, D if used in pregnancy-induced HTN ▶? $
ADULT - HTN: Start 2.5 mg PO daily, usual maintenance dose 2.5–5 mg/d. Edema: Start 2.5 mg PO daily, usual maintenance dose 2.5–10 mg/d.
PEDS - Not approved in children.
FORMS - Generic/Trade: Tabs, scored, 2.5, 5 mg.
NOTES - May dose qod or 3–5 d/wk as maintenance therapy to control edema.
**METOLAZONE** (*Zaroxolyn*) ▶L ♀B, D if used in pregnancy-induced HTN ▶? $$$
ADULT - Edema (heart failure, renal disease): 5–10 mg PO daily, max 10 mg/d in heart failure, 20 mg/d in renal disease. If used with loop diuretic, start with 2.5 mg PO daily. Reduce to lowest effective dose as edema resolves. May be given qod as edema resolves.
PEDS - Not approved in children.
UNAPPROVED PEDS - Edema: 0.2–0.4 mg/kg/d daily or divided bid.
FORMS - Generic/Trade: Tabs 2.5, 5, 10 mg.
NOTES - Generally used for heart failure, not HTN. When used with furosemide or other loop diuretics, administer metolazone 30 min before IV loop diuretic. Cross-allergy may occur if allergic to sulfonamides or thiazides.

| CARDIAC PARAMETERS AND FORMULAS | Normal |
|---|---|
| Cardiac output (CO) = heart rate× stroke volume | 4–8 L/min |
| Cardiac index (CI) = CO/BSA | 2.8–4.2 L/min/m$^2$ |
| MAP (mean arterial press) = [(SBP − DBP)/3] + DBP | 80–100 mm Hg |
| SVR (systemic vasc resis) = (MAP − CVP) × (80)/CO | 800–1200 dyne/sec/cm$^5$ |
| PVR (pulm vasc resis) = (PAM − PCWP) × (80)/CO | 45–120 dyne/sec/cm$^5$ |
| QTc = QT/square root of RR | 0.38–0.42 |
| Right atrial pressure (central venous pressure) | 0–8 mm Hg |
| Pulmonary artery systolic pressure (PAS) | 20–30 mm Hg |
| Pulmonary artery diastolic pressure (PAD) | 10–15 mm Hg |
| Pulmonary capillary wedge pressure (PCWP) | 8–12 mm Hg (post-MI ~16 mm Hg) |

# CARDIOVASCULAR: Nitrates

**NOTE:** Avoid if systolic BP <90 mm Hg or ≥30 mm Hg below baseline, severe bradycardia (<50 bpm), tachycardia (>100 bpm) or right ventricular infarction. Avoid in those who have received erectile dysfunction therapy in the last 24 (sildenafil, vardenafil) to 48 (tadalafil) h.

**AMYL NITRITE** ▶LUNG ♀X ▶- $
ADULT - Angina: 0.3 mL inhaled as needed.
PEDS - Not approved in children.
NOTES - May cause headache and flushing. Flammable. Avoid use in areas with open flames. To avoid syncope, use only when lying down.

**ISOSORBIDE DINITRATE** (*Isordil, Dilatrate-SR, ✦Cedocard SR, Coronex*) ▶L ♀C ▶? $
ADULT - Acute angina: 2.5–10 mg SL or chewed immediately, repeat as needed every 5–10 min up to 3 doses in 30 min. SL and chew Tabs may be used prior to events likely to provoke angina. Angina prophylaxis: Start 5–20 mg PO tid (7 am, noon, & 5 pm), max 40 mg tid. Sustained-release (Dilatrate SR): Start 40 mg PO bid, max 80 mg PO bid (8 am & 2 pm).

**ISOSORBIDE DINITRATE (cont.)**

PEDS - Not approved in children.

UNAPPROVED ADULT - Heart failure: 10–40 mg PO tid, max 80 mg tid. Use in combination with hydralazine.

FORMS - Generic/Trade: Tabs, scored 5, 10, 20, 30 mg. Trade only: Tabs, (Isordil) 40 mg, Cap, extended-release (Dilatate-SR) 40 mg. Generic only: Tab, sustained-release 40 mg, Tab, sublingual 2.5, 5 mg.

NOTES - Headache possible. Use SL or chew Tabs for an acute angina attack. Extended-release tab may be broken, but do not chew or crush, swallow whole; do not use for acute angina. Allow for a nitrate-free period of 10–14 h each d to avoid nitrate tolerance.

**ISOSORBIDE MONONITRATE (ISMO, Monoket, Imdur)** ▶L ♀C ▶? $$

ADULT - Angina: 20 mg PO bid (8 am and 3 pm). Extended-release (Imdur): Start 30–60 mg PO daily, max 240 mg/d.

PEDS - Not approved in children.

FORMS - Generic/Trade: Tabs, non-scored (ISMO, bid dosing) 20 mg, scored (Monoket, bid dosing) 10, 20 mg, extended-release, scored (Imdur, daily dosing) 30, 60, non-scored 120 mg.

NOTES - Headache. Extended-release tab may be broken, but do not chew or crush, swallow whole. Do not use for acute angina.

**NITROGLYCERIN INTRAVENOUS INFUSION (Tridil)** ▶L ♀C ▶? $

ADULT - Perioperative HTN, acute MI/heart failure, acute angina: mix 50 mg in 250 mL D5W (200 mcg/mL), start at 10–20 mcg/min IV (3–6 mL/h), then titrate upward by 10–20 mcg/min every 3–5 min until desired effect is achieved.

PEDS - Not approved in children.

UNAPPROVED ADULT - Hypertensive emergency: Start 10–20 mcg/min IV infusion, titrate up to 100 mcg/min. Antihypertensive effect is usually evident in 2–5 min. Effect may persist for only 3–5 min after infusion is stopped.

UNAPPROVED PEDS - IV infusion: start 0.25–0.5 mcg/kg/min, increase by 0.5–1 mcg/kg/min q3–5 min as needed, max 5 mcg/kg/min.

FORMS - Brand name "Tridil" no longer manufactured, but retained herein for name recognition.

NOTES - Nitroglycerin migrates into polyvinyl chloride (PVC) tubing. Use lower initial doses (5 mcg/min) with non-PVC tubing. Use with caution in inferior/right ventricular myocardial infarction. Nitroglycerin-induced venodilation can cause severe hypotension.

**NITROGLYCERIN OINTMENT (Nitro-BID)** ▶L ♀C ▶? $

ADULT - Angina prophylaxis: Start 0.5 inch q8h applied to non-hairy skin area, maintenance 1–2 inches q8h, max 4 inches q4–6h.

PEDS - Not approved in children.

FORMS - Trade only: Ointment, 2%, tubes 1,30,60g (Nitro-BID).

NOTES - 1 inch ointment is approximately 15 mg nitroglycerin. Allow for a nitrate-free period

of 10–14 h each d to avoid nitrate tolerance. Generally change to oral tabs or transdermal patch for long-term therapy. Do not use topical therapy (ointment, transdermal system) for acute angina.

**NITROGLYCERIN SPRAY (Nitrolingual, NitroMist)** ▶L ♀C ▶? $$$$

ADULT - Acute angina: 1–2 sprays under the tongue at the onset of attack, repeat as needed, max 3 sprays in 15 min. A dose may be given 5–10 min before activities that might provoke angina.

PEDS - Not approved in children.

FORMS - Trade only: Nitrolingual solution, 4.9, 12 mL. 0.4 mg/spray (60 or 200 sprays/canister); NitroMist aerosol 0.4 mg/spray (230 sprays/canister)

NOTES - May be preferred over SL tabs in patients with dry mouth. Patient can see how much medicine is left in the upright bottle. Nitrolingual: replace bottle when fluid is below level of center tube; NitroMist: replace bottle when fluid reaches the bottom of the hole in the side of the container. Before initial use, prime pump: Nitrolingual - spray 5 times into air (away from self and others); NitroMist – spray 10 times into air (away from self and others). Prime at least once every 6 wk if not used: Nitrolingual spray 1 time into the air (away from self and others); NitroMist spray 2 times into the air (away from self and others). Do not shake NitroMist before using.

**NITROGLYCERIN SUBLINGUAL (Nitrostat, NitroQuick)** ▶L ♀C ▶? $

ADULT - Acute angina: 0.4 mg under tongue or between the cheek and gum, repeat dose every 5 min as needed up to 3 doses in 15 min. A dose may be given 5–10 min before activities that might provoke angina.

PEDS - Not approved in children.

FORMS - Generic/Trade: Sublingual tabs, non-scored 0.3, 0.4, 0.6 mg; in bottles of 100 or package of 4 bottles with 25 tabs each.

NOTES - Headache. May produce a burning/tingling sensation when administered, although this should not be used to assess potency. Store in original glass bottle to maintain potency/stability. Traditionally, unused Tabs should be discarded 6 mo after the original bottle is opened; however the Nitrostat product is stable for 24 mo after the bottle is opened or until the expiration date on the bottle, whichever is earlier. If used rarely, prescribe package with 4 bottles with 25 Tabs each.

**NITROGLYCERIN SUSTAINED RELEASE** ▶L ♀C ▶? $

ADULT - Angina prophylaxis: Start 2.5 mg PO bid-tid, then titrate upward as needed.

PEDS - Not approved in children.

FORMS - Generic only: cap, extended-release 2.5, 6.5, 9 mg.

NOTES - Headache. Extended-release tab may be broken, but do not chew or crush, swallow whole. cap should be swallowed whole. Do not use

**(cont.)**

**NITROGLYCERIN SUSTAINED RELEASE** *(cont.)*
extended-release Tabs or Caps for acute angina attack. Allow for a nitrate-free period of 10–14 h each d to avoid nitrate tolerance.

**NITROGLYCERIN TRANSDERMAL** *(Minitran, Nitro-Dur, ✦Trinipatch)* ▶L ♀C ▶? $$
ADULT - Angina prophylaxis: Start with lowest dose and apply 1 patch for 12–14 h each d to non-hairy skin.
PEDS - Not approved in children.

FORMS - Generic/Trade: Transdermal system 0.1, 0.2, 0.4, 0.6 mg/h. Trade only: (Nitro-Dur) 0.3, 0.8 mg/h.
NOTES - Do not use topical therapy (ointment, transdermal system) for acute angina attack. Allow for a nitrate-free period of 10–14 h each d to avoid nitrate tolerance. Elderly are at more risk of hypotension and falling; start at lower doses.

## CARDIOVASCULAR: Pressors/Inotropes

**DOBUTAMINE** *(Dobutrex)* ▶Plasma ♀D ▶- $
ADULT - Inotropic support in cardiac decompensation (heart failure, surgical procedures): 2–20 mcg/kg/min. 70 kg: 5 mcg/kg/min with 1 mg/mL concentration (eg, 250 mg in 250 mL D5W) = 21 mL/h; 5 mcg/kg/min with 2 mg/mL concentration (eg, 200 mg in 100 mL D5W) = 10.5 mL/h.
PEDS - Not approved in children.
UNAPPROVED PEDS - Same as adult. Use lowest effective dose.
NOTES - For short-term use, up to 72 h.

**DOPAMINE** *(Intropin)* ▶Plasma ♀C ▶- $
ADULT - Pressor: Start 5 mcg/kg/min, increase as needed by 5–10 mcg/kg/min increments at 10 min intervals, max 50 mcg/kg/min. 70 kg: 5 mcg/kg/min with 1600 mcg/mL concentration (eg, 400 mg in 250 mL D5W) = 13 mL/h; 5 mcg/kg/min with 3200 mcg/mL concentration (eg, 320 mg in 100 mL D5W) = 6.5 mL/h.
PEDS - Not approved in children.
UNAPPROVED ADULT - Symptomatic bradycardia unresponsive to atropine: 5–20 mcg/kg/min IV infusion.
UNAPPROVED PEDS - Pressor: same as adult.
NOTES - Doses in mcg/kg/min: 2–4 = (traditional renal dose; recent evidence suggests ineffective) dopaminergic receptors; 5–10 = (cardiac dose) dopaminergic and beta1 receptors; >10 = dopaminergic, beta1, and alpha1 receptors.

**EPHEDRINE** ▶K ♀C ▶? $
ADULT - Pressor: 10–25 mg IV slow injection, with repeat doses every 5–10 min as needed, max 150 mg/d. Orthostatic hypotension: 25 mg PO daily-qid. Bronchospasm: 25–50 mg PO q3–4h prn.
PEDS - Not approved in children.
UNAPPROVED PEDS - Pressor: 3 mg/kg/d SC or IV in 4–6 divided doses.
FORMS - Generic only: Caps, 50 mg.

**EPINEPHRINE** *(EpiPen, EpiPen Jr, Twinject, adrenalin)* ▶Plasma ♀C ▶- $
ADULT - Cardiac arrest: 1 mg (1:10,000 solution) IV, repeat every 3–5 min if needed; infusion 1 mg in 250 mL D5W (4 mcg/mL) at 1–4 mcg/min (15–60 mL/h). Anaphylaxis: 0.1–0.5 mg SC/IM (1:1,000 solution), may repeat SC dose every 10–15 min for anaphylactic shock. Acute asthma & hypersensitivity reactions: 0.1 to 0.3 mg of 1:1,000 soln SC or IM. Hypersensitivity reactions: 0.01 mg/kg SC autoinjector.

PEDS - Cardiac arrest: 0.01 mg/kg IV/intraosseous (IO) (max 1 mg/dose) or 0.1 mg/kg ET (max 10 mg/dose), repeat 0.1–0.2 mg/kg IV/IO/ET every 3–5 min if needed. Neonates: 0.01–0.03 mg/kg IV (preferred) or up to 0.1 mg/kg ET, repeat every 3–5 min if needed; IV infusion start 0.1 mcg/kg/min, increase in increments of 0.1 mcg/kg/min if needed, max 1 mcg/kg/min. Anaphylaxis: 0.01 mg/kg (0.01 mL/kg of 1:1000 injection) SC, may repeat SC dose at 20 min to 4 h intervals depending on severity of condition. Acute asthma: 0.01 mL/kg (up to 0.5 mL) of 1:1,000 soln SC or IM; repeat q15 min × 3–4 doses prn. Hypersensitivity reactions: 0.01 mg/kg SC autoinjector.
UNAPPROVED ADULT - Symptomatic bradycardia unresponsive to atropine: 2–10 mcg/min IV infusion. ET administration prior to IV access: 2–2.5 × the recommended IV dose in 10 mL of NS or distilled water.
FORMS - Soln for injection: 1:1,000 (1 mg/mL in 1 mL amps or 10 mL vial). Trade only: EpiPen Autoinjector delivers one 0.3 mg (1:1,000, 0.3 mL) IM dose. EpiPen Jr. Autoinjector delivers one 0.15 mg (1:2,000, 0.3 mL) IM dose. Twinject Auto-injector delivers one 0.15 mg (1:1,000, 0.15 mL) or 0.3 mg (1:1,000, 0.3 mL) IM/SQ dose.
NOTES - Cardiac arrest: ADULT: Use the 1:10,000 injectable solution for IV use in cardiac arrest (10 mL = 1 mg); PEDS: use 1:10,000 for initial IV dose, then 1:1,000 for subsequent dosing or ET doses. Anaphylaxis: Use the 1:1000 injectable solution for SC/IM (0.1 mL = 0.1 mg);. consider EpiPen Jr. in patients weighing <30 kg. Directions for injectable kit use: Remove cap. Place black tip end on thigh & push down to inject. Hold in place for 10 sec. May be injected directly through clothing.

**INAMRINONE** ▶K ♀C ▶? $$$$$
ADULT - Heart failure (NYHA class III,IV): 0.75 mg/kg bolus IV over 2–3 min, then infusion 100 mg in 100 mL NS (1 mg/mL) at 5–10 mcg/kg/min. 70 kg: 5 mcg/kg/min = 21 mL/h. An additional IV bolus of 0.75 mg/kg may be given 30 min after initiating therapy if needed. Total daily dose should not exceed 10 mg/kg.
PEDS - Not approved in children.
UNAPPROVED ADULT - CPR: 0.75 mg/kg bolus IV over 2–3 min, followed by 5–15 mcg/kg/min.

**INAMRINONE** (*cont.*)

UNAPPROVED PEDS - Inotropic support: 0.75 mg/kg IV bolus over 2–3 min, followed by 3–5 mcg/kg/min (neonates) or 5–10 mcg/kg/min (children) maintenance infusion.

NOTES - Thrombocytopenia possible. Children may require higher bolus doses, 3–4.5 mg/kg. Name changed from "amrinone" to avoid medication errors.

**MIDODRINE** (*Orvaten, ProAmatine, ✦Amatine*) ▶LK ♀C ▶? $$$$$

WARNING - May cause significant HTN. Clinical benefits (ie, improved activities of daily living) have not been verified. Use in patients when nonpharmacological treatment fails.

ADULT - Orthostatic hypotension: Start 10 mg PO tid while awake, increase dose as needed to max 40 mg/d. Renal impairment: Start 2.5 mg tid while awake, increase dose as needed.

PEDS - Not approved in children.

FORMS - Generic/Trade: Tabs, scored 2.5, 5, 10 mg.

NOTES - The last daily dose should be no later than 6 pm to avoid supine HTN during sleep.

**MILRINONE** (*Primacor*) ▶K ♀C ▶? $$

ADULT - Systolic heart failure (NYHA class III,IV): Load 50 mcg/kg IV over 10 min, then begin IV infusion of 0.375–0.75 mcg/kg/min. Renal impairment: reduce IV infusion rate (mcg/kg/min) as follows, CrCl 50–41 mL/min, 0.43; CrCl 40–31 mL/min, 0.38; CrCl 30–21 mL/min, 0.33; CrCl 20–11 mL/min, 0.28; CrCl 10–6 mL/min, 0.23; CrCl ≤5 mL/min, 0.2.

PEDS - Not approved in children.

UNAPPROVED PEDS - Inotropic support: Limited data, 50 mcg/kg IV bolus over 10 min, followed by 0.5–1 mcg/kg/min IV infusion, titrate to effect within dosing range.

**NOREPINEPHRINE** (*Levophed*) ▶Plasma ♀C ▶? $

ADULT - Acute hypotension: 4 mg in 500 mL D5W (8 mcg/mL), start IV infusion 8–12 mcg/min, ideally through central line, adjust rate to maintain BP, average maintenance dose 2–4 mcg/min. 3 mcg/min = 22.5 mL/h.

PEDS - Not approved in children.

UNAPPROVED PEDS - Acute hypotension: Start 0.05–0.1mcg/kg/min IV infusion, titrate to desired effect, max dose 2 mcg/kg/min.

NOTES - Avoid extravasation, do not administer IV push or IM.

**PHENYLEPHRINE - INTRAVENOUS** (*Neo-Synephrine*) ▶Plasma ♀C ▶- $

ADULT - Mild to moderate hypotension: 0.1–0.2 mg slow IV injection, do not exceed 0.5 mg in initial dose, repeat dose as needed no less than every 10–15 min; 1–10 mg SC/IM, initial dose should not exceed 5 mg. Infusion for severe hypotension: 20 mg in 250 mL D5W (80 mcg/mL), start 100–180 mcg/min (75–135 mL/h), usual dose once BP is stabilized 40–60 mcg/min.

PEDS - Not approved in children.

UNAPPROVED PEDS - Mild to moderate hypotension: 5–20 mcg/kg IV bolus every 10–15 min as needed; 0.1–0.5 mcg/kg/min IV infusion, titrate to desired effect.

NOTES - Avoid SC or IM administration during shock, use IV route to ensure drug absorption.

---

## CARDIOVASCULAR: Pulmonary Arterial Hypertension

**BOSENTAN** (*Tracleer*) ▶L ♀X ▶-? $$$$$

WARNING - Hepatotoxicity; monitor LFTs prior to starting therapy & monthly thereafter. Contraindicated in pregnancy due to birth defects; women of child bearing age must use reliable contraception and have monthly pregnancy tests. Oral, injectable, transdermal, & implanted contraception must be supplemented with another method. Women of childbearing age need pregnancy test before refills.

ADULT - Pulmonary arterial hypertension (PAH): Start 62.5 mg PO bid for 4 wk, increase to 125 mg bid maintenance dose.

PEDS - Not approved in children.

FORMS - Trade only: Tabs, non-scored 62.5, 125 mg.

NOTES - Available only through access program by calling 866-228-3546. Concomitant glyburide is contraindicated due to increased risk of hepatotoxicity. Ketoconazole and cyclosporine inhibit metabolism of bosentan via cytochrome P450 3A4; concomitant cyclosporine contraindicated. Induces metabolism of other drugs (eg, contraceptives, simvastatin, lovastatin, atorvastatin). Do not use with both CYP2C9 inhibitor (eg, amiodarone, fluconazole) and CYP3A4 inhibitor (eg, ketoconazole, itraconazole, ritonavir); may increase levels of bosentan. May decrease warfarin plasma concentration; monitor INR. Discontinue with signs of pulmonary edema. Monitor hemoglobin after 1 and 3 mo of therapy, then q3 mo.

**EPOPROSTENOL** (*Flolan*) ▶Plasma ♀B ▶? $$$$$

ADULT - Pulmonary arterial hypertension (PAH): Acute dose ranging, 2 ng/kg/min increments via IV infusion until the patient develops symptomatic intolerance (mean maximal dose without symptoms 8.6 ng/kg/min), start continuous IV infusion at 4 ng/kg/min or less than the patient's max-tolerated infusion (MTI) rate for acute dose ranging. If the MTI rate is <5 ng/kg/min, start chronic IV infusion at one-half the MTI.

PEDS - Not approved in children.

NOTES - Administer by continuous IV infusion via a central venous catheter. Temporary peripheral IV infusions may be used until central access is established. Inhibits platelet aggregation; may increase bleeding risk.

**ILOPROST** (*Ventavis*) ▶L ♀C ▶? $$$$$

ADULT - Pulmonary arterial hypertension: Start 2.5 mcg/dose by inhalation (delivered at mouthpiece); if well tolerated increase to 5 mcg/dose by inhalation (delivered at mouthpiece). Use 6–9 times daily (not>than q2h) during waking h.

PEDS - Not approved in children.

**(cont.)**

**ILOPROST** *(cont.)*

NOTES - Only administer with Prodose or I-neb AAD Systems. Each single-use ampule delivers 20 mcg to medication chamber of nebulizer & 2.5 or 5 mcg to mouthpiece; discard remaining solution after each inhalation. Do not mix with other medications. Avoid contact with skin/eyes or oral ingestion. Monitor vital signs when initiating therapy. Do not initiate therapy if SBP < 85 mm Hg. Do not use in patients with moderate to severe hepatic impairment and/or 3x upper limit of transaminase or patients on dialysis. May potentiate bleeding risk for patients on anticoagulants and hypotensive effects of other medications.

**SILDENAFIL** *(Revatio)* ▶LK ♀B ▶? $$$$

ADULT - Pulmonary hypertension: 20 mg PO tid.

PEDS - Not approved in children.

FORMS - Revatio: Tabs 20 mg.

NOTES - Do not use with itraconazole, ketoconazole, ritonavir, pulmonary veno-occlusive disease. Co-administer with CYP3A4 inducers (ie, bosentan, barbiturates, carbamazepine, phenytoin, efavirenz, nevirapine, rifampin, rifabutin) may change levels of either medication; adjust as needed. Use caution with stroke, MI, or life-threatening arrhythmia in last 6 mo; unstable angina; BP > 170/110; or retinitis pigmentosa. Contraindicated in patients given nitrates prior/subsequent 24 h. Caution with alpha blockers due to potential for symptomatic

hypotension. Reports of sudden vision loss due to non-arteritic ischemic optic neuropathy (NAION); prior NAION increases risk. Sudden hearing loss, with or without tinnitus, vertigo or dizziness, reported. Transient global amnesia also reported.

**TREPROSTINIL** *(Remodulin)* ▶KL ♀B ▶? $$$$$

ADULT - Continuous sc (preferred) or central IV infusion in pulmonary arterial HTN with NYHA Class II to IV symptoms: Start 1.25 ng/kg/min based on ideal body weight. Reduce to 0.625 ng/kg/min if initial dose not tolerated. Dose based on clinical response & tolerance. Increase no more than 1.25 ng/kg/min/wk in first 4 wk, then increase no more than 2.5 ng/kg/min/wk. Max 40 ng/kg/min. Transitioning from epoprostenol: Must be done in hospital; initiate at 10% epoprostenol dose; gradually increase dose as epoprostenol dose is decreased (see package insert).

PEDS - Not approved in children.

NOTES - Use cautiously in elderly and with liver or renal dysfunction. Initiate in setting with personnel-equipment for physiological monitoring & emergency care. Administer by continuous infusion using infusion pump. Patient needs access to backup infusion pump and infusion sets. Dilute prior to giving IV; see package insert. May potentiate bleeding risk for patients on anticoagulants. May potentiate hypotensive effects of other medications.

## CARDIOVASCULAR: Thrombolytics

**ALTEPLASE** *(tpa, t-PA, Activase, Cathflo, ◆Activase rt-PA)* ▶L ♀C ▶? $$$$$

ADULT - Acute MI: (patients >67 kg) 15 mg IV bolus, then 50 mg IV over 30 min, then 35 mg IV over the next 60 min; (patients ≤67 kg) 15 mg IV bolus, then 0.75 mg/kg (not to exceed 50 mg) IV over 30 min, then 0.5 mg/kg (not to exceed 35 mg) IV over the next 60 min. Concurrent heparin infusion. Acute ischemic stroke with symptoms ≤3h: 0.9 mg/kg (max 90 mg); give 10% of total dose as an IV bolus, and the remainder IV over 60 min. Multiple exclusion criteria. Acute pulmonary embolism: 100 mg IV over 2h, then restart heparin when PTT ≤twice normal. Occluded central venous access device: 2 mg/mL in catheter for 2 h. May use 2nd dose if needed.

PEDS - Occluded central venous access device: ≥10 kg and <30 kg: Dose equal to 110% of the internal lumen volume, not to exceed 2 mg/2 mL. Other uses not approved in children.

NOTES - Must be reconstituted. Solution must be used within 8h after reconstitution.

**RETEPLASE** *(Retavase)* ▶L ♀C ▶? $$$$$

ADULT - Acute MI: 10 units IV over 2 min; repeat one dose in 30 min.

PEDS - Not approved in children.

NOTES - Must be reconstituted with sterile water for injection to 1 mg/mL concentration. Solution must be used within 4 h after reconstitution.

**STREPTOKINASE** *(Streptase, Kabikinase)* ▶L ♀C ▶? $$$$$

ADULT - Acute MI: 1.5 million units IV over 60 min. Pulmonary embolism: 250,000 units IV loading

### THROMBOLYTIC THERAPY FOR ACUTE MI

*Indications (if high-volume cath lab unavailable):* Clinical history & presentation strongly suggestive of MI within 12 h plus ≥1 of the following: 1 mm ST elevation in ≥2 contiguous leads; new left BBB; or 2 mm ST depression in V1–4 suggestive of true posterior MI.

*Absolute contraindications:* Previous cerebral hemorrhage, known cerebral aneurysm or arteriovenous malformation, known intracranial neoplasm, recent (<3 mo) ischemic stroke (except acute ischemic stroke <3 h), aortic dissection, active bleeding or bleeding diathesis (excluding menstruation), significant closed head or facial trauma (<3 mo).

*Relative contraindications:* Severe uncontrolled HTN (>180/110 mm Hg) on presentation or chronic severe HTN; prior ischemic stroke (>3 mo), dementia, other intracranial pathology; traumatic/prolonged (>10 min) cardiopulmonary resuscitation; major surgery (<3 wk); recent (within 2–4 wk) internal bleeding; puncture of noncompressible vessel; pregnancy; active peptic ulcer disease; current use of anticoagulants. For streptokinase/anistreplase: prior exposure (>5 d ago) or prior allergic reaction.

**STREPTOKINASE** (*cont.*)

dose over 30 min, followed by 100,000 units/h IV infusion for 24 h (maintain infusion for 72 h if concurrent DVT suspected). DVT: 250,000 units IV loading dose over 30 min, followed by 100,000 units/h IV infusion for 24 h. Occluded arteriovenous catheter: 250,000 units instilled into catheter, remove solution containing 250,000 units of drug from catheter after 2 h using 5-mL syringe.

PEDS - Not approved in children.

NOTES - Must be reconstituted. Solution must be used within 8 h of reconstitution. Do not shake vial. Do not repeat use in less than one yr. Do not use with history of severe allergic reaction.

**TENECTEPLASE** (*TNKase*) ▶L ♀C ▶? $$$$$

ADULT - Acute MI: Single IV bolus dose over 5 sec based on body weight; <60 kg, 30 mg; 60–69 kg, 35 mg; 70–79 kg, 40 mg; 80–89 kg, 45 mg; ≥90kg, 50 mg.

PEDS - Not approved in children.

NOTES - Must be reconstituted. Solution must be used within 8h after reconstitution.

**UROKINASE** (*Kinlytic*) ▶L ♀B ▶? $$$$$

ADULT - Pulmonary embolism: 4400 units/kg IV loading dose over 10 min, followed by IV infusion 4400 units/kg/h for 12 h. Occluded IV catheter: 5000 units instilled into the catheter with a tuberculin syringe, remove solution containing 5000 units of drug from catheter after 5 min using a 5-mL syringe. Aspiration attempts may be repeated q5min. If unsuccessful, cap catheter and allow 5000 unit solution to remain in catheter for 30–60 min before again attempting to aspirate solution and residual clot.

PEDS - Not approved in children.

UNAPPROVED ADULT - Acute MI: 2–3 million units IV infusion over 45–90 min. Give one-half the total dose as a rapid initial IV injection over 5 min.

UNAPPROVED PEDS - Arterial or venous thrombosis: 4400 units/kg IV loading dose over 10 min, followed by 4400 units/kg/h for 12–72 h. Occluded IV catheter: same as adult.

NOTES - Must be reconstituted. Do not shake vial.

**ALBUMIN** (*Albuminar, Buminate, Albumarc, ◆Plasbumin*) ▶L ♀C ▶? $$$$$

ADULT - Shock, burns: 500 mL of 5% solution (50 mg/mL) infused as rapidly as tolerated. Repeat infusion in 30 min if response is inadequate. 25% solution may be used with or without dilution if necessary. Undiluted 25% solution should be infused at 1 mL/min to avoid too rapid plasma volume expansion.

PEDS - Shock, burns: 10–20 mL/kg IV infusion at 5–10 mL/min using 50 mL of 5% solution.

UNAPPROVED PEDS - Shock/hypovolemia: 1 g/kg/dose IV rapid infusion. Hypoproteinemia: 1 g/kg/dose IV infusion over 30–120 min.

NOTES - Fever, chills. Monitor for plasma volume overload (dyspnea, fluid in lungs, abnormal increase in BP or CVP). Less likely to cause hypotension than plasma protein fraction, more purified. In treating burns, large volumes of crystalloid solutions (0.9% sodium chloride) are used to maintain plasma volume with albumin. Use 5% solution in pediatric hypovolemic patients. Use 25% solution in pediatric patients with volume restrictions.

**DEXTRAN** (*Rheomacrodex, Gentran, Macrodex*) ▶K ♀C ▶? $$

ADULT - Shock/hypovolemia: Dextran 40, Dextran 70 and 75, up to 20 mL/kg during the first 24 h, up to 10 mL/kg/d thereafter, do not continue for longer than 5 d. The first 500 mL may be infused rapidly with CVP monitoring. DVT/PE prophylaxis during surgery: Dextran 40, 50–100 g IV infusion the d of surgery, continue for 2–3 d post-op with 50 g/d. 50 g/d may be given every 2nd or 3rd d thereafter up to 14 d.

PEDS - Total dose should not exceed 20 mL/kg.

UNAPPROVED ADULT - DVT/PE prophylaxis during surgery: Dextran 70 and 75 solutions have been used.

Other uses: improve circulation with sickle cell crisis, prevent of nephrotoxicity with radiographic contrast media, toxemia of late pregnancy.

NOTES - Monitor for plasma volume overload (dyspnea, fluid in lungs, abnormal increase in BP or CVP) and anaphylactoid reactions. May impair platelet function. Less effective that other agents for DVT/PE prevention.

**HETASTARCH** (*Hespan, Hextend*) ▶K ♀C ▶? $$

ADULT - Shock/hypovolemia: 500–1000 mL IV infusion, total daily dose usually should not exceed 20 mL/kg (1500 mL). Renal impairment: CrCl <10 mL/min, usual initial dose followed by 20–25% of usual dose.

PEDS - Not approved in children.

UNAPPROVED PEDS - Shock/hypovolemia: 10 mL/kg/dose; do not exceed 20 mL/kg/d.

NOTES - Monitor for plasma volume overload (dyspnea, fluid in lungs, abnormal increase in BP or CVP). Little or no antigenic properties compared to dextran.

**PLASMA PROTEIN FRACTION** (*Plasmanate, Protenate, Plasmatein*) ▶L ♀C ▶? $$$

ADULT - Shock/hypovolemia: Adjust initial rate according to clinical response and BP, but rate should not exceed 10 mL/min. As plasma volume normalizes, infusion rate should not exceed 5–8 mL/min. Usual dose 250–500 mL. Hypoproteinemia: 1000–1500 mL/d IV infusion.

PEDS - Shock/hypovolemia: Initial dose 6.6–33 mL/kg infused at a rate of 5–10 mL/min.

NOTES - Fever, chills, hypotension with rapid infusion. Monitor for plasma volume overload (dyspnea, fluid in lungs, abnormal increase in BP or CVP). Less pure than albumin products.

## CARDIOVASCULAR: Other

***BIDIL* (hydralazine + isosorbide dinitrate)** ▶LK ♀C ▶? $$$$$
ADULT - Heart Failure (adjunct to standard therapy in black patients): Start 1 tab PO tid, increase as tolerated to max 2 tabs bid. May decrease to ½ tab tid with intolerable side effects; try to increase dose when side effects subside.
PEDS - Not approved in children.
FORMS - Trade only: Tabs, scored 37.5/20 mg.
NOTES - See component drugs

***CILOSTAZOL* (*Pletal*)** ▶L ♀C ▶? $$$$
WARNING - Contraindicated in heart failure of any severity.
ADULT - Intermittent claudication: 100 mg PO bid on empty stomach. 50 mg PO bid with cytochrome P450 3A4 inhibitors (like ketoconazole, itraconazole, erythromycin, diltiazem) or cytochrome P450 2C19 inhibitors (like omeprazole). Beneficial effect may take up to 12 wk.
PEDS - Not approved in children.
FORMS - Generic/Trade: Tabs 50, 100 mg.
NOTES - Avoid grapefruit juice. Caution with moderate/severe liver impairment or CrCl <25 mL/min. Give with other antiplatelet therapy (aspirin/clopidogrel) when treating lower extremity peripheral arterial disease to reduce cardiovascular risk.

***ISOXSUPRINE* (*Vasodilan*)** ▶KL ♀C ▶? $
ADULT - Adjunctive therapy for cerebral vascular insufficiency and PVD: 10–20 mg PO tid-qid.
PEDS - Not approved in children.
FORMS - Generic/Trade: Tabs, 10,20 mg.
NOTES - Drug has questionable therapeutic effect.

***NESIRITIDE* (*Natrecor*)** ▶K, plasma ♀C ▶? $$$$$
ADULT - Hospitalized patients with decompensated heart failure with dyspnea at rest: 2 mcg/kg IV bolus over 60 sec, then 0.01 mcg/kg/min IV infusion for up to 48 h. Do not initiate at higher doses. Limited experience with increased doses: 0.005 mcg/kg/min increments, preceded by 1 mcg/kg bolus, no more frequently than q3h up to max infusion dose 0.03 mcg/kg/min. 1.5 mg vial in 250mL D5W (6 mcg/mL). 70 kg: 2 mcg/kg bolus = 23.3 mL, 0.01 mcg/kg/min infusion = 7 mL/h.
PEDS - Not approved in children.
NOTES - May increase mortality; meta-analysis showed non-statistically significant increased risk of death within 30 d post-treatment compared with non-inotropic control group. Not indicated for outpatient infusion, for scheduled repetitive use, to improve renal function, or to

enhance diuresis. Contraindicated as primary therapy for cardiogenic shock and when SBP <90 mm Hg. Discontinue if dose-related symptomatic hypotension occurs and support BP prn. May restart infusion with dose reduced by 30% (no bolus dose) once BP stabilized. Do not shake reconstituted vial, and dilute vial prior to administration. Incompatible with most injectable drugs; administer agents using separate IV lines. Do not measure BNP levels while infusing; may measure BNP at least 2–6 h after infusion completion.

***PAPAVERINE* ▶LK ♀C ▶? $
ADULT - Cerebral and peripheral ischemia: Start 150 mg PO bid, increase to max 300 mg bid if needed. Start 30 mg IV/IM, dose range 30–120 mg q3h prn. Give IV doses over 1–2 min.
PEDS - Not approved in children.
FORMS - Generic only: cap, extended-release, 150 mg.

***PENTOXIFYLLINE* (*Trental*)** ▶L ♀C ▶? $$$
ADULT - Intermittent claudication: 400 mg PO tid with meals. For CNS/GI adverse effects, decrease dose to 400 mg PO bid. Beneficial effect may take up to 8 wk. May be less effective in relieving cramps, tiredness, tightness, and pain during exercise.
PEDS - Not approved in children.
FORMS - Generic/Trade: Tabs 400 mg.
NOTES - Contraindicated with recent cerebral/retinal bleed. Increases theophylline levels. Increases INR with warfarin.

***RANOLAZINE* (*Ranexa*)** ▶LK ♀C ▶? $$$$$
ADULT - Chronic angina: 500 mg PO bid, increase to 1000 mg PO bid prn based on clinical symptoms, max 2000 mg daily. Reserve for angina not controlled with other antianginal drugs; use with amlodipine, beta blockers, or nitrates.
PEDS - Not approved in children.
FORMS - Trade only: Tabs, extended release 500, 1000 mg.
NOTES - Get baseline and follow-up EKGs; evaluate effects on QT interval. Contraindicated with pre-existing QT prolongation, hepatic impairment, QT prolonging drugs (eg, Class Ia/III antiarrhythmics, erythromycin, thioridazine, ziprasidone), potent/moderately potent CYP3A4 inhibitors (eg, ketoconazole, HIV protease inhibitors, macrolides, diltiazem, verapamil), grapefruit juice/products, severe renal impairment. May need to reduce doses of co-administered simvastatin, digoxin, or P-gp substrates. Swallow whole; do not crush, break, or chew. May be less effective in women. Instruct patients to report palpitations or fainting spells.

## CONTRAST MEDIA: MRI Contrast—Gadolinium-Based

**NOTE:** Avoid gadolinium-based contrast agents if severe renal insufficiency (GFR <30 mL/min/1.73 m$^2$) due to risk of nephrogenic systemic fibrosis/nephrogenic fibrosing dermopathy. Similarly avoid in acute renal insufficiency of any severity due to hepatorenal syndrome or during the perioperative phase of liver transplant.

***GADOBENATE* (*MultiHance*)** ▶K ♀C ▶? $$$$
ADULT - Non-iodinated, non-ionic IV contrast for MRI.
PEDS - Not approved in children.

***GADODIAMIDE* (*Omniscan*)** ▶K ♀C ▶? $$$$
ADULT - Non-iodinated, non-ionic IV contrast for MRI.
PEDS - Non-iodinated, non-ionic IV contrast for MRI.

**GADODIAMIDE (cont.)**
NOTES - Use caution if renal disease. May falsely lower serum calcium. Not for intrathecal use.

**GADOPENTETATE (Magnevist)** ▶K ♀C ▶? $$$
ADULT - Non-iodinated IV contrast for MRI.
PEDS - >2 yo: Non-iodinated IV contrast for MRI.
NOTES - Use caution in sickle cell and renal disease.

**GADOTERIDOL (Prohance)** ▶K ♀C ▶? $$$$
ADULT - Non-iodinated, non-ionic IV contrast for MRI.

PEDS - >2 yo: Non-iodinated, non-ionic IV contrast for MRI.
NOTES - Use caution in sickle cell and renal disease.

**GADOVERSETAMIDE (OptiMARK)** ▶K ♀C ▶- $$$$
ADULT - Non-iodinated IV contrast for MRI.
PEDS - Not approved in children.
NOTES - Use caution in sickle cell and renal disease.

## CONTRAST MEDIA: MRI Contrast—Other

**FERUMOXIDES (Feridex)** ▶L ♀C ▶? $$$$
ADULT - Non-iodinated, non-ionic, iron-based IV contrast for hepatic MRI.
PEDS - Not approved in children.
NOTES - Contains dextran.

**FERUMOXSIL (GastroMARK)** ▶L ♀B ▶? $$$$
ADULT - Non-iodinated, non-ionic, iron-based, oral

GI contrast for MRI.
PEDS - Not approved in children <16 yo.

**MANGAFODIPIR (Teslascan)** ▶L ♀- ▶- $$$$
ADULT - Non-iodinated IV contrast for MRI.
PEDS - Not approved in children.
NOTES - Contains manganese.

## CONTRAST MEDIA: Radiography Contrast

**NOTE:** Beware of allergic or anaphylactoid reactions. Avoid IV contrast in renal insufficiency or dehydration. Hold metformin (Glucophage) prior to or at the time of iodinated contrast dye use and for 48 h after procedure. Restart after procedure only if renal function is normal.

**BARIUM SULFATE ▶Not Absorbed ♀? ▶+ $**
ADULT - Non-iodinated GI (eg, oral, rectal) contrast.
PEDS - Non-iodinated GI (eg, oral, rectal) contrast.
NOTES - Contraindicated if suspected esophageal, gastric or intestinal perforation. Use with caution in GI obstruction. May cause abdominal distention, cramping, and constipation with oral use.

**DIATRIZOATE (Cystografin, Gastrografin, Hypaque, MD-Gastroview, RenoCal, Reno-DIP, Reno-60, Renografin)** ▶K ♀C ▶? $
WARNING - Not for intrathecal or epidural use.
ADULT - Iodinated, ionic, high osmolality IV or GI contrast.
PEDS - Iodinated, ionic, high osmolality IV or GI contrast.
NOTES - High osmolality contrast may cause tissue damage if infiltrated/extravasated. IV: Hypaque, Renografin, Reno-DIP, RenoCal. GI: Gastrografin, MD-Gastroview.

**IODIXANOL (Visipaque)** ▶K ♀B ▶? $$$
ADULT - Iodinated, non-ionic, iso-osmolar IV contrast.
PEDS - Iodinated, non-ionic, iso-osmolar IV contrast.
NOTES - Not for intrathecal use.

**IOHEXOL (Omnipaque)** ▶K ♀B ▶? $$$
ADULT - Iodinated, non-ionic, low osmolality IV and oral/body cavity contrast.

PEDS - Iodinated, non-ionic, low osmolality IV and oral/body cavity contrast.

**IOPAMIDOL (Isovue)** ▶K ♀? ▶? $$
ADULT - Iodinated, non-ionic, low osmolality IV contrast.
PEDS - Iodinated, non-ionic, low osmolality IV contrast.

**IOPROMIDE (Ultravist)** ▶K ♀B ▶? $$$
ADULT - Iodinated, non-ionic, low osmolality IV contrast.
PEDS - Iodinated, non-ionic, low osmolality IV contrast.

**IOTHALAMATE (Conray, ◆Vascoray)** ▶K ♀B ▶- $
ADULT - Iodinated, ionic, high osmolality IV contrast.
PEDS - Iodinated, ionic, high osmolality IV contrast.
NOTES - High osmolality contrast may cause tissue damage if infiltrated/extravasated.

**IOVERSOL (Optiray)** ▶K ♀B ▶? $$
ADULT - Iodinated, non-ionic, low osmolality IV contrast.
PEDS - Iodinated, non-ionic, low osmolality IV contrast.

**IOXAGLATE (Hexabrix)** ▶K ♀B ▶- $$$
ADULT - Iodinated, ionic, low osmolality IV contrast.
PEDS - Iodinated, ionic, low osmolality IV contrast.

**IOXILAN (Oxilan)** ▶K ♀B ▶- $$$
ADULT - Iodinated, non-ionic, low osmolality IV contrast.
PEDS - Iodinated, non-ionic, low osmolality IV contrast.

## CONTRAST MEDIA: Other

**INDIGOTINDISULFONATE (Indigo Carmine)** ▶K ♀C ▶? $
ADULT - Identification of ureteral tears during surgery: 5 mL IV.
PEDS - Identification of ureteral tears during surgery: Use less than the adult dose.
FORMS - Trade only: 40 mg/5 mL vial.

**ISOSULFAN BLUE (Lymphazurin)** ▶LK ♀? ▶? $
ADULT - Lymphography, identification of lymphatics during cancer surgery: 0.5 to 3 mL SC.
PEDS - Optimal dosing not defined.
FORMS - 1% solution 5 mL vial.

**PENTETATE INDIUM (Indium DTPA)** ▶K ♀C ▶? ?
ADULT - Radionuclide cisternography
PEDS - Not approved in children.

## DERMATOLOGY: Acne Preparations

**NOTE:** For topical agents, wash area prior to application. Wash hands before & after application; avoid eye area.

**ADAPALENE (*Differin*)** ▶Bile ♀C ▶? $$
ADULT - Acne: apply qhs.
PEDS - Not approved in children.
UNAPPROVED PEDS - Acne: apply qhs.
FORMS - Trade only: gel 0.1% & 0.3% (15,45 g) cream 0.1% (15,45 g), soln 0.1% pad (30 mL).
NOTES - During early wk of therapy, acne exacerbation may occur. May cause erythema, scaling, dryness, pruritus, and burning in up to 40% of patients. Therapeutic results take 8–12 wk.

**AZELAIC ACID (*Azelex, Finacea, Finevin*)** ▶K ♀B ▶? $$$
ADULT - Acne (Azelex, Finevin): apply bid. Rosacea (Finacea): apply bid.
PEDS - Not approved in children.
UNAPPROVED ADULT - Melasma: apply bid.
UNAPPROVED PEDS - Acne: apply qhs.
FORMS - Trade only: cream 20%, 30g, 50g (Azelex, Finevin), gel 15% 30, 50g (Finacea).
NOTES - Improvement of acne occurs within 4 wk. Monitor for hypopigmentation esp. in patients with dark complexions. Avoid use of occlusive dressings.

**BENZACLIN (clindamycin + benzoyl peroxide)** ▶K ♀C ▶+ $$$
ADULT - Acne: apply bid.
PEDS - Not approved in children.
UNAPPROVED PEDS - Acne: apply qhs.
FORMS - Trade only: gel clindamycin 1% + benzoyl peroxide 5%; 25, 50 g, gel pump clindamycin 1% + benzoyl peroxide 5%; 50 g.
NOTES - Expires 10 wk after mixing.

**BENZAMYCIN (erythromycin base + benzoyl peroxide)** ▶LK ♀C ▶? $$$
ADULT - Acne: apply bid.
PEDS - Not approved in children.
UNAPPROVED PEDS - Acne: apply qhs.
FORMS - Generic/Trade: gel erythromycin 3% + benzoyl peroxide 5%; 23.3, 46.6 g.
NOTES - Must be refrigerated, expires 3 mo after pharmacy dispensing.

**BENZOYL PEROXIDE (*Benzac, Benzagel 10%, Desquam, Clearasil, ✦Solugel, Benoxyl*)** ▶LK ♀C ▶? $
ADULT - Acne: Cleansers: wash daily-bid. Creams/gels/lotion: apply daily initially, gradually increase to bid-tid if needed.
PEDS - Not approved in children.
UNAPPROVED PEDS - Acne: Cleansers: wash daily-bid. Creams/gels/lotion: apply daily initially, gradually increase to bid-tid if needed.
FORMS - OTC and Rx generic: liquid 2.5,5,10%, bar 5,10%, mask 5%, lotion 5,5.5,10%, cream 5,10%, cleanser 10%, gel 2.5,4,5, 6,10,20%.
NOTES - If excessive drying or peeling occurs, reduce frequency of application. Use with PABA-containing sunscreens may cause transient skin discoloration. May bleach fabric.

**CLENIA (sulfacetamide + sulfur)** ▶K ♀C ▶? $$
ADULT - Acne, rosacea, seborrheic dermatitis: apply cream/gel daily-tid, foaming wash daily-bid.
PEDS - Not approved in children.
FORMS - Generic only: lotion (sodium sulfacetamide 10% & sulfur 5%) 25 g. Trade only (sodium sulfacetamide 10% & sulfur 5%): cream 28 g, foaming wash 170,340 g.
NOTES - Avoid with sulfa allergy, renal failure.

**CLINDAMYCIN - TOPICAL (*Cleocin T, Clindagel, ClindaMax, Evoclin, ✦Dalacin T*)** ▶L ♀B ▶- $
ADULT - Acne: apply daily (Evoclin) or bid (Cleocin T).
PEDS - Not approved in children.
UNAPPROVED ADULT - Rosacea: apply lotion bid.
UNAPPROVED PEDS - Acne: apply bid.
FORMS - Generic/Trade: gel 1% 7.5, 30g, lotion 1% 60 mL, solution 1% 30, 60 mL. Trade only: foam 1% 50, 100 g (Evoclin), gel 1% 40, 75 mL (Clindagel).
NOTES - Concomitant use with erythromycin may decrease effectiveness. Most common adverse effects dryness, erythema, burning, peeling, oiliness and itching. C. difficile associated diarrhea has been reported with topical use.

**DIANE-35 (cyproterone + ethinyl estradiol)** ▶L ♀X ▶- $$
WARNING - Not recommended in women who smoke. Increased risk of thromboembolism, stroke, MI, hepatic neoplasia & gallbladder disease. Nausea, breast tenderness, & breakthrough bleeding are common, transient side effects. Nighttime dosing may minimize nausea. Effectiveness is reduced by hepatic enzyme-inducing drugs such as certain anticonvulsants and barbiturates, rifampin, rifabutin, griseofulvin & protease inhibitors. Antibiotics or products that contain St. John's wort may reduce efficacy.
ADULT - Canada only. In women, severe acne unresponsive to oral antibiotics and other treatments, with associated symptoms of androgenization, including seborrhea and mild hirsutism: 1 tab PO daily for 21 consecutive d, stop for 7 d, repeat cycle.
PEDS - Not approved in children.
FORMS - Rx trade only: blister pack of 21 tabs 2 mg/0.035 mg cyproterone acetate/ethinyl estradiol.
NOTES - Higher thromboembolic risk than other oral contraceptives, therefore only indicated for acne, and not solely for contraception (although effective for the latter). Same warnings, precautions, and contraindications as other oral contraceptives.

**DUAC (clindamycin + benzoyl peroxide, ✦Clindoxyl)** ▶K ♀C ▶+ $$$$
ADULT - Acne: apply qhs
PEDS - Not approved in children.
UNAPPROVED PEDS - Acne: apply qhs.

**DUAC** *(cont.)*

FORMS - Trade only: gel clindamycin 1% + benzoyl peroxide 5%; 45 g.

NOTES - Expires 2 mo after pharmacy dispensing.

**ERYTHROMYCIN - TOPICAL** *(Eryderm, Erycette, Erygel, A/T/S, ♦Sans-Acne, Erysol)* ▶L ♀B ▶? $$

ADULT - Acne: apply bid.

PEDS - Not approved in children.

UNAPPROVED PEDS - Acne: apply bid.

FORMS - Generic only: solution 1.5% 60 mL, 2% 60,120 mL, pads 2%, gel 2% 30,60 g, ointment 2% 25 g.

NOTES - May be more irritating when used with other acne products. Concomitant use with clindamycin may decrease effectiveness.

**ISOTRETINOIN** *(Accutane, Amnesteem, Claravis, Sotret, ♦Clarus)* ▶LK ♀X ▶- $$$$$

WARNING - Physicians pharmacists, and patients must register with the iPledge program in order to prescribe, dispense or take isotretinoin. Contraindicated in pregnant women or in women who may become pregnant. If used in a woman of childbearing age, patient must have severe, disfiguring acne, be reliable, comply with mandatory contraceptive measures, receive written and oral instructions about hazards of taking during pregnancy, have 2 negative pregnancy tests prior to beginning therapy. Must use 2 forms of effective contraception, unless absolute abstinence is chosen or patient has undergone a hysterectomy, from 1 mo prior until 1 mo after discontinuation of therapy. Men should not father children. May cause depression, suicidal thought, and aggressive or violent behavior; monitor for symptoms. Obtain written informed consent. Write prescription for no more than a 1 mo supply. Informed consent documents available from the manufacturer.

ADULT - Severe, recalcitrant cystic acne: 0.5–2 mg/kg/d PO divided bid for 15–20 wk. Typical target dose is 1 mg/kg/d. May repeat 2nd course of therapy after >2 mo off therapy.

PEDS - Not approved in children.

UNAPPROVED ADULT - Prevention of 2nd primary tumors in patients treated for squamous cell carcinoma of the head and neck: 50–100 mg/m²/d PO. Also been used in keratinization disorders.

UNAPPROVED PEDS - Severe, recalcitrant cystic acne: 0.5–2 mg/kg/d PO divided bid for 15–20 wk. Typical target dose is 1 mg/kg/d. Maintenance therapy for neuroblastoma: 100–250 mg/m²/d PO in 2 divided doses.

FORMS - Generic/Trade: caps 10, 20, 40 mg. Generic only (Sotret & Claravis): caps 30 mg.

NOTES - Can only be prescribed by healthcare professionals who have registered with the iPledge program. Prescription must have a "qualification sticker" attached. Prescription can be for a max of a 1 mo supply. May cause headache, cheilitis, drying of mucous membranes including eyes, nose, mouth, hair loss, abdominal pain, pyuria, joint and muscle pain/stiffness, conjunctivitis,

elevated ESR, and changes in serum lipids and LFTs. Effect on bone loss unknown; use caution in patients predisposed to osteoporosis. In children in whom skeletal growth is not complete, do not exceed the recommended dose for the recommended duration of treatment. Pseudotumor cerebri has occurred during therapy; avoid concomitant vitamin A, tetracycline, minocycline. May cause corneal opacities, decreased night vision, and inflammatory bowel disease. May decrease carbamazepine concentrations. Avoid excessive exposure to sunlight.

**ROSULA** *(sulfacetamide + sulfur)* ▶K ♀C ▶? $$$$

ADULT - Acne, rosacea, seborrheic dermatitis: apply cream/gel/aqueous cleanser daily-tid, foaming wash daily-bid.

PEDS - Not approved in children.

FORMS - Trade only: gel (sodium sulfacetamide 10% & sulfur 5%) 45 mL, aqueous cleanser (sodium sulfacetamide 10% & sulfur 5%) 355 mL, soap (sodium sulfacetamide 10% & sulfur 4%) 473 mL.

NOTES - Avoid with sulfa allergy or renal failure.

**SALICYLIC ACID** *(Akurza, Clearasil Cleanser, Stridex Pads)* ▶Not absorbed ♀? ▶? $

ADULT - Acne (OTC): apply/wash area up to three times daily. Removal of excessive keratin in hyperkeratotic disorders (Rx): apply to affected area at bedtime and cover. Hydrate skin before application.

PEDS - Acne: apply/wash area up to three times daily.

FORMS - Generic/Trade: OTC: pads, foam, mask scrub, 0.5%, 1%, 2%. Rx/Trade: cream 6%, 12 oz. (Akurza), lotion 6%, 12 oz. (Akurza)

**SULFACETAMIDE - TOPICAL** *(Klaron, Rosula NS)* ▶K ♀C ▶? $$

ADULT - Acne: apply bid.

PEDS - Not approved in children.

FORMS - Generic/Trade: lotion 10% 59, 118 mL. Trade only (Rosula NS): Single-use pads 10%.

NOTES - Cross-sensitivity with sulfa or sulfite allergy.

**SULFACET-R** *(sulfacetamide + sulfur)* ▶K ♀C ▶? $$

ADULT - Acne, rosacea, seborrheic dermatitis: apply cream/gel daily-tid, foaming wash daily-bid.

PEDS - Not approved in children.

FORMS - Trade (Sulfacet-R) and generic: lotion (sodium sulfacetamide 10% & sulfur 5%) 25 g.

NOTES - Avoid with sulfa allergy or renal failure.

**TAZAROTENE** *(Tazorac, Avage)* ▶L ♀X ▶? $$$$

ADULT - Acne (Tazorac): apply 0.1% cream qhs. Palliation of fine facial wrinkles, mottled hyper- and hypopigmentation, benign facial lentigines (Avage): apply qhs. Psoriasis: apply 0.05% cream qhs, increase to 0.1% prn.

PEDS - Not approved in children.

UNAPPROVED PEDS - Acne: apply 0.1% cream qhs. Psoriasis: apply 0.05% cream qhs.

FORMS - Trade only (Tazorac): Cream 0.05% and 0.1% - 30, 60g, Gel 0.05% and 0.1% - 30, 100g. Trade only (Avage): Cream 0.1% 15, 30g.

(cont.)

**TAZAROTENE** (*cont.*)

NOTES - In psoriasis, may reduce irritation and improve efficacy by using topical corticosteroid in morning and tazarotene at bedtime. Desquamation, burning, dry skin, erythema, pruritus may occur in up to 30% of patients. May cause photosensitivity.

**TRETINOIN - TOPICAL (*Retin-A, Retin-A Micro, Renova, Retisol-A, ◆Stieva-A, Rejuva-A, Vitamin A Acid Cream*)** ▶LK ♀C ▶? $$

ADULT - Acne (Retin A, Retin-A Micro): apply qhs. Wrinkles, hyperpigmentation, tactile roughness (Renova): apply qhs.

PEDS - Not approved in children.

UNAPPROVED ADULT - Used in skin cancer and lamellar ichthyosis, mollusca contagiosa, verrucae plantaris, verrucae planae juvenilis, hyperpigmented lesions in black individuals, ichthyosis

vulgaris, and pityriasis rubra pilaris.

FORMS - Generic/Trade: cream 0.025% 20,45 g, 0.05% 20,45 g, 0.1% 20,45 g, gel 0.025% 15,45 g, 0.1% 15,45 g, liquid 0.05% 28 mL. Trade only: Renova cream 0.02% & 0.05% 40,60 g, Retin-A Micro gel 0.04%, 0.1% 20,45 g.

NOTES - May induce erythema, peeling. Minimize sun exposure. Concomitant use with sulfur, resorcinol, benzoyl peroxide, salicylic acid may result in skin irritation. Gel preps are flammable.

**ZIANA (clindamycin + tretinoin)** ▶LK ♀C ▶? $$$$

ADULT - Acne: Apply qhs.

PEDS - ≥12 yo: Use adult dose.

FORMS - Trade only: gel clindamycin 1.2% + tretinoin 0.025% 30, 60 g.

NOTES - May induce erythema, peeling. Minimize sun exposure.

**AMINOLEVULINIC ACID (*Levulan Kerastick*)** ▶Not absorbed ♀C ▶? $$$

ADULT - Non-hyperkeratotic actinic keratoses: apply solution to lesions on scalp or face; expose to special light source 14–18 h later.

PEDS - Not approved in children.

FORMS - Trade only: 20% solution single use ampules.

NOTES - Solution should be applied by healthcare personnel. Advise patients to avoid sunlight during 14–18 h period before blue light illumination.

**DICLOFENAC - TOPICAL (*Solaraze, Voltaren*)** ▶L ♀B ▶? $$$$$

ADULT - Solaraze: Actinic/solar keratoses: apply bid to lesions × 60–90 d. Voltaren: Osteoarthritis of areas amenable to topical therapy: 2 g (upper extremities) to 4 g (lower extremities) 4 times daily.

PEDS - Not approved in children.

FORMS - Trade only: gel 3% 50 (Solaraze), 100 g (Solaraze, Voltaren).

NOTES - Avoid exposure to sun and sunlamps. Use caution in aspirin-sensitive patients. When using for osteoarthritis (Voltaren), max daily dose 16 g to any single lower extremity joint, 8 g to any single upper extremity joint.

**FLUOROURACIL - TOPICAL (*5-FU, Carac, Efudex, Fluoroplex*)** ▶L ♀X ▶- $$$$$

WARNING - Contraindicated in pregnant women or women who plan to get pregnant during therapy. Avoid application to mucous membranes.

ADULT - Actinic or solar keratoses: apply bid to lesions × 2–6 wk. Superficial basal cell carcinomas: apply 5% cream/solution bid.

PEDS - Not approved in children.

UNAPPROVED ADULT - Condylomata acuminata: a 1% solution in 70% ethanol and the 5% cream has been used.

FORMS - Trade only: Cream 0.5% 30 g (Carac), 5% 25 g (Efudex), 1% 30 g (Fluoroplex). Generic/Trade: Solution 2% & 5% 10 mL (Efudex), Cream 5% 40 g.

NOTES - May cause severe irritation & photosensitivity. Contraindicated in women who are or who may become pregnant during therapy. Avoid application to mucous membranes.

**METHYLAMINOLEVULINATE (*Metvix, Metvixia*)** ▶Not absorbed ♀C ▶? ?

ADULT - Non-hyperkeratotic actinic keratoses of face/scalp: Apply cream 1 mm thick (max 1 g) to lesion and 5·mm surrounding area; cover with dressing for 3h; remove dressing and cream and perform illumination therapy. Repeat in 7 d.

PEDS - Not approved in children.

FORMS - Trade only: cream: 16%, 2 g tube.

NOTES - Use in immunocompetent individuals. Lesion debridement should be performed prior to application of cream. Formulated in peanut and almond oil; has not been tested in patients allergic to peanuts.

**BACITRACIN (◆*Baciguent*)** ▶Not absorbed ♀C ▶? $

ADULT - Minor cuts, wounds, burns or skin abrasions: apply daily-tid.

PEDS - Not approved in children.

UNAPPROVED PEDS - Minor cuts, wounds, burns or skin abrasions: apply daily-tid.

FORMS - OTC Generic/Trade: ointment 500 units/g 1,15,30g.

NOTES - May cause contact dermatitis or anaphylaxis.

**FUSIDIC ACID - TOPICAL (◆*Fucidin*)** ▶L ♀? ▶? $

ADULT - Canada only. Skin infections: Apply tid-qid.

PEDS - Canada only. Skin infections: Apply tid-qid.

FORMS - Canada trade only: cream 2% fusidic acid 5,15,30 g, ointment 2% sodium fusidate 5,15,30 g.

NOTES - Contains lanolin; possible hypersensitivity.

**GENTAMICIN - TOPICAL (*Garamycin*)** ▶K ♀D ▶? $

ADULT - Skin infections: apply tid-qid.

PEDS - Skin infections >1 yo: apply tid-qid.

FORMS - Generic/Trade: ointment 0.1% 15,30 g, cream 0.1% 15,30 g.

**MAFENIDE (*Sulfamylon*) ▶LK ♀C ▶? $$$**
ADULT - Adjunctive treatment of burns: apply daily-bid.
PEDS - Adjunctive treatment of burns: apply daily-bid.
FORMS - Trade only: cream 37, 114, 411 g, 5% topical solution 50 g packets.
NOTES - Can cause metabolic acidosis. Contains sulfonamides.

**METRONIDAZOLE - TOPICAL (*Noritate, MetroCream, MetroGel, MetroLotion, ✦Rosasol*) ▶KL ♀B(- in 1st trimester) ▶- $$$**
ADULT - Rosacea: apply daily (1%) or bid (0.75%).
PEDS - Not approved in children.
UNAPPROVED ADULT - A 1% solution prepared from the oral tabs has been used in the treatment of infected decubitus ulcers.
FORMS - Trade only: Gel (MetroGel) 1% 45,60 g, Cream (Noritate) 1% 30,60 g. Generic/Trade: Gel 0.75% 29g. Cream 0.75% 45 g. Lotion (MetroLotion) 0.75% 59 mL.
NOTES - Results usually noted within 3 wk, with continuing improvement through 9 wk. Avoid using vaginal prep on face due to irritation because of formulation differences.

**MUPIROCIN (*Bactroban, Centany*) ▶Not absorbed ♀B ▶? $$$**
ADULT - Impetigo: apply tid × 3–5 d. Infected wounds: apply tid × 10 d. Nasal methicillin-resistant Staph aureus eradication: 0.5 g in each nostril bid × 5 d.
PEDS - Impetigo (mupirocin cream/ointment): apply tid. Infected wounds: apply tid × 10 d. Nasal form not approved in children <12 yo.
FORMS - Generic/Trade: Cream 2% 15, 30 g, ointment 2% 22 g, 2% nasal ointment 1 g single-use tubes (for MRSA eradication).

**NEOSPORIN CREAM (neomycin + polymyxin) ▶K ♀C ▶? $**
ADULT - Minor cuts, wounds, burns or skin abrasions: apply daily-tid.
PEDS - Not approved in children.
UNAPPROVED PEDS - Minor cuts, wounds, burns or skin abrasions: apply daily-tid.
FORMS - OTC Trade only: neomycin 3.5 mg/g + polymyxin 10,000 units/g 15 g and unit dose 0.94 g.
NOTES - Neomycin component can cause contact dermatitis.

**NEOSPORIN OINTMENT (bacitracin + neomycin + polymyxin) ▶K ♀C ▶? $**
ADULT - Minor cuts, wounds, burns or skin abrasions: apply daily-tid.
PEDS - Not approved in children.
UNAPPROVED PEDS - Minor cuts, wounds, burns or skin abrasions: apply daily-tid.
FORMS - OTC Generic/Trade: bacitracin 400 units/g + neomycin 3.5 mg/g + polymyxin 5,000 units/g 2.4,9.6,14.2,15, 30 g and unit dose 0.94 g.
NOTES - Also known as triple antibiotic ointment. Neomycin component can cause contact dermatitis.

**POLYSPORIN (bacitracin + polymyxin) (✦Polytopic) ▶K ♀C ▶? $**
ADULT - Minor cuts, wounds, burns or skin abrasions: apply daily-tid.
PEDS - Not approved in children.
UNAPPROVED PEDS - Minor cuts, wounds, burns or skin abrasions: apply daily-tid.
FORMS - OTC Trade only: ointment 15,30 g and unit dose 0.9 g, powder 10 g, aerosol 90 g.
NOTES - May cause allergic contact dermatitis and rarely contact anaphylaxis.

**RETAPAMULIN (*Altabax*) ▶Not absorbed ♀B ▶? $$$**
ADULT - Impetigo: apply bid for 5 d.
PEDS - Impetigo (9 mo or older): apply bid for 5 d.
FORMS - Trade only: ointment 1% 5, 10, 15 g.

**SILVER SULFADIAZINE (*Silvadene, ✦Dermazin, Flamazine, SSD*) ▶LK ♀B ▶- $**
ADULT - Burns: apply daily-bid.
PEDS - Not approved in children.
UNAPPROVED ADULT - Has been used for pressure ulcers.
UNAPPROVED PEDS - Burns: apply daily-bid.
FORMS - Generic/Trade: cream 1% 20,50,85,400, 1000g.
NOTES - Avoid in sulfa allergy. Leukopenia, primarily decreased neutrophil count in up to 20% of patients. Significant absorption may occur and serum sulfa concentrations approach therapeutic levels. Avoid in G6PD deficiency. Use caution in pregnancy nearing term, premature infants, infants ≤2 mo and in patients with renal or hepatic dysfunction.

## DERMATOLOGY: Antifungals (Topical)

**BUTENAFINE (*Lotrimin Ultra, Mentax*) ▶L ♀B ▶? $**
ADULT - Treatment of tinea pedis: apply daily for 4 wk or bid × 7 d. Tinea corporis, tinea versicolor, or tinea cruris: apply daily for 2 wk.
PEDS - Not approved in children.
FORMS - Trade only. Rx: cream 1% 15,30 g (Mentax). OTC: cream 1% 12, 24 g (Lotrimin Ultra).
NOTES - Most common adverse effects include contact dermatitis, burning, and worsening of condition. If no improvement in 4 wk, reevaluate diagnosis.

**CICLOPIROX (*Loprox, Penlac, ✦Stieprox shampoo*) ▶K ♀B ▶? $$$$**
ADULT - Tinea pedis, cruris, corporis, and versicolor, candidiasis (cream, lotion): apply bid. Onychomycosis of fingernails/toenails (nail solution): apply daily to affected nails; apply over previous coat; remove with alcohol every 7 d. Seborrheic dermatitis (Loprox shampoo): shampoo twice/wk × 4 wk.
PEDS - Onychomycosis of fingernails/toenails in children ≥12 yo (nail solution): apply daily to

**(cont.)**

**CICLOPIROX** *(cont.)*
affected nails; apply over previous coat; remove with alcohol every 7 d (Penlac). Not approved in children <12 yo.
FORMS - Trade only: gel (Loprox) 0.77% 30, 45, 100 g, shampoo (Loprox) 1% 120 mL. Generic/Trade: nail solution (Penlac) 8% 6.6 mL, cream (Loprox) 0.77% 15, 30, 90 g, lotion (Loprox TS) 0.77% 30, 60 mL.
NOTES - Clinical improvement of tinea usually occurs within first wk. Patients with tinea versicolor usually exhibit clinical and mycological clearing after 2 wk. If no improvement in 4 wk, reevaluate diagnosis. Do not get shampoo in eyes. No safety information available in diabetes or immunocompromise. Shampoo may affect hair color in those with light-colored hair. For nail solution, infected portion of each nail should be removed by health care professional as frequently as monthly. Oral antifungal therapy is more effective for onychomycosis than Penlac.
**CLOTRIMAZOLE - TOPICAL** *(Lotrimin, Mycelex, ✦Canesten, Clotrimaderm)* ▶L ♀B ▶? $
ADULT - Treatment of tinea pedis, cruris, corporis, and versicolor, and cutaneous candidiasis: apply bid.
PEDS - Treatment of tinea pedis, cruris, corporis, versicolor, cutaneous candidiasis: apply bid.
FORMS - Note that Lotrimin brand cream, lotion, solution are clotrimazole, while Lotrimin powders and liquid spray are miconazole. OTC & Rx generic/trade: cream 1% 15, 30, 45, 90 g, solution 1% 10,30 mL. Trade only: lotion 1% 30 mL.
NOTES - If no improvement in 4 wk, reevaluate diagnosis.
**ECONAZOLE** ▶Not absorbed ♀C ▶? $$
ADULT - Treatment of tinea pedis, cruris, corporis, and versicolor: apply daily. Cutaneous candidiasis: apply bid.
PEDS - Not approved in children.
FORMS - Generic only: cream 1% 15, 30, 85g.
NOTES - Treat candidal infections, tinea cruris and tinea corporis for 2 wk and tinea pedis for 1 mo to reduce risk of recurrence.
**KETOCONAZOLE - TOPICAL** *(Extina, Nizoral, Xolegel, ✦Ketoderm)* ▶L ♀C ▶? $$
ADULT - Shampoo (2%): Tinea versicolor: apply to affected area, leave on for 5 min, rinse. Cream: cutaneous candidiasis, tinea corporis, cruris, and versicolor: apply daily. Seborrheic dermatitis: apply cream (2%) bid for 4 wk or gel daily for 2 wk or foam bid for 4 wk. Dandruff: apply shampoo (1%) twice a wk.
PEDS - Not approved in children <12 yr.
UNAPPROVED ADULT - Seborrheic dermatitis: apply cream (2%) daily.
UNAPPROVED PEDS - Shampoo (2%): Tinea versicolor: apply to affected area, leave on for 5 min, rinse. Cream: cutaneous candidiasis, tinea corporis, cruris, and versicolor: apply daily. Seborrheic dermatitis: apply cream (2%) bid. Dandruff: apply shampoo (1%) twice a wk.

FORMS - Generic/Trade: cream 2% 15, 30, 60 g, shampoo 2% (120 mL). Trade only: shampoo 1% (OTC), gel 2%, 15g (Rx, Xolegel) foam 2%, 50, 100 g (Rx, Extina).
NOTES - Treat candidal infections, tinea cruris, corporis and versicolor for 4 wk. Treat seborrheic dermatitis for 4 wk. Treat tinea pedis for 6 wk.
**MICONAZOLE - TOPICAL** *(Monistat-Derm, Micatin, Lotrimin)* ▶L ♀+ ▶? $
ADULT - Tinea pedis, cruris, corporis, and versicolor, cutaneous candidiasis: apply bid.
PEDS - Not approved in children.
UNAPPROVED PEDS - Tinea pedis, cruris, corporis, and versicolor, cutaneous candidiasis: apply bid.
FORMS - Note that Lotrimin brand cream, lotion, solution are clotrimazole, while Lotrimin powders and liquid spray are miconazole. OTC generic: ointment 2% 29 g, spray 2% 105 mL, solution 2% 7.39, 30 mL. Generic/Trade: cream 2% 15,30,90 g, powder 2% 90 g, spray powder 2% 90,100 g, spray liquid 2% 105,113 mL.
NOTES - Symptomatic relief generally occurs in 2–3 d. Treat candida, tinea cruris, tinea corporis for 2 wk, tinea pedis for 1 mo to reduce risk of recurrence.
**NAFTIFINE** *(Naftin)* ▶LK ♀B ▶? $$$
ADULT - Tinea pedis, cruris, and corporis: apply daily (cream) or bid (gel).
PEDS - Not approved in children.
FORMS - Trade only: cream 1% 15, 30, 60, 90 g, gel 1% 20, 40, 60, 90 g.
NOTES - If no improvement in 4 wk, reevaluate diagnosis.
**NYSTATIN - TOPICAL** *(Mycostatin, ✦Nilstat, Nyaderm, Candistatin)* ▶Not absorbed ♀C ▶? $
ADULT - Cutaneous or mucocutaneous Candida infections: apply bid-tid.
PEDS - Cutaneous or mucocutaneous Candida infections: apply bid-tid.
FORMS - Generic/Trade: cream 100,000 units/g 15,30,240 g, ointment 100,000 units/g 15,30 g, powder 100,000 units/g 15 g.
NOTES - Ineffective for dermatophytes/tinea. For fungal infections of the feet, dust feet and footwear with powder.
**OXICONAZOLE** *(Oxistat, Oxizole)* ▶? ♀B ▶? $$$
ADULT - Tinea pedis, cruris, and corporis: apply daily-bid. Tinea versicolor (cream only): apply daily.
PEDS - Cream: Tinea pedis, cruris, and corporis: apply daily-bid. Tinea versicolor: apply daily.
FORMS - Trade only: cream 1% 15, 30, 60 g, lotion 1% 30 mL.
**SERTACONAZOLE** *(Ertaczo)* ▶Not absorbed ♀C ▶? $$
ADULT - Tinea pedis: apply bid.
PEDS - Not approved for children <12 yo.
FORMS - Trade only: cream 2% 15, 30, 60 g.
**TERBINAFINE - TOPICAL** *(Lamisil, Lamisil AT)* ▶L ♀B ▶? $$$
ADULT - Tinea pedis: apply bid. Tinea cruris and corporis: apply daily-bid. Tinea versicolor (solution): apply bid.
PEDS - Not approved in children.

**TERBINAFINE** (*cont.*)
UNAPPROVED ADULT - Cutaneous candidiasis.
UNAPPROVED PEDS - Tinea pedis: apply bid. Tinea cruris and corporis: apply daily-bid. Tinea versicolor (solution): apply bid.
FORMS - Trade only: cream 1% 15,30 g, gel 1% 5,15,30 g OTC: Trade only (Lamisil AT): cream 1% 12,24 g, spray pump solution 1% 30 mL.
NOTES - In many patients, improvement noted within 3–4 d, but continue therapy for a minimum of 1 wk, max of 4 wk. Topical therapy not effective for nail fungus.

**TOLNAFTATE** (*Tinactin, ✚ZeaSorb AF*) ▶? ♀? ▶? $
ADULT - Tinea pedis, cruris, corporis, and versicolor: apply bid. Prevention of tinea pedis (powder and aerosol): apply prn.
PEDS - >2 yo: Tinea pedis, cruris, corporis, and versicolor: apply bid. Prevention of tinea pedis (powder and aerosol): apply prn.
FORMS - OTC Generic/Trade: cream 1% 15,30 g, solution 1% 10,15 mL, powder 1% 45,90 g, spray powder 1% 100,105,150 g, spray liquid 1% 60,120 mL. Trade only: gel 1% 15 g.

**A-200** (pyrethrins + piperonyl butoxide, ✚R&C) ▶L ♀C ▶? $
ADULT - Lice: Apply shampoo, wash after 10 min. Reapply in 5–7 d.
PEDS - Lice: Apply shampoo, wash after 10 min. Reapply in 5–7 d.
FORMS - OTC Generic/Trade: shampoo (0.33% pyrethrins, 4% piperonyl butoxide) 60,120,240 mL.
NOTES - Use caution if allergic to ragweed. Avoid contact with mucous membranes.

**CROTAMITON** (*Eurax*) ▶? ♀C ▶? $$
ADULT - Scabies: massage cream/lotion into entire body from chin down, repeat 24 h later, bathe 48 h later. Pruritus: massage into affected areas prn.
PEDS - Not approved in children.
UNAPPROVED PEDS - Scabies: massage cream/lotion into entire body from chin down, repeat 24h later, bathe 48h later. Pruritus: massage into affected areas prn.
FORMS - Trade only: cream 10% 60 g, lotion 10% 60,480 mL.
NOTES - Patients with scabies should change bed linen and clothing in am after 2nd application and bathe 48h after last application. Consider treating entire family.

**LINDANE** (✚Hexit) ▶L ♀B ▶? $
WARNING - For use only in patients who have failed other agents. Seizures and deaths have been reported with repeat or prolonged use. Use caution with infants, children, elderly, those who weigh <50 kg. Contraindicated in premature infants and patients with uncontrolled seizures.
ADULT - Head/crab lice: Lotion: apply 30–60 mL to affected area, wash off after 12h. Shampoo: apply 30–60 mL, wash off after 4 min. Scabies (lotion): apply 30–60 mL to total body from neck down, wash off after 8–12h.
PEDS - Lindane penetrates human skin and has potential for CNS toxicity. Studies indicate potential toxic effects of topical lindane are greater in young. Max dose for children <6 yo is 30 mL.

FORMS - Generic only: lotion 1% 60, 480 mL, shampoo 1% 60, 480 mL.
NOTES - For lice, reapply if living lice noted after 7 d. After shampooing, comb with fine tooth comb to remove nits. Consider treating entire family.

**MALATHION** (*Ovide*) ▶? ♀B ▶? $$
ADULT - Head lice: apply to dry hair, let dry naturally, wash off in 8–12 h.
PEDS - Head lice in children >6 yo: apply to dry hair, let dry naturally, wash off in 8–12 h.
FORMS - Trade only: lotion 0.5% 59 mL.
NOTES - Do not use hair dryer; flammable. Avoid contact with eyes. Use a fine tooth comb to remove nits and dead lice. Application may be repeated in 7–9 d.

**PERMETHRIN** (*Elimite, Acticin, Nix, ✚Kwellada-P*) ▶L ♀B ▶? $$
ADULT - Scabies (cream): massage cream into entire body (avoid mouth, eyes, nose), wash off after 8–14h. 30 g is typical adult dose. Head lice (liquid): apply to clean, towel-dried hair, saturate hair and scalp, wash off after 10 min.
PEDS - Scabies (cream) >2 mo: massage cream into entire body (avoid mouth, eyes, nose), wash off after 8–14h. Head lice (liquid) in children >2 yo: saturate hair and scalp, wash off after 10 min.
FORMS - Trade only: cream (Elimite, Acticin) 5% 60 g. OTC Generic/Trade: liquid creme rinse (Nix) 1% 60 mL.
NOTES - If necessary, may repeat application in 7 d. Consider treating entire family.

**RID** (pyrethrins + piperonyl butoxide) ▶L ♀C ▶? $
ADULT - Lice: Apply shampoo/mousse, wash after 10 min. Reapply in 5–10 d.
PEDS - Lice: Apply shampoo/mousse, wash after 10 min. Reapply in 5–10 d.
FORMS - OTC Generic/Trade: shampoo 60,120,240 mL. Trade only: mousse 5.5 oz.
NOTES - Use caution if allergic to ragweed. Avoid contact with mucus membranes. Available alone or as part of a RID 1–2–3 kit containing shampoo, egg and nit comb-out gel and home lice control spray for non-washable items.

**ACITRETIN** (*Soriatane*) ▶L ♀X ▶- $$$$$
WARNING - Contraindicated in pregnancy and avoid pregnancy for 3 yr following medication discontinuation. Major human fetal abnormalities have

been reported. Females of child bearing age must avoid alcohol while on medication and for 2 mo following therapy since alcohol prolongs elimination of a teratogenic metabolite. Use in reliable
**(cont.)**

**ACITRETIN** *(cont.)*
females of reproductive potential only if they have severe, unresponsive psoriasis, have received written and oral warnings of the teratogenic potential, are using 2 reliable forms of contraception, and have 2 negative pregnancy tests within 1 wk prior to starting therapy. Contraception should start at least 1 mo prior to therapy and continue for 3 yr following discontinuation. Must have negative monthly pregnancy test during treatment. Therefore, prescribe limited amount and do not allow refill until documented negative pregnancy test. Following discontinuation, repeat pregnancy test every 3 mo. It is unknown whether residual acitretin in seminal fluid poses a risk to the fetus while a male patient is taking the drug or after it is discontinued.
ADULT - Severe psoriasis: initiate at 25–50 mg PO daily.
PEDS - Not approved in children.
UNAPPROVED ADULT - Lichen planus: 30 mg/d PO for 4 wk, then titrate to 10–50 mg/d for 12 wk total. Sjogren-Larsson syndrome: 0.47 mg/kg/d PO. Also used in Darier's disease, palmoplantar pustulosis, non-bullous and bullous ichthyosiform erythroderma, lichen sclerosus et atrophicus of the vulva, palmoplantar lichen nitidus and chemoprevention for high-risk immunosuppressed patients with history of squamous cell carcinomas of the skin.
UNAPPROVED PEDS - Has been used in children with lamellar ichthyosis. Pediatric use is not recommended. Adverse effects on bone growth are suspected.
FORMS - Trade only: cap 10, 25 mg.
NOTES - Transient worsening of psoriasis may occur, and full benefit may take 2–3 mo. Elevated LFTs may occur in 1/3 of patients; monitor LFTs at 1–2 wk intervals until stable and then periodically thereafter. Monitor serum lipid concentrations every 1–2 wk until response to drug is established. May decrease tolerance to contact lenses due to dry eyes. Avoid prolonged exposure to sunlight. May cause hair loss. May cause depression. May cause bone changes, especially with use >6 mo. Many adverse drug reactions.

**ALEFACEPT** *(Amevive)* ▶? ♀B ▶? $$$$$
ADULT - Moderate to severe psoriasis: 7.5 mg IV or 15 mg IM once weekly × 12 doses. May repeat with 1 additional 12-wk course after 12 wk have elapsed from last dose.
PEDS - Not approved in children.
NOTES - Monitor CD4+ T lymphocyte cells weekly; withhold therapy if count <250/mcL and stop altogether if <250/mcL for one mo. Do not give to HIV-positive patients or with other immunosuppressives or phototherapy.

**ANTHRALIN** *(Anthra-Derm, Drithocreme, ✦Anthrascalp, Anthranol, Anthraforte, Dithranol)* ▶? ♀C ▶- $$
ADULT - Chronic psoriasis: apply daily.
PEDS - Not approved in children.

UNAPPROVED PEDS - Chronic psoriasis: apply daily.
FORMS - Trade only: ointment 0.1% 42.5 g, 0.25% 42.5 g, 0.4% 60 g, 0.5% 42.5 g, 1% 42.5 g, cream 0.1% 50 g, 0.2% 50 g, 0.25% 50 g, 0.5% 50 g. Generic/Trade: cream 1% 50 g.
NOTES - Short contact periods (ie, 15–20 min) followed by removal with an appropriate solvent (soap or petrolatum) may be preferred. May stain fabric, skin or hair.

**CALCIPOTRIENE** *(Dovonex)* ▶L ♀C ▶? $$$
ADULT - Moderate plaque psoriasis: apply bid.
PEDS - Not approved in children.
UNAPPROVED ADULT - Has been used for vitiligo.
UNAPPROVED PEDS - Moderate plaque psoriasis: apply bid. Has been used for vitiligo.
FORMS - Trade only: ointment 0.005% 30, 60, 100 g, cream 0.005% 30, 60, 100 g. Generic/Trade: Scalp solution 0.005% 60 mL.
NOTES - Avoid contact with face. Do not exceed 100 g/wk to minimize risk of hypercalcemia, hypercalciuria. Burning, itching, and skin irritation may occur in 10–15% of patients.

**EFALIZUMAB** *(Raptiva)* ▶L ♀C ▶? $$$$$
WARNING - Can cause serious infections or reactivate latent chronic infections. Discontinue if serious infection. Caution if high risk for/history of malignancy. Monitor CBC; can cause severe thrombocytopenia and hemolytic anemia. Can cause worsening of psoriasis during or after treatment.
ADULT - Moderate to severe plaque psoriasis: 0.7 mg/kg SC × 1 then 1 mg/kg SC q wk.
PEDS - Not approved in children.
FORMS - Trade only: single use vials, 125 mg.
NOTES - Monitor platelets upon initiation and monthly thereafter. May decrease to every 3 mo with continued therapy.

**METHOXSALEN** *(8-MOP, Oxsoralen-Ultra)* ▶Skin ♀C ▶? $$$$$
ADULT - Psoriasis: dose based on weight (0.4 mg/kg/dose), 1½ to 2 h before ultraviolet light exposure.
PEDS - Not approved in children.
FORMS - Trade only: soft gelatin cap 10 mg (Oxsoralen-Ultra), hard gelatin cap 10 mg (8-MOP).
NOTES - Oxsoralen-Ultra (soft gelatin cap) cannot be interchanged with 8-MOP (hard gelatin cap) due to significant bioavailability differences and photosensitization onset times. Take with food or milk. Wear ultraviolet light blocking glasses and avoid sun exposure after ingestion and for remainder of d.

**TACLONEX** (calcipotriene + betamethasone) ▶L ♀C ▶? $$$$$
ADULT - Psoriasis vulgaris: Apply daily for up to 4 wk.
PEDS - Not approved in children.
FORMS - Trade only: (calcipotriene 0.005% + betamethasone dipropionate 0.064%) ointment 15, 30, 60, 100g, Topical susp 15, 30, 60g.
NOTES - Do not exceed 100g per wk. Do not use on more than 30% of body surface area. Do not apply to face, groin, or axillae.

## DERMATOLOGY: Antivirals (Topical)

**ACYCLOVIR - TOPICAL (*Zovirax*)** ▶K ♀C ▶? $$$$$
ADULT - Initial episodes of herpes genitalis: apply oint q3h (6 times/d) × 7 d. Non-life threatening mucocutaneous herpes simplex in immunocompromised patients: apply oint q3h (6 times/d) × 7 d. Recurrent herpes labialis: apply cream 5 times/d for 4 d.
PEDS - <12 yo: Not approved. ≥12 yo: Recurrent herpes labialis: apply cream 5 times/d for 4 d.
UNAPPROVED PEDS - Initial episodes of herpes genitalis: apply oint q3h (6 times/d) × 7 d. Non-life threatening mucocutaneous herpes simplex in immunocompromised patients: apply oint q3h (6 times/d) × 7 d.
FORMS - Trade only: ointment 5% 15 g, cream 5% (2 & 5 g).
NOTES - Use finger cot or rubber glove to apply ointment to avoid dissemination. Burning/stinging may occur in up to 28% of patients. Oral form more effective than topical for herpes genitalis.

**DOCOSANOL (*Abreva*)** ▶Not absorbed ♀B ▶? $
ADULT - Oral-facial herpes (cold sores): apply 5x/d until healed.
PEDS - Oral-facial herpes (cold sores), ≥12 yo: Use adult dose.
FORMS - OTC: Trade only: cream 10% 2 g.

**IMIQUIMOD (*Aldara*)** ▶Not absorbed ♀C ▶? $$$$$
ADULT - External genital and perianal warts: apply 3 times weekly at bedtime for up to 16 wk. Wash off after 8 h. Nonhyperkeratotic, nonhypertrophic actinic keratoses on face/scalp in immunocompetent adults: apply to face or scalp (but not both) 2 times weekly for up to 16 wk. Wash off after 8 h. Primary superficial basal cell carcinoma: apply 5 times weekly for 6 wk. Wash off after 8 h.
PEDS - Children >11 yo: External genital and perianal warts: apply 3 times/wk at bedtime. Wash off after 6–10 h.
UNAPPROVED ADULT - Molluscum contagiosum: apply 3 times weekly for 6–10 h.
UNAPPROVED PEDS - Molluscum contagiosum
FORMS - Trade only: cream 5% 250 mg single use packets.
NOTES - May weaken condoms and diaphragms. Avoid sexual contact while cream is on when used for genital/perianal warts. Most common adverse effects include erythema, itching, erosion,
burning, excoriation, edema and pain. Discard partially used packets.

**PENCICLOVIR (*Denavir*)** ▶Not absorbed ♀B ▶? $$
ADULT - Recurrent herpes labialis (cold sores): apply q2h while awake × 4 d.
PEDS - Not approved in children.
UNAPPROVED PEDS - Recurrent herpes labialis: apply q2h while awake × 4 d.
FORMS - Trade only: cream 1% tubes 1.5 g.
NOTES - Start therapy as soon as possible during prodrome. For moderate to severe cases of herpes labialis, systemic treatment with famciclovir or acyclovir may be preferred.

**PODOFILOX (*Condylox*, ◆*Condyline, Wartec*)** ▶? ♀C ▶? $$$
ADULT - External genital warts (gel and solution) and perianal warts (gel only): apply bid for 3 consecutive d of a wk and repeat for up to 4 wk.
PEDS - Not approved in children.
FORMS - Generic/Trade: Solution 0.5% 3.5 mL. Trade only: Gel 0.5% 3.5 g.

**PODOPHYLLIN (*Podocon-25, Podofin, Podofilm*)** ▶? ♀- ▶- $$$
ADULT - Genital wart removal: Initial application: apply to wart and leave on for 30–40 min to determine patient's sensitivity. Thereafter, use minimum contact time necessary (1–4h depending on result). Remove dried podophyllin with alcohol or soap and water.
PEDS - Not approved in children.
FORMS - Not to be dispensed to patients. For hospital/clinic use; not intended for outpatient prescribing. Trade only: Liquid 25% 15 mL
NOTES - Not to be dispensed to patients. Do not treat large areas or numerous warts all at once. Contraindicated in diabetics, pregnancy, patients using steroids or with poor circulation, and on bleeding warts.

**SINECATECHINS (*Veregen*)** ▶Unknown ♀C ▶? $$$$$
ADULT - Apply tid to external genital warts for up to 16 wk.
PEDS - Not approved in children.
FORMS - Trade only: ointment 15% 15g.
NOTES - Botanical drug product. Contains a partially purified fraction of the water extract of green tea leaves. Do not use on open wounds. Do not use in immunocompromised patients. Generic name used to be kunecatechins.

## DERMATOLOGY: Atopic Dermatitis Preparations

**NOTE:** Potential risk of cancer. Should only be used as 2nd-line agent for short-term and intermittent treatment of atopic dermatitis in those unresponsive to or intolerant of other treatments. Long-term safety has not been established. Avoid use in immunocompromised and in children <2 yo. Use minimum amount to control symptoms.

**PIMECROLIMUS (*Elidel*)** ▶L ♀C ▶? $$$$
ADULT - Atopic dermatitis: apply bid.
PEDS - Atopic dermatitis: ≥2 yo: apply bid. Don't use if <2 yo.
FORMS - Trade only: cream 1% 30, 60, 100 g.
NOTES - Long term safety unclear.

**TACROLIMUS - TOPICAL (*Protopic*)** ▶Minimal absorption ♀C ▶? $$$$
ADULT - Atopic dermatitis: apply bid.
PEDS - Children <2yo: not approved. Children 2–15 yo: Atopic dermatitis: apply 0.03% oint bid.

**(cont.)**

**TACROLIMUS** *(cont.)*
  UNAPPROVED ADULT - Vitiligo: apply 0.1% bid.
  Chronic allergic contact dermatitis (ie, nickel-
  induced): apply 0.1% oint bid.

FORMS - Trade only: ointment 0.03% & 0.1% 30,
  60, 100 g.
NOTES - Do not use with an occlusive dressing.
  Continue treatment for 1 wk after clearing of
  symptoms.

## DERMATOLOGY:  Corticosteroids (Topical)

**NOTE:** After long-term use, do not discontinue abruptly; switch to a less potent agent or alternate use of corticosteroids and emollient products. Monitor for hyperglycemia/adrenal suppression if used for long period of time or
over a large area of the body, especially in children. Chronic administration may cause skin atrophy and interfere
with pediatric growth & development.

**ALCLOMETASONE DIPROPIONATE** *(Aclovate)* ▶L ♀C
▶? $$
  ADULT - Inflammatory and pruritic manifestations
    of corticosteroid-responsive dermatoses: apply
    sparingly 2–3 times/d.
  PEDS - Inflammatory and pruritic manifestations of
    corticosteroid-responsive dermatoses in children
    ≥1 yo: apply sparingly 2–3 times/d. Safety and
    efficacy for >3 wk have not been established.
  FORMS - Generic/Trade: Ointment & cream 0.05%
    15, 45, 60 g.
**AMCINONIDE** *(Cyclocort)* ▶L ♀C ▶? $$
  ADULT - Inflammatory and pruritic manifestations
    of corticosteroid-responsive dermatoses: apply
    sparingly 2–3 times/d.
  PEDS - Inflammatory and pruritic manifestations
    of corticosteroid-responsive dermatoses: apply
    sparingly 2–3 times/d.
  FORMS - Generic only: Cream & ointment 0.1% 15,
    30, 60 g, Lotion 0.1% 60 mL.
**AUGMENTED BETAMETHASONE DIPROPIONATE** *(Dipro-
lene, Diprolene AF, ✦Topilene Glycol)* ▶L ♀C ▶? $$
  ADULT - Inflammatory and pruritic manifestations
    of corticosteroid-responsive dermatoses: apply
    sparingly 1–2 times/d.
  PEDS - Not approved in children <12 yo.
  FORMS - Generic/Trade: Diprolene: Ointment 0.05%
    15, 50 g, Lotion 0.05% 30, 60 mL. Diprolene AF:
    Cream 0.05% 15, 50 g. Generic only: Gel 0.05%
    15, 50 g.
  NOTES - Do not use occlusive dressings. Do not use for
    longer than 2 consecutive wk and do not exceed a
    total dose of 45–50 g/wk or 50 mL/wk of the lotion.
**BETAMETHASONE DIPROPIONATE** *(Diprosone, Max-
ivate, ✦Propaderm, TARO-sone)* ▶L ♀C ▶? $
  ADULT - Inflammatory and pruritic manifestations
    of corticosteroid-responsive dermatoses: apply
    sparingly 1–2 times/d.
  PEDS - Inflammatory and pruritic manifestations
    of corticosteroid-responsive dermatoses: apply
    sparingly 1–2 times/d.
  FORMS - Generic only: Ointment & cream 0.05% 15,
    45 g, Lotion 0.05% 60 mL.
  NOTES - Do not use occlusive dressings.
**BETAMETHASONE VALERATE** *(Luxiq foam, Veta-Val,
✦Betaderm)* ▶L ♀C ▶? $
  ADULT - Inflammatory and pruritic manifestations
    of corticosteroid-responsive dermatoses: apply

sparingly 1–2 times/d. Dermatoses of scalp:
  apply small amount of foam to scalp bid.
PEDS - Inflammatory and pruritic manifestations
  of corticosteroid-responsive dermatoses: apply
  sparingly 1–2 times/d.
FORMS - Generic only: Ointment & cream 0.1% 15,
  45 g, Lotion 0.1% 60 mL. Trade only: Foam (Luxiq)
  0.12% 50,100,150 g.
**CLOBETASOL** *(Temovate, Olux, Clobex, Cormax,
✦Dermasone)* ▶L ♀C ▶? $$
  ADULT - Inflammatory and pruritic manifestations
    of corticosteroid-responsive dermatoses: apply
    sparingly 2 times/d. For scalp apply foam 2
    times/d.
  PEDS - Not approved in children.
  FORMS - Generic/Trade: Cream & ointment 0.05%
    15, 30, 45, 60 g, Scalp application 0.05% 25, 50
    mL, Gel 0.05% 15, 30, 60 g. Foam (Olux) 0.05%
    50,100g. Trade only (Clobex): Lotion 0.05% 30,
    60,120 mL, Spray 0.05% 60,125 mL, Shampoo
    0.05% 120 mL.
  NOTES - Adrenal suppression at doses as low as
    2 g/d. Do not use occlusive dressings. Do not
    use for longer than 2 consecutive wk and do not
    exceed a total dose of 50 g/wk.
**CLOCORTOLONE PIVALATE** *(Cloderm)* ▶L ♀C ▶? $$$
  ADULT - Inflammatory and pruritic manifestations
    of corticosteroid-responsive dermatoses: apply
    sparingly 3 times/d.
  PEDS - Inflammatory and pruritic manifestations
    of corticosteroid-responsive dermatoses: apply
    sparingly 3 times/d.
  FORMS - Trade only: Cream 0.1% 15, 30, 45, 90 g.
**DESONIDE** *(DesOwen, Desonate, Tridesilon, Verdeso)*
▶L ♀C ▶? $
  ADULT - Inflammatory and pruritic manifestations
    of corticosteroid-responsive dermatoses: apply
    sparingly 2–3 times/d.
  PEDS - Inflammatory and pruritic manifestations
    of corticosteroid-responsive dermatoses: apply
    sparingly 2–3 times/d.
  FORMS - Generic/Trade: Cream and Ointment
    0.05%, 15, 60 g, Lotion 0.05%, 60,120 mL. Trade
    only: Gel (Desonate) 0.05% 60 g, Foam (Verdeso)
    0.05%, 50,100 g.
  NOTES - Do not use with occlusive dressings.

**DESOXIMETASONE** (*Topicort, Topicort LP, ◆Desoxi*) ▶L ♀C ▶? $$$
ADULT - Inflammatory and pruritic manifestations of corticosteroid-responsive dermatoses: apply sparingly 2 times/d.
PEDS - Safety and efficacy have not been established for Topicort 0.25% ointment. For inflammatory and pruritic manifestations of corticosteroid-responsive dermatoses (cream and gel): apply sparingly 2 times/d.
FORMS - Generic/Trade: Cream and Gel 0.05% 15, 60 g, Cream and Ointment 0.25% 15, 60 g.

**DIFLORASONE** (*Psorcon E, Maxiflor*) ▶L ♀C ▶? $$
ADULT - Inflammatory and pruritic manifestations of corticosteroid-responsive dermatoses: apply sparingly 1–3 times/d.
PEDS - Not approved in children.
FORMS - Generic/Trade: Cream and Ointment 0.05% 15, 30, 60 g.
NOTES - Doses of 30 g/d of diflorasone 0.05% cream for 1 wk resulted in adrenal suppression in some psoriasis patients.

**FLUOCINOLONE** (*Synalar, Capex, Derma-Smoothe/FS, ◆Caprex*) ▶L ♀C ▶? $
ADULT - Inflammatory and pruritic manifestations of corticosteroid-responsive dermatoses: apply sparingly 2–4 times/d. Psoriasis of the scalp (Derma-Smoothe/FS): Massage into scalp, cover with shower cap and leave on ≥4 h or overnight and then wash off.
PEDS - Inflammatory and pruritic manifestations of corticosteroid-responsive dermatoses: apply sparingly 2–4 times/d. Atopic dermatitis: Moisten skin and apply to affected areas twice daily for up to 4 wk (Derma-Smoothe/FS).
FORMS - Generic/Trade: Cream and Ointment 0.025% 15, 30, 60 g, Solution 0.01% 20, 60 mL. Generic only: Cream 0.01% 15, 60 g. Trade only (Derma-Smoothe/FS): Topical oil 0.01% 120 mL, (Capex) Shampoo 0.01% 120 mL.

**FLUOCINONIDE** (*Lidex, Lidex-E, Vanos, ◆Lidemol, Topsyn, Tiamol*) ▶L ♀C ▶? $
ADULT - Inflammatory and pruritic manifestations of corticosteroid-responsive dermatoses: apply sparingly 2–4 times/d. Plaque-type psoriasis: apply 0.1% cream (Vanos) daily-bid × 2 consecutive wk only; no more than 60 g/wk. Atopic dermatitis: apply 0.1% cream (Vanos) once daily.
PEDS - Inflammatory and pruritic manifestations of corticosteroid-responsive dermatoses: apply sparingly 2–4 times/d.
FORMS - Generic/Trade: Cream, Ointment, and Gel 0.05% 15, 30, 60, Solution 0.05% 20, 60 mL. Trade only: Cream 0.1% 30, 60, 120 g (Vanos).

**FLURANDRENOLIDE** (*Cordran, Cordran SP*) ▶L ♀C ▶? $$$
ADULT - Inflammatory and pruritic manifestations of corticosteroid-responsive dermatoses: apply sparingly 2–3 times/d.

PEDS - Inflammatory and pruritic manifestations of corticosteroid-responsive dermatoses: apply sparingly 2–3 times/d.
FORMS - Trade only: Ointment and Cream 0.05% 15, 30, 60 g. Lotion 0.05% 15, 60 mL. Tape 4mcg/cm².

**FLUTICASONE - TOPICAL** (*Cutivate, ◆Flixonase, Flixotide*) ▶L ♀C ▶? $$
ADULT - Eczema: apply sparingly 1–2 times/d. Other inflammatory and pruritic manifestations of corticosteroid-responsive dermatoses: apply sparingly 2 times/d.
PEDS - Children >3 mo old: Eczema: apply sparingly 1–2 times/d. Other inflammatory and pruritic manifestations of corticosteroid-responsive dermatoses: apply sparingly 2 times/d.
FORMS - Generic/Trade: Cream 0.05% 15,30,60 g, Ointment 0.005% 15,30,60 g. Trade only: Lotion 0.05% 60, 120 mL.
NOTES - Do not use with an occlusive dressing.

**HALCINONIDE** (*Halog*) ▶L ♀C ▶? $$
ADULT - Inflammatory and pruritic manifestations of corticosteroid-responsive dermatoses: apply sparingly 2–3 times/d.
PEDS - Inflammatory and pruritic manifestations of corticosteroid-responsive dermatoses: apply sparingly 2–3 times/d.
FORMS - Trade only: Cream and Ointment 0.1% 15, 30, 60 g Solution 0.1% 20, 60 mL.

**HALOBETASOL PROPIONATE** (*Ultravate*) ▶L ♀C ▶? $$
ADULT - Inflammatory and pruritic manifestations of corticosteroid-responsive dermatoses: apply sparingly 1–2 times/d.
PEDS - Not approved in children.
FORMS - Generic/Trade: Cream and Ointment 0.05% 15, 50 g.
NOTES - Do not use occlusive dressings. Do not use for >2 consecutive wk and do not exceed a total dose of 50 g/wk.

**HYDROCORTISONE - TOPICAL** (*Cortizone, Hycort, Hytone, Tegrin-HC, Dermolate, Synacort, Anusol-HC, Proctocream HC, Cortifoam, ◆Cortoderm, Prevex-HC, Cortate, Emo-Cort*) ▶L ♀C ▶? $
ADULT - Inflammatory and pruritic manifestations of corticosteroid-responsive dermatoses: apply sparingly 2–4 times/d. External anal itching: apply cream tid-qid prn or supp bid or rectal foam daily-bid.
PEDS - Inflammatory and pruritic manifestations of corticosteroid-responsive dermatoses: apply sparingly 2–4 times/d.
FORMS - Products available OTC & Rx depending on labeling. 2.5% preparation available Rx only. Generic: ointment 0.5% 30 g, ointment 1% 15, 20,30,60,120 g, ointment 2.5% 20,30 g, cream 0.5% 15,30,60 g, cream 1% 20,30,60,90,120 g, cream 2.5% 15,20,30,60,120 g, lotion 0.25% 120 mL, lotion 0.5% 30,60,120 mL, lotion 1% 60,120 mL, lotion 2% 30 mL, lotion 2.5% 60 mL. Anal preparations: Generic/Trade: cream 1% (Anusol HC-1), 2.5% 30 g (Anusol HC, Proctocream HC), susp 25 mg (Anusol HC), 10% rectal foam (Cortifoam) 15g.

## CORTICOSTEROIDS—TOPICAL

| Potency* | Generic | Trade Name | Forms | Frequency |
|---|---|---|---|---|
| Low | alclometasone dipropionate | Aclovate | 0.05% cream ointment | bid-tid |
| Low | clocortolone pivalate | Cloderm | 0.1% cream | tid |
| Low | desonide | DesOwen, Tridesilon | 0.05% cream lotion ointment | bid-tid |
| Low | hydrocortisone | Hytone, others | 0.5% cream lotion ointment; 1% cream lotion ointment; 2.5% cream lotion ointment | bid-qid |
| Low | hydrocortisone acetate | Cortaid, Corticaine | 0.5% cream ointment, 1% cream ointment spray | bid-qid |
| Medium | betamethasone valerate | Luxiq | 0.1% cream lotion ointment; 0.12% foam (Luxiq) | qd-bid |
| Medium | desoximetasone‡ | Topicort | 0.05% cream | bid |
| Medium | fluocinolone | Synalar | 0.01% cream solution; 0.025% cream ointment | bid-qid |
| Medium | flurandrenolide | Cordran | 0.025% cream ointment; 0.05% cream lotion ointment; tape | bid-qid |
| Medium | fluticasone propionate | Cutivate | 0.005% ointment; 0.05% cream lotion | qd-bid |
| Medium | hydrocortisone butyrate | Locoid | 0.1% cream ointment solution | bid-tid |
| Medium | hydrocortisone valerate | Westcort | 0.2% cream ointment | bid-tid |
| Medium | mometasone furoate | Elocon | 0.1% cream lotion ointment | qd |
| Medium | triamcinolone‡ | Aristocort, Kenalog | 0.025% cream lotion ointment; 0.1% cream lotion ointment; spray | bid-tid |
| High | amcinonide | Cyclocort | 0.1% cream lotion ointment | bid-tid |
| High | betamethasone dipropionate‡ | Maxivate, others | 0.05% cream lotion ointment (non-Diprolene) | qd-bid |
| High | desoximetasone‡ | Topicort | 0.05% gel; 0.25% cream ointment | bid |
| High | diflorasone diacetate‡ | Maxiflor | 0.05% cream ointment | bid |
| High | fluocinonide | Lidex | 0.05% cream gel ointment solution | bid-qid |
| High | halcinonide | Halog | 0.1% cream ointment solution | bid-tid |
| High | triamcinolone‡ | Aristocort, Kenalog | 0.5% cream ointment | bid-tid |
| Very high | betamethasone dipropionate‡ | Diprolene, Diprolene AF | 0.05% cream gel lotion ointment | qd-bid |
| Very high | clobetasol | Temovate, Cormax, Olux | 0.05% cream gel ointment lotion solution spray foam (Olux) | bid |
| Very high | diflorasone diacetate‡ | Psorcon | 0.05% cream ointment | qd-tid |
| Very high | halobetasol propionate | Ultravate | 0.05% cream ointment | qd-bid |

*Potency based on vasoconstrictive assays, which may not correlate with efficacy. Not all available products are listed, including those lacking potency ratings. ‡These drugs have formulations in more than once potency category.

**HYDROCORTISONE ACETATE (Cortaid, Corticaine, Micort-HC Lipocream, ◆Hyderm, Cortamed)** ▶L ♀C ▶? $
ADULT - Inflammatory and pruritic manifestations of corticosteroid-responsive dermatoses: apply sparingly 2–4 times/d.
PEDS - Inflammatory and pruritic manifestations of corticosteroid-responsive dermatoses: apply sparingly 2–4 times/d.

FORMS - OTC Generic/Trade: Ointment 0.5% 15 g, Ointment 1% 15, 30g, Cream 0.5% 15 g, Cream 1% 15, 30, 60 g. Topical spray 1% 60 mL. Rx Trade only: Cream 2.5% 30 g (Micort-HC Lipocream).
**HYDROCORTISONE BUTYRATE (Locoid, Locoid Lipocream)** ▶L ♀C ▶? $$
ADULT - Inflammatory and pruritic manifestations of corticosteroid-responsive dermatoses: apply

**HYDROCORTISONE BUTYRATE** (cont.)
sparingly 2–3 times/d. Seborrheic dermatitis (solution only): apply 2–3 times/d.
PEDS - Inflammatory and pruritic manifestations of corticosteroid-responsive dermatoses: apply sparingly 2–3 times/d. Seborrheic dermatitis (solution only): apply 2–3 times/d.
FORMS - Generic/Trade: Cream and Ointment 0.1% 15, 45 g, Solution 0.1% 20, 60 mL. Trade only: Cream 0.1% (Lipocream) 15, 45, 60 g.

**HYDROCORTISONE PROBUTATE** (*Pandel*) ▶L ♀C ▶? $$
ADULT - Inflammatory and pruritic manifestations of corticosteroid-responsive dermatoses: apply sparingly 1–2 times/d.
PEDS - Not approved in children.
FORMS - Trade only: Cream 0.1% 15, 45, 80 g.

**HYDROCORTISONE VALERATE** (*Westcort*, ✦*Hydroval*) ▶L ♀C ▶? $$
ADULT - Inflammatory and pruritic manifestations of corticosteroid-responsive dermatoses: apply sparingly 2–3 times/d.
PEDS - Safety and efficacy of Westcort ointment have not been established in children. Inflammatory and pruritic manifestations of corticosteroid-responsive dermatoses (cream only): apply sparingly 2–3 times/d.
FORMS - Generic/Trade: Cream and Ointment 0.2% 15, 45, 60 g.

**MOMETASONE - TOPICAL** (*Elocon*, ✦*Elocom*) ▶L ♀C ▶? $
ADULT - Inflammatory and pruritic manifestations of corticosteroid-responsive dermatoses: apply sparingly once daily.
PEDS - Inflammatory and pruritic manifestations of corticosteroid-responsive dermatoses ≥2 yo:

apply sparingly once daily. Safety and efficacy for >3 wk have not been established.
FORMS - Generic/Trade: Cream and Ointment 0.1% 15, 45 g, Lotion 0.1% 30, 60 mL.
NOTES - Do not use an occlusive dressing. Not for ophthalmic use.

**PREDNICARBATE** (*Dermatop*) ▶L ♀C ▶? $$
ADULT - Inflammatory and pruritic manifestations of corticosteroid-responsive dermatoses: apply sparingly 2 times/d.
PEDS - Inflammatory and pruritic manifestations of corticosteroid-responsive dermatoses in children ≥1 yo: apply sparingly 2 times/d. Safety and efficacy for >3 wk have not been established.
FORMS - Generic/Trade: Cream and Ointment 0.1% 15, 60 g.

**TRIAMCINOLONE - TOPICAL** (*Kenalog, Kenalog in Orabase*, ✦*Oracort, Triaderm*) ▶L ♀C ▶? $
ADULT - Inflammatory and pruritic manifestations of corticosteroid-responsive dermatoses: apply sparingly 3–4 times/d. Oral paste: Aphthous ulcers: Using finger, apply about 1/2 cm of paste to oral lesion and a thin film will develop. Apply paste bid-tid, ideally pc & qhs.
PEDS - Inflammatory and pruritic manifestations of corticosteroid-responsive dermatoses: apply sparingly 3–4 times/d.
FORMS - Generic/Trade: Cream and Ointment 0.1% 15, 60, 80 g, Cream 0.5% 20 g, Lotion 0.025% and 0.1% 60 mL, Oral paste (in Orabase) 0.1% 5 g. Generic only: Cream and Ointment 0.025% 15, 80 g, Cream and Ointment 0.5% 15 g. Trade only: Aerosol topical spray 0.147 mg/g-63 g.

---

## DERMATOLOGY: Corticosteroid/Antimicrobial Combinations

*CORTISPORIN* (neomycin + polymyxin + hydrocortisone) ▶LK ♀C ▶? $$$
ADULT - Corticosteroid-responsive dermatoses with secondary infection: apply bid-qid.
PEDS - Not approved in children.
UNAPPROVED PEDS - Corticosteroid-responsive dermatoses with secondary infection: apply bid-qid.
FORMS - Trade only: Cream 7.5 g, Ointment 15 g.
NOTES - Due to concerns about nephrotoxicity and ototoxicity associated with neomycin, do not use over wide areas or for prolonged periods of time.

*FUCIDIN H* (fusidic acid + hydrocortisone) ▶L ♀? ▶? $$
ADULT - Canada only. Atopic dermatitis: apply tid.
PEDS - Canada only. Children >3 yo, atopic dermatitis: apply tid.
FORMS - Canada trade only: cream 2% fusidic acid, 1% hydrocortisone acetate 30 g.

*LOCACORTEN VIOFORM* (flumethasone + cloquinol) ▶? ♀? ▶? $
ADULT - Canada only. Skin: Apply 2–3 times daily. Otic drops: 2–3 gtts bid.
PEDS - Canada only. Children ≥ 2 yo: Skin: Apply 2–3 times daily. Otic drops: 2–3 gtts bid.

FORMS - Trade only: Cream 0.02% flumethasone & 3% cloquinol. Otic drops 0.02% flumethasone & 1% cloquinol, 10 mL.
NOTES - May stain clothing.

*LOTRISONE* (clotrimazole + betamethasone) (✦*Lotriderm*) ▶L ♀C ▶? $$$
ADULT - Tinea pedis, cruris, and corporis: apply bid.
PEDS - Not approved in children.
FORMS - Generic/Trade: cream (clotrimazole 1% + betamethasone 0.05%) 15 g, lotion (clotrimazole 1% + betamethasone 0.05%) 30 mL.
NOTES - Treat tinea cruris and corporis for 2 wk and tinea pedis for 4 wk. Do not use for diaper dermatitis.

*MYCOLOG II* (nystatin + triamcinolone) ▶L ♀C ▶? $
ADULT - Cutaneous candidiasis: apply bid.
PEDS - Not approved in children.
UNAPPROVED PEDS - Sometimes used for diaper dermatitis, but this is not recommended due to risk of adrenal suppression.
FORMS - Generic/Trade: cream 15,30,60,120 g, ointment 15,30,60,120 g.
NOTES - Avoid occlusive dressings.

## DERMATOLOGY: Hemorrhoid Care

**DIBUCAINE (*Nupercainal*)** ▶L ♀? ▶? $
ADULT - Hemorrhoids or other anorectal disorders: apply tid-qid prn.
PEDS - Not approved in children.
UNAPPROVED PEDS - Hemorrhoids or other anorectal disorders; children >2yo or >35 pounds: apply tid-qid prn.
FORMS - OTC Generic/Trade: ointment 1% 30 g.
NOTES - Do not use if <2 yo or <35 pounds.

**PRAMOXINE (*Anusol Hemorrhoidal Ointment, Fleet Pain Relief, Proctofoam NS*)** ▶Not absorbed ♀+ ▶+ $
ADULT - Hemorrhoids: apply ointment, pads, or foam up to 5 times/d prn.
PEDS - Not approved in children.
FORMS - OTC Trade only: ointment (Anusol Hemorrhoidal Ointment), pads (Fleet Pain Relief), aerosol foam (ProctoFoam NS).

***PROCTOFOAM HC* (pramoxine + hydrocortisone)** ▶L ♀C ▶? $$$
ADULT - Inflammatory and pruritic manifestations of corticosteroid-responsive dermatoses of the anal region: apply 3 to 4 times a d.
PEDS - Use with caution. Inflammatory and pruritic manifestations of corticosteroid-responsive dermatoses of the anal region: apply 3 to 4 times a d.
FORMS - Trade only: Topical aerosol foam (1% pramoxine + 1% hydrocortisone) 10g

**STARCH (*Anusol Suppositories*)** ▶Not absorbed ♀+ ▶+ $
ADULT - Hemorrhoids: 1 susp PR up to 6 times/d prn or after each bowel movement.
PEDS - Not approved in children.
FORMS - OTC Trade only: suppositories (51% topical starch; soy bean oil, tocopheryl acetate).

**WITCH HAZEL (*Tucks*)** ▶? ♀+ ▶+ $
ADULT - Hemorrhoids: Apply to anus/perineum up to 6 times/d prn.
PEDS - Not approved in children.
FORMS - OTC Generic/Trade: pads, gel.

## DERMATOLOGY: Other Dermatologic Agents

**ALITRETINOIN (*Panretin*)** ▶Not absorbed ♀D ▶- $$$$$
WARNING - May cause fetal harm if significant absorption were to occur. Women of child-bearing age should be advised to avoid becoming pregnant during treatment.
ADULT - Cutaneous lesions of AIDS-related Kaposi's sarcoma: apply bid-qid.
PEDS - Not approved in children.
FORMS - Trade only: gel 0.1%, 60 g.

**ALUMINUM CHLORIDE (*Drysol, Certain Dri*)** ▶K ♀? ▶? $
ADULT - Hyperhidrosis: apply qhs. For max effect, cover area with plastic wrap held in place with tight shirt and wash area following morning. Once excessive sweating stopped, use once or twice weekly.
PEDS - Not approved in children.
FORMS - Rx: Generic/Trade: solution 20%: 37.5 mL bottle, 35, 60 mL bottle with applicator. OTC: Trade only (Certain Dri): solution 12.5%: 36 mL bottle.
NOTES - To prevent irritation, apply to dry area.

**BECAPLERMIN (*Regranex*)** ▶Minimal absorption ♀C ▶? $$$$$
ADULT - Diabetic neuropathic ulcers: apply daily and cover with saline-moistened gauze for 12 h. Rinse after 12 h and cover with saline gauze without medication.
PEDS - Not approved in children.
FORMS - Trade only: gel 0.01%, 2 & 15 g.
NOTES - Length of gel to be applied calculated by size of wound (length × width × 0.6 = amount of gel in inches). If ulcer does not decrease by 30% in size by 10 wk, or complete healing has not occurred by 20 wk, continued therapy should be reassessed. Ineffective for stasis ulcers and pressure ulcers. FDA investigating possibility of increased cancer risk with use.

**CALAMINE** ▶? ♀? ▶? $
ADULT - Itching due to poison ivy/oak/sumac, insect bites, or minor irritation: apply up to tid-qid prn.
PEDS - Itching due to poison ivy/oak/sumac, insect bites, or minor irritation (>2 yo): apply up to tid-qid prn.
FORMS - OTC Generic only: lotion 120, 240, 480 mL.

**CAPSAICIN (*Zostrix, Zostrix-HP*)** ▶? ♀? ▶? $
ADULT - Pain due to RA, osteoarthritis, and neuralgias such as zoster or diabetic neuropathies: apply to affected area up to tid-qid.
PEDS - Children >2 yo: Pain due to RA, osteoarthritis, and neuralgias such as zoster or diabetic neuropathies: apply to affected area up to tid-qid.
UNAPPROVED ADULT - Psoriasis and intractable pruritus, postmastectomy/ postamputation neuromas (phantom limb pain), vulvar vestibulitis, apocrine chromhidrosis and reflex sympathetic dystrophy.
FORMS - OTC Generic/Trade: cream 0.025% 45,60 g, 0.075% 30,60 g, lotion 0.025% 59 mL, 0.075% 59 mL, gel 0.025% 15,30 g, 0.05% 43 g, roll-on 0.075% 60 mL.
NOTES - Burning occurs in ≥30% patients but diminishes with continued use. Pain more commonly occurs when applied <3–4 times/d. Wash hands immediately after application.

***CARMOL HC* (hydrocortisone acetate + urea)** ▶L ♀C ▶? $
ADULT - Inflammatory and pruritic manifestations of corticosteroid-responsive dermatoses: apply sparingly 2–4 times/d.

**CARMOL HC** (*cont.*)

PEDS - Inflammatory and pruritic manifestations of corticosteroid-responsive dermatoses: apply sparingly 2–4 times/d.

FORMS - Trade only: hydrocortisone acetate 1% + urea 10% cream 30,90g.

**COAL TAR** (*Polytar, Tegrin, Cutar, Tarsum*) ▶? ♀? ▶? $

ADULT - Dandruff, seborrheic dermatitis: apply shampoo at least twice a wk. Psoriasis: apply to affected areas daily to qid or use shampoo on affected areas.

PEDS - Children >2 yo: Dandruff, seborrheic dermatitis: apply shampoo at least twice a wk. Psoriasis: apply to affected areas daily to qid or use shampoo on affected areas.

FORMS - OTC Generic/Trade: shampoo, conditioner, cream, ointment, gel, lotion, soap, oil.

NOTES - May cause photosensitivity for up to 24 h after application.

**DEET** (*Off, Cutter, Repel, Ultrathon, n-n-diethyl-m-toluamide*) ▶L ♀+ ▶+ $

ADULT - Mosquito repellant: 10% to 50% every 2 to 6 h. Higher concentration products do not work better, but have a longer duration of action.

PEDS - Infants and children ≥2 mo: up to 30% spray/lotion every 2 to 6 h.

FORMS - OTC: spray, lotion, towelette: 4.75% to 100%

NOTES - Duration of action varies by concentration. For example, 23.8% DEET provides about 5 h of protection from mosquito bites, 20% DEET provides approximately 4 h of protection, 6.65% DEET provides about 2 h of protection and products with 4.75% DEET provides about 1.5 h of protection. Apply sunscreen prior to application of DEET-containing products.

**DOXEPIN - TOPICAL** (*Zonalon*) ▶L ♀B ▶- $

ADULT - Pruritus associated with atopic dermatitis, lichen simplex chronicus, eczematous dermatitis: apply qid for up to 8 d.

PEDS - Not approved in children.

FORMS - Trade only: cream 5% 30,45 g.

NOTES - Risk of systemic toxicity increased if applied to >10% of body. Can cause contact dermatitis.

**EFLORNITHINE** (*Vaniqa*) ▶K ♀C ▶? $$$

ADULT - Reduction of facial hair: apply to face bid at least 8 h apart.

PEDS - Not approved in children.

FORMS - Trade only: cream 13.9% 30 g.

NOTES - Takes ≥4–8 wk to see an effect.

*EMLA* (prilocaine + lidocaine - topical) ▶LK ♀B ▶? $$

ADULT - Topical anesthesia for minor dermal procedures (eg, IV cannulation, venipuncture) apply 2.5 g over 20–25 cm² area or 1 disc at least 1 h prior to procedure, for major dermal procedures (ie, skin grafting harvesting) apply 2 g per 10 cm² area ≥2h prior to procedure.

PEDS - Prior to circumcision in infants >37 wk gestation: apply a max dose 1g over max of 10 cm². Topical anesthesia: Children age 1–3 mo or <5 kg: apply a max 1 g over max of 10 cm²; age 4–12 mo and >5kg: apply max 2 g over a max of 20

cm²; age 1–6 yo and >10kg: apply max 10g over max of 100 cm²; age 7–12 yo and >20kg: apply max 20g over max of 200 cm².

FORMS - Trade only: cream (2.5% lidocaine + 2.5% prilocaine) 5 g, disc 1 g. Generic/Trade: cream (2.5% lidocaine + 2.5% prilocaine) 30 g.

NOTES - Cover cream with an occlusive dressing. Do not use in children <12 mo if child is receiving treatment with methemoglobin-inducing agents. Do not use on open wounds. Patients with glucose-6-phosphate deficiencies are more susceptible to methemoglobinemia. Use caution with amiodarone, bretylium, sotalol, dofetilide; possible additive cardiac effects. Dermal analgesia increases for up to 3 h under occlusive dressings, and persists for 1–2 h after removal.

**HYALURONIC ACID** (*Bionect, Restylane*) ▶? ♀? ▶? $$$$$

ADULT - Moderate to severe facial wrinkles: inject into wrinkle/fold (Restylane). Protection of dermal ulcers: apply gel/cream/spray to wound bid or tid (Bionect).

PEDS - Not approved in children.

FORMS - Rx: Injection 0.4 mL and 0.7 mL syringe. Cream 0.2% 25 g. Gel 0.2% 30 g. Spray 20 mL.

NOTES - Do not use more than 1.5 mL of injectable form per treatment area. Injectable product contains trace amounts of gram positive bacterial proteins; contraindicated if history of anaphylaxis or severe allergy.

**HYDROQUINONE** (*Eldopaque, Eldoquin, Eldoquin Forte, EpiQuin Micro, Esoterica, Glyquin, Lustra, Melanex, Solaquin, Claripel, ✦Ultraquin*) ▶? ♀C ▶? $$$

ADULT - Temporary bleaching of hyperpigmented skin conditions (ie, chloasma, melasma, freckles, senile lentigines, ultraviolet-induced discoloration from oral contraceptives, pregnancy, or hormone therapy): apply bid to affected area.

PEDS - Not approved in children.

FORMS - OTC Generic/Trade: cream 1.5%, lotion 2%. Rx Generic/Trade: solution 3%, gel 4%, cream 4%.

NOTES - Responses may take 3 wk - 6 mo. Use a sunscreen on treated, exposed areas.

**LACTIC ACID** (*Lac-Hydrin, Amlactin, ✦Dermalac*) ▶? ♀? ▶? $$

ADULT - Ichthyosis vulgaris and xerosis (dry, scaly skin): apply bid to affected area.

PEDS - Ichthyosis vulgaris and xerosis (dry, scaly skin) in children >2 yo: apply bid to affected area.

FORMS - Trade only: lotion 12% 150, 360 mL. Generic/OTC: cream 12% 140, 385 g. AmLactin AP is lactic acid (12%) with pramoxine (1%).

NOTES - Frequently causes irritation in non-intact skin. Minimize exposure to sun, artificial sunlight.

**LIDOCAINE - TOPICAL** (*Xylocaine, Lidoderm, Numby Stuff, LMX, Zingo, ✦Maxilene*) ▶LK ♀B ▶+ $$

WARNING - Contraindicated in allergy to amide-type anesthetics.

(cont.)

**LIDOCAINE - TOPICAL** (*cont.*)

ADULT - Topical anesthesia: apply to affected area prn. Dose varies with anesthetic procedure, degree of anesthesia required and individual patient response. Post-herpetic neuralgia (patch): apply up to 3 patches to affected area at once for up to 12h within a 24h period.

PEDS - Topical anesthesia: apply to affected area prn. Dose varies with anesthetic procedure, degree of anesthesia required and individual patient response. Max 3 mg/kg/dose, do not repeat dose within 2 h. Intradermal powder injection for venipuncture/IV cannulation, 3–18 yo (Zingo): 0.5 mg to site 1–10 min prior.

UNAPPROVED PEDS - Topical anesthesia prior to venipuncture: apply 30 min prior to procedure (ELA-Max 4%).

FORMS - For membranes of mouth and pharynx: spray 10%, ointment 5%, liquid 5%, solution 2,4%, dental patch. For urethral use: jelly 2%. Patch (Lidoderm) 5%. Intradermal powder injection system: 0.5 mg (Zingo). OTC: Trade only: liposomal lidocaine 4% (ELA-Max).

NOTES - Apply patches only to intact skin to cover the most painful area. Patches may be cut into smaller sizes w/scissors prior to removal of the release liner. Store and dispose out of the reach of children & pets to avoid possible toxicity from ingestion.

**MINOXIDIL - TOPICAL** (*Rogaine, Rogaine Forte, Rogaine Extra Strength, Minoxidil for Men, Theroxidil Extra Strength, ♦Minox, Apo-Gain*) ▶K ♀C ▶- $$

ADULT - Androgenetic alopecia in men or women: 1 mL to dry scalp bid.

PEDS - Not approved in children.

UNAPPROVED ADULT - Alopecia areata.

UNAPPROVED PEDS - Alopecia: Apply to dry scalp bid.

FORMS - OTC Trade only: solution 2%, 60 mL, 5%, 60 mL, 5% (Rogaine Extra Strength, Theroxidil Extra Strength - for men only) 60 mL, foam 5% 60g.

NOTES - 5% strength for men only. Alcohol content may cause burning and stinging. Evidence of hair growth usually takes ≥4 mo. If treatment is stopped, new hair will be shed in a few mo.

**MONOBENZONE** (*Benoquin*) ▶Minimal absorption ♀C ▶? $$

ADULT - Extensive vitiligo: apply bid-tid.

PEDS - Not approved if <12 yo.

FORMS - Trade only: cream 20% 35.4 g.

NOTES - Avoid prolonged exposure to sunlight. May take 1–4 mo for depigmentation to occur. Depigmentation is permanent and can cause lifelong increase in photosensitivity.

**OATMEAL** (*Aveeno*) ▶Not absorbed ♀? ▶? $

ADULT - Pruritus from poison ivy/oak, varicella: apply lotion qid prn. Also available in packets to be added to bath.

PEDS - Pruritus from poison ivy/oak, varicella: apply lotion qid prn. Also available in bath packets for tub.

FORMS - OTC Generic/Trade: lotion, packets.

**PANAFIL** (papain + urea + chlorophyllin copper complex) ▶? ♀? ▶? $$$

ADULT - Debridement of acute or chronic lesions: apply to clean wound and cover daily-bid.

PEDS - Not approved in children.

FORMS - Trade only: Ointment: 6, 30 g, spray 33 mL.

NOTES - Longer redressings (2–3 d) are acceptable. May be applied under pressure dressings. Hydrogen peroxide inactivates papain; avoid concomitant use.

**PLIAGIS** (tetracaine + lidocaine - topical) ▶Minimal absorption ♀B ▶? $$$

WARNING - Contraindicated in allergy to amide-type anesthetics.

ADULT - Prior to venipuncture, intravenous cannulation, superficial dermatological procedure: apply 20–30 min prior to procedure (60 min for tattoo removal).

PEDS - Not approved in children.

FORMS - Trade only: cream lidocaine 7% + tetracaine 7%.

**POLY-L-LACTIC ACID** (*Sculptra*) ▶Not absorbed ♀? ▶? $$$$$

ADULT - Restoration of facial fat loss due to HIV lipoatrophy: dose based on degree of correction needed.

PEDS - Not approved in children <18 yo.

**PRAMOSONE** (pramoxine + hydrocortisone) (♦*Pramox HC*) ▶Not absorbed ♀C ▶? $$$

ADULT - Inflammatory and pruritic manifestations of corticosteroid-responsive dermatoses: Apply tid-qid.

PEDS - Apply bid-tid.

FORMS - Trade only: 1% pramoxine/1% hydrocortisone acetate: cream 30, 60 g, oint 30 g, lotion 60, 120, 240 mL. 1% pramoxine/2.5% hydrocortisone acetate: cream 30, 60 g, oint 30 g, lotion 60, 120 mL.

NOTES - Monitor for hyperglycemia/adrenal suppression if used for long period of time or over a large area of the body, especially in children. Chronic administration may interfere with pediatric growth & development.

**SELENIUM SULFIDE** (*Selsun, Exsel, Versel*) ▶? ♀C ▶? $

ADULT - Dandruff, seborrheic dermatitis: Massage 5–10 mL of shampoo into wet scalp, allow to remain 2–3 min, rinse. Apply twice a wk for 2 wk. For maintenance, less frequent administration needed. Tinea versicolor: Apply 2.5% shampoo/lotion to affected area, allow to remain on skin 10 min, rinse. Repeat daily × 7days.

PEDS - Dandruff, seborrheic dermatitis: Massage 5–10 mL of shampoo into wet scalp, allow to remain 2–3 min, rinse. Apply twice a wk for 2 wk. For maintenance, less frequent administration needed. Tinea versicolor: Apply 2.5% lotion/shampoo to affected area, allow to remain on skin 10 min, rinse. Repeat daily × 7days.

FORMS - OTC Generic/Trade: lotion/shampoo 1% 120,210,240, 330 mL, 2.5% 120 mL. Rx Generic/Trade: lotion/shampoo 2.5% 120 mL.

***SOLAG*** **(mequinol + tretinoin)** **(*Solage*)** ▶Not absorbed ♀X ▶? $$$$
ADULT - Solar lentigines: apply bid separated by at least 8 h.
PEDS - Not approved in children.
FORMS - Trade only: soln 30 mL (mequinol 2% + tretinoin 0.01%).
NOTES - Use in non-Caucasians has not been evaluated. Avoid in patients taking photosensitizers. Minimize exposure to sunlight.

**SUNSCREEN** ▶Not absorbed ♀? ▶+ $
ADULT - Apply ≥2 tablespoons for full body coverage 30 min before going outdoors. If you're in the sun between 10 a.m. and 4 p.m., reapply sunscreen q2 h (more often if swimming or sweating).
PEDS - Avoid sun exposure if <6 mo. >6 mo: Apply ≥2 tablespoons for full body coverage 30 min before going outdoors. If you're in the sun between 10 a.m. and 4 p.m., reapply sunscreen q2 h (more often if swimming or sweating). Apply prior to sun exposure.
FORMS - Many formulations available.
NOTES - Sun protection factor (SPF) numbers equal the ratio of doses of ultraviolet radiation (predominantly UVB radiation) that result in sunburn with protection to the doses that result in erythema without protection. SPF 2 equals a 50 percent block, SPF 15 equals a 93 percent block, and SPF 45 equals a 98 percent block.

***SYNERA*** **(tetracaine + lidocaine - topical)** ▶Minimal absorption ♀B ▶? $$
WARNING - Contraindicated in allergy to amide-type anesthetics.

ADULT - Prior to venipuncture, intravenous cannulation, superficial dermatological procedure: apply 20–30 min prior to procedure.
PEDS - Children ≥3 yo: Prior to venipuncture, IV cannulation, superficial dermatological procedure: apply 20–30 min prior to procedure.
FORMS - Trade only: patch lidocaine 70 mg + tetracaine 70 mg.
NOTES - Do not cut patch or remove top cover.

***TRI-LUMA*** **(fluocinolone + hydroquinone + tretinoin)** ▶Minimal absorption ♀C ▶? $$$$
ADULT - Melasma of the face: apply qhs × 4–8 wk.
PEDS - Not approved in children.
FORMS - Trade only: soln 30 g (fluocinolone 0.01% + hydroquinone 4% + tretinoin 0.05%).
NOTES - Minimize exposure to sunlight. Not intended for melasma maintenance therapy.

**UREA (*Carmol 40*)** ▶? ♀B ▶? $
ADULT - Debridement of hyperkeratotic surface lesions: apply 2 times/d.
PEDS - Debridement of hyperkeratotic surface lesions: apply 2 times/d.
FORMS - Trade only: urea 40% cream 30, 90, 200g, lotion 8 oz, gel 15 mL.

***VUSION*** **(miconazole - topical + zinc oxide + white petrolatum)** ▶Minimal absorption ♀C ▶? $$$$$
ADULT - Not approved in adults.
PEDS - Apply to affected diaper area with each change for 7 d.
FORMS - Trade only: ointment 50 g.
NOTES - Use only in documented cases of candidiasis.

**NOTE:** Monitor LFTs & lipids. See OB/GYN section for other hormones.

**FLUOXYMESTERONE (*Halotestin, Androxy*)** ▶L ♀X ▶? ©III $$$$
ADULT - Palliative treatment of androgen-responsive recurrent breast cancer in women who are 1–5 yr postmenopausal: 5–10 mg PO bid-qid × 1–3 mo. Hypogonadism in men: 5–20 mg PO daily.
PEDS - Delayed puberty in males: 2.5–10 mg PO daily × 4–6 mo.
FORMS - Trade only: Tabs (scored) 2, 5, 10 mg. Generic only: Tabs 10 mg.
NOTES - Transdermal or injectable therapy preferred for hypogonadism. Pediatric use by specialists who monitor bone maturation q6 mo. Prolonged high-dose use may cause hepatic adenomas, hepatocellular carcinoma, and peliosis hepatitis.

**METHYLTESTOSTERONE (*Android, Methitest, Testred, Virilon*)** ▶L ♀X ▶? ©III $$$
ADULT - Advancing inoperable breast cancer in women who are 1–5 yr postmenopausal: 50–200 mg/d PO in divided doses. Hypogonadism in men: 10–50 mg PO daily.
PEDS - Delayed puberty in males: 10 mg PO daily × 4–6 mo.
FORMS - Generic only: Caps 10 mg,Tabs 10, 25 mg.

NOTES - Transdermal or injectable therapy preferred to oral for hypogonadism. Pediatric use by specialists who monitor bone maturation q6 mo. Prolonged high-dose use may cause hepatic adenomas, hepatocellular carcinoma, and peliosis hepatitis.

**NANDROLONE (*Deca-Durabolin*)** ▶L ♀X ▶- ©III $$
WARNING - Peliosis hepatitis, liver cell tumors, and lipid changes have occurred secondary to anabolic steroid use.
ADULT - Anemia of renal insufficiency: women 50–100 mg IM q wk, men 100–200 mg IM q wk.
PEDS - Anemia of renal disease age 2- 13 yo: 25- 50 mg IM q3–4 wk.
FORMS - Generic only: Injection 50, 100 & 200 mg/mL.
NOTES - Pediatric use by specialists who monitor bone maturation q6 mo. Long-term use may cause hepatic adenomas, hepatocellular carcinoma, and peliosis hepatitis.

**OXANDROLONE (*Oxandrin*)** ▶L ♀X ▶? ©III $$$$$
WARNING - Peliosis hepatitis, liver cell tumors, and lipid changes have occurred secondary to anabolic steroid use.
ADULT - To promote weight gain following extensive surgery, chronic infection, or severe trauma;

**(cont.)**

**OXANDROLONE** *(cont.)*

in some patients who fail to gain or maintain weight without a physiologic cause; to offset protein catabolism associated with long-term corticosteroid therapy: 2.5 mg PO bid-qid for 2–4 wk. Max 20 mg/d. May repeat therapy intermittently as indicated.

PEDS - Weight gain: ≤0.1 mg/kg or ≤0.045 mg/pound PO divided bid-qid for 2–4 wk. May repeat therapy intermittently as indicated.

FORMS - Generic/Trade: Tabs 2.5, 10 mg.

NOTES - Contraindicated in known or suspected prostate/breast cancer. Not shown to enhance athletic ability. Associated with dyslipidemia. Pediatric use by specialists who monitor bone maturation q6 mo. Long-term use may cause hepatic adenomas, hepatocellular carcinoma, and peliosis hepatitis. May increase anticoagulant effects of warfarin.

**OXYMETHOLONE** *(Anadrol-50)* ▶L ♀X ▶- ©III $$$$$

WARNING - Peliosis hepatitis, liver cell tumors, and lipid changes have occurred secondary to anabolic steroid use.

ADULT - Anemia caused by deficient red cell production: 1–5 mg/kg/d PO. Usual effective dose is 1–2 mg/kg/d PO, but higher doses may be required, & the dose should be individualized.

PEDS - Anemia caused by deficient red cell production: 1–5 mg/kg/d PO. Usual effective dose is 1–2 mg/kg/d PO, but higher doses may be required, & the dose should be individualized.

FORMS - Trade only: Tabs 50 mg (scored).

NOTES - Response is not rapid & may require 3–6 mo. Some patients may need to be maintained on a lower dose following remission. Continued use is usually necessary for congenital aplastic anemia. Contraindicated in known or suspected prostate/breast cancer. Avoid if nephrosis or nephritis. Not shown to enhance athletic ability. Associated with dyslipidemia. Pediatric use by specialists who monitor bone maturation q6 mo. Long-term use may cause hepatic adenomas, hepatocellular carcinoma, and peliosis hepatitis. May increase anticoagulant effects of warfarin. May cause iron deficiency anemia; monitor serum iron & iron binding capacity.

**TESTOSTERONE** *(Androderm, AndroGel, Delatestryl, Depo-Testosterone, Striant, Testim, Testopel, Testro AQ, +Andriol)* ▶L ♀X ▶? ©III $$$$$

ADULT - Hypogonadism in men: injectable enanthate or cypionate- 50–400 mg IM q2–4 wk. Androderm- 5 mg patch qhs to clean, dry area of skin on back, abdomen, upper arms, or thighs. Non-virilized patients start with 2.5 mg patch qhs. AndroGel 1%: Apply 5 g from gel pack or 4 pumps (5 g) from dispenser daily to clean, dry, intact skin of the shoulders, upper arms, or abdomen. May increase dose to 7.5–10 g after 2 wk. Testim: One tube (5 g) daily to the clean, dry intact skin of the shoulders or upper arms. May increase dose to 2 tubes (10 g) after 2 wk. Testopel: 2–6 pellets (150–450 mg testosterone) pellets SC q 3–6 mo. 2 pellets for each 25 mg testosterone propionate required weekly. Buccal- Striant: 30 mg q12 h on upper gum above the incisor tooth; alternate sides for each application.

PEDS - Not approved in children.

FORMS - Trade only: Patch 2.5 & 5 mg/24hr (Androderm). Gel 1% 2.5, 5 g packet & 75 g multidose pump (AndroGel). Gel 1%, 5 g tube (Testim). Pellet 75 mg (Testopel). Buccal: blister packs - 30 mg (Striant). Generic/Trade: Injection 100, 200 mg/mL (cypionate), 200 mg/mL (ethanate).

NOTES - Do not apply Androderm or AndroGel to scrotum. Do not apply Testim to the scrotum or abdomen. Pellet implantation is less flexible for dosage adjustment, therefore, take great care when estimating the amount of testosterone. For testosterone gel form, obtain serum testosterone level 2 wk after initiation, then increase dose if necessary. Inject IM formulations slowly into gluteal muscle; rare reports of cough or respiratory distress following injection. Prolonged high-dose use may cause hepatic adenomas, hepatocellular carcinoma, and peliosis hepatitis. May promote the development of prostatic hyperplasia or prostate cancer. Monitor PSA, hemoglobin to detect polycythemia. Advise patient to regularly inspect the gum region where Striant is applied and report any abnormality; refer for dental consultation as appropriate.

---

## ENDOCRINE & METABOLIC: Bisphosphonates

**NOTE:** Supplemental Vitamin D and calcium are recommended for osteoporosis prevention & treatment. Osteonecrosis of the jaw has been reported with bisphosphonates; generally associated with tooth extraction and/or local infection with delayed healing. Prior to treatment, consider dental exam and appropriate preventive dentistry, particularly with risk factors (eg, cancer, chemotherapy, corticosteroids, poor oral hygiene). Severe musculoskeletal pain has been reported; may occur at any time in therapy.

**ALENDRONATE** *(Fosamax, Fosamax Plus D, +Fosavance)* ▶K ♀C ▶- $$

ADULT - Postmenopausal osteoporosis prevention (5 mg PO daily or 35 mg PO weekly) & treatment (10 mg daily, 70 mg PO weekly or 70 mg/vit D3 2800 IU PO weekly). Treatment of glucocorticoid-induced osteoporosis in men & women: 5 mg PO daily or 10 mg PO daily (postmenopausal women

not taking estrogen). Treatment of osteoporosis in men: 10 mg PO daily, 70 mg PO weekly, or 70 mg/vit D3 2800 IU PO weekly. Paget's disease in men & women: 40 mg PO daily × 6 mo.

PEDS - Not approved in children.

UNAPPROVED ADULT - Prevention of glucocorticoid-induced osteoporosis men & women: 5 mg PO daily or 35 mg PO weekly; 10 mg PO daily or

**ALENDRONATE** *(cont.)*

70 mg PO weekly (postmenopausal women not taking estrogen). Treatment of glucocorticoid-induced osteoporosis in men & women: 35 mg weekly or 70 mg weekly (postmenopausal women not taking estrogen).

FORMS - Generic/Trade (Fosamax): Tabs 5, 10, 35, 40, 70 mg. Trade only: Oral soln 70 mg/75 mL (single dose bottle). Fosamax Plus D: 70 mg + either 2800 or 5600 units of vitamin D3.

NOTES - May cause esophagitis, esophageal ulcers and esophageal erosions, occasionally with bleeding and rarely followed by esophageal stricture or perforation. Monitor frequently for dysphagia, odynophagia, and retrosternal pain. Take 30 min before first food, beverage, or medication of the d with a full glass of water only. Remain in upright position for ≥30 min following dose. Caution if CrCl <35 mL/min.

**CLODRONATE, ✚OSTAC, BONEFOS** ▶K ♀D ▶- $$$$$

ADULT - Canada only. Hypercalcemia of malignancy; management of osteolysis resulting from bone metastases of malignant tumors: IV single dose - 1500 mg slow infusion over ≥4 h. IV multiple dose - 300 mg slow infusion daily over 2–6 h up to 10 d. Oral - following IV therapy, maintenance 1600–2400 mg/d in single or divided doses. Max PO dose 3200 mg/d; duration of therapy is usually 6 mo.

PEDS - Not approved in children.

FORMS - Generic/Trade: Capsules 400 mg.

NOTES - Contraindicated if creat >5 mg/dl or if severe GI tract inflammation. Avoid rapid bolus which may cause severe local reactions, thrombophlebitis, or renal failure. Do not mix with calcium-containing infusions. Ensure adequate hydration prior to infusion. Normocalcemia usually occurs within 2–5 d after initiation of therapy with multiple dose infusion. Monitor serum calcium, renal function in those with renal insufficiency, LFTs & hematological parameters.

**ETIDRONATE** *(Didronel)* ▶K ♀C ▶? $$$$

ADULT - Paget's disease: 5–10 mg/kg PO daily × 6 mo or 11–20 mg/kg daily × 3 mo. Heterotopic ossification with hip replacement: 20 mg/kg/d PO × 1 mo before and 3 mo after surgery. Heterotopic ossification with spinal cord injury: 20 mg/kg/d PO × 2 wk, then 10 mg/kg/d PO × 10 wk.

PEDS - Not approved in children.

FORMS - Generic/Trade: Tabs 200, 400 mg.

NOTES - Divide dose if GI discomfort occurs. Avoid food, vitamins with minerals, or antacids within 2 h of dose.

**IBANDRONATE** *(Boniva)* ▶K ♀C ▶? $$$$

ADULT - Treatment/Prevention of postmenopausal osteoporosis. Oral: 2.5 mg PO daily or 150 mg PO q mo. IV: 3 mg IV every 3 mo.

PEDS - Not approved in children.

FORMS - Trade only: 2.5, 150 mg tabs.

NOTES - May cause esophagitis. Avoid if CrCl <30 mL/min. Oral: Take 1 h before first food/beverage with a full glass of plain water; remain in

upright position 1 h after taking. IV: Administer over 15–30 sec.

**PAMIDRONATE** *(Aredia)* ▶K ♀D ▶? $$$$$

WARNING - Single dose should not exceed 90 mg due to risk of renal impairment/failure.

ADULT - Hypercalcemia of malignancy, moderate (corrected Ca= 12–13.5 mg/dl): 60–90 mg IV single dose infused over 2–24 h. Hypercalcemia of malignancy, severe (Ca >13.5 mg/dl): 90 mg IV single dose infused over 2–24 h. Wait ≥7 d before considering retreatment. Paget's disease: 30 mg IV over 4h daily × 3 d. Osteolytic bone lesions: 90 mg IV over 4 h once monthly. Osteolytic bone metastases: 90 mg IV over 2 h q3–4 wk.

PEDS - Not approved in children.

UNAPPROVED ADULT - Mild hypercalcemia: 30 mg IV single dose over 4 h. Osteoporosis treatment: 30 mg IV q 3 mo. Prevention of bone loss during androgen deprivation treatment for prostate cancer: 60 mg IV q12 wk.

UNAPPROVED PEDS - Osteogenesis imperfecta: 3.0 mg/kg IV over 4 h q4–6 mo.

NOTES - Fever occurs in >20% of patients. Monitor creatinine (prior to each dose), lytes, calcium, phosphate, magnesium and Hb (regularly). Avoid in severe renal impairment and hold dosing if worsening renal function. Longer infusions (>2 h) may reduce renal toxicity. Maintain adequate hydration. Avoid invasive dental procedures.

**RISEDRONATE** *(Actonel, Actonel Plus Calcium)* ▶K ♀C ▶? $$$

ADULT - Prevention & treatment of postmenopausal osteoporosis: 5 mg PO daily, 35 mg PO weekly, 75 mg PO two consecutive d each mo, or 150 mg once monthly. Treatment of osteoporosis in men: 35 mg PO weekly. Prevention & treatment of glucocorticoid-induced osteoporosis: 5 mg PO daily. Paget's disease: 30 mg PO daily × 2 mo.

PEDS - Not approved in children.

UNAPPROVED ADULT - Prevention & treatment of glucocorticoid-induced osteoporosis: 35 mg PO weekly.

FORMS - Generic/Trade: Tabs 5, 30, 35 mg. Trade only: 75, 150 mg; 35/1250 mg (calcium).

NOTES - May cause esophagitis, monitor frequently for dysphagia, odynophagia, and retrosternal pain; take 30 min before first food, beverage, or medication of the d with a full glass of water only. Remain in upright position for ≥30 min following dose.

**TILUDRONATE** *(Skelid)* ▶K ♀C ▶? $$$$$

ADULT - Paget's disease: 400 mg PO daily × 3 mo.

PEDS - Not approved in children.

FORMS - Trade only: Tabs 200 mg.

NOTES - May cause esophagitis; take 30 min before first food, beverage, or medication of the d with a full glass of water only. Remain in upright position for ≥30 min following dose.

**ZOLEDRONIC ACID** *(Reclast, Zometa, ✚Aclasta)* ▶K ♀D ▶? $$$$$

ADULT - Treatment of osteoporosis: 5 mg (Reclast) once yearly IV infusion over ≥15 min.

(cont.)

| CORTICOSTEROIDS | Approximate Equivalent Dose (mg) | Relative Anti-inflammatory Potency | Relative Mineralocorticoid Potency | Biological Half-life (h) |
|---|---|---|---|---|
| betamethasone | 0.6–0.75 | 20–30 | 0 | 36–54 |
| cortisone | 25 | 0.8 | 2 | 8–12 |
| dexamethasone | 0.75 | 20–30 | 0 | 36–54 |
| fludrocortisone | not available | 10 | 125 | 18–36 |
| hydrocortisone | 20 | 1 | 2 | 8–12 |
| methylprednisolone | 4 | 5 | 0 | 18–36 |
| prednisolone | 5 | 4 | 1 | 18–36 |
| prednisone | 5 | 4 | 1 | 18–36 |
| triamcinolone | 4 | 5 | 0 | 12–36 |

**ZOLEDRONIC ACID (cont.)**
Hypercalcemia of malignancy (corrected Ca ≥12 mg/dL, Zometa): 4 mg single dose IV infusion over ≥15 min. Wait ≥7 d before considering retreatment. Paget's Disease (Reclast): 5 mg IV single dose. Multiple myeloma and metastatic bone lesions from solid tumors (Zometa): 4 mg (CrCl >60 mL/min), 3.5mg (CrCl 50–60 mL/min), 3.3 mg (CrCl 40–49 mL/min) or 3 mg (CrCl 30–39 mL/min) IV infusion over ≥15 min q3–4 wk.
PEDS - Not approved in children.
UNAPPROVED ADULT - Osteoporosis: 4 mg (Zometa) once yearly IV infusion over ≥15 min. Paget's Disease (Zometa; approved in Canada): 5 mg IV single dose. Treatment of hormone–refractory prostate cancer metastatic to bone (Zometa): 4 mg IV q 3–4 wk. Prevention of bone loss during androgen-deprivation treatment for non-metastatic prostate cancer (Zometa): 4 mg IV q3 mo for 1 yr.
NOTES - Avoid in severe renal impairment (CrCl <35 mL/min) and hold dosing with worsening renal function. Monitor creatinine (before each dose and interim monitoring in at-risk patients), lytes, calcium, phosphate, magnesium and Hb/HCT (regularly). Avoid single doses >4 mg (Zometa) or > 5 mg (Reclast), infusions <15 min. Fever occurs in >15%. In treatment of Paget's disease, correct pre-existing hypocalcemia with calcium and vitamin D before therapy. Maintain adequate hydration for those with hypercalcemia of malignancy, and give 500 mg calcium supplement and vitamin D 400 IU PO daily to those with multiple myeloma or metastatic bone lesions. Avoid invasive dental procedures. Use with caution in aspirin-sensitive patients.

## ENDOCRINE & METABOLIC: Corticosteroids

NOTE: See also dermatology, ophthalmology.

**BETAMETHASONE (Celestone, Celestone Soluspan, ✦Betaject)** ▶L ♀C ▶- $$$$$
ADULT - Anti-inflammatory/Immunosuppressive: 0.6–7.2 mg/d PO divided bid-qid or up to 9 mg/d IM. 0.25–2.0 mL intraarticular depending on location and size of joint.
PEDS - Dosing guidelines not established.
UNAPPROVED ADULT - Fetal lung maturation, maternal antepartum between 24 & 34 wk gestation: 12 mg IM q24h × 2 doses.
UNAPPROVED PEDS - Anti-inflammatory/ Immunosuppressive: 0.0175–0.25 mg/kg/d PO divided tid-qid. Fetal lung maturation, maternal antepartum: 12 mg IM q24h × 2 doses.
FORMS - Trade only: Syrup 0.6 mg/5 mL.
NOTES - Avoid prolonged use in children due to possible bone growth retardation. If such therapy necessary monitor growth & development.
**CORTISONE (Cortone)** ▶L ♀D ▶- $
ADULT - Adrenocortical insufficiency: 25–300 mg PO daily.
PEDS - Dosing guidelines not established.

UNAPPROVED PEDS - Adrenocortical insufficiency: 0.5–0.75 mg/kg/d PO divided q8h.
FORMS - Generic only: Tabs 5, 10, 25 mg.
**DEXAMETHASONE (Decadron, Dexpak, ✦Dexasone)** ▶L ♀C ▶- $
ADULT - Anti-inflammatory/Immunosuppressive: 0.5–9 mg/d PO/IV/IM divided bid- qid. Cerebral edema: 10–20 mg IV load, then 4 mg IM q6h (off-label IV use common) or 1–3 mg PO tid.
PEDS - Dosage in children <12 yo of age has not been established.
UNAPPROVED ADULT - Initial treatment of immune thrombocytopenic purpura: 40 mg PO daily × 4 d. Fetal lung maturation, maternal antepartum between 24 & 34 wk gestation: 6 mg IM q12h × 4 doses. Bacterial meningitis (controversial): 0.15 mg/kg IV q6h × 2–4 d; start 10–15 min before the first dose of antibiotic. Antiemetic, prophylaxis: 8 mg IV or 12 mg PO prior to chemotherapy; 8 mg PO daily × 2–4 d. Antiemetic, treatment: 10–20 mg PO/IV q4–6h.
UNAPPROVED PEDS - Anti-inflammatory/ immunosuppressive: 0.08–0.3 mg/kg/d PO/IV/IM divided

**DEXAMETHASONE** (*cont.*)

q6–12h. Croup: 0.6 mg/kg PO/IV/IM × 1. Bacterial meningitis: 0.15 mg/kg/dose IV q6h × 16 doses. Bacterial meningitis (controversial): 0.15 mg/kg IV q6h × 2–4 d; start 10–15 min before the first dose of antibiotic. Bronchopulmonary dysplasia in preterm infants: 0.5 mg/kg PO/IV divided q12h × 3 d, then taper. Acute asthma: >2 yo: 0.6 mg/kg to max 16 mg PO daily × 2 d.

FORMS - Generic/Trade: Tabs 0.5, 0.75. Generic only: Tabs 0.25, 1.0, 1.5, 2, 4, 6 mg; elixir 0.5 mg/5 mL; solution 0.5 mg/5 mL, 1 mg/1 mL (concentrate). Trade only: Dexpak (51 total 1.5 mg tabs for a 13 d taper).

NOTES - Avoid prolonged use in children due to possible bone growth retardation. If such therapy necessary monitor growth & development.

**FLUDROCORTISONE** (*Florinef*) ▶L ♀C ▶? $

ADULT - Adrenocortical insufficiency/ Addison's disease: 0.1 mg PO 3 times weekly to 0.2 mg PO daily. Salt-losing adrenogenital syndrome: 0.1–0.2 mg PO daily.

PEDS - Not approved in children.

UNAPPROVED ADULT - Postural hypotension: 0.05–0.4 mg PO daily.

UNAPPROVED PEDS - Adrenocortical insufficiency: 0.05–0.2 mg PO daily.

FORMS - Generic only: Tabs 0.1 mg.

NOTES - Usually given in conjunction with cortisone or hydrocortisone for adrenocortical insufficiency.

**HYDROCORTISONE** (*Cortef, Cortenema, Solu-Cortef*) ▶L ♀C ▶- $

ADULT - Adrenocortical insufficiency: 20–240 mg/d PO divided tid-qid or 100–500 mg IV/IM q2–10h prn (sodium succinate). Ulcerative colitis: 100 mg retention enema qhs (laying on side for ≥1 h) for 21 d. May use for 2–3 mo for severe cases; when course extends >3 wk then discontinue gradually by decreasing frequency to every other night for 2–3 wk.

PEDS - Dosing guidelines not established.

UNAPPROVED PEDS - Chronic adrenocortical insufficiency: 0.5–0.75 mg/kg/d PO divided q8h or 0.25–0.35 mg/kg/d IM daily. Acute adrenocortical insufficiency: infants & young children 1–2 mg/kg IV bolus, then 25–150 mg/d divided q6–8 h. Older children 1–2 mg/kg IV bolus, then 150–250 mg/d IV q6–8 h.

FORMS - Generic/Trade: Tabs 5, 10, 20 mg, Enema 100 mg/60 mL.

NOTES - Agent of choice for adrenocortical insufficiency because of mixed glucocorticoid and mineralocorticoid properties at doses >100 mg/d.

**METHYLPREDNISOLONE** (*Solu-Medrol, Medrol, Depo-Medrol*) ▶L ♀C ▶- $

ADULT - Anti-inflammatory/ Immunosuppressive: Parenteral (Solu-Medrol) 10- 250 mg IV/IM q4h prn. Oral (Medrol) 4- 48 mg PO daily. Medrol Dosepak tapers 24 to 0 mg PO over 7d. IM/ joints (Depo-Medrol) 4- 120 mg IM q1–2 wk. Multiple sclerosis flare: 200 mg PO/IV daily × 1 wk followed by 80 mg PO daily × 1 mo.

PEDS - Dosing guidelines not established.

UNAPPROVED ADULT - Optic neuritis: 1 g IV daily (or in divided doses) × 3 d, then PO prednisone 1 mg/kg/d × 11 d (followed by a 3-d taper). Multiple sclerosis flare: 1 g IV daily (or in divided doses) × 3–5 d. May follow with PO prednisone 1 mg/kg/d for 14 d, then taper off. Spinal cord injury: 30 mg/kg IV over 15 min, followed in 45 min by 5.4 mg/kg/h IV infusion for 23 h (if initiated within 3 h of injury) or for 47 h (if initiated 3–8h after injury).

UNAPPROVED PEDS - Anti-inflammatory/ Immunosuppressive: 0.5–1.7 mg/kg/d PO/IV/IM divided q6–12h. Spinal cord injury: 30 mg/kg IV over 15 min, followed in 45 min by 5.4 mg/kg/h IV infusion × 23 h.

FORMS - Trade only: Tabs 2, 16, 32 mg. Generic/Trade: Tabs 4, 8 mg. Medrol Dosepak (4 mg-21 tabs).

NOTES - Other dosing regimens have been used for MS and optic neuritis. Avoid initial treatment of optic neuritis with oral steroids, as it may increase the risk of new episodes.

**PREDNISOLONE** (*Flo-Pred, Prelone, Pediapred, Orapred, Orapred ODT*) ▶L ♀C ▶+ $$

ADULT - Anti-inflammatory/ Immunosuppressive: 5–60 mg/d PO; individualize to severity of disease and response. Multiple sclerosis: 200 mg IV daily × 1 wk, then 80 mg qod × 1 mo.

PEDS - Anti-inflammatory/immunosuppressive: 0.14–2 mg/kg/d PO divided tid-qid (4 to 60 mg/m²/d); individualize to severity of disease and response. Acute asthma: 1–2 mg/kg/d divided daily-bid × 3–10d. Nephrotic syndrome: 60 mg/m²/d divided tid × 4 wk; then 40 mg/m²/d qod × 4 wk.

UNAPPROVED PEDS - Early active RA: 10 mg/d PO.

FORMS - Generic/Trade: Syrup 15 mg/5 mL (Prelone; wild cherry flavor). Solution 5 mg/5 mL (Pediapred, raspberry flavor), 15 mg/5 mL (Orapred; grape flavor). Trade only: Orally disintegrating tabs 10, 15, 30 mg (Orapred ODT); Suspension 5mg/5 mL, 15 mg/5 mL (Flo-Pred; cherry flavor). Generic only: Tabs 5 mg. Syrup 5 mg/5 mL.

**PREDNISONE** (*Deltasone, Sterapred, ✦Winpred*) ▶L ♀C ▶+ $

ADULT - Anti-inflammatory/ Immunosuppressive: 5–60 mg/d PO daily or divided bid-qid.

PEDS - Dosing guidelines not established.

UNAPPROVED PEDS - Anti-inflammatory/ Immunosuppressive: 0.05–2 mg/kg/d divided daily-qid.

FORMS - Trade only: Sterapred (5 mg tabs: tapers 30 to 5 mg PO over 6d or 30 to 10 mg over 12d), Sterapred DS (10 mg tabs: tapers 60 to 10 mg over 6d, or 60 to 20 mg PO over 12d) taper packs. Generic only: Tabs 1, 2.5, 5, 10, 20, 50 mg. Solution 5 mg/5 mL & 5 mg/mL (Prednisone Intensol).

NOTES - Conversion to prednisolone may be impaired in liver disease.

**TRIAMCINOLONE** (*Aristospan, Kenalog, Trivaris*) ▶L ♀C ▶- $
ADULT - Anti-inflammatory/ Immunosuppressive: 4–48 mg/d PO divided daily-qid. 2.5–60 mg IM daily (Kenalog, Trivaris). Intraarticular: small joints 2.5–5 mg (Kenalog, Trivaris), 2–6 mg (Aristospan); large joints 5–15 mg (Kenalog, Trivaris); 10–20 mg (Aristospan). Intravitreal: 4 mg (Trivaris).
PEDS - Dosing guidelines not established.

UNAPPROVED PEDS - Anti-inflammatory/ Immunosuppressive: 0.117–1.66 mg/kg/d PO divided qid.
FORMS - Trade only: Injection 10 mg/mL & 40 mg/ mL (Kenalog), 5 mg/mL & 20 mg/mL (Aristospan), 8 mg (80 mg/mL) syringe (Trivaris).
NOTES - Parenteral form not for IV use. Kenalog & Atistospan contain benzyl alcohol; do not use in neonates. Due to Trivaris availability in a syringe, multiple injections may be required for dose.

## ENDOCRINE & METABOLIC: Diabetes-Related—Alphaglucosidase Inhibitors

**ACARBOSE** (*Precose, ✦Glucobay*) ▶Gut/K ♀B ▶- $$$
ADULT - Diabetes: initiate therapy with 25 mg PO tid with the first bite of each meal. Start with 25 mg PO daily to minimize GI adverse effects. May increase to 50 mg PO tid after 4–8 wk. Usual range is 50–100 mg PO tid. Max dose for patients ≤60 kg is 50 mg tid, >60 kg is 100 mg tid.
PEDS - Not approved in children.
UNAPPROVED ADULT - Type 2 DM prevention: 100 mg PO tid or to max tolerated dose.
FORMS - Generic/Trade: Tabs 25, 50, 100 mg.
NOTES - Acarbose alone should not cause hypoglycemia. If hypoglycemia occurs, treat with oral glucose rather than sucrose (table sugar). Adverse

GI effects (eg, flatulence, diarrhea, abdominal pain) may occur with initial therapy.
**MIGLITOL** (*Glyset*) ▶K ♀B ▶- $$$
ADULT - Diabetes: Initiate therapy with 25 mg PO tid with the first bite of each meal. Use 25 mg PO daily to start if GI adverse effects. May increase dose to 50 mg PO tid after 4–8 wk, max 300 mg/d.
PEDS - Not approved in children.
FORMS - Trade only: Tabs 25, 50, 100 mg.
NOTES - Miglitol administered alone should not cause hypoglycemia. If hypoglycemia occurs, treat with oral glucose rather than sucrose (table sugar). Adverse GI effects (ie, flatulence, diarrhea, abdominal pain) may occur with initial therapy.

## ENDOCRINE & METABOLIC: Diabetes-Related—Combinations

**NOTE:** Metformin-containing products may cause life-threatening lactic acidosis, usually in setting of decreased tissue perfusion, hypoxia, hepatic dysfunction, or impaired renal clearance. Hold prior to IV contrast agents and for 48 h after. Avoid if ethanol abuse, heart failure (requiring treatment), hepatic or renal insufficiency (creat ≥1.4 mg/dl in women, ≥1.5 mg/dl in men), or hypoxic states (cardiogenic shock, septicemia, acute MI). Glitazone-containing products may cause edema, weight gain, new heart failure, or exacerbate existing heart failure (avoid in NYHA Class III or IV). Monitor for signs of heart failure (rapid weight gain, dyspnea, edema) following initiation or dose increase. If occurs, manage fluid retention and consider discontinuation or dosage decrease. Rosiglitazone (Avandia) is not recommended with nitrates or insulin, and its labeling includes boxed warning regarding increased risk of myocardial ischemic events and notes that studies are currently inconclusive. Avoid if liver disease or ALT >2.5 × normal. Monitor LFTs before therapy & periodically thereafter. Discontinue if ALT >3x upper normal limit. Full effect may not be apparent for up to 12 wk. May cause resumption of ovulation in premenopausal anovulatory women; recommend contraception use.

**ACTOPLUS MET** (pioglitazone + metformin) ▶KL ♀C ▶? $$$$
ADULT - Type 2 DM: 1 tab PO daily-bid. If inadequate control with metformin monotherapy, start 15/500 or 15/850 PO daily-bid. If inadequate control with pioglitazone monotherapy, start 15/500 bid or 15/850 daily. Max 45/2550 mg/d.
PEDS - Not approved in children.
FORMS - Trade only: Tabs 15/500, 15/850 mg.
NOTES - Initial GI upset may be minimized by starting with lower dose of metformin component. Reports of fracture risk in women.
**AVANDAMET** (rosiglitazone + metformin) ▶KL ♀C ▶? $$$$$
ADULT - Type 2 DM, initial therapy (drug naive): Start 2/500 mg PO daily or bid. If inadequate control with metformin alone, select tab strength based on adding 4 mg/d rosiglitazone to existing

metformin dose. If inadequate control with rosiglitazone alone, select tab strength based on adding 1000 mg/d metformin to existing rosiglitazone dose. Max 8/2000 mg/d.
PEDS - Not approved in children.
FORMS - Trade only: Tabs 2/500, 4/500, 2/1000, 4/1000 mg.
NOTES - May be given concomitantly with sulfonylureas. Initial GI upset may be minimized by starting with lower dose of metformin component.
**AVANDARYL** (rosiglitazone + glimepiride) ▶LK ♀C ▶? $$$$
ADULT - Type 2 DM, initial therapy (drug naive): Start 4/1 mg PO daily. If switching from monotherapy with a sulfonylurea or glitazone, consider 4/2 mg PO daily. Max 8/4 mg per d. Give with breakfast or the first main meal of the d. Use low starting dose of 4/1 mg and titrate more slowly in elderly, malnourished and in renal and hepatic impairment.

**AVANDARYL** (cont.)
PEDS - Not approved in children.
FORMS - Trade only: Tabs 4/1, 4/2, 4/4, 8/2, 8/4 mg rosiglitazone/glimepiride.

**DUETACT** (pioglitazone + glimepiride) ▶LK ♀C ▶- $$$$
ADULT - Type 2 DM: Start 30/2 mg PO daily. May start up to 30/4 mg PO daily if prior glimepiride therapy, or up to 30/2 mg PO daily if prior pioglitazone therapy; max 30/4 mg per d. Give with breakfast or the first main meal of the d. In the elderly, the malnourished, or those with renal/hepatic impairment, precede therapy with trial of glimepiride 1 mg/d and then titrate Duetact more slowly.
PEDS - Not approved in children.
FORMS - Trade only: Tabs 30/2, 30/4 mg pioglitazone/glimepiride.
NOTES - Reports of fracture risk in women.

**GLUCOVANCE** (glyburide + metformin) ▶KL ♀B ▶? $$$
ADULT - Type 2 DM, initial therapy (drug naive): Start 1.25/250 mg PO daily or bid with meals; max 10/2000 mg daily. Inadequate control with a sulfonylurea or metformin alone: Start 2.5/500 or 5/500 mg PO bid with meals; max 20/2000 mg daily.
PEDS - Not approved in children.
FORMS - Generic/Trade: Tabs 1.25/250, 2.5/500, 5/500 mg
NOTES - May add thiazolidinedione if glycemic control is not obtained.

**JANUMET** (sitagliptin + metformin) ▶K ♀B ▶? $$$$
ADULT - Type 2 DM: Start 1 tab PO bid. Individualize based on patient's current therapy. If inadequate control with metformin monotherapy, start 50/500 or 50/1000 bid based on current metformin dose. If inadequate control on sitagliptin monotherapy, start 50/500 bid. Max 100/2000 mg daily. Give with meals.
PEDS - Not approved in children.
FORMS - Trade only: Tabs 50/500, 50/1000 mg sitagliptin/metformin.
NOTES - Not for use in Type 1 DM or DKA. Assess renal function and hematologic parameters prior to initiating and at least annually thereafter.

**METAGLIP** (glipizide + metformin) ▶KL ♀C ▶? $$$
ADULT - Type 2 DM, initial therapy (drug naive): Start 2.5/250 mg PO daily to 2.5/500 mg PO bid with meals; max 10/2000 mg daily. Inadequate control with a sulfonylurea or metformin alone: Start 2.5/500 or 5/500 mg PO bid with meals; max 20/2000 mg daily.
PEDS - Not approved in children.
FORMS - Generic/Trade: Tabs 2.5/250, 2.5/500, 5/500 mg.
NOTES - May add thiazolidinedione if glycemic control is not obtained.

---

### DIABETES NUMBERS*

| *Criteria for diagnosis*: | *Self-monitoring glucose goals* | |
|---|---|---|
| Pre-diabetes: Fasting glucose 100–125 mg/dL | | |
| Diabetes:† Fasting glucose ≥126 mg/dL, random glucose with symptoms: ≥200 mg/dL, or ≥200 mg/dL 2 h after 75 g oral glucose load | Preprandial | 90–130 mg/dL |
| | Postprandial | <180 mg/dL |
| Estimated average glucose (eAG): eAG (mg/dL) = (28.7 × A1C) – 46.7 | A1C General goal <7%; Normal <6% | |

*Complications prevention & management*: Aspirin‡ (75–162 mg/d) in Type 1 & 2 adults for primary prevention (those with an increased cardiovascular risk, including >40 yo or with additional risk factors) and secondary prevention (those with any vascular disease); statin therapy to achieve 30–40% LDL reduction regardless of baseline LDL (for those with any vascular disease, those >40 yo and additional risk factor, or those <40 yo but LDL >100 mg/dL); ACE inhibitor or ARB if hypertensive or micro-/macro-albuminuria; pneumococcal vaccine (revaccinate one time if age ≥65 and previously received vaccine at age <65 and >5 yr ago). *At every visit*: Measure weight & BP (goal <130/80 mm Hg); visual foot exam; review self-monitoring glucose record; review/adjust meds; review self-management skills, dietary needs, and physical activity; smoking cessation counseling. *Twice a year*: A1C in those meeting treatment goals with stable glycemia (quarterly if not); dental exam. *Annually*: Fasting lipid profile [goal LDL <100 mg/dL; cardiovascular disease consider LDL <70mg/dL, HDL >40 mg/dL (>50 mg/dL in women), TG <150 mg/dL], q2 yr with low-risk lipid values; creatinine; albumin to creatinine ratio spot collection; dilated eye exam; flu vaccine; comprehensive foot exam.

*See recommendations at: care.diabetesjournals.org. Reference: *Diabetes Care* 2008;30 (Suppl 1):S12–S54. Glucose values are plasma. †Confirm diagnosis with glucose testing on subsequent day. ‡Avoid aspirin if <21 yo due to Reye's Syndrome risk; use if <30 yo has not been studied. LDL is primary target of therapy.

---

### ENDOCRINE & METABOLIC: Diabetes-Related —"Glitazones" (Thiazolidinediones)

**NOTE:** May cause edema, weight gain, new heart failure or exacerbate existing heart failure (contraindicated in NYHA Class III or IV). Monitor for signs of heart failure (rapid weight gain, dyspnea, edema) following initiation or dose increase. If occurs, manage fluid retention and consider discontinuation or dosage decrease. Rosiglitazone (Avandia) is not recommended with nitrates or insulin, and its labeling includes boxed warning regarding increased risk of myocardial ischemic events and notes that studies are currently inconclusive. Avoid if liver disease or ALT >2.5 × normal. Monitor LFTs before therapy & periodically thereafter. Discontinue if ALT

(cont.)

>3x upper normal limit. Full effect may not be apparent for up to 12 wk. May cause resumption of ovulation in premenopausal anovulatory women; recommend contraception use.

**PIOGLITAZONE (*Actos*)** ▶L ♀C ▶- $$$$
ADULT - Diabetes monotherapy or in combination with a sulfonylurea, metformin, or insulin: Start 15–30 mg PO daily, may adjust dose after 3 mo to max 45 mg/d.
PEDS - Not approved in children.
FORMS - Trade only: Tabs 15, 30, 45 mg.
NOTES - Reports of fracture risk in women.

**ROSIGLITAZONE (*Avandia*)** ▶L ♀C ▶- $$$$
ADULT - Diabetes monotherapy or in combination with metformin or sulfonylurea: Start 4 mg PO daily or divided bid, may increase after 8–12 wk to max 8 mg/d.
PEDS - Not approved in children <18 yo.
FORMS - Trade only: Tabs 2, 4, 8 mg.

## ENDOCRINE & METABOLIC: Diabetes-Related—Insulins

**NOTE:** Adjust insulin dosing to achieve glycemic control. See table "diabetes numbers" for goals.

**INSULIN - INJECTABLE COMBINATIONS (*Humalog Mix 75/25, Humalog Mix 50/50, Humulin 70/30, Humulin 50/50, Novolin 70/30, Novolog Mix 70/30*)** ▶LK ♀B/C ▶+ $$$$
ADULT - Doses vary, but typically total insulin 0.3–1 unit/kg/d SC in divided doses (Type 1), and 0.5–1.5 unit/kg/d SC in divided doses (Type 2). Generally, 50% of insulin requirements are provided by basal insulin (intermediate- or long-acting) and the remainder from rapid or short-acting insulin.
PEDS - Not approved in children
UNAPPROVED PEDS - Diabetes: maintenance: total insulin 0.5–1 unit/kg/d SC, but doses vary.
FORMS - Trade only: Insulin lispro protamine susp/insulin lispro (Humalog Mix 75/25, Humalog Mix 50/50). Insulin aspart protamine/insulin aspart (Novolog Mix 70/30). NPH and regular mixtures (Humulin 70/30, Novolin 70/30 or Humulin 50/50). Insulin available in pen form: Novolin 70/30 InnoLet, Novolog Mix 70/30 FlexPen, Humulin 70/30, Humalog Mix 75/25 KwikPen, Humalog Mix 50/50 KwikPen.
NOTES - Administer rapid-acting insulin mixtures (Humalog, NovoLog) within 15 min before meals. Administer regular insulin mixtures 30 min before meals.

INSULIN—INJECTABLE INTERMEDIATE/LONG-acting (*Novolin N, Humulin N, Lantus, Levemir*) ▶ LK ♀B/C ▶+ $$$$
ADULT - Doses vary, but typically total insulin 0.3–0.5 unit/kg/d SC in divided doses (Type 1), and 1–1.5 unit/kg/d SC in divided doses (Type 2). Generally, 50–70% of insulin requirements are provided by rapid or short-acting insulin and the remainder from intermediate- or long-acting insulin. Lantus: Start 10 units SC daily (same time everyday) in insulin naive patients, adjust to usual dose of 2–100 units/d. When transferring from twice daily NPH human insulin, the initial Lantus dose should be reduced by ~20% from the previous total daily NPH dose, then adjust dose based on patient response. Levemir: Type 2 DM (inadequately controlled on oral meds): Start 0.1–0.2 units/kg once daily; or 10 units SC daily or BID. When transferring from basal insulin (Lantus, NPH) in type 1 or 2 DM, change on a

unit-to-unit basis; more Levemir may be required than NPH insulin.
PEDS - Diabetes: maintenance: total insulin 0.5–1 unit/kg/d SC, but doses vary. Generally, 50–70% of insulin requirements are provided by rapid-acting insulin and the remainder from intermediate- or long-acting insulin. Age 6–15 yo (Lantus): Start 10 units SC daily (same time everyday) in insulin naive patients, adjust to usual dose of 2–100 units/d. When transferring from twice daily NPH human insulin, the initial Lantus dose should be reduced by ~20% from the previous total daily NPH dose, then adjust dose based on patient response. Levemir (Type 1 DM): When transferring from NPH, change on a unit-to-unit basis; more Levemir may be required than NPH.
FORMS - Trade only: Injection NPH (Novolin N, Humulin N). Insulin glargine (Lantus). Insulin detemir (Levemir). Insulin available in pen form: Novolin N InnoLet, Humulin N Pen, Lantus OptiClik (reusable), Lantus SoloStar (prefilled-disposable), Levemir InnoLet, Levemir FlexPen. Premixed preparations of NPH and regular insulin also available.
NOTES - May mix NPH with aspart, lispro, glulisine or regular. Draw up rapid/short-acting insulin first. Do not mix Lantus (glargine) or Levemir (detemir) with other insulins.

**INSULIN - INJECTABLE SHORT/RAPID-ACTING (*Apidra, Novolin R, NovoLog, Humulin R, Humalog, ♦NovoRapid*)** ▶LK ♀B/C ▶+ $$$
ADULT - Doses vary, but typically total insulin 0.3–0.5 unit/kg/d SC in divided doses (Type 1), and 1–1.5 unit/kg/d SC in divided doses (Type 2). Generally, 50–70% of insulin requirements are provided by rapid or short-acting insulin and the remainder from intermediate- or long-acting insulin.
PEDS - Diabetes age >3 yo (Humalog) or >2 (NovoLog): Doses vary, but typically total insulin maintenance dose 0.5–1 unit/kg/d SC in divided doses. Generally, 50–70% of insulin requirements are provided by rapid-acting insulin and the remainder from intermediate- or long-acting insulin. Apidra not approved in children.

| INJECTABLE INSULINS* | | Onset (h) | Peak (h) | Duration (h) |
|---|---|---|---|---|
| Rapid/short-acting: | Insulin aspart (NovoLog) | <0.2 | 1–3 | 3–5 |
| | Insulin glulisine (Apidra) | 0.30–0.4 | 1 | 4–5 |
| | Insulin lispro (Humalog) | 0.25–0.5 | 0.5–2.5 | ≤5 |
| | Regular (Novolin R, Humulin R) | 0.5–1 | 2–3 | 3–6 |
| Intermediate/long-acting: | NPH (Novolin N, Humulin N) | 2–4 | 4–10 | 10–16 |
| | Insulin detemir (Levemir) | not available | flat action profile | up to 23† |
| | Insulin glargine (Lantus) | 2–4 | peakless | 24 |
| Mixtures: | Insulin aspart protamine suspension/aspart (NovoLog Mix 70/30, NovoLog Mix 50/50) | 0.25 | 1–4 (biphasic) | up to 24 |
| | Insulin lispro protamine suspension/insulin lispro (HumaLog Mix 75/25, HumaLog Mix 50/50) | <0.25 | 1–3 (biphasic) | 10–20 |
| | NPH/Reg (Humulin 70/30, Humulin 50/50, Novolin 70/30) | 0.5–1 | 2–10 (biphasic) | 10–20 |

*These are general guidelines, as onset, peak, and duration of activity are affected by the site of injection, physical activity, body temperature, and blood supply. † Dose dependent duration of action, range from 6 to 23 h.

**INSULIN - INJECTABLE SHORT/RAPID-ACTING (cont.)**
UNAPPROVED ADULT - Severe hyperkalemia: 5–10 units regular insulin plus concurrent dextrose IV. Profound hyperglycemia (eg, DKA): 0.1 unit/kg regular insulin IV bolus, then begin IV infusion 100 units in 100 mL NS (1 unit/mL) at 0.1 units/kg/h. 70 kg: 7 units/h (7 mL/h). Titrate to clinical effect.
UNAPPROVED PEDS - Profound hyperglycemia (eg, DKA): 0.1 unit/kg regular insulin IV bolus, then IV infusion 100 units in 100 mL NS (1 unit/mL) at 0.1 units/kg/h. Titrate to clinical effect. Severe hyperkalemia: 0.1 units/kg regular insulin IV with glucose over 30 min. May repeat in 30–60 min or start 0.1 units/kg/h.
FORMS - Trade only: Injection regular (Novolin R, Humulin R). Insulin glulisine (Apidra). Insulin lispro (Humalog). Insulin aspart (NovoLog). Insulin available in pen form: Novolin R InnoLet, Humulin R, Apidra OptiClik, Humalog KwikPen, Novolog FlexPen.
NOTES - Administer rapid-acting insulin (Humalog, NovoLog, Apidra) within 15 min before or immediately after a meal. Administer regular insulin 30 min before meals. May mix with NPH. Draw up rapid/short-acting insulin first.

## ENDOCRINE & METABOLIC: Diabetes-Related—Meglitinides

NOTE: No clinical studies have established conclusive evidence of decreased macrovascular outcomes with anti-diabetic drugs.

**NATEGLINIDE (Starlix)** ▶L ♀C ▶? $$$$
ADULT – Diabetes, monotherapy or in combination with metformin or thiazolidinedione: 120 mg PO tid ≤30 min before meals; use 60 mg PO tid in patients who are near goal A1C.
PEDS - Not approved in children.
FORMS - Trade only: Tabs 60, 120 mg.
NOTES - Not to be used as monotherapy in patients inadequately controlled with glyburide or other anti-diabetic agents previously. Patients with severe renal impairment are at risk for hypoglycemic episodes.

**REPAGLINIDE (Prandin, ✦Gluconorm)** ▶L ♀C ▶? $$$$
ADULT - Diabetes: 0.5- 2 mg PO tid within 30 min before a meal. Allow 1 wk between dosage adjustments. Usual range is 0.5–4 mg PO tid-qid, max 16 mg/d.
PEDS - Not approved in children.
FORMS - Trade only: Tabs 0.5, 1, 2 mg.
NOTES - May take dose immediately preceding meal to as long as 30 min before the meal. Gemfibrozil and itraconazole increase blood repaglinide levels and may result in an increased risk of hypoglycemia.

## ENDOCRINE & METABOLIC: Diabetes-Related—Sulfonylureas—1st Generation

**CHLORPROPAMIDE (Diabinese)** ▶LK ♀C ▶- $$
ADULT - Initiate therapy with 100–250 mg PO daily. Titrate after 5–7 d by increments of 50–125 mg at intervals of 3–5 d to obtain optimal control. Max 750 mg/d.
PEDS - Not approved in children.
FORMS - Generic/Trade: Tabs 100, 250 mg.
NOTES - Clinical use in the elderly has not been properly evaluated. Elderly are more prone to hypoglycemia and/or hyponatremia possibly from

(cont.)

**CHLORPROPAMIDE** *(cont.)*
renal impairment or drug interactions. May cause disulfiram-like reaction with alcohol.

**TOLAZAMIDE** *(Tolinase)* ▶LK ♀C ▶? $$
ADULT - Initiate therapy with 100 mg PO daily in patients with FBS <200 mg/dl, and in patients who are malnourished, underweight, or elderly. Initiate therapy with 250 mg PO daily in patients with FBS >200 mg/dl. Give with breakfast or the first main meal of the d. If daily doses exceed 500 mg, divide the dose bid. Max 1,000 mg/d.

PEDS - Not approved in children.
FORMS - Generic/Trade: Tabs 100, 250, 500 mg.

**TOLBUTAMIDE** ▶LK ♀C ▶+ $
ADULT - Start 1g PO daily. Maintenance dose is usually 250 mg to 2 g PO daily. Total daily dose may be taken in the morning, divide doses if GI intolerance occurs. Max 3 g/d.

PEDS - Not approved in children.
FORMS - Generic only: Tabs 500 mg.

---

## ENDOCRINE & METABOLIC: Diabetes-Related—Sulfonylureas—2nd Generation

**GLICLAZIDE** *(★Diamicron, Diamicron MR)* ▶KL ♀C ▶? $
ADULT - Canada only, diabetes type 2: Immediate release: Start 80–160 mg PO daily, max 320 mg PO daily (≥160 mg in divided doses). Modified release: Start 30 mg PO daily, max 120 mg PO daily.

PEDS - Not approved in children.
FORMS - Generic/Trade: Tab 80 mg (Diamicron). Trade only: Tabs, modified release 30 mg (Diamicron MR).
NOTES - Immediate and modified release not equipotent; 80 mg of immediate release can be changed to 30 mg of modified release.

**GLIMEPIRIDE** *(Amaryl)* ▶LK ♀C ▶- $$
ADULT - Diabetes: initiate therapy with 1–2 mg PO daily. Start with 1 mg PO daily in elderly, malnourished patients or those with renal or hepatic insufficiency. Give with breakfast or the first main meal of the d. Titrate in increments of 1–2 mg at 1–2 wk intervals based on response. Usual maintenance dose is 1–4 mg PO daily, max 8 mg/d.

PEDS - Not approved in children.
FORMS - Generic/Trade: Tabs 1, 2, 4 mg. Generic only: Tabs 8 mg.

**GLIPIZIDE** *(Glucotrol, Glucotrol XL)* ▶LK ♀C ▶? $
ADULT - Diabetes: initiate therapy with 5 mg PO daily. Give 2.5 mg PO daily to geriatric patients or those with liver disease. Adjust dose in increments of 2.5–5 mg to a usual maintenance dose of 10–20 mg/d, max 40 mg/d. Doses >15 mg should be divided bid. Extended release (Glucotrol XL): initiate therapy with 5 mg PO daily. Usual dose is 5–10 mg PO daily, max 20 mg/d.

PEDS - Not approved in children.
FORMS - Generic/Trade: Tabs 5, 10 mg; Extended release tabs 2.5, 5, 10 mg.
NOTES - Max effective dose is generally 20 mg/d.

**GLYBURIDE** *(Micronase, DiaBeta, Glynase PresTab, ★Euglucon)* ▶LK ♀B ▶? $
ADULT - Diabetes: initiate therapy with 2.5–5 mg PO daily. Start with 1.25 mg PO daily in elderly or malnourished patients or those with renal or hepatic insufficiency. Give with breakfast or the first main meal of the d. Titrate in increments of ≤2.5 mg at weekly intervals based on response. Usual maintenance dose is 1.25–20 mg PO daily or divided bid, max 20 mg/d. Micronized tabs: initiate therapy with 1.5–3 mg PO daily. Start with 0.75 mg PO daily in elderly, malnourished patients or those with renal or hepatic insufficiency. Give with breakfast or the first main meal of the d. Titrate in increments of ≤1.5 mg at weekly intervals based on response. Usual maintenance dose is 0.75–12 mg PO daily, max 12 mg/d. May divide dose bid if >6 mg/d.

PEDS - Not approved in children.
FORMS - Generic/Trade: Tabs (scored) 1.25, 2.5, 5 mg. Micronized Tabs (scored) 1.5, 3, 4.5, 6 mg.
NOTES - Max effective dose is generally 10 mg/d.

---

## ENDOCRINE & METABOLIC: Diabetes-Related—Other

**A1C HOME TESTING** *(Metrika A1CNow)* ▶None ♀+ ▶+ $
ADULT - Use for home A1C testing.
PEDS - Use for home A1C testing.
FORMS - Fingerstick blood.
NOTES - Result displays in 8 min.

**DEXTROSE** *(Glutose, B-D Glucose, Insta-Glucose, Dex-4)* ▶L ♀C ▶? $
ADULT - Hypoglycemia: 0.5–1 g/kg (1–2 mL/kg) up to 25 g (50 mL) of 50% solution by slow IV injection. Hypoglycemia in conscious diabetics: 10–20 g PO q10–20 min prn.
PEDS - Hypoglycemia in neonates: 0.25–0.5 g/kg/dose (5–10 mL of 25% dextrose in a 5 kg infant). Severe hypoglycemia or older infants may require larger doses up to 3 g (12 mL of 25% dextrose) followed by a continuous IV infusion of 10% dextrose. Non-neonates may require 0.5–1.0 g/kg.
FORMS - OTC Generic/Trade: Chewable tabs 4 g (Dex-4), 5 g (Glutose). Trade only: Oral gel 40%.
NOTES - Do not exceed an infusion rate of 0.5 g/kg/h.

**EXENATIDE** *(Byetta)* ▶K ♀C ▶? $$$$$
ADULT - Type 2 DM adjunctive therapy when inadequate control on metformin, a sulfonylurea, or a glitazone (alone or in combination): 5 mcg SC bid (within 1 h before the morning and evening meals, or 1 h before the two main meals of the d ≥6h apart). May increase to 10 mcg SC bid after 1 mo.
PEDS - Not approved in children.
FORMS - Trade only: prefilled pen (60 doses each) 5 mcg/dose, 1.2 mL; 10 mcg/dose, 2.4 mL.

**EXENATIDE** (*cont.*)

NOTES - Protect from light. Prior to initial use, keep refrigerated. After initial use, store at temperature ≤77 degrees; do not freeze. Discard pen 30 d after 1st use. May give SC in upper arm, abdomen, or thigh. Avoid use if renal insufficiency (CrCl <30 mL/min) or severe gastrointestinal disease, including gastroparesis. Discontinue and do not rechallenge if pancreatitis occurs. Do not substitute for insulin in the insulin-dependent. Concurrent use with insulin, meglitinides or alpha-glucosidase inhibitors has not been studied. Risk of hypoglycemia is higher when used with sulfonylurea, therefore, consider reduction in sulfonylurea dose. Take medications that require rapid gastrointestinal absorption ≥1 h prior to exenatide. May promote slight weight loss. May potentiate warfarin.

**GLUCAGON** (*GlucaGen*) ▶LK ♀B ▶? $$$

ADULT - Hypoglycemia in adults: 1 mg IV/IM/SC. If no response within 15 min, may repeat dose 1-2 times. Diagnostic aid for GI tract radiography: 1 mg IV/IM/SC.

PEDS - Hypoglycemia in children >20 kg: same as adults. Hypoglycemia in children <20 kg: 0.5 mg IV/IM/SC or 20-30 mcg/kg. If no response in 5-20 min, may repeat dose 1-2 times.

UNAPPROVED ADULT - The following indications are based upon limited data. Esophageal obstruction caused by food: 1 mg IV over 1-3 min. Symptomatic bradycardia/hypotension, especially with beta blocker therapy: 3-10 mg IV bolus (0.05 mg/kg general recommendation) may repeat in 10 min; may be followed by continuous infusion of 1-5 mg/h or 0.07 mg/kg/h. Infusion rate should be titrated to the desired response.

FORMS - Trade only: injection 1 mg.

NOTES - Should be reserved for refractory/severe cases or when IV/IM dextrose cannot be administered. Advise patients to educate family members and co-workers how to administer a dose. Give supplemental carbohydrates when patient responds.

**GLUCOSE HOME TESTING** (*Accu-Chek Active, Accu-Check Advantage, Accu-Check Aviva, Accu-Check Compact, Accu-Check Compact Plus, Accu-Check Complete, Accu-Check Voicemate, FreeStyle Flash, FreeStyle Freedom, FreeStyle Freedom Lite, FreeStyle Lite, OneTouch Ultra, OneTouch UltraMini, OneTouch UltraSmart, Precision Xtra, ReliOn, Sidekick, True Track Smart System, Clinistix, Clinitest, Diastix, Tes-Tape*) ▶None ♀+ ▶+ $$

ADULT - Use for home glucose monitoring.

PEDS - Use for home glucose monitoring.

FORMS - Plasma: Accu-Check meters, FreeStyle meters, OneTouch meters, Precision Xtra, ReliOn, Sidekick, True Track. Urine: Clinistix, Clinitest, Diastix, Tes-Tape.

NOTES - Product list is not all-inclusive; check with manufacturers for current products. Accu-Check Active, Accu-Check Aviva, Accu-Check Compact, Accu-Check Compact Plus, FreeStyle meters, OneTouch Ultra, OneTouch UltraSmart, ReliOn Sidekick, Precision Xtra, and True Track can be used on alternate site testing (eg, forearm) prior to or ≥2 h after meal or exercise. Accu-Check Voicemate has voice prompts for visually impaired. Precision Xtra allows for ketone testing. Sidekick is 50-strip disposable meter.

**METFORMIN** (*Glucophage, Glucophage XR, Glumetza, Fortamet, Riomet*) ▶K ♀B ▶? $

ADULT - Diabetes: Immediate-release: Start 500 mg PO daily-bid or 850 mg PO daily with meals. Increase by 500 mg q wk or 850 mg q2 wk to a max of 2550 mg/d. Higher doses may be divided tid with meals. Extended release: Glucophage XR: 500 mg PO daily with evening meal; increase by 500 mg q wk to max 2000 mg/d (may divide bid). Glumetza: 1000 mg PO daily with evening meal; increase by 500 mg q wk to max 2000 mg/d (may divide bid). Fortamet: 500-1000 mg daily with evening meal; increase by 500 mg q wk to max 2500 mg/d.

PEDS - Diabetes ≥10 yo: Start 500 mg PO daily-bid (Glucophage) with meals, increase by 500 mg q wk to max 2000 mg/d in divided doses (10-16 yo). Glucophage XR & Fortamet are indicated in ≥17 yo.

UNAPPROVED ADULT - Polycystic ovary syndrome: 500 mg PO tid or 850 mg PO bid. Prevention/delay Type 2 DM (with lifestyle modifications): 850 mg PO daily for 1 mo, then increase to 850 mg PO bid.

FORMS - Generic/Trade: Tabs 500, 850,1000 mg, extended release 500, 750 mg. Trade only, extended release: Fortamet 500, 1000 mg; Glumetza 500, 1000 mg. Trade only: oral soln 500 mg/5 mL (Riomet).

NOTES - May reduce the risk of progression to Type 2 diabetes in those with impaired glucose tolerance, but less effectively than intensive lifestyle modification. Metformin-containing products may cause life-threatening lactic acidosis, usually in setting of decreased tissue perfusion, hypoxia, hepatic dysfunction, unstable congestive heart failure or impaired renal clearance. Hold prior to IV contrast agents and for 48 h after. Avoid if ethanol abuse, hepatic or renal insufficiency (creat ≥1.4 mg/dl in women, ≥1.5 mg/dl in men), or hypoxic states (cardiogenic shock, septicemia, acute MI).

**PRAMLINTIDE** (*Symlin, Symlinpen*) ▶K ♀C ▶? $$$$

WARNING - May cause severe insulin-induced hypoglycemia especially in Type 1 DM, usually within 3 h. Avoid if hypoglycemic unawareness, gastroparesis, GI motility medications, alpha-glucosidase inhibitors, A1C >9%, poor compliance, or hypersensitivity to the metacresol preservative. Appropriate patient selection, careful patient instruction and insulin dose adjustments (reduction in pre-meal short-acting insulin of 50%) are critical for reducing the hypoglycemia risk.

(cont.)

**PRAMLINTIDE** (cont.)

ADULT - Type 1 DM with mealtime insulin therapy: Initiate 15 mcg SC immediately before major meals & titrate by 15 mcg increments (if significant nausea has not occurred for ≥3 d) to maintenance 30–60 mcg as tolerated. If significant nausea, decrease to 30 mcg. Type 2 DM with mealtime insulin therapy: Initiate 60 mcg SC immediately before major meals and increase to 120 mcg as tolerated (if significant nausea not occurred for 3–7 d.) If significant nausea, decrease dose to 60 mcg.

PEDS - Not approved in children.

FORMS - Trade only: 600 mcg/mL in 5 mL vials, 1000 mcg/mL pen injector (Symlinpen) 1.5 & 2.7 mL.

NOTES - Keep unopened vials refrigerated. Opened vials can be kept at room temperature or refrigerated up to 28 d. May give SC in abdomen or thigh. Take medications that require rapid onset 1 h prior or 2 h after. Careful patient selection and skilled health care supervision are critical for safe and effective use. Monitor pre-/post-meal and bedtime glucose. Decrease initial pre-meal short-acting insulin doses by 50% including fixed-mix insulin (ie, 70/30). Do not mix with insulin. Use new needle & syringe for each dose.

**SITAGLIPTIN (Januvia)** ▶K ♀B ▶? $$$$

ADULT - Type 2 DM: 100 mg PO daily. If CrCl 30–49 mL/min reduce dose to 50 mg daily; if CrCl <30 mL/min then 25 mg daily.

PEDS - Not approved in children.

FORMS - Trade only: Tabs 25, 50, 100 mg.

NOTES - Not for use in Type 1 DM or DKA. Assess renal function periodically. Not studied in combination with insulin. When adding to sulfonylurea therapy, consider reducing dose of sulfonylurea to decrease risk of hypoglycemia.

## ENDOCRINE & METABOLIC: Diagnostic Agents

**CORTICOTROPIN (H.P. Acthar Gel)** ▶K ♀C ▶- $$$$$

ADULT - Diagnostic testing of adrenocortical function: 80 units IM or SC. Acute exacerbation of multiple sclerosis: 80–120 units IM daily IM × 2–3 wk.

UNAPPROVED PEDS - Various dosing regimens have been used for infantile spasms.

NOTES - Has limited therapeutic value in conditions responsive to corticosteroids therapy, corticosteroids should be the treatment of choice. Prolonged use in children may inhibit skeletal growth. Cosyntropin preferred for diagnostic testing as it is less allergenic and more potent.

**COSYNTROPIN (Cortrosyn, ✦Synacthen)** ▶L ♀C ▶? $

ADULT - Rapid screen for adrenocortical insufficiency: 0.25 mg IM/ IV over 2 min; measure serum cortisol before & 30–60 min after.

PEDS - Rapid screen for adrenocortical insufficiency: 0.25 mg (0.125 mg if <2 yo) IM/IV over 2 min; measure serum cortisol before & 30–60 min after.

**METYRAPONE (Metopirone)** ▶KL ♀C ▶? $$

WARNING - May cause acute adrenal insufficiency.

ADULT - Diagnostic aid for testing hypothalamic-pituitary adrenocorticotropic hormone (ACTH) function: Specialized single- and multiple-test dose available.

PEDS - Diagnostic aid for testing hypothalamic-pituitary adrenocorticotropic hormone (ACTH) function: Specialized single- and multiple-test dose available.

UNAPPROVED ADULT - Cushing's syndrome: dosing varies.

FORMS - Trade only: Caps 250 mg. Only available from manufacturer due to limited supply: 1-800-988-7768.

NOTES - Ability of adrenals to respond to exogenous ACTH should be demonstrated before metyrapone is employed as a test. In the presence of hypo- or hyperthyroidism, response to the test may be subnormal. May suppress aldosterone synthesis. May cause dizziness & sedation.

## ENDOCRINE & METABOLIC: Enzymes

**AGALSIDASE BETA (Fabrazyme)** ▶? ♀B ▶? $$$$$

ADULT - Fabry disease: 1 mg/kg infused q 2 wk. Initial infusion rate <0.25 mg/min. If tolerated, increase rate in increments of 0.05–0.08 mg/min each subsequent infusion. Pretreat with antipyretic and antihistamine.

PEDS - Not approved in children.

FORMS - Trade only: 5 & 35 mg single-use vial.

NOTES - When an infusion reaction occurs, may decrease infusion rate, temporarily stop the infusion and/or give additional antipyretic, antihistamine and/or steroids; medical support should be readily available. Immunogenicity may develop within 3 mo; consider testing for IgE in suspected patients; determine risk & benefits of continued treatment with anti-Fabrazyme IgE. Orphan drug; available through specialty distributor; encourage patient to enroll in the Fabry disease registry.

**ALGLUCERASE (Ceredase)** ▶K ♀C ▶? $$$$$

ADULT - Type 1 Gaucher disease: Dose ranges from 1.15 units/kg IV 3 times a wk to 60 units/kg administered once a wk or every 4 wk (most data are available on 60 units/kg every 2 wk); the dosage depends on the patient and the clinical response. Infuse over 1–2 h.

PEDS - Type 1 Gaucher disease: Dose ranges from 1.15 units/kg IV 3 times a wk to 60 units/kg administered as once a wk or every 4 wk (most data is available on the 60 units/kg every 2 wk); the dosage depends on the patient and the clinical response. Infuse over 1–2 h.

**ALGLUCERASE** (cont.)

NOTES - Orphan drug for Type 1 Gaucher patients with anemia, thrombocytopenia, bone disease, hepatomegaly or splenomegaly. Monitor IgG antibody periodically.

**ALGLUCOSIDASE ALFA (*Myozyme*)** ▶? ♀B ▶? $$$$$

WARNING - Infusion-related hypersensitivity may occur.

ADULT - Not approved for juvenile-onset or adult-onset Pompe disease.

PEDS - Infantile-onset Pompe disease: 20 mg/kg infused every 2 wk with specialized weight-based infusion rate.

FORMS - Trade only: Single use vial, 50 mg.

NOTES - Decrease infusion rate or give additional antipyretic and/or antihistamine when an infusion reaction occurs; stop infusion when severe hypersensitivity or anaphylactic reactions occur. Greater risk of infusion reactions during concurrent acute illness. Encourage patient to enroll in the Pompe disease registry.

**GALSULFASE (*Naglazyme*)** ▶? ♀B ▶? $$$$$

ADULT - Mucopolysaccharidosis IV: 1 mg/kg IV once weekly administered as infusion over 4 or more h. Initial infusion rate 6 mL/h for first h, increase as tolerated to 80 mL/h. Pretreat with antihistamine.

PEDS - Mucopolysaccharidosis IV, ≥5 yo: 1 mg/kg IV once weekly administered as infusion over ≥4 h. Initial infusion rate 6 mL/h for first h, increase as tolerated to 80 mL/h. Pretreat with antihistamine.

NOTES - When an infusion reaction occurs, may decrease infusion rate, temporarily stop the infusion and/or give additional antipyretic, antihistamine and/or steroids.

**HYALURONIDASE (*Amphadase*)** ▶Serum ♀C ▶? $$

ADULT - Absorption and dispersion of injected drugs: Add 50–300 U (typically 150 U) to the injection solution. Hypodermoclysis: Administer 50–300 U after clysis or 150 U under the skin prior to clysis which will facilitate absorption of >1 L of solution. Subcutaneous urography: 75 U injected SC over each scapula, followed by injection of contrast media.

PEDS - Absorption and dispersion of injected drugs: Add 50–300 U (typically 150 U) to the injection solution. Hypodermoclysis, <3 yo: 50–300 U to a small volume of solution (up to 200 mL); premature infant/neonatal - daily dosage should not exceed 25 mL/kg, rate of administration should <2 mL/min. Subcutaneous urography: 75 U injected SC over each scapula, followed by injection of contrast media.

FORMS - Trade only: 2 mL vial; 150 U/mL

NOTES - Not recommended for IV use. Do not use in infected or acutely inflamed areas including bites or stings. Do not use to enhance absorption & dispersion of alpha agonists (eg, dopamine). Incompatible with furosemide, benzodiazepines & phenytoin; assess potential physical or chemical incompatibilities with other drugs. May enhance side effects of co-administered drug.

Larger amounts may be needed when administering large doses of salicylates, cortisone, ACTH, estrogens, or antihistamines. Use the same precaution as parenteral fluid therapy during hypodermoclysis.

**IDURSULFASE (*Elaprase*)** ▶? ♀C ▶? $$$$$

WARNING - Infusion-related hypersensitivity may occur. Medical support should be available during administration.

ADULT - Hunter Syndrome (mucopolysaccharidosis II): 0.5 mg/kg infused q wk IV over 1 to 3 h. Initial infusion rate 8 mL/h for first 15 min, increase rate as tolerated to 100 mL/h.

PEDS - Hunter Syndrome (mucopolysaccharidosis II): ≥5 yo: 0.5 mg/kg infused q wk IV over 1 to 3 h. Initial infusion rate 8 mL/h for first 15 min, increase rate as tolerated to 100 mL/h.

NOTES - Decrease infusion rate or discontinue if an infusion reaction occurs. If prior infusion reaction, pretreat with antihistamine and/or corticosteroids and slow rate of administration. Delay administration if concomitant acute respiratory or febrile illness. Orphan drug; available through specialty distributor; encourage patient to complete Hunter Outcome Survey.

**IMIGLUCERASE (*Cerezyme*)** ▶K ♀C ▶? $$$$$

ADULT - Type 1 Gaucher disease: 2.5 units/kg IV three times a wk to 60 units/kg IV q2 wk. Dose individualized to each patient.

PEDS - Type 1 Gaucher disease, 2–16 yo: Dose ranges from 2.5 units/kg IV three times a wk to 60 units/kg IV q2 wk. Dose individualized to each patient.

NOTES - Orphan drug for Type 1 Gaucher patients with anemia, thrombocytopenia, bone disease, hepatomegaly, or splenomegaly. Monitor IgG antibody periodically during the 1st yr of treatment. Caution if prior alglucerase hypersensitivity.

**LARONIDASE (*Aldurazyme*)** ▶? ♀B ▶? $$$$$

WARNING - Infusion-related hypersensitivity may occur.

ADULT - Hurler and Hurler-Scheie forms of mucopolysaccharidosis I and for patients with the Scheie form who have moderate to severe symptoms: 0.58 mg/kg infused q wk with specialized weight-based infusion rate. Pretreat 60 min prior to infusion with antipyretics and/or antihistamines.

PEDS - Hurler and Hurler-Scheie forms of mucopolysaccharidosis I and for patients with the Scheie form who have moderate to severe symptoms >5 yo: 0.58 mg/kg infused q wk with specialized weight-based infusion rate. Pretreat 60 min prior to infusion with antipyretics and/or antihistamines.

FORMS - Trade only: 2.9 mg single-use vial.

NOTES - Decrease infusion rate or give additional antipyretic and/or antihistamine when an infusion reaction occurs; stop infusion when severe hypersensitivity or anaphylactic reactions occur. Orphan drug; available through specialty distributor; encourage patient to enroll in the mucopolysaccharidosis I registry.

## ENDOCRINE & METABOLIC: Gout-Related

**ALLOPURINOL (*Aloprim, Zyloprim*)** ▶K ♀C ▶+ $
  ADULT - Mild gout or recurrent calcium oxalate stones: 200–300 mg PO daily (start with 100 mg PO daily). Moderately severe gout: 400–600 mg PO daily. Secondary hyperuricemia: 600–800 mg PO daily. Doses in excess of 300 mg should be divided. Max 800 mg/d. Reduce dose in renal insufficiency (CrCl 10–20 mL/ min = 200 mg/d, CrCl <10 mL/min = 100 mg/d). Prevention of hyperuricemia secondary to chemotherapy and unable to tolerate PO: 200–400 mg/m²/d as a single IV infusion or in equally divided infusions q6–12h. Max 600 mg/d. Reduce dose in renal insufficiency (CrCl 10–20 mL/min = 200 mg/d, CrCl 3–10 mL/min = 100 mg/d, CrCl < 3ml/min 100 mg/d at extended intervals). Initiate 24–48h before chemotherapy.
  PEDS - Secondary hyperuricemia: age <6 yo = 150 mg PO daily; age 6–10 yo = 300 mg PO daily or 1 mg/kg/d divided q6h to a max of 600 mg/d. Prevention of hyperuricemia secondary to chemotherapy and unable to tolerate PO: Initiate with 200 mg/m²/d as a single IV infusion or in equally divided infusions q6–12h.
  FORMS - Generic/Trade: Tabs 100, 300 mg.
  NOTES - May precipitate acute gout; consider using NSAIDs or colchicine prophylactically. Start with 100 mg PO daily and increase weekly to target serum uric acid of <6 mg/dL. Incidence of rash and allopurinol hypersensitivity syndrome is increased in renal impairment. Discontinue if rash or allergic symptoms, do not restart after severe rash. Drug interaction with warfarin and azathioprine. Normal serum uric acid levels are usually achieved after 1–3 wk of therapy. Ensure hydration before IV administration.

**COLBENEMID (colchicine + probenecid)** ▶KL ♀C ▶? $$$
  ADULT - Chronic gouty arthritis: start 1 tab PO daily × 1 wk, then 1 tab PO bid.
  PEDS - Not approved in children.
  FORMS - Generic only: Tabs 0.5 mg colchicine + 500 mg probenecid.
  NOTES - Maintain alkaline urine.

**COLCHICINE** ▶L ♀C ▶? $
  ADULT - Older FDA-approved dosing no longer recommended; see "unapproved adult" section.

  PEDS - Not approved in children.
  UNAPPROVED ADULT - Rapid treatment of acute gouty arthritis: 0.6 mg PO q1h for up to 3h (max 3 tabs). Gout prophylaxis: 0.6 mg PO bid if CrCl ⩾50 mL/min, 0.6 mg PO daily if CrCl 35–49 mL/min, 0.6 mg PO q2–3 d if CrCl 10–34 mL/min. Familial Mediterranean fever: 1 mg in divided doses daily, may increase to 2–3 mg/d if needed. Acute/recurrent pericarditis in addition to usual therapy: 1 mg PO bid × 1 d, then 0.5 mg PO bid × 3 mo; give once daily if <70 kg or intolerance.
  FORMS - Generic only: Tabs 0.6 mg.
  NOTES - Colchicine is most effective when initiated on the first d of gouty arthritis. IV route no longer recommended due to serious adverse effects including death.

**PROBENECID (*Benuryl*)** ▶KL ♀B ▶? $
  ADULT - Gout: 250 mg PO bid × 7 d, then 500 mg PO bid. May increase by 500 mg/d q4 wk not to exceed 2 g/d. Adjunct to penicillin: 2 g/d PO in divided doses. Reduce dose to 1 g/d in renal impairment.
  PEDS - Adjunct to penicillin in children 2–14 yo: 25 mg/kg PO initially, then 40 mg/kg/d divided qid. For children >50 kg, use adult dose. Contraindicated in children <2 yo.
  FORMS - Generic only: Tabs 500 mg.
  NOTES - Decrease dose if GI intolerance occurs. Maintain alkaline urine. Begin therapy 2–3 wk after acute gouty attack subsides.

**RASBURICASE (*Elitek, ◆Fasturtec*)** ▶L ♀C ▶- $$$$$
  WARNING - May cause hypersensitivity reactions including anaphylaxis, hemolysis (G6PD-deficient patients), methemoglobinemia, interference with uric acid measurements
  ADULT - Not approved in adults.
  PEDS - Uric acid elevation prevention in children (1 mo-17 yr) with leukemia, lymphoma, and solid tumor malignancies receiving anti-cancer therapy: 0.15 or 0.20 mg/kg IV over 30 min daily × 5 d. Initiate chemotherapy 4 to 24 h after the first dose.
  NOTES - Safety and efficacy have been established only for one 5 d treatment course. Hydrate IV if at risk for tumor lysis syndrome. Screen for G6PD deficiency in high risk patients.

| INTRAVENOUS SOLUTIONS | | | | | | | | |
| Solution | Dextrose | Calories/ Liter | Na | K | Ca | Cl | Lactate | Osm |
| --- | --- | --- | --- | --- | --- | --- | --- | --- |
| 0.9 NS | 0 g/L | 0 | 154 meq/L | 0 meq/L | 0 meq/L | 154 meq/L | 0 meq/L | 310 meq/L |
| LR | 0 g/L | 9 | 130 meq/L | 4 meq/L | 3 meq/L | 109 meq/L | 28 meq/L | 273 meq/L |
| D5 W | 50 g/L | 170 | 0 meq/L | 0 meq/L | 0 meq/L | 0 meq/L | 0 meq/L | 253 meq/L |
| D5 0.2 NS | 50 g/L | 170 | 34 meq/L | 0 meq/L | 0 meq/L | 34 meq/L | 0 meq/L | 320 meq/L |
| D5 0.45 NS | 50 g/L | 170 | 77 meq/L | 0 meq/L | 0 meq/L | 77 meq/L | 0 meq/L | 405 meq/L |
| D5 0.9 NS | 50 g/L | 170 | 154 meq/L | 0 meq/L | 0 meq/L | 154 meq/L | 0 meq/L | 560 meq/L |
| D5 LR | 50 g/L | 179 | 130 meq/L | 4 meq/L | 2.7 meq/L | 109 meq/L | 28 meq/L | 527 meq/L |

**SULFINPYRAZONE (*Anturane*, *✦Anturan*)** ▶K ♀? ▶? $$
ADULT - Gout: start 100–200 mg PO bid with meals, titrate over 1 wk to 400–800 mg/d.
PEDS - Not approved in children.

FORMS - Generic only: Tabs 100 mg. Caps 200 mg.
NOTES - May precipitate an acute gouty flare; continue treatment throughout exacerbation. Maintain adequate fluid intake and alkaline urine.

## ENDOCRINE & METABOLIC: Minerals

**CALCIUM ACETATE (*PhosLo*)** ▶K ♀+ ▶? $$$
ADULT - Hyperphosphatemia in end-stage renal failure: initially 2 tabs/caps PO tid with each meal. Titrate dose based on serum phosphorus.
PEDS - Not approved in children.
UNAPPROVED PEDS - Titrate to response.
FORMS - Generic/Trade: Gelcaps 667 mg (169 mg elem Ca).
NOTES - Higher doses more effective, but may cause hypercalcemia, especially if given with vitamin D. Most patients require 3–4 tabs/meal.

**CALCIUM CARBONATE (*Caltrate, Mylanta Children's, Os-Cal, Oyst-Cal, Tums, Surpass, Viactiv, ✦Calsan*)** ▶K ♀+ (? 1st trimester) ▶? $
ADULT - Supplement: 1–2 g elem Ca/d or more PO with meals divided bid-qid. Prevention of osteoporosis: 1000–1500 mg elem Ca/d PO divided bid-tid with meals. The adequate intake in most adults is 1000–1200 mg elem Ca/d. Antacid: 1000–3000 mg (2–4 tab) PO q2h prn or 1–2 pieces gum chewed prn, max 7000 mg/d.
PEDS - Hypocalcemia: Neonates: 50–150 mg elem Ca/kg/d PO in 4–6 divided doses; Children: 45–65 mg elem Ca/kg/d PO divided qid. Adequate intake for children (in elem calcium): <6 mo: 210 mg/d when fed human milk and 315 mg/d when fed cow's milk; 6–12 mo: 270 mg/d when fed human milk+solid food and 335 mg/d when fed cow's milk+solid food; 1–3 yo: 500 mg/d; 4–8 yo: 800 mg/d; 9–18 yo 1300 mg/d.
UNAPPROVED ADULT - May lower BP in patients with HTN. May reduce PMS symptoms such as fluid retention, pain, and negative affect.
FORMS - OTC Generic/Trade: tab 500, 650, 750, 1000, 1250, 1500 mg, chew tab 400, 500, 750,850, 1000, 1177, 1250 mg, cap 1250 mg, gum 300, 450 mg, susp 1250 mg/5 mL. Calcium carbonate is 40% elem Ca and contains 20 mEq of elem Ca/g calcium carbonate. Not more than 500–600 mg elem Ca/dose. Available in combination with sodium fluoride, vitamin D and/or vitamin K. Trade examples: Caltrate 600 + D = 600 mg elemental Ca/200 units vit D, Os-Cal 500 + D = 500 mg elemental Ca/200 units vit D, Os-Cal Extra D = 500 mg elemental Ca/400 units vit D, Tums (regular strength) = 200 mg elemental Ca, Tums (ultra) = 400 mg elemental Ca, Viactiv (chew) 500 mg elemental Ca+ 100 units vit D + 40 mcg vit K.
NOTES - Decreases absorption of levothyroxine, tetracycline, and fluoroquinolones.

**CALCIUM CHLORIDE** ▶K ♀+ ▶+ $
ADULT - Hypocalcemia: 500–1000 mg slow IV q1–3 d. Magnesium intoxication: 500 mg IV. Hyperkalemic ECG changes: dose based on ECG.

PEDS - Hypocalcemia: 0.2 mL/kg IV up to 10 mL/d. Cardiac resuscitation: 0.2 mL/kg IV.
UNAPPROVED ADULT - Has been used in calcium channel blocker toxicity and to treat or prevent calcium channel blocker-induced hypotension.
UNAPPROVED PEDS - Has been used in calcium channel blocker toxicity.
FORMS - Generic only: injectable 10% (1000 mg/10 mL) 10 mL ampules, vials, syringes.
NOTES - Calcium chloride contains 14.4 mEq Ca/g versus calcium gluconate 4.7 mEq Ca/g. For IV use only; do not administer IM or SC. Avoid extravasation. Administer no faster than 0.5–1 mL/min. Use cautiously in patients receiving digoxin; inotropic and toxic effects are synergistic and may cause arrhythmias. Usually not recommended for hypocalcemia associated with renal insufficiency because calcium chloride is an acidifying salt.

**CALCIUM CITRATE (*Citracal*)** ▶K ♀+ ▶+ $
ADULT - 1–2 g elem Ca/d or more PO with meals divided bid-qid. Prevention of osteoporosis: 1000–1500 mg elem Ca/d PO divided bid-tid with meals. The adequate intake in most adults is 1000–1200 mg elem Ca/d.
PEDS - Not approved in children.
FORMS - OTC: Trade only (mg elem Ca): 200 & 250 mg with 200 units vitamin D and 250 mg with 125 units vitamin D and 80 mg of magnesium. Chew tabs 500 mg with 200 units vitamin D. OTC: Generic/Trade: Tabs 200 mg, 315 mg with 200 units vitamin D.
NOTES - Calcium citrate is 21% elem Ca. Not more than 500–600 mg elem Ca/dose. Decreases absorption of levothyroxine, tetracycline and fluoroquinolones.

**CALCIUM GLUCONATE** ▶K ♀+ ▶+ $
ADULT - Emergency correction of hypocalcemia: 7–14 mEq slow IV prn. Hypocalcemic tetany: 4.5–16 mEq IM prn. Hyperkalemia with cardiac toxicity: 2.25–14 mEq IV while monitoring ECG. May repeat after 1–2 min. Magnesium intoxication: 4.5–9 mEq IV, adjust dose based on patient response. If IV not possible, give 2–5 mEq IM. Exchange transfusions: 1.35 mEq calcium gluconate IV concurrent with each 100 mL of citrated blood. Oral calcium gluconate: 1–2 g elem Ca/d or more PO with meals divided bid-qid. Prevention of osteoporosis: 1000–1500 mg elem Ca/d PO with meals in divided doses.
PEDS - Emergency correction of hypocalcemia: Children: 1–7 mEq IV prn. Infants: 1 mEq IV prn. Hypocalcemic tetany: Children: 0.5–0.7 mEq/kg IV tid-qid. Neonates: 2.4 mEq/kg/d IV in divided doses. Exchange transfusions: Neonates:

**(cont.)**

**CALCIUM GLUCONATE** (*cont.*)
0.45 mEq IV/100 mL of exchange transfusions. Oral calcium gluconate: Hypocalcemia: Neonates: 50–150 mg elem Ca/kg/d PO in 4–6 divided doses; children: 45–65 mg elem Ca/kg/d PO divided qid.
UNAPPROVED ADULT - Has been used in calcium channel blocker toxicity and to treat or prevent calcium channel blocker-induced hypotension.
UNAPPROVED PEDS - Has been used in calcium channel blocker toxicity.
FORMS - Generic only: Injectable 10% (1000 mg/10 mL, 4.65mEq/10 mL) 1, 10, 50, 100, 200 mL. OTC Generic only: Tab 50, 500, 650, 975,1000 mg. Chew tab 650 mg.
NOTES - Calcium gluconate is 9.3% elem Ca and contains 4.6 mEq elem Ca/g calcium gluconate. Administer IV calcium gluconate not faster than 0.5–2 mL/min. Use cautiously in patients receiving digoxin; inotropic and toxic effects are synergistic and may cause arrhythmias.

**FERRIC GLUCONATE COMPLEX** (*Ferrlecit*) ▶KL ♀B ▶? $$$$$
WARNING - Potentially fatal hypersensitivity reactions rarely reported with sodium ferric gluconate complex. Facilities for CPR must be available during dosing.
ADULT - Iron deficiency in chronic hemodialysis patients: 125 mg elem iron IV over 10 min or diluted in 100 mL NS IV over 1 h. Most hemodialysis patients require 1 g of elem iron over 8 consecutive hemodialysis session.
PEDS - Iron deficiency in chronic hemodialysis ≥6 yo: 1.5 mg/kg elem iron diluted in 25 mL NS & administered IV over 1 h at 8 sequential dialysis sessions. Max 125 mg/dose.
UNAPPROVED ADULT - Iron deficiency: 125 mg elem iron IV over 10 min or diluted in 100 mL NS IV over 1 h.
NOTES - Serious hypotensive events occur in 1.3% of patients.

**FERROUS GLUCONATE** (*Fergon*) ▶K ♀+ ▶+ $
ADULT - Iron deficiency: 800–1600 mg ferrous gluconate (100–200 mg elem iron) PO divided tid. RDA (elem iron): adult males (≥19 yo): 8 mg; adult premenopausal females (19–50 yo) 18 mg; adult females (≥51 yo): 8 mg; pregnancy: 27 mg; lactation: 14–18 yo: 10 mg; 19–50 yo: 9 mg. Upper limit: 45 mg/d.
PEDS - Mild-moderate iron deficiency: 3 mg/kg/d of elem iron PO in 1–2 divided doses; severe iron deficiency: 4–6 mg/kg/d PO in 3 divided doses. RDA (elem iron): <6 mo: 0.27 mg; 7–12 mo:

11 mg; 1–3 yo: 7 mg; 4–8 yo: 10 mg; 9–13 yo: 8 mg; males 14–18 yo: 11 mg; females 14–18 yo: 15 mg.
UNAPPROVED ADULT - Adjunct to epoetin to maximize hematologic response: 200 mg elem iron/d PO.
UNAPPROVED PEDS - Adjunct to epoetin to maximize hematologic response: 2–3 mg/kg elem iron/d PO.
FORMS - OTC Generic/Trade: Tab (ferrous gluconate) 240. Generic only: Tab 27, 300, 324, 325 mg.
NOTES - Ferrous gluconate is 12% elem iron. For iron deficiency, 4–6 mo of therapy generally necessary to replete stores even after hemoglobin has returned to normal. Do not take within 2 h of antacids, tetracyclines, levothyroxine or fluoroquinolones. May cause black stools, constipation or diarrhea.

**FERROUS SULFATE** (*Fer-in-Sol, Feosol, ✦Ferodan, Slow-Fe*) ▶K ♀+ ▶+ $
ADULT - Iron deficiency: 500–1000 mg ferrous sulfate (100–200 mg elem iron) PO divided tid. Liquid: 5–10 mL tid. For iron supplementation RDA see ferrous gluconate.
PEDS - Mild-moderate iron deficiency: 3 mg/kg/d of elem iron PO in 1–2 divided doses; severe iron deficiency: 4–6 mg/kg/d PO in 3 divided doses. For Iron supplementation RDA see ferrous gluconate.
UNAPPROVED ADULT - Adjunct to epoetin to maximize hematologic response: 200 mg elem iron/d PO.
UNAPPROVED PEDS - Adjunct to epoetin to maximize hematologic response: 2–3 mg/kg elem iron/d PO.
FORMS - OTC Generic/Trade (mg ferrous sulfate): Tabs, extended-release 160 mg; tabs 324 & 325 mg; drops 75 mg/0.6 mL. OTC Generic only: Tabs, extended-release 50 mg; elixir 220 mg/5 mL.
NOTES - Iron sulfate is 20% elem iron. For iron deficiency, 4–6 mo of therapy generally necessary. Do not take within 2 h of antacids, tetracyclines, levothyroxine or fluoroquinolones. May cause black stools, constipation or diarrhea.

**FLUORIDE** (*Luride, ✦Fluor-A-Day, Fluotic*) ▶K ♀? ▶? $
ADULT - Prevention of dental cavities: 10 mL of topical rinse swish and spit daily.
PEDS - Prevention of dental caries: Dose based on age and fluoride concentrations in water. See chart.
FORMS - Generic only: chew tab 0.5,1 mg, tab 1 mg, drops 0.125 mg, 0.25 mg, and 0.5 mg/

| FLUORIDE SUPPLEMENTATION | | | |
|---|---|---|---|
| Age | <0.3 ppm in drinking water | 0.3–0.6 ppm in drinking water | >0.6 ppm in drinking water |
| 0–0.5 yo | No supplementation necessary | No supplementation necessary | No supplementation necessary |
| 0.5–3 yo | 0.25 mg PO qd | No supplementation necessary | No supplementation necessary |
| 3–6 yo | 0.5 mg PO qd | 0.25 mg PO qd | No supplementation necessary |
| 6–16 yo | 1 mg PO qd | 0.5 mg PO qd | No supplementation necessary |

**FLUORIDE** (*cont.*)

dropperful, lozenges 1 mg, solution 0.2 mg/mL, gel 0.1%, 0.5%, 1.23%, rinse (sodium fluoride) 0.05,0.1,0.2%).

NOTES - In communities without fluoridated water, fluoride supplementation should be used until 13–16 yr of age. Chronic overdosage of fluorides may result in dental fluorosis (mottling of tooth enamel) and osseous changes. Use rinses and gels after brushing and flossing and before bedtime.

**IRON DEXTRAN** (*InFed, DexFerrum, ◆Dexiron, Infufer*) ▶KL ♀- ▶? $$$$

WARNING - Parenteral iron therapy has resulted in anaphylactic reactions. Potentially fatal hypersensitivity reactions have been reported with iron dextran injection. Facilities for CPR must be available during dosing. Use only when clearly warranted.

ADULT - Iron deficiency: Dose based on patient weight and hemoglobin. Total dose (mL) = 0.0442 × (desired hgb - observed hgb) × weight (kg) + [0.26 × weight (kg)]. For weight, use lesser of lean body weight or actual body weight. Iron replacement for blood loss: replacement iron (mg) = blood loss (mL) × hematocrit. Max daily IM dose 100 mg.

PEDS - Not recommended for infants <4 mo of age. Iron deficiency in children >5 kg: Dose based on patient weight and hemoglobin. Dose (mL) = 0.0442 × (desired hgb - observed hgb) × weight (kg) + [0.26 × weight (kg)]. For weight, use lesser of lean body weight or actual body weight. Iron replacement for blood loss: replacement iron (mg) = blood loss (mL) × hematocrit. Max daily IM dose: infants <5 kg: 25 mg; children 5–10 kg: 50 mg; children >10 kg 100 mg.

UNAPPROVED ADULT - Adjunct to epoetin to maximize hematologic response. Total dose (325–1500 mg) as a single, slow (6 mg/min) IV infusion has been used.

UNAPPROVED PEDS - Adjunct to epoetin to maximize hematologic response.

NOTES - A 0.5 mL IV test dose (0.25 mL in infants) over ≥30 sec should be given at least 1 h before therapy. Infuse ≤50 mg/min. For IM administration, use Z-track technique.

**IRON POLYSACCHARIDE** (*Niferex, Niferex-150, Nu-Iron 150*) ▶K ♀+ ▶+ $$

ADULT - Iron deficiency: 50–200 mg PO divided daily-tid. For iron supplementation RDA see ferrous gluconate.

PEDS - Mild-moderate iron deficiency: 3 mg/kg/d of elem iron PO in 1–2 divided doses. Severe iron deficiency: 4–6 mg/kg/d PO in 3 divided doses. For iron supplementation RDA see ferrous gluconate.

UNAPPROVED ADULT - Adjunct to epoetin to maximize hematologic response: 200 mg elem iron/d PO.

UNAPPROVED PEDS - Adjunct to epoetin to maximize hematologic response: 2–3 mg/kg elem iron/d PO.

FORMS - OTC Trade only: Cap 60 mg (Niferex). OTC Generic/Trade: Cap 150 mg (Niferex-150, Nu-Iron 150), liquid 100 mg/5 mL (Niferex). 1 mg iron polysaccharide = 1 mg elemental iron.

NOTES - For iron deficiency, 4–6 mo of therapy generally necessary. Do not take within 2 h of antacids, tetracyclines, levothyroxine, or fluoroquinolones. May cause black stools, constipation or diarrhea.

**IRON SUCROSE** (*Venofer*) ▶KL ♀B ▶? $$$$$

WARNING - Potentially fatal hypersensitivity reactions have been rarely reported with iron sucrose injection. Facilities for CPR must be available during dosing.

ADULT - Iron deficiency in chronic hemodialysis patients: 5 mL (100 mg elem iron) IV over 5 min or diluted in 100 mL NS IV over ≥15 min. Iron deficiency in non-dialysis chronic kidney disease patients: 10 mL (200 mg elem iron) IV over 5 min or 500 mg diluted in 250 mL NS IV over 4 h.

PEDS - Not approved in children.

UNAPPROVED ADULT - Iron deficiency: 5 mL (100 mg elem iron) IV over 5 min or diluted in 100 mL NS IV over ≥15 min.

NOTES - Most hemodialysis patients require 1 g of elem iron over 10 consecutive hemodialysis sessions. Non-dialysis patients require 1 g of elemental iron divided and given over 14 d.

**MAGNESIUM CHLORIDE** (*Slow-Mag*) ▶K ♀A ▶+ $

ADULT - Dietary supplement: 2 tabs PO daily. RDA (elem Mg): Adult males: 400 mg if 19–30 yo, 420 mg if >30 yo. Adult females: 310 mg if 19–30 yo, 320 mg if >30 yo.

PEDS - Not approved in children.

UNAPPROVED ADULT - Hypomagnesemia: 300 mg elem magnesium PO divided qid.

UNAPPROVED PEDS - Hypomagnesemia: 10–20 mg elem magnesium/kg/dose PO qid. For RDA (elem Mg) see magnesium gluconate.

FORMS - OTC Trade only: enteric coated tab 64 mg. 64 mg tab Slow-Mag = 64 mg elem magnesium.

NOTES - May cause diarrhea. May accumulate in renal insufficiency.

**MAGNESIUM GLUCONATE** (*Almora, Magtrate, Maganate, ◆Maglucate*) ▶K ♀A ▶+ $

ADULT - Dietary supplement: 500–1000 mg/d PO divided tid. RDA (elem Mg): Adult males: 19–30 yo: 400 mg; >30 yo: 420 mg. Adult females: 19–30 yo: 310 mg; >30 yo: 320 mg.

PEDS - Not approved in children.

UNAPPROVED ADULT - Hypomagnesemia: 300 mg elem magnesium PO divided qid. Unproven efficacy for oral tocolysis following IV magnesium sulfate.

UNAPPROVED PEDS - Hypomagnesemia: 10–20 mg elem magnesium/kg/dose PO qid. RDA (elem Mg): Age 0–6 mo: 30 mg/d; 7–12 mo: 75 mg/d; 1–3 yo: 80 mg; 4–8 yo: 130 mg; 9–13 yo: 240 mg; 14–18 yo (males): 410 mg; 14–18 yo (females): 360 mg.

FORMS - OTC Generic only: tab 500 mg, liquid 54 mg elem Mg/5 mL.

(cont.)

**MAGNESIUM GLUCONATE** *(cont.)*

NOTES - 500 mg tabs of magnesium gluconate contain 27–29 mg elem magnesium. May cause diarrhea. Use caution in renal failure; may accumulate.

**MAGNESIUM OXIDE** *(Mag-200, Mag-Ox 400)* ▶K ♀A ▶+ $

ADULT - Dietary supplement: 400–800 mg PO daily. RDA (elem Mg): Adult males: 19–30 yo: 400 mg; >30 yo 420 mg. Adult females: 19–30 yo: 310 mg; >30yo: 320 mg.

PEDS - Not approved in children.

UNAPPROVED ADULT - Hypomagnesemia: 300 mg elem magnesium PO qid. Has also been used as oral tocolysis following IV magnesium sulfate (unproven efficacy) and in the prevention of calcium-oxalate kidney stones.

UNAPPROVED PEDS - Hypomagnesemia: 10–20 mg elem magnesium/kg/dose PO qid. For RDA (elem Mg) see magnesium gluconate.

FORMS - OTC Generic/Trade: cap 140,250,400, 420,500 mg.

NOTES - Magnesium oxide is approximately 60% elem magnesium. May accumulate in renal insufficiency.

**MAGNESIUM SULFATE** ▶K ♀A ▶+ $

ADULT - Hypomagnesemia: mild deficiency: 1g IM q6h × 4 doses; severe deficiency: 2 g IV over 1 h (monitor for hypotension). Hyperalimentation: maintenance requirements not precisely known; adults generally require 8–24 mEq/d. Seizure prevention in pre-eclampsia or eclampsia: 4–6 g IV over 30 min, then 1–2 g IV per h. 5 g in 250 mL D5W (20 mg/mL), 2 g/h = 100 mL/h. 4–5 g of a 50% soln IM q4h prn.

PEDS - Not approved in children.

UNAPPROVED ADULT - Preterm labor: 6 g IV over 20 min, then 1–3 g/h titrated to decrease contractions. Has been used as an adjunctive bronchodilator in very severe acute asthma (2 g IV over 10–20 min), and in chronic fatigue syndrome. Torsades de pointes: 1–2 g IV in D5W over 5–60 min.

UNAPPROVED PEDS - Hypomagnesemia: 25–50 mg/kg IV/IM q4–6h for 3–4 doses, max single dose 2 g. Hyperalimentation: maintenance requirements not precisely known; infants require 2–10 mEq/d. Acute nephritis: 20–40 mg/kg (in 20% solution) IM prn. Adjunctive bronchodilator in very severe acute asthma: 25–100 mg/kg IV over 10–20 min.

NOTES - 1000 mg magnesium sulfate contains 8 mEq elem magnesium. Do not give faster than 1.5 mL/min (of 10% solution) except in eclampsia or seizures. Use caution in renal insufficiency; may accumulate. Monitor urine output, patellar reflex, respiratory rate and serum magnesium level. Concomitant use with terbutaline may lead to fatal pulmonary edema. IM administration must be diluted to a 20% soln. If needed, may reverse toxicity with calcium gluconate 1 g IV.

**PHOSPHORUS** *(Neutra-Phos, K-Phos)* ▶K ♀C ▶? $

ADULT - Dietary supplement: 1 cap/packet (Neutra-Phos) PO qid or 1–2 tab (K-Phos) PO qid after meals and at bedtime. Severe hypophosphatemia (<1 mg/dl): 0.08–0.16 mmol/kg IV over 6 h. In TPN, 310–465 mg/d (10–15 mM) IV is usually adequate, although higher amounts may be necessary in hypermetabolic states. RDA for adults is 800 mg.

PEDS - RDA (elem phosphorus): 0–6 mo: 100 mg; 6–12 mo: 275 mg; 1–3 yo: 460 mg; 4–8 yo: 500 mg; 9–18: 1,250 mg. Severe hypophosphatemia (<1 mg/dl): 0.25–0.5 mmol/kg IV over 4–6 h. Infant TPN: 1.5–2 mmol/kg/d in TPN.

FORMS - OTC: Trade only: (Neutra-Phos, Neutra-Phos K) tab/cap/packet 250 mg (8 mmol) phosphorus. Rx: Trade only: (K-Phos) tab 250 mg (8 mmol) phosphorus.

NOTES - Dissolve caps/tabs/powder in 75 mL water prior to ingestion.

**POTASSIUM** *(Cena-K, Effer-K, K+8, K+10, Kaochlor, Kaon, Kaon Cl, Kay Ciel, Kaylixir, K+Care, K+Care ET, K-Dur, K-G Elixir, K-Lease, K-Lor, Klor-con, Klorvess, Klorvess Effervescent, Klotrix, K-Lyte, K-Lyte Cl, K-Norm, Kolyum, K-Tab, K-vescent, Micro-K, Micro-K LS, Slow-K, Ten-K, Tri-K)* ▶K ♀C ▶? $

ADULT - Hypokalemia: 20–40 mEq/d or more PO/IV. Intermittent infusion: 10–20 mEq/dose IV over 1–2 h prn. Consider monitoring for infusions >10 mEq/h. Prevention of hypokalemia: 20–40 mEq/d PO daily-bid.

PEDS - Not approved in children.

UNAPPROVED ADULT - Diuretic-induced hypokalemia: 20–60 mEq/d PO.

UNAPPROVED PEDS - Hypokalemia: 2.5 mEq/kg/d given IV/PO daily-bid. Intermittent infusion: 0.5–1 mEq/kg/dose IV at 0.3–0.5 mEq/kg/h prn. Infusions faster than 0.5 mEq/kg/h require continuous monitoring.

FORMS - Injectable, many different products in a variety of salt forms (ie, chloride, bicarbonate, citrate, acetate, gluconate), available in tabs, caps, liquids, effervescent tabs, packets. Potassium gluconate is available OTC.

### POTASSIUM (oral forms)

**Effervescent Granules:** 20 mEq: Klorvess Effervescent, K-vescent

**Effervescent Tablets:** 25 mEq: Effer-K, K+Care ET, K-Lyte, K-Lyte/Cl, Klor-Con/EF 50 mEq: K-Lyte DS, K-Lyte/Cl 50

**Liquids:** 20 mEq/15 mL: Cena-K, Kaochlor S-F, K-G Elixir, Kaochlor 10%, Kay Ciel, Kaon, Kaylixir, Klorvess, Kolyum, Potasalan, Twin-K 30 mEq/15 mL: Rum-K 40 mEq/15 mL: Cena-K, Kaon-Cl 20% 45 mEq/15 mL: Tri-K

**Powders:** 15 mEq/pack: K+Care 20 mEq/pack: Gen-K, K+Care, Kay Ciel, K-Lor, Klor-Con 25 mEq/pack: K+Care, Klor-Con 25

**Tablets/Capsules:** 8 mEq: K+8, Klor-Con 8, Slow-K, Micro-K 10 mEq: K+10, K-Norm, Kaon-Cl 10, Klor-Con 10, Klotrix, K-Tab, K-Dur 10, Micro-K 10 20 mEq: Klor-Con M20, K-Dur 20

## PEDIATRIC REHYDRATION SOLUTIONS

| Brand | Glucose | Calories/ Liter | Na* | K* | Cl* | Cit- rate* | Phos* | Ca* | Mg* |
|---|---|---|---|---|---|---|---|---|---|
| CeraLyte 50 (premeasured powder packet) | 0 g/L | 160 | 50 | 20 | 40 | 30 | 0 | 0 | 0 |
| CeraLyte 70 (premeasured powder packet) | 0 g/L | 160 | 70 | 20 | 60 | 30 | 0 | 0 | 0 |
| CeraLyte 90 (premeasured powder packet) | 0 g/L | 160 | 90 | 20 | 80 | 30 | 0 | 0 | 0 |
| Infalyte | 30 g/L | 140 | 50 | 25 | 45 | 34 | 0 | 0 | 0 |
| Kao Lectrolyte (premeasured powder packet) | 20 g/L | 90 | 50 | 20 | 40 | 30 | 0 | 0 | 0 |
| Lytren (Canada) | 20 g/L | 80 | 50 | 25 | 45 | 30 | 0 | 0 | 0 |
| Naturalyte | 25 g/L | 100 | 45 | 20 | 35 | 48 | 0 | 0 | 0 |
| Pedialyte and Pedialyte Freezer Pops | 25 g/L | 100 | 45 | 20 | 35 | 30 | 0 | 0 | 0 |
| Rehydralyte | 25 g/L | 100 | 75 | 20 | 65 | 30 | 0 | 0 | 0 |
| Resol | 20 g/L | 80 | 50 | 20 | 50 | 34 | 5 | 4 | 4 |

*mEq/L

**POTASSIUM** (cont.)
NOTES - Use potassium chloride for hypokalemia associated with alkalosis; use potassium bicarbonate, citrate, acetate, or gluconate when associated with acidosis.

**ZINC ACETATE** (*Galzin*) ▶Minimal absorption ♀A ▶- $
ADULT - RDA (elemental Zn): Adult males: 11 mg daily. Adult females: 8–12 mg daily. Zinc deficiency: 25–50 mg (elemental) daily. Wilson's disease, previously treated with chelating agent: 25–50 mg (elemental) tid.
PEDS - RDA (elem Zn): Age 7 mo–3 yo: 3 mg/d; 4–8 yo: 5 mg; 9–13 yo: 8 mg; 14–18 yo (males): 8 mg; 14–18 yo (females): 9–14 mg. Zinc deficiency: 0.5–1 mg elemental zinc mg/kg/d divided bid-tid. Wilson's disease (≥10 yo): 25–50 mg (elemental) tid.
FORMS - Trade: cap 25, 50 mg elemental zinc.
NOTES - Poorly absorbed; take 1 h before or 2–3 h after meals. Decreases absorption of tetracycline and fluoroquinolones.

**ZINC SULFATE** (*Orazinc, Zincate*) ▶Minimal absorption ♀A ▶- $
ADULT - RDA (elemental Zn): Adult males: 11 mg daily. Adult females: 8–12 mg daily. Zinc deficiency: 25–50 mg (elemental) daily.
PEDS - RDA (elemental Zn): Age 7 mo–3 yo: 3 mg/d; 4–8 yo: 5 mg; 9–13 yo: 8 mg; 14–18 yo (males): 8 mg; 14–18 yo (females): 9–14 mg. Zinc deficiency: 0.5–1 mg elemental zinc mg/kg/d divided bid-tid.
UNAPPROVED ADULT - Wound healing in zinc deficiency: 200 mg TID.
FORMS - OTC Generic/Trade: tab 66, 110, 200 mg; Rx: cap 220 mg.
NOTES - Zinc sulfate is 23% elemental Zn. Decreases absorption of tetracycline and fluoroquinolones. Poorly absorbed; increased absorption on empty stomach; however administration with food decreases GI upset.

## ENDOCRINE & METABOLIC: Nutritionals

**BANANA BAG** ▶KL ♀+ ▶+ $
UNAPPROVED ADULT - Alcoholic malnutrition (one formula): Add thiamine 100 mg + folic acid 1 mg + IV multivitamins to 1 liter NS and infuse over 4h. Magnesium sulfate 2g may be added. "Banana bag" is jargon and not a valid drug order; also known as "rally pack"; specify individual components.

**FAT EMULSION** (*Intralipid, Liposyn*) ▶L ♀C ▶? $$$$$
WARNING - Deaths have occurred in preterm infants after infusion of IV fat emulsions. Autopsy results showed intravascular fat accumulation in the lungs. Strict adherence to total daily dose and administration rate is mandatory. Premature and small for gestational age infants have poor clearance of IV fat emulsion. Monitor infant's ability to eliminate fat (ie, triglycerides or plasma free fatty acid levels).

(cont.)

**FAT EMULSION** (cont.)

ADULT - Calorie and essential fatty acids source: As part of TPN, fat emulsion should be no more than 60% of total calories; when correcting essential fatty acid deficiency, 8–10% of caloric intake should be supplied by lipids. Initial infusion rate 1 mL/min IV (10% fat emulsion) or 0.5 mL/min (20% fat emulsion) IV for first 15–30 min. If tolerated increase rate. If using 10% fat emulsion infuse 500 mL first d and increase the next d. Max daily dose 2.5 g/kg. If using 20% fat emulsion, infuse up to 250 mL (Liposyn II) or up to 500 mL (Intralipid) first d and increase the next d. Max daily dose 2.5 g/kg.

PEDS - Calorie and essential fatty acids source: As part of TPN, fat emulsion should be no more than 60% of total calories; when correcting essential fatty acid deficiency, 8–10% of caloric intake should be supplied by lipids. Initial infusion rate 0.1 mL/min IV (10% fat emulsion) or 0.05 mL/min (20% fat emulsion) for first 10–15 min. If tolerated increase rate up to 1 mL/kg/h (10% fat emulsion) or 0.5 mL/kg/h (20% fat emulsion). Max daily dose 3g/kg. For premature infants, start at 0.5 g/kg/d and increase based on infant's ability to eliminate fat.

NOTES - Do not use in patients with severe egg allergy; contains egg yolk phospholipids. Use caution in severe liver disease, pulmonary disease, anemia, blood coagulation disorders, when there is the danger of fat embolism or in jaundiced or premature infants. Monitor CBC, blood coagulation, LFTs, plasma lipid profile and platelet count.

**FORMULAS - INFANT** (*Enfamil, Similac, Isomil, Nursoy, Prosobee, Soyalac, Alsoy, Nutramigen Lipil*) ▶L ♀+ ▶+ $

ADULT - Not used in adults.

PEDS - Infant meals.

FORMS - OTC: Milk-based (Enfamil, Similac, SMA); soy-based (Isomil, Nursoy, ProSobee, Soyalac, Alsoy).

**LEVOCARNITINE** (*Carnitor*) ▶KL ♀B ▶? $$$$$

ADULT - Prevention of levocarnitine deficiency in dialysis patients: 10–20 mg/kg IV at each dialysis session. Titrate dose based on serum concentration.

PEDS - Prevention of deficiency in dialysis patients: 10–20 mg/kg IV at each dialysis session. Titrate dose based on serum concentration.

FORMS - Generic/Trade: Tabs 330 mg, Oral solution 1 g /10 mL

NOTES - Adverse neurophysiologic effects may occur with long term, high doses of oral levocarnitine in patients with renal dysfunction. Only the IV formulation is indicated in patients receiving hemodialysis.

**OMEGA-3 FATTY ACID** (*fish oil, Lovaza, Promega, Cardio-Omega 3, Sea-Omega, Marine Lipid Concentrate, MAX EPA, SuperEPA 1200*) ▶L ♀C ▶? $$

ADULT - Lovaza, adjunct to diet to reduce high triglycerides (≥500 mg/dL): 4 caps PO daily or divided bid.

PEDS - Not approved in children.

UNAPPROVED ADULT - Hypertriglyceridemia: 2–4 g EPA+DHA content daily under physician's care. Secondary prevention of CHD: 1–2 g EPA+DHA content daily. Adjunctive treatment in RA: 20 g/d PO. Psoriasis: 10–15 g/d PO. Prevention of early restenosis after coronary angioplasty in combination with dipyridamole and aspirin: 18 g/d PO

FORMS - Trade: (Lovaza) 1 g cap (total 840 mg EPA+DHA). Generic/Trade: cap, shown as EPA+DHA content, 240 (Promega Pearls), 300 (Cardi-Omega 3, Max EPA), 320 (Sea-Omega), 400 (Promega), 500 (Sea-Omega), 600 (Marine Lipid Concentrate, SuperEPA 1200), 875 mg (SuperEPA 2000).

NOTES - Lovaza is only FDA approved fish oil, previously known as Omacor. Dose dependent GI upset, may increase LDL-cholesterol, excessive bleeding, hyperglycemia. Marine Lipid Concentrate, Super EPA 1200 mg cap contains EPA 360 mg + DHA 240 mg, daily dose = 5–8 Caps. Treatment doses lowers triglycerides by 30–50%. Caps may contain omega-6 fatty acids and/or vitamin E; content varies with product. May potentiate warfarin. Monitor blood sugar in Type 2 diabetes. Caution in seafood allergy.

**RALLY PACK** ▶KL ♀C ▶- $

UNAPPROVED ADULT - Alcoholic malnutrition (one formula): Add thiamine 100 mg + folic acid 1 mg + IV multivitamins to 1 liter NS and infuse over 4h. Magnesium sulfate 2g may be added. "Rally pack" is jargon and not a valid drug order; also known as "Banana Bag"; specify individual components.

## ENDOCRINE & METABOLIC: Phosphate Binders

**LANTHANUM CARBONATE** (*Fosrenol*) ▶Not absorbed ♀C ▶? $$$$$

ADULT - Treatment of hyperphosphatemia in end stage renal disease: Start 750–1500 mg/d PO in divided doses with meals. Titrate dose every 2–3 wk in increments of 750 mg/d until acceptable serum phosphate reached. Most require 1500–3000 mg/d to reduce serum phosphate <6.0 mg/dL. Chew tabs completely before swallowing.

PEDS - Not approved in children.

FORMS - Trade only: chewable tabs 250, 500, 750, 1000 mg.

NOTES - Caution if acute peptic ulcer, ulcerative colitis, Crohn's disease or bowel obstruction. Avoid medications known to interact with antacids within 2 h. May be radio-opaque enough to appear on abdominal x-ray.

**SEVELAMER** (*Renagel, Renvela*) ▶Not absorbed ♀C ▶? $$$$$

ADULT - Hyperphosphatemia in kidney disease on dialysis: start 800–1600 mg PO tid with meals, adjust according to serum phosphorus concentration.

**SEVELAMER** (cont.)
PEDS - Not approved in children.
FORMS - Trade only: sevelamer hydrochloride (Renagel): Tabs 400, 800 mg; sevelamer carbonate (Renvela): Tab 800 mg.
NOTES - Titrate by one tab/per meal at 2 wk intervals to keep phosphorus ≤5.5 mg/dl; highest daily dose in studies: Renagel, 13 grams; Renvela,14 grams. Decreases absorption of ciprofloxacin; may decrease absorption of anti-arrhythmic & anti-seizure medications; administer these meds 1h before or 3h. Caution in GI motility disorders, including severe constipation.

## ENDOCRINE & METABOLIC: Thyroid Agents

**LEVOTHYROXINE** (L-Thyroxine, Levolet, Levo-T, Levothroid, Levoxyl, Novothyrox, Synthroid, Thyro-Tabs, Tirosint, Unithroid, T4, ✦Eltroxin, Euthyrox) ▶L ♀A ▶+ $
WARNING - Do not use for obesity/weight loss.
ADULT - Hypothyroidism: Start 100–200 mcg PO daily (healthy adults) or 12.5–50 mcg PO daily (elderly or CV disease), increase by 12.5–25 mcg/d at 3–8 wk intervals. Usual maintenance dose 100–200 mcg PO daily, max 300 mcg/d.
PEDS - Hypothyroidism 0–6 mo: 8–10 mcg/kg/d PO; 6–12 mo: 6–8 mcg/kg/d PO; 1–5 yo: 5–6 mcg/kg/d PO; 6–12 yo: 4–5 mcg/kg/d PO; >12 yo: 2–3 mcg/kg/d PO, max 300 mcg/d.
UNAPPROVED ADULT - Hypothyroidism: 1.6 mcg/kg/d PO; start with lower doses (25 mcg PO daily) in elderly and patients with cardiac disease.
FORMS - Generic/Trade: Tabs 25, 50, 75, 88, 100, 112, 125, 137, 150, 175, 200, 300 mcg. Trade only: Caps: 25, 50, 75, 100, 125, 150 mcg in 7 d blister packs, Tabs: 13 mcg (Tirosint).
NOTES - May crush tabs for infants and children. May give IV or IM at ½ oral dose in adults and ½ - ¾ oral dose in children; then adjust based on tolerance and therapeutic response. Generics are not necessarily bioequivalent to brand products; reevaluate thyroid function when switching.
**LIOTHYRONINE** (T3, Cytomel, Triostat) ▶L ♀A ▶? $$
WARNING - Do not use for obesity/weight loss.
ADULT - Mild hypothyroidism: 25 mcg PO daily, increase by 12.5–25 mcg/d at 1–2 wk intervals to desired response. Usual maintenance dose 25–75 mcg PO daily. Goiter: 5 mcg PO daily, increase by 5–10 mcg/d at 1–2 wk intervals. Usual maintenance dose 75 mcg PO daily. Myxedema: 5 mcg PO daily, increase by 5–10 mcg/d at 1–2 wk intervals. Usual maintenance dose 50–100 mcg/d.
PEDS - Congenital hypothyroidism: 5 mcg PO daily, increase by 5 mcg/d at 3–4 d intervals to desired response.
FORMS - Trade only: Tabs 5, 25, 50 mcg.
NOTES - Start therapy at 5 mcg/d in children & elderly and increase by 5 mcg increments only. Rapidly absorbed from the GI tract. Monitor T3 and TSH. Elderly may need lower doses due to potential decreased renal function
**METHIMAZOLE** (Tapazole) ▶L ♀D ▶+ $$$
ADULT - Mild hyperthyroidism: 5 mg PO tid. Moderate hyperthyroidism: 10 mg PO tid. Severe hyperthyroidism: 20 mg PO tid (q8h intervals). Maintenance dose = 5–30 mg/d.
PEDS - Hyperthyroidism: 0.4 mg/kg/d PO divided q8h. Maintenance dose = ½ initial dose, max 30 mg/d.
UNAPPROVED ADULT - Start 10–30 mg PO daily, then adjust.
FORMS - Generic/Trade: Tabs 5, 10. Generic only: Tabs 15, 20 mg.
NOTES - Monitor CBC for evidence of marrow suppression if fever, sore throat, or other signs of infection. Propylthiouracil preferred over methimazole in pregnancy.
**POTASSIUM IODIDE** (Iosat, Thyro-Block, Thyrosafe, Thyroshield) ▶L ♀D ▶- $
WARNING - Do not use for obesity.
ADULT - Thyroidectomy preparation: 50–250 mg PO tid × 10–14 d prior to surgery. Thyroid storm: 1 mL (Lugol's) PO tid at least 1h after initial propylthiouracil or methimazole dose. Thyroid blocking in radiation emergency: 130 mg PO daily × 10 d or as directed by state health officials.
PEDS - Thyroid blocking in radiation emergency age 3–18 yr: 65 mg (one-half of a 130 mg tab) PO daily, or 130 mg PO daily in adolescents >70 kg. 1 mo to 3 yr: 32 mg (one-quarter of a 130 mg tab) PO daily. Birth to 1 mo: 16 mg (one-eighth of a 130 mg tab) PO daily. Duration is until risk of exposure to radioiodines no longer exists.
FORMS - Trade only OTC: Tabs 130 mg (Iosat, Thyroblock). Generic OTC tab 65 mg (Thyrosafe). Generic only OTC Soln: 65 mg/mL (Thyroshield).
**PROPYLTHIOURACIL** (PTU, ✦Propyl Thyracil) ▶L ♀D (but preferred over methimazole) ▶+ $
ADULT - Hyperthyroidism: 100–150 mg PO tid. Severe hyperthyroidism and/or large goiters: 200–400 mg PO tid. Continue initial dose for approximately 2 mo. Adjust dose to desired response. Usual maintenance dose 100–150 mg/d. Thyroid storm: 200 mg PO q4–6h × 1 d, decrease dose gradually to usual maintenance dose.
PEDS - Hyperthyroidism in children age 6–10 yo: 50 mg PO daily-tid. Children ≥10 yo: 50–100 mg PO tid. Continue initial dose for 2 mo, then maintenance dose is 1/3 to 2/3 initial dose.
UNAPPROVED PEDS - Hyperthyroidism in neonates: 5–10 mg/kg/d PO divided q8h. Children: 5–7 mg/kg/d PO divided q8h.
FORMS - Generic only: Tabs 50 mg.

(cont.)

**PROPYLTHIOURACIL** (cont.)
NOTES - Monitor CBC for marrow suppression if fever, sore throat, or other signs of infection. Vasculitic syndrome with positive anti-neutrophilic cytoplasmic antibodies (ANCA) reported requiring discontinuation. Propylthiouracil preferred over methimazole in pregnancy.

**SODIUM IODIDE I-131** (*Hicon, Iodotope, Sodium Iodide I-131 Therapeutic*) ▶K ♀X ▶- $$$$$
ADULT - Specialized dosing for hyperthyroidism and thyroid carcinoma.
PEDS - Not approved in children.
FORMS - Generic/Trade: Capsules & oral solution: radioactivity range varies at the time of calibration. Hicon is a kit containing caps and a concentrated oral solution for dilution and cap preparation.
NOTES - Avoid if preexisting vomiting or diarrhea. Discontinue antithyroid therapy ≥3 d before starting. Low serum chloride or nephrosis may increase uptake; renal insufficiency may decrease excretion and thus increase radiation exposure. Ensure adequate hydration before and after administration. Follow low iodine diet for 1–2 wk before treatment. Women should have negative pregnancy test prior to treatment and advise not to conceive for ≥6 mo.

**THYROID - DESICCATED** (*Thyroid USP, Armour Thyroid*) ▶L ♀A ▶? $
WARNING - Do not use for obesity.
ADULT - Obsolete; use thyroxine instead. Hypothyroidism: Start 30 mg PO daily, increase by 15 mg/d at 2–3 wk intervals to a max dose of 180 mg/d.
PEDS - Congenital hypothyroidism: 15 mg PO daily. Increase at 2 wk intervals.

FORMS - Generic/Trade: Tabs 15, 30, 60, 90, 120, 180, 300 mg. Trade only: Tabs 240 mg.
NOTES - 60 mg thyroid desiccated is roughly equivalent to 100 mcg levothyroxine. Combination of levothyroxine (T4) and liothyronine (T3); content varies (range 2:1 to 5:1).

**THYROLAR** (**levothyroxine + liothyronine**) ▶L ♀A ▶? $
WARNING - Do not use for obesity.
ADULT - Hypothyroidism: 1 PO daily, starting with small doses initially (¼ - ½ strength), then increase at 2 wk intervals.
PEDS - Not approved in children.
FORMS - Trade only: Tabs T4/T3 12.5/3.1 (¼ strength), 50/12.5 (#1), 100/25 (#2), 150/37.5 (#3) mcg.
NOTES - Combination of levothyroxine (T4) and liothyronine (T3).

**THYROTROPIN ALFA** (*Thyrogen*) ▶K ♀C ▶? $$$$$
ADULT - Diagnostic aid: 0.9 mg IM q24 h × 2 doses. Thyroid cancer remnant ablation: 0.9 mg IM q24 h × 2 doses.
PEDS - Not approved in children.
NOTES - Give IM only. For radioiodine imaging or remnant ablation, radioiodine administration should be given 24 h after the final thyrotropin injection. Perform diagnostic scanning 48h after radioiodine administration (72 h after final thyrotropin injection). Serum Tg testing should be 72h after final thyrotropin injection. Increases serum thyroid hormone concentrations; caution in patients with heart disease or significant residual thyroid tissue. Consider pretreatment with glucocorticoids if local tumor expansion may compromise vital anatomic structures. Caution in patients with prior bovine TSH therapy.

## ENDOCRINE & METABOLIC: Vitamins

**ASCORBIC ACID** (*vitamin C, ✦Redoxon*) ▶K ♀C ▶? $
ADULT - Prevention of scurvy: 70–150 mg/d PO. Treatment of scurvy: 300–1000 mg/d PO. RDA females: 75 mg/d; males: 90 mg/d. Smokers: add 35 mg/d more than nonsmokers.
PEDS - Prevention of scurvy: Infants: 30 mg/d PO. Treatment of scurvy: Infants: 100–300 mg/d PO. Adequate daily intake for infants 0–6 mo: 40 mg; 7–12 mo: 50 mg. RDA for children: 1–3 yo: 15 mg; 4–8 yo: 25 mg; 9–13 yo: 45 mg; 14–18 yo: 75 mg (males), 65 mg (females).
UNAPPROVED ADULT - Urinary acidification with methenamine: >2 g/d PO. Idiopathic methemoglobinemia: 150 mg/d or more PO. Wound healing: 300–500 mg/d or more PO for 7–10 d. Severe burns: 1–2 g/d PO.
FORMS - OTC: Generic only: tab 25,50,100,250, 500,1000 mg, chew tab 100,250,500 mg, time-released tab 500 mg, 1000,1500 mg, time-released cap 500 mg, lozenge 60 mg, liquid 35 mg/0.6 mL, oral solution 100 mg/mL, syrup 500 mg/5 mL.
NOTES - Use IV/IM/SC ascorbic acid for acute deficiency or when oral absorption is uncertain. Avoid

excessive doses in diabetics, patients prone to renal calculi, those undergoing stool occult blood tests (may cause false-negative), those on sodium restricted diets and those taking anticoagulants (may decrease INR). Doses in adults >2 g/d may cause osmotic diarrhea.

**CALCITRIOL** (*Rocaltrol, Calcijex*) ▶L ♀C ▶? $$
ADULT - Hypocalcemia in chronic renal dialysis: Oral: 0.25 mcg PO daily, increase by 0.25 mcg q 4–8 wk until normocalcemia achieved. Most hemodialysis patients require 0.5–1 mcg/d PO. Hypocalcemia and/or secondary hyperparathyroidism in chronic renal dialysis IV: 1–2 mcg, 3 times a wk; increase dose by 0.5–1 mcg every 2–4 wk. If PTH decreased <30% then increase dose; if PTH decreased 30–60% then maintain current dose; if PTH decreased >60% then decrease dose; if PTH 1.5–3 times the upper normal limit then maintain current dose. Hypoparathyroidism: 0.25 mcg PO qam; increase q 2–4 wk if inadequate response. Most adults respond to 0.5–2 mcg/d PO. Secondary hyperparathyroidism in pre-dialysis patients: 0.25 mcg PO qam; may increase dose to 0.5 mcg qam.

**CALCITRIOL (cont.)**

PEDS - Hypoparathyroidism 1–5 yo: 0.25–0.75 mcg PO qam. If ≥6 yo then 0.25 mcg PO qam; increase dose in 2–4 wk; usually respond to 0.5–2 mcg/d PO. Secondary hyperparathyroidism in pre-dialysis patients ≥3 yo: 0.25 mcg qam; may increase dose to 0.5 mcg qam. If <3 yo: 0.01–0.015 mcg/kg/d PO.

UNAPPROVED ADULT - Psoriasis vulgaris: 0.5 mcg/d PO or 0.5 mcg/g petrolatum topically daily.

FORMS - Generic/Trade: Cap 0.25, 0.5 mcg. Oral soln 1 mcg/mL. Injection 1,2 mcg/mL.

NOTES - Calcitriol is the activated form of vitamin D. During titration period, monitor serum calcium at least twice weekly. Successful therapy requires an adequate daily calcium intake. Topical preparation must be compounded (not commercially available).

***CEREFOLIN* (L-methylfolate + riboflavin + pyridoxine + cyanocobalamin)** ▶KL ♀C ▶+ $$

ADULT - Nutritional supplement for hyperhomocysteinemia: 1–2 tab PO daily.

PEDS - Not approved in children.

FORMS - Trade only: Each tab contains 5.635 mg of L-methylfolate + 5 mg riboflavin + 50 mg pyridoxine + 1 mg cyanocobalamin.

NOTES - Folic acid doses >0.1 mg may obscure pernicious anemia; preventable with the concurrent cyanocobalamin in product.

***CEREFOLIN WITH NAC* (L-methylfolate + methylcobalamin + acetylcysteine)** ▶KL ♀B ▶- $$

ADULT - Nutritional supplement for neurovascular oxidative stress or hyperhomocysteinemia: 1 cap PO daily.

PEDS - Not approved in children.

FORMS - Trade only: L-methylfolate 5.6 mg + methylcobalamin 2 mg + N-acetylcysteine 600 mg cap.

NOTES - Folic acid doses >0.1 mg may obscure pernicious anemia; preventable with the concurrent cyanocobalamin in product.

**CYANOCOBALAMIN (*vitamin B12, CaloMist, Nascobal*)** ▶K ♀C ▶+ $

ADULT - See also "unapproved adult" dosing. Maintenance of nutritional deficiency following IM correction: 500 mcg intranasal weekly (Nascobal: 1 spray one nostril once weekly) or 50–100 mcg intranasal daily (CaloMist: 1–2 sprays each nostril daily). Pernicious anemia: 100 mcg IM/SC daily, for 6–7 d, then qod for 7 doses, then q3–4 d for 2–3 wk, then q mo. Other patients with vitamin B12 deficiency: 30 mcg IM daily for 5–10 d, then 100–200 mcg IM q mo. RDA for adults is 2.4 mcg.

PEDS - Nutritional deficiency: 100 mcg/24 h deep IM/SC × 10–15 d then at least 60 mcg/mo IM/ deep SC. Pernicious anemia: 30–50 mcg/24 h for ≥14 d to total dose of 1000–5000 mcg deep IM/ SC then 100 mcg/mo deep IM/SC. Adequate daily intake for infants: 0–6 mo: 0.4 mcg; 7–11 mo: 0.5 mcg. RDA for children: 1–3 yo: 0.9 mcg; 4–8 yo: 1.2 mcg; 9–13 yo: 1.8 mcg; 14–18 yo: 2.4 mcg.

UNAPPROVED ADULT - Pernicious anemia & nutritional deficiency states: 1000–2000 mcg PO daily for 1–2 wk, then 1000 mcg PO daily. Prevention and treatment of cyanide toxicity associated with nitroprusside.

UNAPPROVED PEDS - Prevention/treatment of nitroprusside-associated cyanide toxicity.

FORMS - OTC Generic only: tab 100, 500, 1000, 5000 mcg; lozenges 100, 250, 500 mcg. Rx Trade only: nasal spray 500 mcg/spray (Nascobal 2.3 mL), 25 mcg/spray (CaloMist, 18mL).

NOTES - Prime nasal pump before use per package insert directions. Although official dose for deficiency states is 100–200 mcg IM q mo, some give 1000 mcg IM periodically. Oral supplementation is safe & effective for B12 deficiency even when intrinsic factor is not present. Monitor B12, folate, iron and CBC.

***DIATX* (folic acid + niacinamide + cobalamin + pantothenic acid + pyridoxine + d-biotin + thiamine + ascorbic acid + riboflavin)** ▶LK ♀? ▶? $$$

ADULT - Nutritional supplement for end stage renal failure, dialysis, hyperhomocysteinemia or inadequate dietary vitamin intake: 1 tab PO daily.

PEDS - Not approved in children.

FORMS - Trade only: Each tab contains folic acid 5 mg + niacinamide 20 mg + cobalamin 1 mg + pantothenic acid 10 mg + pyridoxine 50 mg + d-biotin 300 mcg + thiamine 1.5 mg + vitamin C 60 mg + riboflavin 1.5 mg. Diatreatment Fe: adds 100 mg ferrous fumarate per tab. Diatreatment Zn adds 25 mg of zinc oxide per tab.

NOTES - Cobalamin component appears to prevent masking of pernicious anemia by folic acid.

**DOXERCALCIFEROL (*Hectorol*)** ▶L ♀B ▶? $$$$

ADULT - Secondary hyperparathyroidism on dialysis: Oral: If PTH >400 pg/mL then start 10 mcg PO 3x/ wk; if PTH >300 pg/mL then increase by 2.5 mcg/dose q8 wk as necessary; if PTH 150–300 pg/mL then maintain current dose; if PTH <100 pg/mL then stop × 1 wk, then resume at a dose at least 2.5 mcg lower. Max 60 mcg/ wk. IV: If PTH >400 pg/mL then 4 mcg IV 3x/ wk; if PTH decreased by <50% & >300 pg/mL then increase by 1–2 mcg q8 wk as necessary; if PTH decreased by >50% & >300 pg/mL then maintain current dose; if PTH 150–300 pg/mL then maintain current dose; if PTH <100 pg/mL then stop x1 wk, then resume at a dose that is at least 1 mcg lower. Max 18 mcg/wk. Secondary hyperparathyroidism not on dialysis: If PTH >70 pg/mL (Stage 3) or >110 pg/mL (Stage 4) then start 1 mcg PO daily; if PTH >70 pg/mL (Stage 3) or >110 pg/mL (Stage 4) then increase by 0.5 mcg/dose q2 wk; if PTH 35–70 pg/mL (Stage 3) or 70–110 pg/mL (Stage 4) then maintain current dose; if <35 pg/mL (Stage 3) or <70 pg/mL (Stage 4) then stop x1 wk, then resume at a dose that is at least 0.5mcg lower. Max 3.5 mcg/d.

PEDS - Not approved in children.

(cont.)

**DOXERCALCIFEROL** *(cont.)*
FORMS - Trade only: Caps 0.5, 2.5 mcg.
NOTES - Monitor PTH, serum calcium and phosphorus weekly during dose titration; may need to monitor patients with hepatic insufficiency more closely.

**FOLGARD** (folic acid + cyanocobalamin + pyridoxine) ▶K ♀? ▶? $
ADULT - Nutritional supplement: 1 tab PO daily.
PEDS - Not approved in children.
FORMS - Trade only: folic acid 0.8 mg + cyanocobalamin 0.115 mg + pyridoxine 10 mg tab.
NOTES - Folic acid doses >0.1 mg may obscure pernicious anemia, preventable with the concurrent cyanocobalamin.

**FOLIC ACID** *(folate, Folvite)* ▶K ♀A ▶+ $
ADULT - Megaloblastic anemia: 1 mg PO/IM/IV/SC daily. When symptoms subside and CBC normalizes, give maintenance dose of 0.4 mg PO daily and 0.8 mg PO daily in pregnant and lactating females. RDA for adults 0.4 mg, 0.6 mg for pregnant females, and 0.5 mg for lactating women. Max recommended daily dose 1 mg.
PEDS - Megaloblastic anemia: Infants: 0.05 mg PO daily, maintenance of 0.04 mg PO daily; Children: 0.5–1 mg PO daily, maintenance of 0.4 mg PO daily. Adequate daily intake for infants: 0–6 mo: 65 mcg; 7–12 mo: 80 mcg. RDA for children: 1–3 yo: 150 mcg; 4–8 yo: 200 mcg; 9–13 yo: 300 mcg, 14–18 yo: 400 mcg.
UNAPPROVED ADULT - For hyperhomocysteinemia: 0.5–1 mg PO daily.
FORMS - OTC Generic only: Tab 0.4,0.8 mg. Rx Generic 1 mg.
NOTES - Folic acid doses >0.1 mg/d may obscure pernicious anemia. Prior to conception all women should receive 0.4 mg/d to reduce the risk of neural tube defects in infants. Consider high dose (up to 4 mg) in women with prior history of infant with neural tube defect. Use oral route except in cases of severe intestinal absorption.

**FOLTX** (folic acid + cyanocobalamin + pyridoxine) ▶K ♀A ▶+ $
ADULT - Nutritional supplement for end stage renal failure, dialysis, hyperhomocysteinemia, homocystinuria, nutrient malabsorption or inadequate dietary intake: 1 tab PO daily.
PEDS - Not approved in children.
FORMS - Trade only: folic acid 2.5 mg/ cyanocobalamin 2 mg/ pyridoxine 25 mg tab.
NOTES - Folic acid doses >0.1 mg may obscure pernicious anemia, preventable with the concurrent cyanocobalamin.

**METANX** (L-methylfolate + pyridoxal phosphate + methylcobalamin) ▶K ♀C ▶? $$$
ADULT - Nutritional supplement for endothelial dysfunction or hyperhomocysteinemia: 1–2 tab PO daily.
PEDS - Not approved in children.
FORMS - Trade only: Each tab contains 2.8 mg L-methylfolate + 25 mg pyridoxal phosphate + 2 mg methylcobalamin.

NOTES - Folic acid doses >0.1 mg may obscure pernicious anemia; preventable with the concurrent cyanocobalamin in product.

**MULTIVITAMINS** *(MVI)* ▶LK ♀+ ▶+ $
ADULT - Dietary supplement: Dose varies by product.
PEDS - Dietary supplement: Dose varies by product.
FORMS - OTC & Rx: Many different brands and forms available with and without iron (tab, cap, chew tab, drops, liquid).
NOTES - Do not take within 2 h of antacids, tetracyclines, levothyroxine or fluoroquinolones.

**NEPHROCAP** (ascorbic acid + folic acid + niacin + thiamine + riboflavin + pyridoxine + pantothenic acid + biotin + cyanocobalamin) ▶K ♀? ▶? $
ADULT - Nutritional supplement for chronic renal failure, uremia, impaired metabolic functions of the kidney & to maintain levels when the dietary intake of vitamins is inadequate or excretion & loss are excessive: 1 cap PO daily. If on dialysis, take after treatment.
PEDS - Not approved in children.
FORMS - Generic/Trade: vitamin C 100 mg/folic acid 1 mg/ niacin 20 mg/ thiamine 1.5 mg/ riboflavin 1.7 mg/ pyridoxine 10 mg/ pantothenic acid 5 mg/ biotin 150 mcg/ cyanocobalamin 6 mcg
NOTES - Folic acid doses >0.1 mg/d may obscure pernicious anemia (preventable with the concurrent cyanocobalamin).

**NEPHROVITE** (ascorbic acid + folic acid + niacin + thiamine + riboflavin + pyridoxine + pantothenic acid + biotin + cyanocobalamin) ▶K ♀? ▶? $
ADULT - Nutritional supplement for chronic renal failure, dialysis, hyperhomocysteinemia or inadequate dietary vitamin intake: 1 tab PO daily. If on dialysis, take after treatment.
PEDS - Not approved in children.
FORMS - Generic/Trade: vitamin C 60 mg/folic acid 1 mg/ niacin 20 mg/ thiamine 1.5 mg/ riboflavin 1.7 mg/ pyridoxine 10 mg/ pantothenic acid 10 mg/ biotin 300 mcg/ cyanocobalamin 6 mcg
NOTES - Folic acid doses >0.1 mg/d may obscure pernicious anemia (preventable with the concurrent cyanocobalamin).

**NIACIN** *(vitamin B3, nicotinic acid, Niacor, Nicolar, Slo-Niacin, Niaspan)* ▶K ♀C ▶? $
ADULT - Niacin deficiency: 100 mg PO daily. Pellagra: up to 500 mg PO daily. RDA is 16 mg for males and 14 mg for females. Hyperlipidemia: Start 50–100 mg PO bid-tid with meals, increase slowly, usual maintenance range 1.5–3 g/d, max 6 g/d. Extended-release (Niaspan): Start 500 mg qhs with a low-fat snack for 4 wk, increase as needed every 4 wk to max 2000 mg.
PEDS - Safety and efficacy not established for doses which exceed nutritional requirements. Adequate daily intake for infants: 0–6 mo: 2 mg; 7–12 mo: 3 mg. RDA for children: 1–3 yo: 6 mg; 48 yo: 8 mg; 9–13 yo: 12 mg; 14–18 yo: 16 mg (males) and 14 mg (females).
FORMS - OTC: Generic only: tab 50,100,250,500 mg, timed-release cap 125,250,400 mg, timed-

**NIACIN** (*cont.*)

release tab 250,500 mg, liquid 50 mg/5 mL. Trade only: 250,500,750 mg (Slo-Niacin). Rx: Trade only: tab 500 mg (Niacor), timed-release cap 500 mg, timed-release tab 500,750,1000 mg (Niaspan, $$$$).

NOTES - Start with low doses and increase slowly to minimize flushing (usually <2h); 325 mg aspirin 30–60 min prior to niacin ingestion will minimize flushing. Use caution in diabetics, patients with gout, peptic ulcer, liver, or gallbladder disease. Extended-release formulations not listed here may have greater hepatotoxicity.

**PARICALCITOL** (*Zemplar*) ▶L ♀C ▶? $$$$$

ADULT - Prevention/treatment of secondary hyperparathyroidism with renal insufficiency: If PTH ≤500 pg/mL then start 1 mcg PO daily or 2 mcg PO 3 times/wk. If PTH >500 pg/mL then start 2 mcg PO daily or 4 mcg PO 3 times/wk. Can increase PO dose by 1 mcg daily or 2 mcg 3/wk based on PTH in 2–4 wk intervals. Prevention/treatment of secondary hyperparathyroidism with renal failure (CrCl <15 mL/min): Initially 0.04–0.1 mcg/kg (2.8–7 mcg) IV 3 times/wk during dialysis. Can increase IV dose 2–4 mcg based on PTH in 2–4 wk intervals. PO/IV: If PTH level decreased <30% then increase dose; if PTH level decreased 30–60% then maintain current dose; if PTH level decreased >60% then decrease dose.

PEDS - Prevention/treatment of secondary hyperparathyroidism with renal failure (CrCl <15 mL/min): 0.04–0.1 mcg/kg (2.8–7 mcg) IV 3 times/wk at dialysis; increase dose by 2–4 mcg or 0.04 mcg/kg q 2–4 wk until desired PTH level is achieved. Max dose 0.24 mcg/kg (16.8 mcg).

FORMS - Trade only: Caps 1, 2, 4 mcg.

NOTES - Monitor serum PTH, calcium and phosphorous. IV doses up to 0.24 mcg/kg (16.8 mcg) have been administered.

**PHYTONADIONE** (*vitamin K, Mephyton, AquaMephyton*) ▶L ♀C ▶+ $

WARNING - Severe reactions, including fatalities, have occurred during and immediately after IV injection, even with diluted injection and slow administration. Restrict IV use to situations where other routes of administration are not feasible.

ADULT - Excessive oral anticoagulation: Dose varies based on INR. INR 5–9: 1–2.5 mg PO (≤5 mg PO may be given if rapid reversal necessary); INR >9 with no bleeding: 5–10 mg PO; Serious bleeding & elevated INR: 10 mg slow IV infusion. Hypoprothrombinemia due to other causes: 2.5–25 mg PO/IM/SC. Adequate daily intake 120 mcg (males) and 90 mcg (females).

PEDS - Hemorrhagic disease of the newborn: Prophylaxis: 0.5–1 mg IM 1 h after birth; Treatment: 1 mg SC/IM.

UNAPPROVED PEDS - Nutritional deficiency: Children: 2.5–5m g PO daily or 1–2 mg IM/SC/IV. Excessive oral anticoagulation: Infants: 1–2 mg

IM/SC/IV q4–8 h; Children: 2.5–10 mg PO/IM/SC/IV, may be repeated 12–48 h after PO dose or 6–8 h after IM/SC/IV dose.

FORMS - Trade only: Tab 5 mg.

NOTES - Excessive doses of vitamin K in a patient receiving warfarin may cause warfarin resistance for up to a wk. Avoid IM administration in patients with a high INR.

**POTASSIUM P-AMINOBENZOATE** (*Potaba*) ▶K ♀? ▶? $$$$$

ADULT - "Possibly effective" for scleroderma, morphea, linear scleroderma, pemphigus, Peyronie's disease: 12 g/d PO given in 4–6 divided doses. Dermatomyositis: Start 15–20 g/d. Tabs & caps 500 mg are given at the rate of 4 tabs or caps 6 times daily, or 6 given qid, usually with meals, and at bedtime with a snack. Tabs must be taken with an adequate amount of liquid to prevent GI upset.

PEDS - "Possibly effective" in the treatment of scleroderma, dermatomyositis, morphea, linear scleroderma, pemphigus, Peyronie's disease: 1 g/d PO in divided doses for each 10 lbs. of body weight. Tabs must be taken with an adequate amount of liquid to prevent GI upset.

FORMS - Trade only: tabs & caps 500 mg, powder envules 2g (pure drug powder)

NOTES - Avoid concurrent sulfonamides. Caution in renal impairment. Therapy usually requires the maintenance of adequate dosage for 2–3 mo. If anorexia & nausea occur, discontinue until resumption of normal food intake to prevent hypoglycemia. May cause rash.

**PYRIDOXINE** (*vitamin B6*) ▶K ♀A ▶+ $

ADULT - Dietary deficiency: 10–20 mg PO daily for 3 wk. Prevention of deficiency due to isoniazid in high-risk patients: 10–25 mg PO daily. Treatment of neuropathies due to INH: 50–200 mg PO daily. INH overdose (>10 g): Give an equal amount of pyridoxine: 4 g IV followed by 1 g IM q 30 min. RDA for adults: 19–50 yo: 1.3 mg; >50 yo: 1.7 mg (males), 1.5 mg (females). Max recommended: 100 mg/d.

PEDS - Not approved in children. Adequate daily intake for infants: 0–6 mo: 0.1 mg; 7–12 mo: 0.3 mg. RDA for children: 1–3 yo: 0.5 mg; 4–8 yo: 0.6 mg; 9–13 yo: 1 mg; 14–18 yo: 1.3 (boys) and 1.2 mg (girls).

UNAPPROVED ADULT - PMS: 50–500 mg/d PO. Hyperoxaluria type I and oxalate kidney stones: 25–300 mg/d PO. Prevention of oral contraceptive-induced deficiency; 25–40 mg PO daily. Hyperemesis of pregnancy: 10–50 mg PO q8h. Has been used in hydrazine poisoning.

UNAPPROVED PEDS - Dietary deficiency: 5–10 mg PO daily for 3 wk. Prevention of deficiency due to isoniazid: 1–2 mg/kg/d PO daily. Treatment of neuropathies due to INH: 10–50 mg PO daily. Pyridoxine-dependent epilepsy: neonatal: 25–50 mg/dose IV; older infants and children: 100 mg/dose IV for 1 dose then 100 mg PO daily.

**(cont.)**

**PYRIDOXINE** (*cont.*)
FORMS - OTC Generic only: Tab 25,50,100 mg, timed-release tab 100 mg.

**RIBOFLAVIN** (*vitamin B2*) ▶K ♀A ▶+ $
ADULT - Deficiency: 5–25 mg/d PO. RDA for adults is 1.3 mg (males) and 1.1 mg (females), 1.4 mg for pregnant women and 1.6 mg for lactating women.
PEDS - Deficiency: 5–10 mg/d PO. Adequate daily intake for infants: 0–6 mo: 0.3 mg; 7–12 mo: 0.4 mg. RDA for children: 1–3 yo: 0.5 mg; 4–8 yo: 0.6 mg; 9–13 yo: 0.9 mg; 14–18 yo: 1.3 mg (males) and 1 mg (females).
UNAPPROVED ADULT - Prevention of migraine headaches: 400 mg PO daily.
FORMS - OTC Generic only: tab 25,50,100 mg.
NOTES - May cause yellow/orange discoloration of urine.

**THIAMINE** (*vitamin B1*) ▶K ♀A ▶+ $
ADULT - Beriberi: 10–20 mg IM 3 times/wk for 2 wk. Wet beriberi with myocardial infarction: 10–30 mg IV tid. Wernicke encephalopathy: 50–100 mg IV and 50–100 mg IM for 1 dose then 50–100 mg IM daily until patient resumes normal diet. Give before starting glucose. RDA for adults is 1.2 mg (males) and 1.1 mg (females).
PEDS - Beriberi: 10–25 mg IM daily or 10–50 mg PO daily for 2 wk then 5–10 mg PO daily for 1 mo. Adequate daily intake infants: 0–6 mo: 0.2 mg; 7–12 mo: 0.3 mg. RDA for children: 1–3 yo: 0.5 mg; 4–8 yo: 0.6 mg; 9–13 yo: 0.9 mg; 14–18 yo: 1.2 mg (males), 1.0 mg (females).
FORMS - OTC Generic only: tab 50,100,250,500 mg, enteric coated tab 20 mg.

**TOCOPHEROL** (*vitamin E*, *✦Aquasol E*) ▶L ♀A ▶? $
ADULT - RDA is 22 units (natural, d-alpha-tocopherol) or 33 units (synthetic, d,l-alpha-tocopherol) or 15 mg (alpha-tocopherol). Max recommended 1000 units (alpha-tocopherol).
PEDS - Adequate daily intake (alpha-tocopherol): infants 0–6 mo: 4 mg; 7–12 mo: 6 mg. RDA for children (alpha-tocopherol): 1–3 yo: 6 mg; 4–8 yo: 7 mg; 9–13 yo: 11 mg; 14–18 yo: 15 mg.
UNAPPROVED ADULT - Alzheimer's disease: 1000 units PO bid (controversial based on limited data & efficacy).
UNAPPROVED PEDS - Nutritional deficiency: Neonates: 25–50 units PO daily; Children: 1 units/kg PO daily. Cystic fibrosis: 5–10 units/kg PO daily (use water soluble form), max 400 units/d.
FORMS - OTC Generic only: tab 200,400 units, cap 73.5, 100, 147, 165, 200, 330, 400, 500, 600, 1000 units, drops 50 mg/mL.
NOTES - Natural vitamin E (d-alpha-tocopherol) recommended over synthetic (d,l-alpha-tocopherol). Do not exceed 1500 units natural vit E/d. Higher doses may increase risk of bleeding. Large randomized trials have failed to demonstrate cardioprotective effects.

**VITAMIN A** ▶L ♀A (C if exceed RDA, × in high doses) ▶+ $
ADULT - Treatment of deficiency states: 100,000 units IM daily × 3 d, then 50,000 units IM daily × 2 wk. RDA: 1000 mcg RE (males), 800 mcg RE (females). Max recommended daily dose in non-deficiency 3000 mcg (see notes).
PEDS - Treatment of deficiency states: Infants: 7,500 - 15,000 units IM daily × 10 d; children 1–8 yo: 17,500 - 35,000 units IM daily × 10 d. Kwashiorkor: 30 mg IM of water-soluble palmitate followed by 5,000–10,000 units PO daily × 2 mo. Xerophthalmia: >1 yo: 110 mg retinyl palmitate PO or 55 mg IM plus 110 mg PO next d. Administer another 110 mg PO prior to discharge. Vitamin E (40 units) should be co-administered to increase efficacy of retinol. RDA for children: 0–6 mo: 400 mcg (adequate intake); 7–12 mo: 500 mcg; 1–3 yo: 300 mcg; 4–8 yo: 400 mcg; 9–13 yo: 600 mcg; 14–18 yo: 900 mcg (males), 700 mcg (females).
UNAPPROVED ADULT - Test for fat absorption: 7000 units/kg (2100 RE/kg) PO × 1. Measure serum vitamin A concentrations at baseline and 4 h after ingestion. Dermatologic disorders such as follicularis keratosis: 50,000 - 500,000 units PO daily × several wk.
UNAPPROVED PEDS - Tried in reduction of malaria episodes in children >12 mo & to reduce the mortality in HIV-infected children.
FORMS - OTC: Generic only: cap 10,000, 15,000 units. Trade only: tab 5,000 units. Rx: Generic: 25,000 units. Trade only: soln 50,000 units/mL.
NOTES - 1 RE (retinol equivalent) = 1 mcg retinol or 6 mcg beta-carotene. Continued Vitamin A/retinol intake of ≥2000 mcg/d may increase risk of hip fracture in postmenopausal women.

**VITAMIN D** (*vitamin D2, ergocalciferol, Calciferol, Drisdol*, *✦Osteoforte*) ▶L ♀A (C if exceed RDA) ▶+ $
ADULT - Familial hypophosphatemia (Vitamin D Resistant Rickets): 12,000–500,000 units PO daily. Hypoparathyroidism: 50,000–200,000 units PO daily. Adequate daily intake adults: 19–50 yo: 5 mcg (200 units); 51–70 yo: 10 mcg (400 units); >70 yo: 15 mcg (600 units). Max recommended daily dose in non-deficiency 50 mcg (2000 units).
PEDS - Adequate daily intake infants and children: 5 mcg (200 units). Hypoparathyroidism: 1.25–5 mg PO daily.
UNAPPROVED ADULT - Osteoporosis prevention: 400–800 units PO daily with calcium supplements. Fanconi syndrome: 50,000–200,000 units PO daily. Osteomalacia: 1000–5000 units PO daily. Anticonvulsant-induced osteomalacia: 2000–50,000 units PO daily. Vitamin D deficiency: 50,000 units PO q wk to q mo.
UNAPPROVED PEDS - Familial hypophosphatemia: 400,000–800,000 units PO daily, increased by 10,000–20,000 units/d q 3–4 mo as needed.

**VITAMIN D** (cont.)

Hypoparathyroidism: 50,000–200,000 units PO daily. Fanconi syndrome: 250–50,000 units PO daily.

FORMS - OTC: Generic: 200 units, 400 units, 800 units, 1000 units, 2000 units (cap/tab).Trade only: soln 8000 units/mL. Rx: Trade only: cap 50,000 units, inj 500,000 units/mL.

NOTES - 1 mcg ergocalciferol = 40 units vitamin D. IM or high-dose oral therapy may be necessary if malabsorption exists. Familial hypophosphatemia also requires phosphate supplementation; hypoparathyroidism also requires calcium supplementation.

## ENDOCRINE & METABOLIC: Other

**AMINOGLUTETHIMIDE (Cytadren)** ▶K ♀D ▶? $$$$

WARNING - Used only as an interim measure until more definitive therapy such as surgery can be undertaken; only small numbers of patients have been treated >3 mo. Benefits are limited in ACTH-dependent Cushing's syndrome as high levels of ACTH overcome the drug's effect. Avoid alcohol. May cause adrenocortical hypofunction; may give hydrocortisone & mineralocorticoid supplements if indicated; dexamethasone should not be used. May cause orthostatic hypotension; monitor BP.

ADULT - Cushing's syndrome: 250 mg PO q6h (should be initiated in hospital). Increase dose in increments of 250 mg at intervals of 1–2 wk if cortisol suppression is inadequate. Max dose 2 g/d.

PEDS - Not approved in children.

UNAPPROVED ADULT - Advanced breast cancer in postmenopausal women: Start 250 mg PO daily, then increase every couple of d to bid, tid, then to qid. Metastatic prostate carcinoma: Start 250 mg PO bid, then increase to 250 mg qid as tolerated. Response may take 4–6 wk.

FORMS - Trade only: Tab 250 mg.

NOTES - Monitor plasma cortisol levels (or to avoid daily variation instead monitor urinary free cortisol or other steroid metabolites) to determine if suppression is adequate. May need glucocorticoid & mineralocorticoid replacement if oversuppression. Dose reduction or temporary discontinuation may be required if adverse effects occurs. Discontinue if skin rash persists >5–8 d or becomes severe; may start at lower dose if rash is mild or moderate. Obtain baseline and monitor periodically hematologic studies, thyroid function tests, LFTs and electrolytes. Decreases effects of warfarin, dexamethasone, digoxin, medroxyprogesterone & theophylline.

**AMMONUL (sodium phenylacetate + sodium benzoate)** ▶KL ♀C ▶? $$$$$

ADULT - Acute hyperammonemia with encephalopathy in urea cycle enzyme deficiency: 55 mL/m² IV over 90–120 min, followed by maintenance 55 mL/m² over 24 h. Stop when hyperammonemia resolved or oral nutrition and medications are tolerated.

PEDS - Acute hyperammonemia with encephalopathy in urea cycle enzyme deficiency: If ≤20 kg, then 2.5 mL/kg IV over 90–120 min, followed by maintenance 2.5mL/kg over 24 h. If >20 kg, then 55 mL/m² IV over 90–120 min, followed by

maintenance 55 mL/m² over 24 h. Consider co-administration of arginine in hyperammonemic infants. Stop when hyperammonemia resolved or oral nutrition and medications are tolerated.

FORMS - Single-use vial 50 mL (10% sodium phenylacetate & 10% sodium benzoate).

NOTES - Administer through a central line. Closely monitor if renal insufficiency. Monitor plasma ammonia level, neurological status, electrolytes, blood pH, blood pCO2 and clinical response. May cause hypokalemia. Consider co-administration of antiemetic. Penicillin and probenecid may affect renal secretion.

**BETAINE (Cystadane)** ▶? ♀C ▶? $$$$$

ADULT - Treatment of homocystinuria: 3 g PO bid; mix with 4–6 oz of fluid. Dosage may be gradually increased until homocystine level is undetectable or present only in small amounts; dosages up to 20 g/d have been used in some patients.

PEDS - Treatment of homocystinuria: <3 yo - Start 100 mg/kg/d, then increase weekly by 100 mg/kg increments; mix with 4–6 oz of fluid. >3 yo - 3 g PO bid; mix with 4–6 oz of fluid. Dosage may be gradually increased until homocysteine level is undetectable or present only in small amounts; dosages up to 20 g/d have been used in some patients.

FORMS - Trade only: 180 g/bottle (1 scoop = 1 g betaine)

NOTES - Response to therapy occurs within a wk & steady state within a mo. May take with vitamin B6 & B12 & folate.

**BROMOCRIPTINE (Parlodel)** ▶L ♀B ▶- $$$$$

ADULT - Hyperprolactinemia: Start 1.25–2.5 mg PO qhs, then increase q3–7 d to usual effective dose of 2.5–15 mg/d, max 40 mg/d. Acromegaly: Usual effective dose is 20–30 mg/d, max 100 mg/d. Doses >20 mg/d can be divided bid. Also approved for Parkinson's Disease, but rarely used. Take with food to minimize dizziness and nausea.

PEDS - Not approved in children.

UNAPPROVED ADULT - Neuroleptic malignant syndrome: 2.5–5 mg PO 2–6 times/d. Hyperprolactinemia: 2.5–7.5 mg/d vaginally if GI intolerance occurs with PO dosing.

FORMS - Generic/Trade: Tabs 2.5 mg. Caps 5 mg.

NOTES - Take with food to minimize dizziness and nausea. Ergots have been associated with potentially life-threatening fibrotic complications. Seizures, stroke, HTN, arrhythmias, and MI have been reported. Should not be used for post-partum lactation suppression. Contraindicated in

(cont.)

**BROMOCRIPTINE** (cont.)

Raynaud's Syndrome. Avoid concomitant use of other ergot medications.

**CABERGOLINE (Dostinex)** ▶L ♀B ▶– $$$$$

ADULT - Hyperprolactinemia: initiate therapy with 0.25 mg PO twice weekly. Increase by 0.25 mg twice weekly at 4 wk intervals up to a max of 1 mg twice weekly.

PEDS - Not approved in children.

UNAPPROVED ADULT - Acromegaly: 0.5 mg PO twice/wk. Increase as needed up to 3.5 mg/wk based on plasma IGF-I levels.

FORMS - Generic/Trade: Tabs 0.5 mg.

NOTES - Monitor serum prolactin levels. Use with caution in hepatic insufficiency or valvular disease. Postmarketing reports of pathological gambling, increased libido and hypersexuality.

**CALCITONIN (Miacalcin, Fortical, ◆Calcimar, Caltine)** ▶Plasma ♀C ▶? $$$$

ADULT - Osteoporosis: 100 units SC/IM daily or 200 units (1 spray) intranasal daily (alternate nostrils). Paget's disease: 50–100 units SC/IM daily or 3 times weekly. Hypercalcemia: 4 units/kg SC/IM q12h. May increase after 2 d to max of 8 units/kg q6h.

PEDS - Not approved in children.

UNAPPROVED ADULT - Acute osteoporotic vertebral fracture pain: 100 units SC/IM daily or 200 units intranasal daily (alternate nostrils).

UNAPPROVED PEDS - Osteogenesis imperfecta age 6 mo–15 yo: 2 units/kg SC/IM three times weekly with oral calcium supplements.

FORMS - Trade only: nasal spray 200 units/activation in 3.7 mL bottle (minimum of 30 doses/bottle).

NOTES - Skin test before using injectable product: 1 unit intradermally and observe for local reaction. Hypocalcemic effect diminishes in 2–7 d, therefore, only useful during acute short-term management of hypercalcemia.

**CINACALCET (Sensipar)** ▶LK ♀C ▶? $$$$$

ADULT - Treatment of secondary hyperparathyroidism in dialysis patients: 30 mg PO daily. May titrate q 2–4 wk through sequential doses of 60, 90, 120 & 180 mg daily to target intact parathyroid hormone level of 150–300 pg/mL. Treatment of hypercalcemia in parathyroid carcinoma: 30 mg PO bid. May titrate q 2–4 wk through sequential does of 60 mg bid, 90 mg bid & 90 mg tid-qid as necessary to normalize serum calcium levels.

PEDS - Not approved in children.

UNAPPROVED ADULT - Primary hyperparathyroidism: 30 mg PO bid. May titrate q2–8 wk up to 45 mg bid to maintain serum calcium ≤10.3 mg/dL.

FORMS - Trade only: Tab 30, 60, 90 mg.

NOTES - Monitor serum calcium & phosphorus 1 wk after initiation or dose adjustment, then monthly after a maintenance dose has been established. Intact parathyroid hormone should be checked 1–4 wk after initiation or dose adjustment, and then 1–3 mo after a maintenance dose has been established. For parathyroid carcinoma, monitor serum calcium within 1 wk after initiation or dose adjustment, then q 2 mo after a maintenance dose has been established. Withhold if serum calcium falls below <7.5 mg/dL or if signs & symptoms of hypocalcemia. May restart when calcium level reaches 8.0 mg/dL or when signs & symptoms of hypocalcemia resolve. Re-initiate using the next lowest dose. Use calcium-containing phosphate binder and/or vitamin D to raise calcium if it falls between 7.5–8.4 mg/dL. Reduce dose or discontinue if intact parathyroid hormone level is <150–300 pg/mL to prevent adynamic bone disease. Do not check parathyroid hormone levels within 12 h after administration of a dose. Inhibits metabolism by CYP2D6; may increase levels of flecainide, vinblastine, thioridazine, tricyclic antidepressants. Dose adjustment may be needed when initiating/discontinuing a strong CYP3A4 inhibitor (ie, ketoconazole, erythromycin & itraconazole). Closely monitor parathyroid hormone & serum calcium if moderate to severe hepatic impairment.

**CONIVAPTAN (Vaprisol)** ▶LK ♀C ▶? $$$$$

WARNING - Avoid concurrent use of CYP 3A4 inhibitors (ketoconazole, itraconazole, clarithromycin, ritonavir, indinavir). Discontinue if hypovolemia, hypotension, or rapid rise in serum sodium (>12 mEq/L/24 h) occurs.

ADULT - Euvolemic or hypervolemic hyponatremia: Loading dose of 20 mg IV over 30 min, then continuous infusion 20 mg over 24 h for 1–4 d. Titrate to desired serum sodium. Max dose 40 mg daily as continuous infusion.

PEDS - Not approved in children.

NOTES - Not indicated in hyponatremia of heart failure. Requires frequent monitoring of serum sodium, volume, and neurologic status. Administer through large veins and change infusion site daily to minimize irritation. May increase digoxin levels.

**DESMOPRESSIN (DDAVP, Stimate, ◆Minirin, Octostim)** ▶LK ♀B ▶? $$$$

WARNING - Adjust fluid intake downward to decrease potential water intoxication and hyponatremia; use cautiously in those at risk.

ADULT - Diabetes insipidus: 10–40 mcg (0.1–0.4 mL) intranasally daily or divided bid-tid or 0.05–1.2 mg PO daily or divided bid-tid or 0.5–1 mL (2–4 mcg) SC/IV daily in 2 divided doses. Hemophilia A, von Willebrand's disease: 0.3 mcg/kg IV over 15–30 min; 300 mcg intranasally if ≥50 kg (1 spray in each nostril), 150 mcg intranasally if <50 kg (single spray in 1 nostril). Primary nocturnal enuresis: 0.2–0.6 mg PO qhs.

PEDS - Diabetes insipidus 3 mo–12 yo: 5–30 mcg (0.05–0.3 mL) intranasally daily-bid or 0.05 mg PO daily. Hemophilia A, von Willebrand's disease (age ≥3 mo for IV, age ≥11 mo - 12 yo for nasal spray): 0.3 mcg/kg IV over 15–30 min; 300 mcg intranasally if ≥50 kg (1 spray in each nostril), 150 mcg intranasally if <50 kg (single spray

**DESMOPRESSIN** *(cont.)*

in 1 nostril). Primary nocturnal enuresis ⩾6 yo: 0.2–0.6 mg PO qhs.

UNAPPROVED ADULT - Uremic bleeding: 0.3 mcg/kg IV single dose or q12h (onset 1–2h; duration 6–8h after single dose). Intranasal is 20 mcg/d (onset 24–72 h; duration 14 d during 14-d course).

UNAPPROVED PEDS - Hemophilia A and type 1 von Willebrand's disease: 2–4 mcg/kg intranasally or 0.2–0.4 mcg/kg IV over 15–30 min.

FORMS - Trade only: Stimate nasal spray 150 mcg/0.1 mL (1 spray), 2.5 mL bottle (25 sprays). Generic/Trade (DDAVP nasal spray): 10 mcg/0.1 mL (1 spray), 5 mL bottle (50 sprays). Note difference in concentration of nasal solutions. Rhinal Tube: 2.5 mL bottle with 2 flexible plastic tube applicators with graduation marks for dosing. Generic only: Tabs 0.1, 0.2 mg.

NOTES - Monitor serum sodium. Restrict fluid intake 1 h before to 8 h after PO administration. Hold PO treatment for enuresis during acute illnesses that may cause fluid/electrolyte imbalances. Start at lowest dose with diabetes insipidus. IV/SC doses are approximately 1/10th the intranasal dose. Anaphylaxis reported with both IV and intranasal forms. Do not give if type IIB von Willebrand's disease. Changes in nasal mucosa may impair absorption of nasal spray. Refrigerate nasal spray - stable for 3 wk at room temperature. 10 mcg = 40 units desmopressin.

**GALLIUM** *(Ganite)* ▶K ♀C ▶? $$$$$

ADULT - Hypercalcemia of malignancy: 200 mg/m²/d × 5 d. Shorten course if hypercalcemia is corrected. If mild hypercalcemia with few symptoms, consider 100 mg/m²/d × 5 d. Administer as slow IV infusion over 24 h.

PEDS - Not approved in children.

NOTES - Monitor creatinine (contraindicated if >2.5 mg/dL), urine output, calcium and phosphorous. Avoid concurrent nephrotoxic drugs (eg, aminoglycosides, amphotericin B). Ensure adequate hydration prior to infusion.

**LANREOTIDE** *(Somatuline Depot)* ▶LK ♀C ▶? $$$$$

ADULT - Acromegaly unresponsive to other therapies: Start 90 mg every 4 wk via deep SC injection. Adjust dose based on GH and/or IGF-1 levels. Range 60–120 mg every 4 wk.

PEDS - Not approved in children.

FORMS - Trade only: 60, 90 and 120 mg single-use syringes.

NOTES - Orphan drug. Starting dose in renal or hepatic impairment is 60 mg. Monitor glucose closely in patients with diabetes. Check GH and IGF levels after 3 mo and refer to manufacturer's guideline for specific adjustment.

**MECASERMIN** *(Increlex)* ▶LK ♀C ▶? $$$$$

ADULT - Not studied in adults.

PEDS - Growth failure with severe primary insulin-like growth factor-1 deficiency or with neutralizing antibodies to growth hormone in gene deletion: Start 0.04 to 0.08 mg/kg SC bid. As tolerated, increase at weekly intervals by 0.04 mg/kg per

dose to max of 0.12 mg/kg bid. Administer within 20 min of meal or snack. Omit dose if patient will skip meal.

FORMS - Trade only: 40 mg multiple dose vial.

NOTES - Monitor pre-prandial glucose at initiation and until stable dose. Reduce dose if hypoglycemia occurs despite adequate food intake. Do not use with closed epiphyses or malignancy. Do not give IV. Contains benzyl alcohol.

**MIGLUSTAT** *(Zavesca)* ▶K ♀X ▶- $$$$$

ADULT - Treatment of mild to moderate type 1 Gaucher's disease when enzyme replacement therapy is not an option: 100 mg PO tid; may reduce dose to 100 mg PO daily-bid if adverse effects occur. Reduce dose in renal insufficiency (CrCl 50–70 mL/min = 100 mg PO bid; 30–50 mL/min = 100 mg PO daily; avoid use if <30ml/min).

PEDS - Not approved in children.

FORMS - Trade only: gelatin caps 100 mg

NOTES - Requires effective birth control for both men & women; including 3 mo after stopping therapy for men. Tremors may occur but usually resolve within 1–3 mo of treatment; may need to reduce dose and/or discontinue. Avoid high-carbohydrate foods if diarrhea occurs. Diarrhea frequently decreases over time. May cause peripheral neuropathy; perform neurological evaluation at baseline and q 6 mo. Consider discontinuation if significant diarrhea/weight loss unresponsive to diet modification.

**NITISINONE** *(Orfadin)* ▶? ♀C ▶? $$$$$

WARNING - Elevation of plasma tyrosine level, transient thrombocytopenia and leukopenia.

ADULT - Hereditary tyrosinemia type I: 1–2 mg/kg/d PO divided bid.

PEDS - Hereditary tyrosinemia type I: 1–2 mg/kg/d PO divided bid.

FORMS - Trade only: caps 2, 5, 10 mg.

NOTES - Orphan drug; keep tyrosine levels <500 micromoles/L; regular liver monitoring by imaging and LFTs, alpha-fetoprotein, serum tyrosine, phenylalanine, and urine succinylacetone (may use to guide dosing).

**PEGVISOMANT** *(Somavert)* ▶? ♀B ▶? $$$$$

ADULT - Acromegaly unresponsive to other therapies: Load 40 mg SC on d 1, then maintenance 10 mg SC daily. Max 30 mg/d.

PEDS - Not approved in children.

FORMS - Trade only: 10,15,20 mg single-dose vials. Available only from manufacturer.

NOTES - Orphan drug. May cause elevations of growth hormone levels and pituitary tumor growth; periodically image sella turcica. May increase glucose tolerance. May cause IGF-1 deficiency, monitor IGF-1 4–6 wk after initiation or dose change and q6 mo after IGF-1 normalizes. May elevate LFTs; obtain baseline LFTs then check monthly × 6 mo, quarterly for the next 6 mo and biannually for the next yr. Refer to manufacturer's guideline when initiating with abnormal LFTs.

**(cont.)**

**PEGVISOMANT** (*cont.*)
Dose adjustment should be every 4–6 wk in 5-mg increment and based on IGF-1.

**SAPROPTERIN (*Kuvan*)** ▶? ♀C ▶? $$$$$
ADULT - Phenylketonuria: Start 10 mg/kg PO daily. Regularly monitor blood phenylalanine levels and adjust to 5–20 mg/kg PO daily according to response.
PEDS - Not approved in children.
UNAPPROVED PEDS - Phenylketonuria, ages 4–16: Start 10 mg/kg PO daily. Regularly monitor blood phenylalanine levels and adjust to 5–20 mg/kg PO daily according to response. Frequent monitoring recommended.
FORMS - Trade only: Tab 100 mg.
NOTES - Use in conjunction with phenylalanine-restricted diet. Take with food to increase absorption; dissolve tabs in 4–8 oz water or apple juice and take within 15 min. Caution with phosphodiesterase inhibitors, levodopa and folate metabolism inhibitors.

**SODIUM POLYSTYRENE SULFONATE (*Kayexalate*)** ▶Fecal excretion ♀C ▶? $$$$
ADULT - Hyperkalemia: 15 g PO daily-qid or 30–50 g retention enema (in sorbitol) q6h prn. Retain for 30 min to several h. Irrigate with tap water after enema to prevent necrosis.
PEDS - Hyperkalemia: 1 g/kg PO q6h.
UNAPPROVED PEDS - Hyperkalemia: 1 g/kg PR q2–6h.
FORMS - Generic only: Suspension 15 g/60 mL. Powdered resin.
NOTES - 1 g binds approximately 1 mEq of potassium. Avoid in bowel obstruction or constipation.

**SOMATROPIN (*human growth hormone, Genotropin, Humatrope, Norditropin, Norditropin NordiFlex, Nutropin, Nutropin AQ, Nutropin Depot, Omnitrope, Protropin, Serostim, Serostim LQ, Saizen, Tev-Tropin, Valtropin, Zorbtive*)** ▶LK ♀B/C ▶? $$$$$
WARNING - Avoid in patients with Prader-Willi syndrome who are severely obese, have severe respiratory impairment or sleep apnea, or unidentified respiratory infection; fatalities have been reported.
ADULT - Growth hormone deficiency (Genotropin, Humatrope, Nutropin, Nutropin AQ, Norditropin, Nutropin, Nutropin AQ, Omnitrope, Saizen, Valtropin): doses vary according to product. AIDS wasting or cachexia (Serostim, Serostim LQ): 0.1 mg/kg SC daily, max 6 mg daily. Short bowel syndrome (Zorbtive): 0.1 mg/kg SC daily, max 8 mg daily.
PEDS - Growth hormone deficiency (Genotropin, Humatrope, Norditropin, Nutropin, Nutropin AQ, Nutropin Depot, Omnitrope, Tev-Tropin, Saizen): Doses vary according to product used. Turner syndrome (Genotropin, Humatrope, Norditropin, Nutropin, Nutropin AQ, Valtropin): Doses vary according to product used. Growth failure in Prader-Willi syndrome (Genotropin): individualized dosing. Idiopathic short stature (Genotropin, Humatrope): individualized dosing. SHOX deficiency

(Humatrope): individualized dosing. Short stature in Noonan syndrome (Norditropin): individualized dosing. Growth failure in chronic renal insufficiency (Nutropin, Nutropin AQ): individualized dosing.
FORMS - Single dose vials (powder for injection with diluent). Tev-Tropin: 5mg vial (powder for injection with diluent, stable for 14 d when refrigerated). Genotropin: 1.5, 5.8, 13.8 mg cartridges. Humatrope: 6, 12, 24 mg pen cartridges, 5mg vial (powder for injection with diluent, stable for 14 d when refrigerated). Nutropin AQ: 10 mg multiple dose vial & 5, 10, 20 mg/pen cartridges. Norditropin: 5,10,15 mg pen cartridges. Norditropin NordiFlex: 5, 10, 15 mg prefilled pens. Omnitrope: 1.5, 5.8 mg vial (powder for injection with diluent). Saizen: pre-assembled reconstitution device with autoinjector pen. Serostim: 4, 5, 6 mg single dose vials, 4 & 8.8 mg multidose vials and 8.8 mg cartridges for autoinjector. Valtropin: 5 mg single dose vials, 5 mg prefilled syringe. Zorbtive: 8.8 mg vial (powder for injection with diluent, stable for 14 d when refrigerated).
NOTES - Do not use in children with closed epiphyses. Contraindicated in active malignancy or acute critical illness. Monitor glucose for insulin resistance; use with caution if diabetes or risk for diabetes. Transient and dose-dependent fluid retention may occur in adults. May cause hypothyroidism. Monitor thyroid function periodically. Evaluate patients with Prader-Willi syndrome for upper airway obstruction and sleep apnea prior to treatment; control weight and monitor for signs & symptoms of respiratory infection. Avoid if pre-proliferative or proliferative diabetic retinopathy. Perform funduscopic exam initially & then periodically.

**TERIPARATIDE (*Forteo*)** ▶LK ♀C ▶- $$$$$
WARNING - Possibility of osteosarcoma; avoid in those at risk (eg, Paget's disease, prior skeletal radiation).
ADULT - Treatment of postmenopausal women or men with primary or hypogonadal osteoporosis and high risk for fracture: 20 mcg SC daily in thigh or abdomen for ≤2 yr.
PEDS - Not approved in children.
FORMS - Trade only: 28-dose pen injector (20 mcg/dose).
NOTES - Take with calcium and vitamin D. Pen-like delivery device requires education, and should be discarded 28 d after first injection even if not empty.

**TRIENTINE (*Syprine*)** ▶K ♀C ▶? $$$$
ADULT - Treatment of Wilson's disease and intolerance of penicillamine: 750–1250 mg/d PO divided bid-qid. Max 2000 mg/d. Take 1h before or 2h after meals.
PEDS - 500–750 mg/d PO divided bid-qid. Max 1500 mg/d if ≤12 yo.
FORMS - Trade only: caps 250 mg.
NOTES - Limited clinical experience – optimal dose or dosing intervals not established. Determine

**TRIENTINE** (*cont.*)
    long-term maintenance dosage at 6–12 mo inter-
    vals. Monitor for iron deficiency anemia. Give at
    least 1h apart from any other drug, food, or milk.
    Do not open/chew; swallow whole with water.
**VASOPRESSIN** (*Pitressin, ADH, ✦Pressyn AR*) ▶LK ♀C
▶? $$$$$
    ADULT - Diabetes insipidus: 5–10 units IM/SC bid-
    qid prn
    PEDS - Not approved in children.
    UNAPPROVED ADULT - Cardiac arrest: 40 units IV;
    may repeat if no response after 3 min. Septic
    shock: 0.01–0.1 units/min IV infusion, usual

dose <0.04 units/min. Bleeding esophageal varices: 0.2–0.4 units/min initially (max
0.9 units/min).
UNAPPROVED PEDS - Diabetes insipidus: 2.5–10
units IM/SC bid-qid prn. Bleeding esophageal
varices: start 0.002–0.005 units/kg/min IV,
increase prn to 0.01 units/kg/min. Growth hormone and corticotropin provocative test: 0.3
units/kg IM, max 10 units.
NOTES - Monitor serum sodium. Injectable form may
be given intranasally. May cause tissue necrosis
with extravasation.

## ENT: Antihistamines—Non-sedating

**NOTE:** Antihistamines ineffective when treating the common cold.

**DESLORATADINE** (*Clarinex, ✦Aerius*) ▶LK ♀C ▶+ $$$
    ADULT - Allergic rhinitis/urticaria: 5 mg PO daily.
    PEDS - Allergic rhinitis/urticaria: ≥12 yo: Use adult
    dose. 6-11 yo: 2.5 mg PO daily. 12 mo - 5 yo: ½
    teaspoonful (1.25 mg) PO daily. 6-11 mo: 2 mL
    (1 mg) PO daily.
    FORMS - Trade only: Tabs 5 mg. Fast-dissolve
    RediTabs 2.5 & 5 mg. Syrup 0.5 mg/mL
    NOTES - Increase dosing interval in liver or renal
    insufficiency to every other d. Use a measured
    dropper for syrup.
**FEXOFENADINE** (*Allegra*) ▶LK ♀C ▶+ $$$
    ADULT - Allergic rhinitis, urticaria: 60 mg PO bid
    or 180 mg PO daily. 60 mg PO daily if decreased
    renal function.
    PEDS - Allergic rhinitis, urticaria: ≥12 yo: use adult
    dose. 6-11 yo: 30 mg PO bid or orally disintegrat-
    ing tab bid. 30 mg PO daily if decreased renal
    function.

FORMS - Generic/Trade: Tabs 30, 60, 180 mg, Caps
60 mg. Trade only: Susp 30mg/5 mL, orally disintegrating tab 30 mg.
NOTES - Avoid taking with fruit juice due to a large
decrease in bioavailability. Do not remove orally
disintegrating tab from its blister package until
time of administration.
**LORATADINE** (*Claritin, Claritin Hives Relief, Claritin
RediTabs, Alavert, Tavist ND*) ▶LK ♀B ▶+ $
    ADULT - Allergic rhinitis/urticaria: 10 mg PO daily.
    PEDS - Allergic rhinitis/urticaria ≥6 yo: Use adult
    dose. 2-5 yo: 5 mg PO daily (syrup).
    FORMS - OTC: Generic/Trade: Tabs 10 mg. Fast-
    dissolve tabs (Alavert, Claritin RediTabs) 5, 10
    mg. Syrup 1 mg/mL. Rx: Trade only: Chew tab 5
    mg (Claritin).
    NOTES - Decrease dose in liver failure or renal insuf-
    ficiency. Fast-dissolve tabs dissolve on tongue
    without water. ND = non-drowsy (Tavist).

## ENT: Antihistamines—Other

**NOTE:** Antihistamines ineffective when treating the common cold. Contraindicated in narrow angle glaucoma,
BPH, stenosing peptic ulcer disease, & bladder obstruction. Use half the normal dose in the elderly. May cause
drowsiness and/or sedation, which may be enhanced with alcohol, sedatives, and other CNS depressants. Deaths
have occurred in children <2 yo attributed to toxicity from cough and cold medications; the FDA does not recommend their use in this age group.

**CARBINOXAMINE** (*Palgic*) ▶L ♀C ▶- $$$
    ADULT - Allergic/vasomotor rhinitis/urticaria: 4-8
    mg PO tid-qid.
    PEDS - Allergic/vasomotor rhinitis/urticaria: ≥6 yo:
    4-6 mg PO tid-qid. 3-6 yo: 2-4 mg PO tid-qid. 2-3
    yo: 2 mg PO tid-qid.
    FORMS - Trade only: Tabs 4 mg. Generic/Trade: Oral
    soln 4 mg/5 mL.
    NOTES - Decrease dose in hepatic impairment.
**CETIRIZINE** (*Zyrtec, ✦Reactine, Aller-Relief*) ▶LK
♀B ▶- $$$
    ADULT - Allergic rhinitis/urticaria: 5-10 mg PO
    daily.
    PEDS - Allergic rhinitis/urticaria: 6-11 yo: Use adult
    dose. 2-5 yo: 2.5 mg PO daily-bid or 5 mg PO
    daily. 6-23 mo: 2.5 mg PO daily. If >12 mo, may
    increase to 2.5 mg PO bid.

FORMS - OTC: Generic/Trade: Tabs 5, 10 mg. Syrup 5
mg/5 mL. Chewable tabs, grape-flavored 5, 10 mg.
NOTES - Decrease dose in renal or hepatic
impairment.
**CHLORPHENIRAMINE** (*Chlor-Trimeton, Aller-Chlor*)
▶LK ♀B ▶- $
    ADULT - Allergic rhinitis: 4 mg PO q4-6h. 8 mg PO
    q8-12h (timed release) or 12 mg PO q12h (timed
    release). Max 24 mg/d.
    PEDS - Allergic rhinitis ≥12 yo: Use adult dose.
    6-11 yo: 2 mg PO q4-6h. Max 12 mg/d.
    UNAPPROVED PEDS - Allergic rhinitis 2-5 yo: 1 mg
    PO q4-6h. Max 6 mg/d. Timed release 6-11 yo: 8
    mg PO q12h prn.
    FORMS - OTC: Trade only: Tabs, extended-release 12
    mg. Generic/Trade: Tabs 4 mg. Syrup 2 mg/5 mL.
    Tabs, extended release 8 mg.

**CLEMASTINE** (*Tavist-1*) ▶LK ♀B ▶- $
ADULT - Allergic rhinitis: 1.34 mg PO bid. Max 8.04 mg/d. Urticaria/angioedema: 2.68 mg PO daily-tid. Max 8.04 mg/d.
PEDS - Allergic rhinitis ≥12 yo: Use adult dose. 6-12 yo: 0.67 mg PO bid. Max 4.02 mg/d. Urticaria/angioedema ≥12 yo: Use adult dose. 6-12 yo: 1.34 mg PO bid. Max 4.02 mg/d.
UNAPPROVED PEDS - Allergic rhinitis <6 yo: 0.05 mg/kg/d (as clemastine base) PO divided bid-tid. Max dose 1 mg/d.
FORMS - OTC: Generic/Trade: Tabs 1.34 mg. Rx: Generic/Trade: Tabs 2.68 mg, Syrup 0.67 mg/5 mL. Rx: Generic only: Syrup 0.5mg/5 mL.
NOTES - 1.34 mg = 1 mg clemastine base

**CYPROHEPTADINE** (*Periactin*) ▶LK ♀B ▶- $
ADULT - Allergic rhinitis/urticaria: Start 4 mg PO tid, usual effective dose is 12-16 mg/d. Max 32 mg/d.
PEDS - Allergic rhinitis/urticaria: 2-6 yo: Start 2 mg PO bid-tid. Max 12 mg/d. 7-14 yo: Start 4 mg PO bid-tid. Max 16 mg/d.
UNAPPROVED ADULT - Appetite stimulant: 2-4 mg PO tid 1h ac. Prevention of cluster headaches: 4 mg/d. Treatment of acute serotonin syndrome: 12 mg PO/NG followed by 2 mg q2h until symptoms clear, then 8 mg q6h maintenance while syndrome remains active.
FORMS - Generic only: Tabs 4 mg. Syrup 2 mg/5 mL.

**DEXCHLORPHENIRAMINE** (*Polaramine*) ▶LK ♀? ▶- $$
ADULT - Allergic rhinitis/urticaria: 2 mg PO q4-6h. Timed release tabs: 4 or 6 mg PO at qhs or q8-10h.
PEDS - Allergic rhinitis/urticaria: Immediate release tabs & syrup: ≥12 yr: Use adult dose. 6-11 yo: 1 mg PO q4-6h. 2-5 yo: 0.5 mg PO q4-6h. Timed Release tabs: 6-12 yo: 4 mg PO daily, preferably at qhs.
FORMS - Generic only: Tabs, immediate release 2 mg, timed release 4, 6 mg. Syrup 2 mg/5 mL.

**DIPHENHYDRAMINE** (*Benadryl, Banophen, Allermax, Diphen, Diphenhist, Dytan, Siladryl, Sominex, ◆Allerdryl, Nytol*) ▶LK ♀B ▶- $
ADULT - Allergic rhinitis, urticaria, hypersensitivity reactions: 25-50 mg PO/IM/IV q4-6h. Max 300-400 mg/d. Motion sickness: 25-50 mg PO pre-exposure & q4-6h prn. Drug-induced parkinsonism: 10-50 mg IV/IM. Antitussive: 25 mg PO q4h. Max 100 mg/d. EPS: 25-50 mg PO tid-qid

or 10-50 mg IV/IM tid-qid. Insomnia: 25-50 mg PO qhs.
PEDS - Hypersensitivity reactions: ≥12 yo: Use adult dose. 6-11 yo: 12.5-25 mg PO q4-6h or 5 mg/kg/d PO/IV/IM divided qid. Max 150 mg/d. Antitussive (syrup): 6-12 yo: 12.5 mg PO q4h. Max 50 mg/d. 2-5 yo: 6.25 mg PO q4h. Max 25 mg/d. EPS: 12.5-25 mg PO tid-qid or 5 mg/kg/d IV/IM divided qid, max 300 mg/d. Insomnia age ≥12 yo: 25-50 mg PO qhs.
FORMS - OTC: Trade only: Tabs 25, 50 mg, Chew tabs 12.5 mg. OTC & Rx: Generic only: Caps 25, 50 mg, softgel cap 25 mg. OTC: Generic/Trade: Solution 6.25 or 12.5 mg per 5 mL. Rx: Trade only: (Dytan) Suspension 25 mg/mL, Chew tabs 25 mg.
NOTES - Anticholinergic side effects are enhanced in the elderly, and may worsen dementia or delirium. Avoid use with donepezil, rivastigmine, galantamine, or tacrine.

**HYDROXYZINE** (*Atarax, Vistaril*) ▶L ♀C ▶- $$
ADULT - Pruritus: 25-100 mg IM/PO daily-qid or prn.
PEDS - Pruritus: <6 yo: 50 mg/d PO divided qid. ≥6 yo: 50-100 mg/d PO divided qid.
FORMS - Generic only: Tabs 10, 25, 50, 100 mg, Caps 100 mg, Syrup 10 mg/5 mL. Generic/Trade: Caps 25, 50 mg, Suspension 25 mg/5 mL (Vistaril). (Caps = Vistaril, Tabs = Atarax)
NOTES - Atarax (hydrochloride salt), Vistaril (pamoate salt).

**LEVOCETIRIZINE** (*Xyzal*) ▶K ♀B ▶- $$$
ADULT - Allergic rhinitis/urticaria: 5 mg PO daily.
PEDS - Allergic rhinitis/urticaria: 6-11 yo: 2.5 mg PO daily.
FORMS - Trade only: Tabs 5 mg, scored, oral soln 2.5 mg/5 mL.
NOTES - Decrease dose in renal impairment.

**MECLIZINE** (*Antivert, Bonine, Medivert, Meclicot, Meni-D, ◆Bonamine*) ▶L ♀B ▶? $
ADULT - Motion sickness: 25-50 mg PO 1 h prior to travel, then 25-50 mg PO daily.
PEDS - Not approved in children.
UNAPPROVED ADULT - Vertigo: 25 mg PO daily-qid prn.
FORMS - Rx/OTC/Generic/Trade: tabs 12.5, 25 mg. Chew tabs 25 mg. Rx/Trade only: tabs 50 mg.
NOTES - FDA classifies meclizine as "possibly effective" for vertigo. May cause dizziness and drowsiness.

## ENT: Antitussives/Expectorants

**BENZONATATE** (*Tessalon, Tessalon Perles*) ▶L ♀C ▶? $$
ADULT - Cough: 100-200 mg PO tid. Max 600 mg/d.
PEDS - Cough, >10 yo: Use adult dose.
FORMS - Generic/Trade: Softgel caps: 100, 200 mg.
NOTES - Swallow whole. Do not chew. Numbs mouth; possible choking hazard.

**DEXTROMETHORPHAN** (*Benylin, Delsym, Dexalone, Robitussin Cough, Vick's 44 Cough*) ▶L ♀+ ▶+ $
ADULT - Cough: 10- 20 mg PO q4h or 30 mg PO q6-8h. 60 mg PO q12h (Delsym).

PEDS - Cough >12 yo: Use adult dose. 6-12 yo: 5-10 mg PO q4h or 15 mg PO q6-8h. 30 mg PO q12h (sustained action liquid). 2-5 yo: 2.5-5 mg PO q4h or 7.5 mg PO q6-8h. 15 mg PO q12h (sustained action liquid).
FORMS - OTC: Trade only: Caps 15 mg (Robitussin) & 30 mg (DexAlone), Suspension, extended release 30 mg/5 mL (Delsym). Generic/Trade: Syrup 5, 7.5, 10, 15 mg/5 mL. Generic only: Lozenges 5, 10 mg.

**DEXTROMETHORPHAN** (cont.)

NOTES - Contraindicated with MAOIs due to potential for serotonin syndrome.

**GUAIFENESIN** (*Robitussin, Hytuss, Guiatuss, Mucinex*) ▶L ♀C ▶+ $

ADULT - Expectorant: 100-400 mg PO q4h or 600-1200 mg PO q12h (extended release). Max 2.4g/d.

PEDS - Expectorant >12 yo: Use adult dose. 6-11 yo: 100-200 mg PO q4h. Max 1.2g/d. 2-5 yo: 50-100 mg PO q4h. Max 600 mg/d.

UNAPPROVED PEDS - Expectorant: 12-23 mo: 50 mg PO q4h. Max 300 mg/d. 6-11 mo: 25 mg PO q4h. Max 150 mg/d.

FORMS - Rx-Generic/Trade: Extended release tabs 600, 1200 mg. OTC-Generic/Trade: Liquid & Syrup 100 mg/5 mL. OTC-Trade only: Caps 200 mg (Hytuss), Extended release tabs 600 mg (Mucinex). OTC-Generic only: Tabs 100, 200, 400 mg.

NOTES - Lack of convincing studies to document efficacy.

## ENT: Combination Products—OTC

**NOTE:** Decongestants in some ENT combination products can increase BP, aggravate anxiety or cause insomnia (use caution). Some contain sedating antihistamines. Sedation can be enhanced by alcohol and other CNS depressants. Some states have restricted or ended OTC sale of pseudoephedrine and pseudoephedrine combination products or reclassified it as a scheduled drug due to the potential for diversion to methamphetamine labs. Deaths have occurred in children <2 yo attributed to toxicity from cough and cold medications; the FDA does not recommend their use in this age group.

*ACTIFED COLD & ALLERGY* (phenylephrine + chlorpheniramine) ▶L ♀C ▶+ $

ADULT - Allergic rhinitis/nasal congestion: 1 tab PO q4-6h. Max 4 tabs/d.

PEDS - Allergic rhinitis/nasal congestion: >12 yo: Use adult dose. 6-12 yo: 1/2 tab PO q4-6h. Max 2 tabs/d.

FORMS - OTC: Trade only: Tabs 10 mg phenylephrine/4 mg chlorpheniramine

*ACTIFED COLD & SINUS* (pseudoephedrine + chlorpheniramine + acetaminophen) ▶L ♀C ▶+ $$

ADULT - Allergic rhinitis/nasal congestion/headache: 2 caplets PO q6h. Max 8 caplets/d.

PEDS - Allergic rhinitis/nasal congestion/headache: >12 yo: Use adult dose.

FORMS - OTC: Trade only: Tabs 30 mg pseudoephedrine/2 mg chlorpheniramine/500 mg acetaminophen.

*ALAVERT D-12* (pseudoephedrine + loratadine) ▶LK ♀B ▶- $

ADULT - Allergic rhinitis/nasal congestion: 1 tab PO bid.

PEDS - Not approved in children.

FORMS - OTC: Generic/Trade: Tabs, 12-h extended release tabs, 120 mg pseudoephedrine/5 mg loratadine.

NOTES - Decrease dose to 1 tab PO daily with CrCl <30 mL/min. Avoid in hepatic insufficiency.

*ALEVE COLD & SINUS* (naproxen + pseudoephedrine) ▶L ♀C (D in 3rd trimester) ▶+ $

ADULT - Nasal/sinus congestion, fever & pain: 1 cap PO q12h.

PEDS - Nasal/sinus congestion, fever & pain: >12 yo: Use adult dose.

FORMS - OTC: Generic/Trade: Extended release caplets: 220 mg naproxen sodium/120 mg pseudoephedrine.

*ALLERFRIM* (pseudoephedrine + triprolidine) ▶L ♀C ▶+ $

ADULT - Allergic rhinitis/nasal congestion: 1 tab or 10 mL PO q4-6h. Max 4 tabs/d or 40 mL/d.

PEDS - Allergic rhinitis/nasal congestion: >12 yo: Use adult dose. 6-12 yo: 1/2 tab or 5 mL PO q4-6h. Max 2 tabs/d or 20 mL/d.

FORMS - OTC: Trade only: Tabs 60 mg pseudoephedrine/2.5 mg triprolidine. Syrup 30 mg pseudoephedrine/1.25 mg triprolidine/5 mL.

*APRODINE* (pseudoephedrine + triprolidine) ▶L ♀C ▶+ $

ADULT - Allergic rhinitis/nasal congestion: 1 tab or 10 mL PO q4-6h. Max 4 tabs/d or 40 mL/d.

PEDS - Allergic rhinitis/nasal congestion: >12 yo: Use adult dose. 6-12 yo: 1/2 tab or 5 mL PO q4-6h. Max 2 tabs/d or 20 mL/d.

FORMS - OTC: Trade only: Tabs 60 mg pseudoephedrine/2.5 mg triprolidine. Syrup 30 mg pseudoephedrine/1.25 mg triprolidine/5 mL.

*BENADRYL ALLERGY & COLD* (phenylephrine + diphenhydramine + acetaminophen) ▶L ♀C ▶- $

ADULT - Allergic rhinitis/nasal congestion/headache: 2 tabs PO q4h. Max 12 tabs/d.

PEDS - Allergic rhinitis/nasal congestion/headache: >12 yo: Use adult dose. 6-12 yo: 1 tab PO q4h. Max 5 tabs/d.

FORMS - OTC: Trade only: Tabs 5/12.5/325 mg of phenylephrine/diphenhydramine/acetaminophen

*BENADRYL-D ALLERGY & SINUS* (phenylephrine + diphenhydramine) ▶L ♀C ▶- $

ADULT - Allergic rhinitis/nasal congestion: 1 tab PO q4h. Max 6 tabs/d.

PEDS - Allergic rhinitis/nasal congestion: >12 yo: Use adult dose.

FORMS - OTC: Trade only: Tabs 10/25 mg phenylephrine/diphenhydramine.

*CHERACOL D COUGH* (guaifenesin + dextromethorphan) (◆*Benylin DME*) ▶L ♀C ▶? $

ADULT - Cough: 10 mL PO q4h

PEDS - Cough ≥12 yo: Use adult dose. 6-11 yo: 5 mL PO q4h. Max 30 mL/d. 2- 5 yo: 2.5 mL PO q4h. Max 15 mL/d.

FORMS - OTC: Generic/Trade: Syrup 100 mg guaifenesin/10 mg dextromethorphan/5 mL.

***CHILDREN'S ADVIL COLD*** (ibuprofen + pseudoephedrine) ▶L ♀C (D in 3rd trimester) ▶ + $
ADULT - Not approved for use in adults
PEDS - Nasal congestion/sore throat/fever: 6-11 yo: 10 mL PO q6h. 2-5 yo: 5 mL PO q6h.
FORMS - OTC: Trade only: Suspension: 100 mg ibuprofen/15 mg pseudoephedrine/5 mL. Grape flavor, alcohol-free.
NOTES - Shake well before using. Do not use for >7 d for cold, sinus, & flu symptoms.

***CLARITIN-D 12 H*** (pseudoephedrine + loratadine) ▶LK ♀B ▶ + $
ADULT - Allergic rhinitis/nasal congestion: 1 tab PO bid.
PEDS - Not approved in children.
FORMS - OTC: Generic/Trade: Tabs, 12-h extended-release tabs: 120 mg pseudoephedrine/5 mg loratadine.
NOTES - Decrease dose to 1 tab PO daily with CrCl <30 mL/min. Avoid in hepatic insufficiency.

***CLARITIN-D 24 H*** (pseudoephedrine + loratadine) ▶LK ♀B ▶ + $
ADULT - Allergic rhinitis/nasal congestion: 1 tab PO/d.
PEDS - Not approved in children.
FORMS - OTC: Generic/Trade: Tabs, 24-h extended release tabs: 240 mg pseudoephedrine/10 mg loratadine.
NOTES - Decrease dose to 1 tab PO every other d with CrCl <30 mL/min. Avoid in hepatic insufficiency.

***CORICIDIN HBP CONGESTION & COUGH*** (guaifenesin + dextromethorphan) ▶LK ♀B ▶ + $$
ADULT - Productive cough: 1-2 softgels PO q4h. Max 12 softgels/d.
PEDS - Productive cough: ≥12 yo: Use adult dose.
FORMS - OTC: Trade only: Softgels 200 mg guaifenesin/10 mg dextromethorphan.

***CORICIDIN HBP COUGH & COLD*** (chlorpheniramine + dextromethorphan) ▶LK ♀B ▶ + $
ADULT - Rhinitis/cough: 1 tab q6h. Max 4 doses/d.
PEDS - Rhinitis/cough: ≥12 yo: Use adult dose.
FORMS - OTC: Trade only: Tabs 4 mg chlorpheniramine/30 mg dextromethorphan.

***DIMETAPP COLD & ALLERGY*** (phenylephrine + brompheniramine) ▶LK ♀C ▶ - $$
ADULT - Allergic rhinitis/nasal congestion: 20 mL PO q4h. Max 4 doses/d.
PEDS - Allergic rhinitis/nasal congestion: ≥12 yo: Use adult dose. 6-11 yo: 10ml PO q4h.
FORMS - OTC: Trade only: Liquid 2.5 mg phenylephrine/1 mg brompheniramine/5 mL.
NOTES - Grape flavor, alcohol-free.

***DIMETAPP DM COLD & COUGH*** (pseudoephedrine + brompheniramine + dextromethorphan) ▶LK ♀C ▶ - $
ADULT - Nasal congestion/cough: 20 mL PO q4h. Max 6 doses/d.
PEDS - Nasal congestion/cough: ≥12 yo: Use adult dose. 6-11 yo: 10 mL PO q4h. Max: 6 doses/d.
FORMS - OTC: Trade only: Elixir 2.5 mg phenylephrine/1 mg brompheniramine/5 mg dextromethorphan/5 mL.
NOTES - Red grape flavor, alcohol-free.

***DIMETAPP NIGHTTIME FLU*** (phenylephrine + dextromethorphan + acetaminophen + chlorpheniramine) ▶LK ♀C ▶ - $
ADULT - Nasal congestion/runny nose/fever/cough/sore throat: 20 mL PO q4h. Max of 5 doses/d.
PEDS - Nasal congestion/runny nose/fever/cough/sore throat ≥12 yo: Use adult dose. 6-11 yo: 10 mL PO q4h. Max: 5 doses/d.
FORMS - OTC: Trade only: Syrup 2.5 mg phenylephrine/5 mg dextromethorphan/160 mg acetaminophen/1 mg chlorpheniramine/5 mL.
NOTES - Bubble gum flavor, alcohol-free.

***DRIXORAL COLD & ALLERGY*** (pseudoephedrine + dexbrompheniramine) ▶LK ♀C ▶ - $
ADULT - Allergic rhinitis/nasal congestion: 1 tab PO q12h.
PEDS - Allergic rhinitis/nasal congestion ≥12 yo: Use adult dose.
FORMS - OTC: Trade only: Tabs, sustained-action 120 mg pseudoephedrine/6 mg dexbrompheniramine.

***GUIATUSS PE*** (pseudoephedrine + guaifenesin) ▶L ♀C ▶ - $
ADULT - Nasal congestion/cough: 10 mL PO q4h. Max 40 mL/d.
PEDS - Nasal congestion/cough: ≥12 yo: Use adult dose. 6-11 yo: 5 mL PO q4h. 2-5 yo: 2.5 mL PO q4h. Max 4 doses/d.
FORMS - OTC: Trade only: Syrup 30 mg pseudoephedrine/100 mg guaifenesin/5 mL.
NOTES - PE = pseudoephedrine

***MUCINEX D*** (guaifenesin + pseudoephedrine) ▶L ♀C ▶? $
WARNING - Multiple strengths; write specific product on Rx.
ADULT - Cough/congestion: 2 tabs (600/60) PO q12h; max 4 tabs/24h. 1 tab (1200/120) PO q12h; max 2 tabs/24h.
PEDS - Cough: ≥12 yo: Use adult dose.
FORMS - OTC: Trade only: Tabs, extended release: 600/60 & 1200/120 mg guaifenesin/pseudoephedrine.
NOTES - Do not crush, chew or break the tab. Take with a full glass of water.

***MUCINEX DM*** (guaifenesin + dextromethorphan) ▶L ♀C ▶? $
WARNING - Multiple strengths; write specific product on Rx.
ADULT - Cough: 1-2 tabs (600/30) PO q12h; max 4 tabs/24 h. 1 tab (1200/60) PO q12h; max 2 tabs/24 h.
PEDS - Cough: ≥12 yo: Use adult dose.
FORMS - OTC: Trade only: Tabs, extended release: 600/30 & 1200/60 mg guaifenesin/dextromethorphan.
NOTES - DM = dextromethorphan. Do not crush, chew or break the tab. Take with a full glass of water.

***ROBITUSSIN CF*** (phenylephrine + guaifenesin + dextromethorphan) ▶L ♀C ▶ - $
ADULT - Nasal congestion/cough: 10 mL PO q4h.

**ROBITUSSIN CF** *(cont.)*

PEDS - Nasal congestion/cough: ≥12 yo: Use adult dose. 6-11 yo: 5 mL PO q4h. 2-5 yo: 2.5 mL PO q4h.

FORMS - OTC: Generic/Trade: Syrup 5 mg phenylephrine/100 mg guaifenesin/10 mg dextromethorphan/5 mL.

NOTES – CF = COUGH FORMULA.

**ROBITUSSIN DM (guaifenesin + dextromethorphan)** ▶L ♀C ▶+ $

ADULT - Cough: 10 mL PO q4h. Max 60 mL/d.

PEDS - Cough: ≥12 yo: Use adult dose. 6-11 yo: 5 mL PO q4h. Max 30 mL/d. 2-5 yo: 2.5 mL PO q4h. Max 15 mL/d.

FORMS - OTC: Generic/Trade: Syrup 100 mg guaifenesin/10 mg dextromethorphan/5 mL.

NOTES - Alcohol-free. DM = dextromethorphan.

**ROBITUSSIN PE (phenylephrine + guaifenesin)** ▶L ♀C ▶- $

ADULT - Nasal congestion/cough: 10 mL PO q4h. Max 6 doses/d.

PEDS - Nasal congestion/cough: ≥12 yo: Use adult dose. 6-11 yo: 5 mL PO q4h. 2-5 yo: 2.5 mL PO q4h. Max 6 doses/d.

FORMS - OTC: Trade only: Syrup 5 mg phenylephrine/100 mg guaifenesin/5 mL.

NOTES - PE = phenylephrine

**TRIAMINIC CHEST AND NASAL CONGESTION (phenylephrine + guaifenesin)** ▶LK ♀C ▶- $

ADULT - Child-only preparation.

PEDS - Chest/nasal congestion: Give PO q4h to max 6 doses/24h: 6-12 yo: 10 mL/dose. 2-6 yo: 5 mL/dose.

FORMS - OTC: Yellow label -Trade only: Syrup 2.5 mg phenylephrine/50 mg guaifenesin/5 mL, tropical flavor.

**TRIAMINIC COLD & ALLERGY (phenylephrine + chlorpheniramine)** ▶LK ♀C ▶- $

ADULT - Child-only preparation.

PEDS - Allergic rhinitis/nasal congestion: 6-12 yo: 10 mL PO q4h to max 6 doses/24h.

FORMS - OTC: Orange label -Trade only: Syrup 2.5 mg phenylephrine/1 mg chlorpheniramine/5 mL, orange flavor.

**TRIAMINIC COUGH & SORE THROAT (dextromethorphan + acetaminophen)** ▶LK ♀C ▶- $

ADULT - Child-only preparation.

PEDS - Cough/sore throat: Give PO q4h to max 5 doses/24h: 6-12 yo: 10 mL or 2 softchew tabs per dose. 2-6 yo: 5 mL or 1 softchew tab per dose.

FORMS - OTC: Purple label - Trade only: Syrup & softchew tabs 5 mg dextromethorphan/160 mg acetaminophen/5 mL or tab, grape flavor.

**TRIAMINIC DAY TIME COLD & COUGH (phenylephrine + dextromethorphan)** ▶LK ♀C ▶- $

ADULT - Child-only preparation.

PEDS - Nasal congestion/cough: Give PO q4h to max 6 doses/24h: 6-12 yo: 10 mL or 2 strips per dose. 2-6 yo: 5 mL or 1 strip per dose.

FORMS - OTC: Red label - Trade only: Syrup, thin strips 2.5 mg phenylephrine/5 mg dextromethorphan/5 mL, cherry flavor

NOTES - Allow strips to dissolve on the tongue.

**TRIAMINIC FLU COUGH AND FEVER (acetaminophen + chlorpheniramine + dextromethorphan)** ▶LK ♀C ▶- $

ADULT - Child-only preparation.

PEDS - Fever/cough: 6-12 yo: 10 mL PO q6h to max 4 doses/24h.

FORMS - OTC: Pink label - Trade only: Syrup 160mg acetaminophen/1 mg chlorpheniramine/7.5 mg dextromethorphan/5 mL, bubble gum flavor.

**TRIAMINIC NIGHT TIME COLD & COUGH (phenylephrine + diphenhydramine)** ▶LK ♀C ▶- $

ADULT - Child-only preparation.

PEDS - Nasal congestion/cough: 6-12 yo: 10 mL PO q4h to max 6 doses/24h.

FORMS - OTC: Blue label - Trade only: Syrup 2.5 mg pheynylephrine/6.25 mg diphenhydramine/5 mL, grape flavor.

---

## ENT: Combination Products—Rx Only

**NOTE:** Decongestants in some ENT combination products can increase BP, aggravate anxiety or cause insomnia (use caution). Some contain sedating antihistamines. Sedation can be enhanced by alcohol and other CNS depressants. Deaths have occurred in children <2 yo attributed to toxicity from cough and cold medications; the FDA does not recommend their use in this age group.

**ALLEGRA-D 12-H (fexofenadine + pseudoephedrine)** ▶LK ♀C ▶+ $$$$

ADULT - Allergic rhinitis/nasal congestion: 1 tab PO q12h.

PEDS - Not approved in children.

FORMS - Trade only: Tabs, extended release 60/120 mg fexofenadine/pseudoephedrine.

NOTES - Decrease dose to 1 tab PO daily with decreased renal function. Take on an empty stomach. Avoid taking with fruit juice due to a large decrease in bioavailability.

**ALLEGRA-D 24-H (fexofenadine + pseudoephedrine)** ▶LK ♀C ▶+ $$$$

ADULT - Allergic rhinitis/nasal congestion: 1 tab PO daily.

PEDS - Not approved in children.

FORMS - Trade only: Tabs, extended release 180/240 mg fexofenadine/pseudoephedrine.

NOTES - Decrease dose to 1 tab PO every other d in patient with decreased renal function. Take on an empty stomach. Avoid taking with fruit juice because of a large decrease in bioavailability.

**ALLERX (pseudoephedrine + methscopolamine + chlorpheniramine)** ▶LK ♀C ▶- $$$

ADULT - Allergic rhinitis/vasomotor rhinitis/nasal congestion: One yellow AM tab q am and one blue PM tab q pm.

*(cont.)*

**ALLERX** (cont.)
PEDS - Allergic rhinitis/vasomotor rhinitis/nasal congestion: >12 yo: Use adult dose.
FORMS - Trade only: Tabs, AM (yellow): 120 mg pseudophedrine/2.5 mg methscopolamine. PM (blue): 8 mg chlorpheniramine/2.5 mg methscopolamine.
NOTES - Contraindicated in severe hypertension, CAD, MAOI therapy, narrow angle glaucoma, urinary retention, & peptic ulcer. Caution in elderly, hepatic and renal disease.

**BROMFENEX** (pseudoephedrine + brompheniramine) ▶LK ♀C ▶- $
ADULT - Allergic rhinitis/nasal congestion: 1 cap PO q12h. Max 2 caps/d.
PEDS - Allergic rhinitis/nasal congestion: >12 yo: Use adult dose. 6-11 yo: 1 cap PO daily.
FORMS - Generic/Trade: Caps, sustained release 120 mg pseudoephedrine/12 mg brompheniramine.

**BROMFENEX PD** (pseudoephedrine + brompheniramine) ▶LK ♀C ▶- $
ADULT - Allergic rhinitis/nasal congestion: 1-2 caps PO q12h. Max 4 caps/d.
PEDS - Allergic rhinitis/nasal congestion: >12 yo: 1 cap PO q12h. Max 2 caps/d.
FORMS - Generic/Trade: Caps, sustained release 60 mg pseudoephedrine/6 mg brompheniramine.
NOTES - PD = pediatric.

**CARBODEC DM** (pseudoephedrine + carbinoxamine + dextromethorphan) ▶L ♀C ▶- $
ADULT - Allergic rhinitis/nasal congestion/cough: 5 mL PO qid.
PEDS - Allergic rhinitis/nasal congestion/cough >6 yo: 5 mL PO qid. 18 mo-5 yo: 2.5 mL PO q6h. Infant drops: Give PO qid: 1-3 mo: 0.25 mL. 4-6 mo: 0.5 mL. 7-9 mo: 0.75 mL. 10 mo-17 mo: 1 mL.
FORMS - Generic only: Syrup, 60/4/15 mg pseudoephedrine/carbinoxamine/dextromethorphan/5 mL. Drops, 25/2/4 mg/mL, grape flavor 30 mL w/ dropper, sugar-free.
NOTES - Carbinoxamine has potential for sedation similar to diphenhydramine. DM = dextromethorphan.

**CHERATUSSIN AC** (guaifenesin + codeine) ▶L ♀C ▶? ©V $
ADULT - Cough: 10 mL PO q4h. Max 60 mL/d.
PEDS - Cough ≥12 yo: Use adult dose. 6-11 yo: 5 mL PO q4h. Max 30 mL/d. 2-5 yo: 2.5-5 mL PO q4h. Max 30 mL/d. 6-23 mo: 1.25-2.5 mL PO q4h. Max 15 mL/d.
FORMS - Generic/Trade: Syrup 100 mg guaifenesin/10 mg codeine/5 mL. Sugar-free.

**CHERATUSSIN DAC** (pseudoephedrine + guaifenesin + codeine) ▶L ♀C ▶? ©V $
ADULT - Nasal congestion/cough: 10 mL PO q4h. Max 40 mL/d.
PEDS - Nasal congestion/cough ≥12 yo: Use adult dose. 6-11 yo: 5 mL PO q4h. Max 20 mL/d.
FORMS - Generic/Trade: Syrup 30 mg pseudoephedrine/100 mg guaifenesin/10 mg codeine/5 mL. Sugar-free.
NOTES - DAC = decongestant and codeine.

**CHLORDRINE SR** (pseudoephedrine + chlorpheniramine) ▶LK ♀C ▶- $
ADULT - Allergic rhinitis/nasal congestion: 1 cap PO q12h. Max 2 caps/d.
PEDS - Allergic rhinitis/nasal congestion >12 yo: Use adult dose. 6-11 yo: 1 cap PO daily.
FORMS - Generic only: Caps, sustained release 120 mg pseudoephedrine/8 mg chlorpheniramine.

**CLARINEX-D 12 H** (pseudoephedrine + desloratadine) ▶LK ♀C ▶+ $$$$
ADULT - Allergic rhinitis: 1 tab PO q12h.
PEDS - Allergic rhinitis >12 yo: Use adult dose.
FORMS - Trade only: Tabs, extended release 120 mg pseudoephedrine/2.5 mg desloratadine.
NOTES - Swallow tabs whole. Avoid with liver or renal insufficiency.

**CLARINEX-D 24 H** (pseudoephedrine + desloratadine) ▶LK ♀C ▶+ $$$$
ADULT - Allergic rhinitis: 1 tab PO daily.
PEDS - Allergic rhinitis ≥12 yo: Use adult dose.
FORMS - Trade only: Tabs, extended release pseudoephedrine + desloratadine, 120/2.5, 240/5 mg.
NOTES - Instruct patients to swallow the tab whole. Increase dosing interval in renal insufficiency to every other d. Avoid with liver insufficiency.

**DECONAMINE** (pseudoephedrine + chlorpheniramine) ▶LK ♀C ▶- $$
WARNING - Multiple strengths; write specific product on Rx.
ADULT - Allergic rhinitis/nasal congestion: 1 tab or 10 mL PO tid-qid. Max 6 tabs or 60 mL/d. Sustained release: 1 cap PO q12h. Max 2 caps/d.
PEDS - Allergic rhinitis/nasal congestion: >12 yo: Use adult dose. 6-11 yo: ½ tab or 5 mL PO tid-qid. Max 3 tabs or 30 mL/d.
FORMS - Trade only: Tabs 60/4 mg pseudoephedrine/chlorpheniramine, scored. Syrup 30/2 mg per 5 mL. Chew tab 15/1 mg. Generic/Trade: Caps, sustained release 120/8 mg (Deconamine SR).

**DECONSAL II** (phenylephrine + guaifenesin) ▶L ♀C ▶- $$
ADULT - Nasal congestion/cough: 1-2 tabs PO q12h. Max 4 tabs/d.
PEDS - Nasal congestion/cough: >12 yo: Use adult dose. 6-12 yo: 1 tab PO q12h, max 2 tabs/d. 2-5 yo: ½ tab PO q12h. Max 1 tab/d.
FORMS - Trade only: Caps, sustained release 20 mg phenylephrine/375 mg guaifenesin.

**DIMETANE-DX COUGH SYRUP** (pseudoephedrine + brompheniramine + dextromethorphan) ▶L ♀C ▶- $$$
ADULT - Nasal congestion/rhinitis/cough: 10 mL PO q4h prn.
PEDS - Nasal congestion/rhinitis/cough: >12 yo: Use adult dose. 6-11 yo: 5 mL PO q4h. 2-5 yo: 2.5 mL PO q4h. 22-40 kg: 2.5 mL PO qid prn. 12-22 kg: 1.25 mL PO qid prn.
FORMS - Trade only: Liquid 30 mg pseudoephedrine/2 mg brompheniramine/10 mg dextromethorphan/5 mL, butterscotch flavor. Sugar-free.

*DURATUSS* (phenylephrine + guaifenesin) ▶L ♀C ▶- $
ADULT - Nasal congestion/cough: 1 tab PO q12h.
PEDS - Nasal congestion/cough: >12 yo: Use adult dose. 6-12 yo: ½ tab PO q12h.
FORMS - Generic/Trade: Tabs, long-acting 25 mg phenylephrine/900 mg guaifenesin.

*DURATUSS GP* (phenylephrine + guaifenesin) ▶L ♀C ▶- $
ADULT - Nasal congestion/cough: 1 tab PO q12h.
PEDS - Not approved in children.
FORMS - Generic/Trade: Tabs, long-acting 25 mg phenylephrine /1200 mg guaifenesin.

*DURATUSS HD* (hydrocodone + phenylephrine + guaifenesin) ▶L ♀C ▶- ©III $$$
ADULT - Cough/nasal congestion: 10 mL PO q4-6h.
PEDS - Cough/nasal congestion: >12 yo: Use adult dose. 6-12 yo: 5 mL PO q4-6h.
FORMS - Generic/Trade: Elixir 2.5 mg hydrocodone/10 mg phenylephrine /225 mg guaifenensin/5 mL. 5% alcohol.

*ENTEX LA* (phenylephrine + guaifenesin) ▶L ♀C ▶- $$
ADULT - Nasal congestion/cough: 1 tab PO q12h.
PEDS - Nasal congestion/cough: ≥11 yo: Use adult dose. 6-11 yo: ½ tab PO q12h.
FORMS - Generic/Trade: Tabs, long-acting 30/600 mg phenylephrine/guaifenesin. Caps, long-acting 30/400 mg.
NOTES - Do not crush or chew.

*ENTEX LIQUID* (phenylephrine + guaifenesin) ▶L ♀C ▶- $$$
ADULT - Nasal congestion/cough: 5-10 mL PO q4-6h. Max 40 mL/d.
PEDS - Nasal congestion/cough: ≥12 yo: Use adult dose. 6-11 yo: 5 mL PO q4-6h. Max 20 mL/d. 2-5 yo: 2.5 mL PO q4-6h. Max 10 mL/d.
FORMS - Generic/Trade: Liquid 7.5 mg phenylephrine/100 mg guaifenesin/5 mL. Punch flavor, alcohol-free.

*ENTEX PSE* (pseudoephedrine + guaifenesin) ▶L ♀C ▶- $
ADULT - Nasal congestion/cough: 1 tab PO q12h.
PEDS - Nasal congestion/cough: >12 yo: Use adult dose. 6-12 yo: ½ tab PO q12h.
FORMS - Generic/Trade: Tabs, long-acting 120 mg pseudoephedrine/600 mg guaifenesin, scored.
NOTES - PSE = pseudoephedrine.

*GANI-TUSS NR* (guaifenesin + codeine) ▶L ♀C ▶? ©V $
ADULT - Cough: 10 mL PO q4h. Max 60 mL/d.
PEDS - Cough ≥12 yo: Use adult dose. 6-11 yo: 5 mL PO q4h. Max 30 mL/d. 2-5 yo: 2.5-5 mL PO q4h. Max 30 mL/d. 6-23 mo: 1.25-2.5 mL PO q4h. Max 15 mL/d.
FORMS - Generic/Trade: Syrup 100 mg guaifenesin/10 mg codeine/5 mL. Sugar-free.

*GUAIFENEX DM* (guaifenesin + dextromethorphan) ▶L ♀C ▶? $
ADULT - Cough: 1-2 tabs PO q12h. Max 4 tabs/d.
PEDS - Cough ≥12 yo: Use adult dose. 6-12 yo: 1 tab PO q12h. Max 2 tabs/d. 2-6 yo: ½ tab PO q12h. Max 1 tab/d.

FORMS - Generic/Trade: Tabs, sustained release 600 mg guaifenesin/30 mg dextromethorphan, scored.
NOTES - DM = dextromethorphan.

*GUAIFENEX PSE* (pseudoephedrine + guaifenesin) ▶L ♀C ▶- $
WARNING - Multiple strengths; write specific product on Rx.
ADULT - Nasal congestion/cough: PSE 60: 1-2 tabs PO q12h. Max 4 tabs/d. PSE 120: 1 tab PO q12h.
PEDS - Nasal congestion/cough: PSE 60: >12 yo: Use adult dose. 6-12 yo: 1 tab PO q12h. Max 2 tabs/d. 2-6 yo: ½ tab PO q12h. Max 1 tab/d. PSE 120: >12 yo: Use adult dose. 6-12 yo: ½ tab PO q12h.
FORMS - Generic/Trade: Tabs, extended release 60/600 mg pseudoephedrine/guaifenesin, scored (Guaifenex PSE 60). Trade only: Tabs, extended release 120/600 mg (Guaifenex PSE 120).
NOTES - PSE = pseudoephedrine.

*GUAITEX II SR/PSE* (pseudoephedrine + guaifenesin) ▶L ♀C ▶- $
WARNING - Multiple strengths; write specific product on Rx.
ADULT - Nasal congestion/cough: 1-2 tabs PO q12h. Max 4 tabs/d (Guaitex II SR). 1 tab PO q12h. Max 2 tabs/d (Guaitex PSE).
PEDS - Nasal congestion/cough: >12 yo: Use adult dose. 6-12 yo: 1 tab PO q12h. Max 2 tabs/d. 2-5 yo: ½ tab PO q12h. Max 1 tab/d (Guaitex II SR). >12 yo: Use adult dose. 6-12 yo: ½ tab PO q12h (Guaitex PSE).
FORMS - Generic/Trade: Tabs, sustained release 60 mg pseudoephedrine/600 mg guaifenesin (Guaitex II SR). Trade only: Tabs, long-acting 120 mg pseudoephedrine/600 mg guaifenesin (Guaitex PSE).
NOTES - PSE=pseudoephedrine.

*GUIATUSS AC* (guaifenesin + codeine) ▶L ♀C ▶? ©V $
ADULT - Cough: 10 mL PO q4h. Max 60 mL/d.
PEDS - Cough ≥12 yo: Use adult dose. 6-11 yo: 5 mL PO q4h. Max 30 mL/d.
FORMS - Generic/Trade: Syrup 100 mg guaifenesin/10 mg codeine/5 mL. Sugar-free.
NOTES - AC = and codeine

*GUIATUSSIN DAC* (pseudoephedrine + guaifenesin + codeine) ▶L ♀C ▶- ©V $
ADULT - Nasal congestion/cough: 10 mL PO q4h. Max 40 mL/d.
PEDS - Nasal congestion/cough ≥12 yo: Use adult dose. 6-11 yo: 5 mL PO q4h. Max 20 mL/d.
FORMS - Generic/Trade: Syrup 30 mg pseudoephedrine/100 mg guaifenesin/10 mg codeine/5 mL. Sugar-free.
NOTES - DAC = decongestant and codeine.

*HALOTUSSIN AC* (guaifenesin + codeine) ▶L ♀C ▶? ©V $
ADULT - Cough: 10 mL PO q4h. Max 60 mL/d.
PEDS - Cough ≥12 yo: Use adult dose. 6-11 yo: 5 mL PO q4h. Max 30 mL/d.

(cont.)

**HALOTUSSIN AC** (cont.)

FORMS - Generic/Trade: Syrup 100 mg guaifenesin/10 mg codeine/5 mL. Sugar-free.

NOTES - AC = and codeine

**_HALOTUSSIN DAC_** (pseudoephedrine + guaifenesin + codeine) ▶L ♀C ▶- ⊙V $

ADULT - Nasal congestion/cough: 10 mL PO q4h. Max 40 mL/d.

PEDS - Nasal congestion/cough: ≥12 yo: Use adult dose. 6-11 yo: 5 mL PO q4h. Max 20 mL/d.

FORMS - Generic/Trade: Syrup 30 mg pseudoephedrine/100 mg guaifenesin/10 mg codeine/5 mL. Sugar-free.

NOTES - DAC = decongestant and codeine.

**_HISTINEX HC_** (phenylephrine + chlorpheniramine + hydrocodone) ▶L ♀C ▶- ⊙III $

ADULT - Allergic rhinitis/congestion/cough: 10 mL PO q4h. Max 40 mL/d.

PEDS - Allergic rhinitis/congestion/cough: >12 yo: Use adult dose. 6-12 yo: 5 mL PO q4h. Max 20 mL/d.

FORMS - Generic/Trade: Syrup 5 mg phenylephrine/2 mg chlorpheniramine/2.5 mg hydrocodone/5 mL. Alcohol- and sugar-free.

**_HISTUSSIN D_** (pseudoephedrine + hydrocodone) ▶L ♀C ▶- ⊙III $$

ADULT - Nasal congestion/cough: 5 mL PO qid prn.

PEDS - Nasal congestion/cough: 22-40 kg: 2.5 mL PO qid prn. 12-22 kg: 1.25 mL PO qid prn.

FORMS - Generic/Trade: Liquid 60 mg pseudoephedrine/5 mg hydrocodone/5 mL, cherry/black raspberry flavor.

**_HISTUSSIN HC_** (phenylephrine + dexbrompheniramine + hydrocodone) ▶L ♀C ▶- ⊙III $$

ADULT - Allergic rhinitis/congestion/cough: 10 mL PO q4h. Max 40 mL/d.

PEDS - Allergic rhinitis/congestion/cough: >12 yo: Use adult dose. 6-12 yo: 5 mL PO q4h. Max 20 mL/d.

FORMS - Generic/Trade: Syrup 5 mg phenylephrine/1 mg dexbrompheniramine/2.5 mg hydrocodone/5 mL.

**_HUMIBID DM_** (guaifenesin + guaiacolsulfonate + dextromethorphan) ▶L ♀C ▶? $

ADULT - Cough: 1 cap PO q12h. Max 2 caps/d.

PEDS - Cough: ≥12 yo: Use adult dose. 6-12 yo: 1 cap PO daily.

FORMS - Trade only: Caps, sustained release 400 mg guaifenesin/200 mg guaiacolsulfonate/50 mg dextromethorphan.

NOTES - DM = dextromethorphan.

**_HUMIBID LA_** (guaifenesin + guaiacolsulfonate) ▶L ♀C ▶+ $

ADULT - Expectorant: 1 tab PO q12h (extended release). Max 2 tabs/d.

PEDS - Expectorant >12 yo: Use adult dose.

FORMS - Trade only: Tabs, extended release 600 mg guaifenesin/300 mg guaiacolsulfonate.

**_HYCOCLEAR TUSS_** (hydrocodone + guaifenesin) ▶L ♀C ▶- ⊙III $

ADULT - Cough: 5 mL PO pc & qhs. Max 6 doses/d.

PEDS - Cough: >12 yo: Use adult dose. 6-12 yo: 2.5 mL PO pc & qhs. Max 6 doses/d.

FORMS - Generic/Trade: Syrup 5 mg hydrocodone/100 mg guaifenesin/5 mL. Generic is alcohol and sugar free.

**_HYCODAN_** (hydrocodone + homatropine) ▶L ♀C ▶- ⊙III $

ADULT - Cough: 1 tab or 5 mL PO q4-6h. Max 6 doses/d.

PEDS - Cough >12 yo: Use adult dose. 6-12 yo: 2.5 mg (based on hydrocodone) PO q4-6h prn. Max 15 mg/d.

FORMS - Generic/Trade: Syrup 5 mg hydrocodone/1.5 mg homatropine methylbromide/5 mL. Tabs 5/1.5 mg.

NOTES - May cause drowsiness/sedation. Dosing based on hydrocodone content.

**_HYCOTUSS_** (hydrocodone + guaifenesin) ▶L ♀C ▶- ⊙III $

ADULT - Cough: 5 mL PO pc & qhs. Max 6 doses/d.

PEDS - Cough: >12 yo: Use adult dose. 6-12 yo: 2.5 mL PO pc & qhs. Max 6 doses/d.

FORMS - Generic/Trade: Syrup 5 mg hydrocodone/100 mg guaifenesin/5 mL. Generic is alcohol and sugar free.

**_NOVAFED A_** (pseudoephedrine + chlorpheniramine) ▶LK ♀C ▶- $

ADULT - Allergic rhinitis/nasal congestion: 1 cap PO q12h. Max 2 caps/d.

PEDS - Allergic rhinitis/nasal congestion: >12 yo: Use adult dose. 6-12 yo: 1 cap PO daily.

FORMS - Generic/Trade: Caps, sustained release 120 mg pseudoephedrine/8 mg chlorpheniramine.

**_PALGIC DS_** (pseudoephedrine + carbinoxamine) ▶L ♀C ▶- $$

ADULT - Allergic rhinitis/nasal congestion: 10 mL PO qid.

PEDS - Allergic rhinitis/nasal congestion: Give up to the following PO qid: 1-3 mo: 1.25 mL. 3-6 mo: 2.5 mL. 6-9 mo: 3.75 mL. 9-18 mo: 3.75-5 mL. 18 mo-6 yo: 5 mL. >6 yo use adult dose.

FORMS - Generic/Trade: Syrup, 25 mg pseudoephedrine/2 mg carbinoxamine/5 mL. Alcohol & sugar-free.

NOTES - Carbinoxamine has potential for sedation similar to diphenhydramine.

**_PHENERGAN VC_** (phenylephrine + promethazine) ▶LK ♀C ▶? $

WARNING - Promethazine contraindicated if <2 yo due to risk of fatal respiratory depression; caution in older children.

ADULT - Allergic rhinitis/congestion: 5 mL PO q4-6h. Max 30 mL/d.

PEDS - Allergic rhinitis/congestion: ≥12 yo: Use adult dose. 6-11 yo: 2.5-5 mL PO q4-6h. Max 20 mL/d. 2-5 yo: 1.25-2.5 mL PO q4-6h. Max 15 mL/d.

FORMS - Trade unavailable. Generic only: Syrup 6.25 mg promethazine/5 mg phenylephrine/5 mL.

NOTES - VC = vasoconstrictor.

**PHENERGAN VC W/CODEINE** (phenylephrine + promethazine + codeine) ▶LK ♀C ▶? ©V $
 WARNING - Promethazine contraindicated if <2 yo due to risk of fatal respiratory depression; caution in older children.
 ADULT - Allergic rhinitis/congestion/cough: 5 mL PO q4-6h. Max 30 mL/d.
 PEDS - Allergic rhinitis/congestion/cough: ≥12 yo: Use adult dose. 6-11 yo: 2.5-5 mL PO q4-6h. Max 20 mL/d. 2-5 yo: 1.25-2.5 mL PO q4-6h. Max 10 mL/d.
 FORMS - Trade unavailable. Generic only: Syrup 5 mg phenylephrine/6.25 mg promethazine/10 mg codeine/5 mL.

**PHENERGAN WITH CODEINE** (promethazine + codeine) ▶LK ♀C ▶? ©V $
 WARNING - Promethazine contraindicated if <2 yo due to risk of fatal respiratory depression; caution in older children.
 ADULT - Allergic rhinitis/cough: 5 mL PO q4-6h. Max 30 mL/d.
 PEDS - Allergic rhinitis/cough: ≥12 yo: Use adult dose. 6-11 yo: 2.5-5 mL PO q4-6h. Max 20 mL/d. 2-5 yo: 1.25-2.5 mL PO q4-6h. Max 10 mL/d.
 FORMS - Trade unavailable. Generic only: Syrup 6.25 mg promethazine/10 mg codeine/5 mL.

**PHENERGAN/DEXTROMETHORPHAN** (promethazine + dextromethorphan) ▶LK ♀C ▶? $
 WARNING - Promethazine contraindicated if <2 yo due to risk of fatal respiratory depression; caution in older children.
 ADULT - Allergic rhinitis/cough: 5 mL PO q4-6h. Max 30 mL/d.
 PEDS - Allergic rhinitis/cough: ≥12 yo: Use adult dose. 6-11 yo: 2.5-5 mL PO q4-6h. Max 20 mL/d. 2-5 yo: 1.25-2.5 mL PO q4-6h. Max 10 mL/d.
 FORMS - Trade unavailable. Generic only: Syrup 6.25 mg promethazine/15 mg dextromethorphan/5 mL.

**PSEUDO-CHLOR** (pseudoephedrine + chlorpheniramine) ▶LK ♀C ▶- $
 ADULT - Allergic rhinitis/nasal congestion: 1 cap PO q12h. Max 2 caps/d.
 PEDS - Allergic rhinitis/nasal congestion: >12 yo: Use adult dose.
 FORMS - Generic/Trade: Caps, sustained release 120 mg pseudoephedrine/8 mg chlorpheniramine.

**ROBITUSSIN AC** (guaifenesin + codeine) ▶L ♀C ▶? ©V $
 ADULT - The "Robitussin AC" brand is no longer produced; corresponding generics include Cheratussin AC, Gani-Tuss NR, Guiatuss AC, and Halotussin AC.
 PEDS - The "Robitussin AC" brand is no longer produced; corresponding generics include Cheratussin AC, Gani-Tuss NR, Guiatuss AC, and Halotussin AC.
 FORMS - The "Robitussin AC" brand is no longer produced; corresponding generics include Cheratussin AC, Gani-Tuss NR, Guiatuss AC, and Halotussin AC.

**ROBITUSSIN DAC** (pseudoephedrine + guaifenesin + codeine) ▶L ♀C ▶- ©V $
 ADULT - The "Robitussin DAC" brand is no longer produced; corresponding generics include Cheratussin DAC, Guiatuss DAC, and Halotussin DAC.
 PEDS - The "Robitussin DAC" brand is no longer produced; corresponding generics include Cheratussin DAC, Guiatuss DAC, and Halotussin DAC.
 FORMS - The "Robitussin DAC" brand is no longer produced; corresponding generics include Cheratussin DAC, Guiatuss DAC, and Halotussin DAC.

**RONDEC** (phenylephrine + chlorpheniramine) ▶L ♀C ▶- $$
 ADULT - Allergic rhinitis/nasal congestion: 5 mL syrup PO qid.
 PEDS - Allergic rhinitis/nasal congestion >12 yo: Use adult dose. 6-12 yo: 2.5 mL syrup PO qid. 2-5 yo: 1.25 mL PO qid.
 FORMS - Trade only: Syrup 12.5 mg phenylephrine /4 mg chlorpheniramine/5 mL, bubble-gum flavor. Alcohol- & sugar-free.

**RONDEC DM** (phenylephrine + chlorpheniramine + dextromethorphan) ▶L ♀C ▶- $$
 ADULT - Allergic rhinitis/nasal congestion/cough: 5 mL syrup PO qid.
 PEDS - Allergic rhinitis/nasal congestion/cough >12 yo: Use adult dose. 6-12 yo: 2.5 mL syrup PO qid. 2-5 yo: 1.25 mL syrup PO qid.
 FORMS - Trade only: Syrup 12.5mg phenylephrine /4 mg chlorpheniramine/15 mg dextromethorphan/5 mL, grape flavor. Alcohol- & sugar-free.
 NOTES - DM = dextromethorphan.

**RONDEC INFANT DROPS** (phenylephrine + chlorpheniramine) ▶L ♀C ▶- $$
 PEDS - Allergic rhinitis/nasal congestion: Give PO qid: 6-12 mo: 0.75 mL. 13-24 mo: 1 mL.
 FORMS - Trade only: Drops 3.5 mg phenylephrine/1 mg chlorpheniramine/mL, bubble-gum flavor, 30 mL. Alcohol- & sugar-free.

**RYNA-12 S** (phenylephrine + pyrilamine) ▶L ♀C ▶- $$
 PEDS - Nasal congestion, allergic rhinitis, sinusitis: >6 yo: 5-10 mL PO q12h. 2-6 yo 2.5-5 mL PO q12h.
 FORMS - Generic/Trade: Suspension 5 mg phenylephrine/30 mg pyrilamine/5 mL strawberry-currant flavor with graduated oral syringe.

**RYNATAN** (phenylephrine + chlorpheniramine) ▶LK ♀C ▶- $$
 ADULT - Allergic rhinitis/nasal congestion: 1-2 tabs PO q12h.
 PEDS - Allergic rhinitis/nasal congestion: ≥12 yo: 1 tab PO q12h.
 FORMS - Trade only: Tabs, extended release: 25/9 mg phenylephrine/chlorpheniramine. Chew tabs 5/4.5 mg.

**RYNATAN PEDIATRIC SUSPENSION** (phenylephrine + chlorpheniramine) ▶L ♀C ▶- $$$
 PEDS - Nasal congestion, allergic rhinitis, sinusitis >6 yo: 5-10 mL PO q12h. 2-6 yo 2.5-5 mL PO q12h.

(cont.)

**RYNATAN PEDIATRIC SUSPENSION (cont.)**
FORMS - Trade only: Suspension 5 mg phenyleph-
rine/4.5 mg chlorpheniramine/5 mL strawberry-
currant flavor.

***SEMPREX-D* (pseudoephedrine + acrivastine)** ▶LK
♀C ▶- $$
ADULT - Allergic rhinitis/nasal congestion: 1 cap PO
q4-6h. Max 4 caps/d.
PEDS - Not approved in children.
FORMS - Trade only: Caps 60 mg pseudoephedrine/8
mg acrivastine.

***DICEL* (pseudoephedrine + chlorpheniramine)** ▶L
♀C ▶- $$
ADULT - Allergic rhinitis/nasal congestion: 10-20
mL PO q12h. Max 40 mL/d.
PEDS - Allergic rhinitis/nasal congestion: ≥12
yo: Use adult dose. 6-11 yo: 5-10 mL PO q12h.
Max 20 mL/d. 2-5 yo: 2.5-5 mL PO q12h. Max 10
mL/d.
FORMS - Generic/Trade: Suspension 75 mg pseu-
doephedrine/5 mg chlorpheniramine/5 mL,
strawberry-banana flavor.

***TANAFED DMX* (pseudoephedrine + dexchlorphe-
niramine + dextromethorphan)** ▶L ♀C ▶- $$
ADULT - Allergic rhinitis/nasal congestion: 10-20
mL PO q12h. Max 40 mL/d.
PEDS - Allergic rhinitis/nasal congestion: ≥12 yo:
Use adult dose. 6-11 yo: 5-10 mL PO q12h. Max 20
mL/d. 2-5 yo: 2.5-5 mL PO q12h. Max 10 mL/d.
FORMS - Generic/Trade: Suspension 75 mg
pseudoephedrine/2.5 mg dexchlorpheniramine/25
mg dextromethorphan/5 mL, strawberry-banana
flavor.

***TUSS-HC* (phenylephrine + chlorpheniramine +
hydrocodone)** ▶L ♀C ▶- ©III $
ADULT - Allergic rhinitis/congestion/cough: 10 mL
PO q4h. Max 40 mL/d.
PEDS - Allergic rhinitis/congestion/cough: >12 yo:
Use adult dose. 6-12 yo: 5 mL PO q4h. Max 20
mL/d.

FORMS - Generic/Trade: Syrup 5 mg phenylephrine/
2 mg chlorpheniramine/2.5 mg hydrocodone/
5 mL.

***TUSSICAPS* (chlorpheniramine + hydrocodone)** ▶L
♀C ▶- ©III $$
ADULT - Allergic rhinitis/cough: 1 full strength cap
PO q12h. Max 2 caps/d.
PEDS - Allergic rhinitis/congestion/cough: >12 yo:
Use adult dose. 6-12 yo: 1 half strength cap PO
q12h. Max 2 caps/d.
FORMS - Trade only: Caps, extended release 4/5
mg (half strength) & 8/10 mg (full strength)
chlorpheniramine/hydrocodone.

***TUSSIONEX* (chlorpheniramine + hydrocodone)** ▶L
♀C ▶- ©III $$$
ADULT - Allergic rhinitis/cough: 5 mL PO q12h. Max
10 mL/d.
PEDS - Allergic rhinitis/cough: 6-12 yo: 2.5 mL PO
q12h. Max 5 mL/d.
FORMS - Generic/Trade: Extended release susp
8 mg chlorpheniramine/10 mg hydrocodone/
5 mL.

***ZEPHREX-LA* (pseudoephedrine + guaifenesin)** ▶L
♀C ▶- $
ADULT - Nasal congestion/cough: 1 tab PO q12h.
PEDS - Nasal congestion/cough: >12 yo: Use adult
dose. 6-12 yo: ½ tab PO q12h.
FORMS - Trade only: Tabs, extended release 120 mg
pseudoephedrine/600 mg guaifenesin.

***ZYRTEC-D* (cetirizine + pseudoephedrine)** ▶LK ♀C
▶- $$
ADULT - Allergic rhinitis/nasal congestion: 1 tab
PO q12h.
PEDS - Not approved in children.
FORMS - OTC Generic/Trade: Tabs, extended release
5 mg cetirizine/120 mg pseudoephedrine.
NOTES - Decrease dose to 1 tab PO daily with
decreased renal or hepatic function. Take on an
empty stomach.

## ENT: Decongestants

**NOTE:** See ENT: Nasal Preparations for nasal spray decongestants (oxymetazoline, phenylephrine). Systemic decongestants are sympathomimetic and may aggravate HTN, anxiety and insomnia. Use cautiously in such patients.
Some states have restricted or ended OTC sale of pseudoephedrine or reclassified it as schedule III or V drug due to
the potential for diversion to methamphetamine labs. Deaths have occurred in children <2 yo attributed to toxicity
from cough and cold medications; the FDA does not recommend their use in this age group.

**PHENYLEPHRINE (*Sudafed PE*)** ▶L ♀C ▶+ $
ADULT - Nasal congestion: 10 mg PO q4h prn. Max
6 doses/d.
PEDS - Nasal congestion, >12 yo: Use adult dose.
FORMS - OTC: Trade only: Tabs 10 mg.
NOTES - Avoid with MAO inhibitors.
**PSEUDOEPHEDRINE (*Sudafed, Sudafed 12 Hour,
Efidac/24, Dimetapp Decongestant Infant Drops,
PediaCare Infants' Decongestant Drops, Triaminic
Oral Infant Drops, ✦Pseudofrin*)** ▶L ♀C ▶+ $
ADULT - Nasal Congestion: 60 mg PO q4-6h. 120
mg PO q12h (extended release). 240 mg PO daily
(extended release). Max 240 mg/d.

PEDS - Nasal Congestion >12 yo: Use adult dose.
6-11 yo: 30 mg PO q4-6h. Max 120 mg/d. 2-5
yo: 15 mg PO q4-6h. Max 60 mg/d. Dimetapp,
PediaCare, & Triaminic Infant Drops: 2-3 yo: Give
1.6 mL PO q4-6h prn. Max 4 doses/d.
FORMS - OTC: Generic/Trade: Tabs 30, 60 mg, Tabs,
extended release 120 mg (12 h), Infant drops 7.5
mg/0.8 mL, Solution 15 & 30 mg/5 mL. Trade
only: Chew tabs 15 mg, Tabs, extended release
240 mg (24 h).
NOTES - 12 to 24-h extended release dosage forms
may cause insomnia; use a shorter-acting form
if this occurs.

## ENT: Ear Preparations

*AURALGAN* (benzocaine + antipyrine) ▶Not absorbed ♀C ▶? $
ADULT - Otitis media, adjunct: Instill 2-4 drops (or enough to fill the ear canal) tid-qid or q1-2h prn. Cerumen removal: Instill 2-4 drops (or enough to fill the ear canal) tid × 2-3 d to detach cerumen, then prn for discomfort. Insert cotton plug moistened with soln after instillation.
PEDS - Otitis media, adjunct: Use adult dose. Cerumen removal: Use adult dose.
FORMS - Generic/Trade: Otic soln 10 & 15 mL.

**CARBAMIDE PEROXIDE** (*Debrox, Murine Ear*) ▶Not absorbed ♀? ▶? $
ADULT - Cerumen impaction: Instill 5-10 drops into ear bid × 4 d.
PEDS - Not approved in children.
FORMS - OTC: Generic/Trade: Otic soln 6.5%, 15 & 30 mL.
NOTES - Drops should remain in ear >15 min. Do not use for >4 d. Remove excess wax by flushing with warm water using a rubber bulb ear syringe.

*CIPRO HC OTIC* (ciprofloxacin + hydrocortisone) ▶Not absorbed ♀C ▶- $$$$
ADULT - Otitis externa: Instill 3 drops into affected ear(s) bid × 7 d.
PEDS - Otitis externa ≥1 yo: Use adult dose.
FORMS - Trade only: Otic susp 10 mL.
NOTES - Shake well. Contains benzyl alcohol.

*CIPRODEX OTIC* (ciprofloxacin + dexamethasone) ▶Not absorbed ♀C ▶- $$$$
ADULT - Otitis externa: Instill 4 drops into affected ear(s) bid × 7 d.
PEDS - Otitis externa & otitis media w/ tympanostomy tubes, ≥6 mo: Instill 4 drops into affected ear(s) bid × 7 d.
FORMS - Trade only: Otic susp 5 & 7.5 mL.
NOTES - Shake well. Warm susp by holding bottle in hands for 1-2 min before instilling.

*CORTISPORIN OTIC* (hydrocortisone + polymyxin + neomycin) (*Pediotic*) ▶Not absorbed ♀? ▶? $
ADULT - Otitis externa: Instill 4 drops in affected ear(s) tid-qid up to 10 d.
PEDS - Otitis externa: Instill 3 drops in affected ear(s) tid-qid up to 10 d.
FORMS - Generic/Trade: Otic soln or susp 7.5 & 10 mL.
NOTES - Caveats with perforated TMs or tympanostomy tubes: (1) Risk of neomycin ototoxicity, especially if use prolonged or repeated; (2) Use susp rather than acidic soln.

*CORTISPORIN TC OTIC* (hydrocortisone + neomycin + thonzonium + colistin) ▶Not absorbed ♀? ▶? $$$
ADULT - Otitis externa: Instill 5 drops in affected ear(s) tid-qid up to 10 d.

PEDS - Otitis externa: Instill 4 drops in affected ear(s) tid-qid up to 10 d.
FORMS - Trade only: Otic susp, 10 mL.

*DOMEBORO OTIC* (acetic acid + aluminum acetate) ▶Not absorbed ♀? ▶? $
ADULT - Otitis externa: Instill 4-6 drops in affected ear(s) q2-3h.
PEDS - Otitis externa: Instill 2-3 drops in affected ear(s) q3-4h.
FORMS - Generic only: Otic soln 60 mL.
NOTES - Insert a saturated wick. Keep moist × 24 h.

**FLUOCINOLONE - OTIC** (*DermOtic*) ▶L ♀C ▶? $$
ADULT - Chronic eczematous external otitis: Instill 5 drops in affected ear(s) bid for 7-14 d.
PEDS - Chronic eczematous external otitis: ≥ 2 yo: Use adult dose.
FORMS - Trade only: Otic oil 0.01% 20 mL.
NOTES - Contains peanut oil.

**OFLOXACIN - OTIC** (*Floxin Otic*) ▶Not absorbed ♀C ▶- $$$
ADULT - Otitis externa: Instill 10 drops in affected ear(s) daily × 7 d. Chronic suppurative otitis media: 10 drops in affected ear(s) bid × 14 d.
PEDS - Otitis externa >12 yo: Use adult dose. 1-12 yo: Instill 5 drops in affected ear(s) daily × 7 d. Chronic suppurative otitis media >12 yo: Use adult dose. Acute otitis media with tympanostomy tubes 1-12 yo: Instill 5 drops in affected ear(s) bid × 10 d.
FORMS - Generic/Trade: Otic soln 0.3% 5, 10 mL. Trade only: "Singles": single-dispensing containers 0.25 mL (5 drops), 2 per foil pouch.

*SWIM-EAR* (isopropyl alcohol + anhydrous glycerins) ▶Not absorbed ♀? ▶? $
ADULT - Otitis externa, prophylaxis: Instill 4-5 drops in ears after swimming, showering, or bathing.
PEDS - Otitis externa, prophylaxis: Use adult dose.
FORMS - OTC: Trade only: Otic soln 30 mL.

*VOSOL HC* (acetic acid + propylene glycol + hydrocortisone) ▶Not absorbed ♀? ▶? $
ADULT - Otitis externa: Instill 5 drops in affected ear(s) tid-qid. Insert cotton plug moistened with 3-5 drops q4-6h for the first 24 h.
PEDS - Otitis externa >3 yo: Instill 3-4 drops in affected ear(s) tid-qid. Insert cotton plug moistened with 3-4 drops q4-6h for the first 24 h.
FORMS - Generic/Trade: Otic soln 2%-3%-1% 10 mL.
NOTES - VoSoL HC adds hydrocortisone 1%.

## ENT: Mouth & Lip Preparations

**AMLEXANOX** (*Aphthasol, OraDisc A*) ▶LK ♀B ▶? $
ADULT - Aphthous ulcers: Apply ¼ inch paste or mucoadhesive patch to ulcer in mouth qid after oral hygiene for up to 10 d.
PEDS - Aphthous ulcers >12 yo: use adult dose.

FORMS - Trade only: Oral paste 5%, 5 g tube. Mucoadhesive patch 2 mg, #20.
NOTES - Mucoadhesive patch should be applied ≥80 min before bedtime to ensure its erosion before sleep. Up to 3 patches may be applied

**(cont.)**

**AMLEXANOX** (*cont.*)
at one time. Avoid food or liquid for 1 h after application.

**CEVIMELINE** (*Evoxac*) ▶L ♀C ▶- $$$$
WARNING - May alter cardiac conduction/heart rate; caution in heart disease. May worsen broncho-spasm in asthma/COPD.
ADULT - Dry mouth due to Sjogren's syndrome: 30 mg PO tid.
PEDS - Not approved in children.
FORMS - Trade only: Caps 30 mg.
NOTES - Contraindicated in narrow-angle glaucoma, acute iritis & severe asthma. May potentiate beta-blockers.

**CHLORHEXIDINE GLUCONATE** (*Peridex, Periogard, ◆Denticare*) ▶Fecal excretion ♀B ▶? $
ADULT - Gingivitis: Bid as an oral rinse, morning & evening after brushing teeth. Rinse with 15 mL of undiluted soln for 30 sec. Do not swallow. Spit after rinsing.
PEDS - Not approved in children.
FORMS - Generic/Trade: Oral rinse 0.12% 473-480 mL bottles.

*DEBACTEROL* (sulfuric acid + sulfonated phenolics) ▶Not absorbed ♀C ▶+ $$
ADULT - Aphthous stomatitis, mucositis: Apply to dry ulcer. Rinse with water.
PEDS - Not approved in children <12 yo.
FORMS - Trade only: 1 mL prefilled, single-use applicator.
NOTES - One application per ulcer treatment. Dry ulcer area with cotton swab. Apply to ulcer and ring of normal mucosa around it for 5 to 10 sec. Rinse and spit. Return of ulcer pain right after rinsing indicates incomplete application; can be reapplied immediately one time. Avoid eye contact. If excess irritation, rinse with dilute bicarbonate soln.

*GELCLAIR* (maltodextrin + propylene glycol) ▶Not absorbed ♀+ ▶+ $$$
ADULT - Aphthous ulcers, mucositis, stomatitis: Rinse mouth with 1 packet tid or prn.
PEDS - Not approved in children.
FORMS - Trade only: 21 packets/box.
NOTES - Mix packet with 3 tablespoons of water. Swish for 1 min, then spit. Do not eat or drink for 1 h after treatment.

**LIDOCAINE - VISCOUS** (*Xylocaine*) ▶LK ♀B ▶+ $
WARNING - Avoid swallowing during oral or lingual use due to GI absorption & toxicity. Measure dose exactly. May apply to small areas in mouth with a cotton-tipped applicator.

ADULT - Mouth or lip pain: 15-20 mL topically or swish & spit q3h. Max 8 doses/d.
PEDS - Use with extreme caution, as therapeutic doses approach potentially toxic levels. Use the lowest effective dose. Mouth or lip pain >3 yo: 3.75-5 mL topically or swish and spit up to q3h.
FORMS - Generic/Trade: soln 2%, 20 mL unit dose, 100 mL bottle.
NOTES - High risk of adverse effects and overdose in children. Consider benzocaine as a safer alternative. Clearly communicate the amount, frequency, max daily dose, & mode of administration (eg, cotton pledget to individual lesions, 1/2 dropper to each cheek q4h, or 20 min before meals). Do not prescribe on a "PRN" basis without specified dosing intervals.

*MAGIC MOUTHWASH* (diphenhydramine + Mylanta + sucralfate) ▶LK ♀B(- in 1st trimester) ▶- $$$
ADULT - See components
PEDS - Not approved in children.
UNAPPROVED ADULT - Stomatitis: 5 mL PO swish & spit or swish & swallow tid before meals and prn.
UNAPPROVED PEDS - Stomatitis: Apply small amounts to lesions prn.
FORMS - Compounded susp. A standard mixture is 30 mL diphenhydramine liquid (12.5 mg/5 mL)/60 mL Mylanta or Maalox/4 g Carafate.
NOTES - Variations of this formulation are available. The dose and decision to swish and spit or swallow may vary with the indication and/or ingredient. Some preparations may contain: Kaopectate, nystatin, tetracycline, hydrocortisone, 2% lidocaine, cherry syrup (for children). Check local pharmacies for customized formulations. Avoid diphenhydramine formulations that contain alcohol - may cause stinging of mouth sores.

**PILOCARPINE** (*Salagen*) ▶L ♀C ▶- $$$$
ADULT - Dry mouth due to radiation of head & neck: 5 mg PO tid. May increase to 10 mg PO tid. Dry mouth due to Sjogren's syndrome: 5 mg PO qid. Hepatic dysfunction: 5 mg PO bid.
PEDS - Not approved in children.
UNAPPROVED ADULT - Dry mouth due to Sjogren's syndrome: 2% pilocarpine eye drops: Swish & swallow 4 drops diluted in water tid ($).
FORMS - Generic/Trade: Tabs 5, 7.5 mg.
NOTES - Contraindicated in narrow-angle glaucoma, acute iritis & severe asthma. May potentiate beta-blockers.

---

## ENT: Nasal Preparations—Corticosteroids

**NOTE:** Decrease to the lowest effective dose for maintenance therapy. Tell patients to prime pump before 1st use and shake well before each subsequent use.

**BECLOMETHASONE** (*Vancenase, Vancenase AQ Double Strength, Beconase AQ*) ▶L ♀C ▶? $$$$
ADULT - Allergic rhinitis/nasal polyp prophylaxis: Vancenase: 1 spray in each nostril bid-qid. Beconase AQ: 1-2 spray(s) in each nostril bid.

Vancenase AQ Double Strength: 1-2 spray(s) in each nostril daily.
PEDS - Allergic rhinitis/nasal polyp prophylaxis: Vancenase: >12 yo: adult dose. 6-12 yo: 1 spray in each nostril tid. Beconase AQ: >6 yo

**BECLOMETHASONE** (*cont.*)

1-2 spray(s) in each nostril bid. Vancenase AQ Double Strength: >6 yo: 1-2 spray(s) in each nostril daily.

FORMS - Trade only: Vancenase 42 mcg/spray, 80 or 200 sprays/bottle. Beconase AQ 42 mcg/spray, 200 sprays/bottle. Vancenase AQ Double Strength 84 mcg/spray, 120 sprays/bottle.

NOTES - AQ (aqueous) formulation may cause less stinging.

**BUDESONIDE - NASAL** (*Rhinocort Aqua*) ▶L ♀B ▶? $$$

ADULT - Allergic rhinitis: 1-4 sprays per nostril daily.

PEDS - Allergic rhinitis ≥6 yo: 1-2 sprays per nostril daily.

FORMS - Trade only: Nasal inhaler 120 sprays/bottle.

NOTES - CYP3A4 inhibitors such as ketoconazole, erythromycin, ritonavir, etc significantly increase systemic concentrations, possibly causing adrenal suppression.

**CICLESONIDE** (*Omnaris*) ▶L ♀C ▶? $

ADULT - Allergic rhinitis: 2 sprays per nostril daily.

PEDS - Allergic rhinitis, seasonal ≥6 yo, perennial ≥12 yo: Use adult dose.

FORMS - Trade only: Nasal spray, 50 mcg/spray, 120 sprays/bottle.

**FLUNISOLIDE** (*Nasalide, Nasarel, ✦Rhinalar*) ▶L ♀C ▶? $$

ADULT - Allergic rhinitis: 2 sprays per nostril bid, may increase to tid. Max 8 sprays/nostril/d.

PEDS - Allergic rhinitis 6-14 yo: 1 spray per nostril tid or 2 sprays per nostril bid. Max 4 sprays/nostril/d.

FORMS - Generic/Trade: Nasal soln 0.025%, 200 sprays/bottle. Nasalide with pump unit. Nasarel with meter pump & nasal adapter.

**FLUTICASONE - NASAL** (*Flonase, Veramyst*) ▶L ♀C ▶? $$$

ADULT - Allergic rhinitis: 2 sprays per nostril daily or 1 spray per nostril bid, decrease to 1 spray per nostril daily when appropriate. Seasonal allergic rhinitis alternative: 2 sprays per nostril daily prn.

PEDS - Allergic rhinitis: >4 yo: 1-2 sprays per nostril daily. Max 2 sprays/nostril/d. Seasonal allergic rhinitis alternative: >12 yo: 2 sprays per nostril daily prn.

FORMS - Generic/Trade: Flonase: Nasal spray 0.05%, 120 sprays/bottle. Trade only: (Veramyst): Nasal spray susp: 27.5 mcg/spray, 120 sprays/bottle.

NOTES - CYP3A4 inhibitors such as ketoconazole, erythromycin, ritonavir, etc significantly increase systemic concentrations, possibly causing adrenal suppression.

**MOMETASONE - NASAL** (*Nasonex*) ▶L ♀C ▶? $$$

ADULT - Allergic rhinitis: 2 sprays per nostril daily.

PEDS - Allergic rhinitis >12 yo: Use adult dose. 2-11 yo: 1 spray per nostril daily.

FORMS - Trade only: Nasal spray, 120 sprays/bottle.

**TRIAMCINOLONE - NASAL** (*Nasacort AQ, Nasacort HFA, Tri-Nasal*) ▶L ♀C ▶- $$$

ADULT - Allergic rhinitis: Nasacort HFA, Tri-Nasal: Start 2 sprays per nostril daily, may increase to 2 sprays/nostril bid. Max 4 sprays/nostril/d. Nasacort AQ: 2 sprays per nostril daily.

PEDS - Allergic rhinitis: ≥12 yo: Use adult dose. 6-12 yo: 1-2 sprays per nostril daily (Nasacort & Nasacort AQ).

FORMS - Trade only: Nasal inhaler 55 mcg/spray, 100 sprays/bottle (Nasacort HFA). Nasal spray, 55 mcg/spray, 120 sprays/bottle (Nasacort AQ). Nasal spray 50 mcg/spray, 120 sprays/bottle (Tri-Nasal).

NOTES - AQ (aqueous) formulation may cause less stinging. Decrease to lowest effective dose after allergy symptom improvement.

---

## ENT: Nasal Preparations—Other

**NOTE:** For ALL nasal sprays except saline, oxymetazoline, & phenylephrine, tell patients to prime pump before 1st use and shake well before each subsequent use.

**AZELASTINE - NASAL** (*Astelin*) ▶L ♀C ▶? $$$

ADULT - Allergic/vasomotor rhinitis: 1-2 sprays/nostril bid.

PEDS - Allergic rhinitis: >12 yo: Use adult dose. ≥5 yo: 1 spray/nostril bid. Vasomotor rhinitis ≥12 yo: Use adult dose.

FORMS - Trade only: Nasal spray, 200 sprays/bottle.

**CROMOLYN - NASAL** (*NasalCrom*) ▶LK ♀B ▶+ $

ADULT - Allergic rhinitis: 1 spray per nostril tid-qid up to 6 times/d.

PEDS - Allergic rhinitis ≥2 yo: Use adult dose.

FORMS - OTC: Generic/Trade: Nasal inhaler 200 sprays/bottle 13 & 26 mL.

NOTES - Therapeutic effects may not be seen for 1-2 wk.

**IPRATROPIUM - NASAL** (*Atrovent Nasal Spray*) ▶L ♀B ▶? $$

ADULT - Rhinorrhea due to allergic/non-allergic rhinitis: 2 sprays (0.03%) per nostril bid-tid or 2 sprays (0.06%) per nostril qid. Rhinorrhea due to common cold: 2 sprays (0.06%) per nostril tid-qid.

PEDS - Rhinorrhea due to allergic/non-allergic rhinitis ≥6 yo: Use adult dose (0.03%) or ≥5 yo: Use adult dose (0.06%). Rhinorrhea due to common cold ≥5 yo: 2 sprays (0.06%) per nostril tid.

UNAPPROVED ADULT - Vasomotor rhinitis: 2 sprays (0.06%) in each nostril tid-qid.

FORMS - Generic/Trade: Nasal spray 0.03%, 345 sprays/bottle & 0.06%, 165 sprays/bottle.

**LEVOCABASTINE - NASAL** (*✦Livostin Nasal Spray*) ▶L (but minimal absorption) ♀C ▶- $$

ADULT - Canada only. Allergic rhinitis: 2 sprays per nostril bid; increase prn to 2 sprays per nostril tid-qid.

PEDS - Not approved in children <12 yo.

FORMS - Trade only: nasal spray 0.5 mg/mL, plastic bottles of 15 mL. Each spray delivers 50 mcg.

**(cont.)**

**LEVOCABASTINE - NASAL** *(cont.)*
NOTES - Nasal spray is devoid of CNS effects. Safety/efficacy in patients >65 yo has not been established.

**OLOPATADINE - NASAL** *(Patanase)* ▶L ♀C ▶? $$$
ADULT - Allergic rhinitis: 2 sprays/nostril bid.
PEDS - Allergic rhinitis ≥12 yo: Use adult dose.
FORMS - Trade only: Nasal spray, 240 sprays/bottle.

**OXYMETAZOLINE** *(Afrin, Dristan 12 Hr Nasal, Nostrilla, Vicks Sinex 12 Hr)* ▶L ♀C ▶? $
ADULT - Nasal congestion: 2-3 sprays or drops (0.05%) per nostril bid prn rhinorrhea for ≤3 d.
PEDS - Nasal congestion ≥6 yo: 2-3 sprays or drops (0.05%) per nostril bid prn rhinorrhea for ≤3 d. 2-5 yo: 2-3 drops (0.025%) per nostril bid × 3 d.
FORMS - OTC: Generic/Trade: Nasal spray 0.05% 15 & 30 mL, Nose drops 0.025% & 0.05% 20 mL with dropper.
NOTES - Overuse (>3-5 d) may lead to rebound congestion. If this occurs, taper to use in one nostril only, alternating sides, then discontinue. Substituting an oral decongestant or nasal steroid may also be useful.

**PHENYLEPHRINE - NASAL** *(Neo-Synephrine, Vicks Sinex)* ▶L ♀C ▶? $
ADULT - Nasal congestion: 2-3 sprays or drops (0.25 or 0.5%) per nostril q4h prn × 3 d. Use 1% soln for severe congestion.

PEDS - Nasal congestion: >12 yo: Use adult dose. 6-12 yo: 2-3 drops or sprays (0.25%) per nostril q4h prn × 3 d. 1-5 yo: 2-3 drops (0.125% or 0.16%) per nostril q4h prn × 3 d. 6-11 mo: 1-2 drops (0.125% or 0.16%) per nostril q4h prn × 3 d.
FORMS - OTC: Generic/Trade: Nasal drops/spray 0.25, 0.5, 1% (15 mL).
NOTES - Overuse (>3-5 d) may lead to rebound congestion. If this occurs, taper to use in one nostril only, alternating sides, then discontinue. Substituting an oral decongestant or nasal steroid may also be useful.

**SALINE NASAL SPRAY** *(SeaMist, Entsol, Pretz, NaSal, Ocean, ✦HydraSense)* ▶Not metabolized ♀A ▶+ $
ADULT - Nasal dryness: 1-3 sprays per nostril prn.
PEDS - Nasal dryness: 1-3 drops per nostril prn.
FORMS - Generic/Trade: Nasal spray 0.4, 0.5, 0.65, 0.75%, Nasal drops 0.4 & 0.65%. Trade only: Preservative Free-Nasal spray 3% (Entsol).
NOTES - May be prepared at home by combining: 1/4 teaspoon salt with 8 ounces (1 cup) warm water. Add 1/4 teaspoon baking soda (optional) and put in spray bottle, ear syringe, or any container with a small spout. Discard after one wk.

## ENT: Other

***CETACAINE*** (benzocaine + tetracaine + butamben) ▶LK ♀C ▶? $$
WARNING - Do not use on the eyes. Hypersensitivity (rare). Methemoglobinemia (rare).
ADULT - Topical anesthesia of mucous membranes: Spray: Apply for 1 sec or less. Liquid or gel: Apply with cotton applicator directly to site.
PEDS - Use adult dose.

FORMS - Trade only: (14%-2%-2%) Spray 56 mL. Topical liquid 56 mL. Topical gel 5 & 29 g.
NOTES - Do not hold cotton applicator in position for extended time due to increased risk of local reactions. Do not use multiple applications. Max anesthesia occurs 1 min after application; duration 30 min. May result in potentially dangerous methemoglobinemia; use minimum amount needed.

## GASTROENTEROLOGY: Antidiarrheals

**BISMUTH SUBSALICYLATE** *(Pepto-Bismol, Kaopectate)* ▶K ♀D ▶? $
WARNING - Avoid in children and teenagers with chickenpox or flu due to possible association with Reye's syndrome.
ADULT - Diarrhea: 2 tabs or 30 mL (262 mg/15 mL) PO q 30 min-60 min up to 8 doses/d.
PEDS - Diarrhea: 100 mg/kg/d divided into 5 doses. Age 3–6 yo: 1/3 tab or 5 mL (262 mg/15 mL) every 30 min-60 min prn up to 8 doses/d. 6–9 yo: 2/3 tab or 10 mL (262 mg/15 mL) every 30 min-1 h prn up to 8 doses/d. 9–12 yo: 1 tab or 15 mL (262 mg/15 mL) every 30 min-1 h prn up to 8 doses/d.
UNAPPROVED ADULT - Prevention of traveler's diarrhea: 2.1g/d or 2 tab qid before meals and qhs. Has been used as part of a multi-drug regimen for Helicobacter pylori.
UNAPPROVED PEDS - Chronic infantile diarrhea: Age 2–24 mo: 2.5 mL (262 mg/15 mL) PO q4h.

24–48 mo: 5 mL (262 mg/15 mL) q4h. 48–70 mo: 10 mL (262 mg/15 mL) q4h.
FORMS - OTC Generic/Trade: chew tab 262 mg, susp 262, 525, 750 mg/15 mL. Generic only: susp 130 mg/15 mL. Trade only: caplets 262 mg (Pepto-Bismol), susp 87 mg/5 mL (Kaopectate Children's Liquid), caplets 750mg (Kaopectate).
NOTES - Use with caution in patients already taking salicylates or warfarin, children recovering from chickenpox or flu. Decreases absorption of tetracycline. May darken stools or tongue.

***IMODIUM ADVANCED*** (loperamide + simethicone) ▶L ♀B ▶+ $
ADULT - Diarrhea: 2 caplets PO initially, then 1 caplet PO after each unformed stool to a max of 4 caplets/24 h.
PEDS - Diarrhea: 1 caplet PO initially, then ½ caplet PO after each unformed stool to a max of 2 caplets/d (if 6–8 yo or 48–59 lbs) or 3 caplets/d (if 9–11 yo or 60–95 lbs).

**IMODIUM ADVANCED** *(cont.)*
FORMS - OTC Generic/trade: caplet & chew tab 2 mg loperamide/125 mg simethicone.
NOTES - Not for C. difficile associated diarrhea, toxigenic bacterial diarrhea, or most childhood diarrhea (difficult to exclude toxigenic).

***LOMOTIL* (diphenoxylate + atropine)** ▶L ♀C ▶- ©V $
ADULT - Diarrhea: 2 tabs or 10 mL PO qid.
PEDS - Diarrhea: 0.3–0.4 mg diphenoxylate/kg/24h in 4 divided doses. Age <2 yo: not recommended. 2 yo: 1.5–3 mL PO qid; 3 yo: 2–3 mL PO qid; 4 yo: 2–4 mL PO qid; 5 yo: 2.5–4.5 mL PO qid; 6–8 yo: 2.5–5 mL PO qid; 9–12 yo: 3.5–5 mL PO qid.
FORMS - Generic/Trade: soln 2.5/0.025 mg diphenoxylate/atropine per 5 mL, tab 2.5/0.025 mg.
NOTES - Give with food to decrease GI upset. May cause atropinism in children, esp. with Down syndrome, even at recommended doses. Can cause delayed toxicity. Has been reported to cause severe respiratory depression, coma, brain damage, death after overdose in children. Naltrexone reverses toxicity. Do not use for C. difficile associated diarrhea, toxigenic bacterial diarrhea, or most childhood diarrhea (difficult to exclude toxigenic).

**LOPERAMIDE** (*Imodium, Imodium AD, ↔Loperacap, Diarr-eze*) ▶L ♀B ▶+ $
WARNING - Discontinue if abdominal distention or ileus. Caution in children due to variable response. Diarrhea may need concurrent fluid/electrolyte repletion.
ADULT - Diarrhea: 4 mg PO initially, then 2 mg after each unformed stool to max 16 mg/d.
PEDS - Diarrhea (first d): Age 2–5 yo (13–20 kg): 1 mg PO tid. 6–8 yo (20–30 kg): 2 mg PO bid. 9–12 yo (>30 kg): 2 mg PO tid. After first d, give 1 mg/10 kg PO after each loose stool; daily dose not to exceed daily dose of first d.
UNAPPROVED ADULT - Chronic diarrhea or ileostomy drainage : 4 mg initially then 2 mg after each stool until symptoms are controlled, then reduce dose for maintenance treatment, average adult maintenance dose 4–8 mg daily as a single dose or in divided doses.
UNAPPROVED PEDS - Chronic diarrhea: limited information. Average doses of 0.08–0.24 mg/kg/d PO in 2–3 divided doses.
FORMS - Rx Generic/Trade: cap 2 mg, tab 2 mg. OTC Generic/Trade: tab 2 mg, liquid 1 mg/5 mL.
NOTES - Not for C. difficile associated diarrhea, toxigenic bacterial diarrhea, or most childhood diarrhea (difficult to exclude toxigenic).

***MOTOFEN* (difenoxin + atropine)** ▶L ♀C ▶- ©IV $
ADULT - Diarrhea: 2 tabs PO initially, then 1 after each loose stool q3–4 h prn. Max of 8 tabs/24h.
PEDS - Not approved in children. Contraindicated in children <2 yo.
FORMS - Trade only: tab difenoxin 1 mg + atropine 0.025 mg.
NOTES - Do not use for C. difficile associated diarrhea, toxigenic bacterial diarrhea, or most childhood diarrhea (difficult to exclude toxigenic). May cause atropinism in children, esp. with Down's syndrome, even at recommended doses. Can cause delayed toxicity. Has been reported to cause severe respiratory depression, coma, brain damage, death after overdose in children. Difenoxin is the primary metabolite of diphenoxylate.

**OPIUM** (*opium tincture, paregoric*) ▶L ♀B (D with long-term use) ▶? ©II (opium tincture), III (paregoric) $$
ADULT - Diarrhea: 5–10 mL paregoric PO daily-qid or 0.3–0.6 mL PO opium tincture qid.
PEDS - Diarrhea: 0.25–0.5 mL/kg paregoric PO daily-qid or 0.005–0.01 mL/kg PO opium tincture q3–4h, max 6 doses/d.
FORMS - Trade only: opium tincture 10% (deodorized opium tincture, 10 mg morphine equivalent per mL). Generic only: paregoric (camphorated opium tincture, 2 mg morphine equivalent/5 mL).
NOTES - Opium tincture contains 25 times more morphine than paregoric. Do not use for C. difficile associated diarrhea, toxigenic bacterial diarrhea, or most childhood diarrhea.

---

## GASTROENTEROLOGY: Anti-Emetics—5-HT3 Receptor Antagonists

**DOLASETRON** (*Anzemet*) ▶LK ♀B ▶? $$$
ADULT - Prevention of N/V with chemo: 1.8 mg/kg up to 100 mg IV/PO single dose 30 min (IV) or 60 min (PO) before chemo. Prevention/treatment of post-op N/V: 12.5 mg IV as a single dose 15 min before end of anesthesia or as soon as N/V starts. Alternative for prevention 100 mg PO 2 h before surgery.
PEDS - Prevention of N/V with chemo in children 2–16 yo: 1.8 mg/kg up to 100 mg IV/PO single dose 30 min (IV) or 60 min (PO) before chemo. Prevention/treatment of post-op N/V in children 2–16 yo: 0.35 mg/kg IV as single dose 15 min before end of anesthesia or as soon as N/V starts. Max 12.5 mg. Prevention alternative 1.2 mg/kg PO to max of 100 mg 2 h before surgery.
UNAPPROVED ADULT - N/V due to radiotherapy: 40 mg IV as a single dose. Alternatively, 0.3 mg/kg IV as a single dose.
FORMS - Trade only: Tab 50,100 mg.
NOTES - Use caution in patients of any age who have or may develop prolongation of QT interval (ie, hypokalemia, hypomagnesemia, concomitant antiarrhythmic therapy, cumulative high-dose anthracycline therapy).

**GRANISETRON** (*Kytril*) ▶L ♀B ▶? $$$
ADULT - Prevention of N/V with chemo: 10 mcg/kg over 5 min IV 30 min prior to chemo. Oral: 1 mg PO bid × 1 d only. Radiation-induced N/V: 2 mg PO 1 h before first irradiation fraction of each d. Prevention/treatment post-op N/V: 1 mg IV.

(cont.)

**GRANISETRON** (cont.)

PEDS - Children 2–16 yo: Prevention of N/V with chemo: 10 mcg/kg IV 30 min prior to chemo. Oral form not approved in children.
FORMS - Generic/Trade: Tab 1 mg. Oral soln 2 mg/ 10 mL (30 mL).

**ONDANSETRON** (*Zofran*) ▶L ♀B ▶? $$$$$

ADULT - Prevention of N/V with chemo: 32 mg IV as a single dose over 15 min, or 0.15 mg/kg IV 30 min prior to chemo and repeated at 4 and 8 h after first dose. Alternatively, 8 mg PO 30 min before moderately emetogenic chemo and 8 h later. Can be given q12h for 1–2 d after completion of chemo. For single-d highly emetogenic chemo, 24 mg PO 30 min before chemo. Prevention of post-op nausea: 4 mg IV over 2–5 min or 4 mg IM or 16 mg PO 1 h before anesthesia. Prevention of N/V associated with radiotherapy: 8 mg PO tid.
PEDS - Prevention of N/V with chemo: IV: Age >6 mo: 0.15 mg/kg 30 min prior to chemo and repeated at 4 and 8 h after first dose. PO: Children 4–11 yo: 4 mg 30 min prior to chemo and repeated at 4 and 8 h after first dose. Can be given q8h for 1–2 d after completion of chemo. Children ≥12

yo: 8 mg PO 30 min before chemo and 8 h later. Prevention of post-op N/V: 1 mo-12 yo: 0.1 mg/kg IV over 2–5 min × 1 if ≤40kg; 4 mg IV over 2–5 min × 1 if >40 kg.
UNAPPROVED ADULT - Has been used in hyperemesis associated with pregnancy.
UNAPPROVED PEDS - Use with caution if <4 yo based on BSA: <0.3 m²: 1 mg PO tid. 0.3–0.6 m²: 2 mg PO tid. 0.6–1 m²: 3 mg PO tid. >1 m²: 4 mg PO tid. Use caution in infants <6 mo of age.
FORMS - Generic/Trade: Tab 4, 8, 24 mg, orally disintegrating tab 4, 8 mg, solution 4 mg/5 mL. Generic only: Tab 16 mg, orally disintegrating tab 16, 24 mg.
NOTES - Max oral dose if severe liver disease is 8 mg/d. Use following abdominal surgery or in those receiving chemotherapy may mask a progressive ileus or gastric distension.

**PALONOSETRON** (*Aloxi*) ▶L ♀B ▶? $$$$$

ADULT - Prevention of N/V with chemo: 0.25 mg IV over 30 sec, 30 min prior to chemo. Prevention of postoperative N/V: 0.075 mg IV over 10 sec just prior to anesthesia.
PEDS - Not approved in children.

---

## GASTROENTEROLOGY: Anti-Emetics—Other

**APREPITANT** (*Emend, Fosaprepitant*) ▶L ♀B ▶? $$$$$

ADULT - Prevention of N/V with moderately to highly emetogenic chemo, in combination with dexamethasone and ondansetron: 125 mg PO on d 1 (1 h prior to chemo), then 80 mg PO qam on d 2 & 3. Alternative for first dose only is 115 mg IV (fosaprepitant form) over 15 min given 30 min prior to chemo. Prevention of postoperative N/V: 40 mg PO within 3 h prior to anesthesia.
PEDS - Not approved in children.
FORMS - Trade only (aprepitant): cap 40, 80, 125 mg. IV prodrug form is fosaprepitant.
NOTES - Use caution with other medications metabolized by CYP3A4 hepatic enzyme system and an inducer of the CYP2C9 hepatic enzyme system. Contraindicated with pimozide. May decrease efficacy of oral contraceptives; women should use alternate/back-up method. Monitor INR in patients receiving warfarin. Fosaprepitant is a prodrug of aprepitant.

*DICLECTIN* (doxylamine + pyridoxine) ▶LK ♀A ▶? $

ADULT - Canada only. Nausea/vomiting in pregnancy. 2 tabs PO qhs. May add 1 tab in am and 1 tab in afternoon, if needed.
PEDS - Not approved in children.
FORMS - Trade only: delayed-release tab doxylamine 10 mg + pyridoxine 10 mg.

**DIMENHYDRINATE** (*Dramamine, ✦Gravol*) ▶LK ♀B ▶- $

ADULT - Nausea: 50–100 mg/dose PO/IM/IV q4–6h prn. Max PO dose 400 mg/24h, max IM dose 300 mg/24h.
PEDS - Nausea: Age <2 yo: not recommended. 2–6 yo: 12.5–25 mg PO q6–8h or 5 mg/5kg/24h divided q6h. Max daily PO dose: 75 mg/24h. Children

6–12 yo: 25–50 mg PO q6–8h. Max daily PO dose 150 mg/24h.
FORMS - OTC: Generic/Trade: Tab 50 mg. Trade only: chew tab 50 mg. Generic only: solution 12.5 mg/5ml.
NOTES - May cause drowsiness. Use with caution in conditions which may be aggravated by anticholinergic effects (ie, prostatic hypertrophy, asthma, narrow-angle glaucoma).

**DOMPERIDONE** (✦*Motilium*) ▶L ♀? ▶- $

ADULT - Canada only. Postprandial dyspepsia: 10–20 mg PO tid-qid, 30 min before a meal.
PEDS - Not approved in children.
UNAPPROVED ADULT - Has been used for diabetic gastroparesis, chemotherapy/radiation induced N/V. Has also been used to increase milk production in lactating mothers although this is not currently recommended due to safety concerns.
UNAPPROVED PEDS - Use in children generally not recommended except for chemotherapy or radiation-induced N/V: 200–400 mcg/kg PO q4–8h.
FORMS - Canada only. Trade/generic: tabs 10, 20 mg.
NOTES - Similar in efficacy to metoclopramide but less likely to cause extrapyramidal symptoms.

**DOXYLAMINE** (*Unisom Nighttime Sleep Aid, others*) ▶L ♀A ▶- $

PEDS - Not approved in children.
UNAPPROVED ADULT - N/V associated with pregnancy: 12.5 mg PO bid; often used in combination with pyridoxine.
FORMS - OTC Generic/Trade: tab 25 mg.

**DRONABINOL** (*Marinol*) ▶L ♀C ▶- ©III $$$$$

ADULT - Nausea with chemo: 5 mg/m² PO 1–3 h before chemo then 5 mg/m²/dose q2–4h after

**DRONABINOL** *(cont.)*

chemo for 4–6 doses/d. Dose can be increased to max 15 mg/m². Anorexia associated with AIDS: Initially 2.5 mg PO bid before lunch and dinner. Max 20 mg/d.

PEDS - Not approved in children.

UNAPPROVED PEDS - Nausea with chemo: 5 mg/m² PO 1–3 h before chemo then 5 mg/m²/dose q2–4h after chemo for 4–6 doses/d. Dose can be increased to max 15 mg/m².

FORMS - Trade only: cap 2.5, 5, 10 mg.

NOTES - Patient response varies; individualize dosing (start with low doses in elderly). Additive CNS effects with alcohol, sedatives, hypnotics, psychomimetics. Caution if history of seizures.

**DROPERIDOL** *(Inapsine)* ▶L ♀C ▶? $

WARNING - Cases of fatal QT prolongation and/or torsades de pointes have occurred in patients receiving droperidol at or below recommended doses (some without risk factors for QT prolongation). Reserve for non-response to other treatments, and perform 12-lead ECG prior to administration and continue ECG monitoring 2–3 h after treatment. Use with extreme caution (if at all) if prolonged baseline QT.

ADULT - Antiemetic premedication: 0.625–2.5 mg IV or 2.5 mg IM then 1.25 mg prn.

PEDS - Preop: Age 2–12 yo: 0.088–0.165 mg/kg IV. Post-op antiemetic: 0.01–0.03 mg/kg/dose IV q 6–8h prn. Usual dose 0.05–0.06 mg/kg/dose; max of 0.1 mg/kg.

UNAPPROVED ADULT - Chemo-induced nausea: 2.5–5 mg IV/IM q 3–4h prn.

UNAPPROVED PEDS - Chemo-induced nausea: 0.05–0.06 mg/kg/dose IV/IM q 4–6h prn.

NOTES - Has no analgesic or amnestic effects. Consider lower doses in geriatric, debilitated, or high-risk patients such as those receiving other CNS depressants. May cause hypotension or tachycardia, extrapyramidal reactions, drowsiness.

**METOCLOPRAMIDE** *(Reglan, ✦Maxeran)* ▶K ♀B ▶? $

ADULT - Gastroesophageal reflux: 10–15 mg PO qid 30 min before meals and qhs. Diabetic gastroparesis: 10 mg PO/IV/IM 30 min before meals and bedtime. Prevention of chemo-induced emesis: 1–2 mg/kg 30 min before chemo and then q2h for 2 doses then q3h for 3 doses prn. Prevention of post-op nausea: 10–20 mg IM/IV near end of surgical procedure, may repeat q3–4 h prn. Intubation of small intestine: 10 mg IV. Radiographic exam of upper GI tract: 10 mg IV.

PEDS - Intubation of small intestine: Age <6 yo: 0.1 mg/kg IV. 6–14 yo: 2.5–5 mg IV. Radiographic exam of upper GI tract: Age <6 yo: 0.1 mg/kg IV; 6–14 yo: 2.5–5 mg IV.

UNAPPROVED ADULT - Prevention/treatment of chemo-induced emesis: 3 mg/kg over 1h followed by continuous IV infusion of 0.5 mg/kg/h for 12h. Migraine treatment: 10 mg IV. Migraine adjunct: 10 mg PO 5–10 min before ergotamine/analgesic/sedative.

UNAPPROVED PEDS - Gastroesophageal reflux: 0.4–0.8 mg/kg/d in 4 divided doses. Prevention

of chemo-induced emesis: 1–2 mg/kg 30 min before chemo and then q3h prn, max of 5 doses/d or 5–10 mg/kg/d.

FORMS - Generic/Trade: tabs 5,10 mg, Generic only: soln 5 mg/5 mL.

NOTES - To reduce incidence and severity of akathisia, consider giving IV doses over 15 min. If extrapyramidal reactions occur (especially with high IV doses) give diphenhydramine IM/IV. Adjust dose in renal dysfunction. May cause drowsiness, agitation, seizures, hallucinations, galactorrhea, hyperprolactinemia, constipation, diarrhea. Increases cyclosporine and ethanol absorption. Do not use if bowel perforation or mechanical obstruction present. Levodopa decreases metoclopramide effects. Tardive dyskinesia in <1% with long-term use.

**NABILONE** *(Cesamet)* ▶L ♀C ▶- ©II $$$$

ADULT - Nausea/vomiting in cancer chemotherapy patients with poor response to other agents: 1 to 2 mg PO bid, 1 to 3 h before chemotherapy. Max dose 6 mg/d in 3 divided doses.

PEDS - Not approved in children.

FORMS - Trade only: cap 1 mg.

NOTES - Contraindicated in known sensitivity to marijuana or other cannabinoids, current or past psychiatric reactions. Additive CNS effects with alcohol, sedatives, hypnotics, psychomimetics. Additive cardiac effects with amphetamines, antihistamines, anticholinergic medications.

**PHOSPHORATED CARBOHYDRATES** *(Emetrol)* ▶L ♀A ▶+ $

ADULT - Nausea: 15–30 mL PO q15 min until nausea subsides or up to 5 doses.

PEDS - Nausea: 2–12 yo: 5–10 mL q15 min until nausea subsides or up to 5 doses.

UNAPPROVED ADULT - Morning sickness: 15–30 mL PO upon rising, repeat q3h prn. Motion sickness or nausea due to drug therapy or anesthesia: 15 mL/dose.

UNAPPROVED PEDS - Regurgitation in infants: 5–10 mL PO 10–15 min prior to each feeding. Motion sickness or nausea due to drug therapy or anesthesia: 5 mL/dose.

FORMS - OTC Generic/Trade: Solution containing dextrose, fructose, and phosphoric acid.

NOTES - Do not dilute. Do not ingest fluids before or for 15 min after dose. Monitor blood glucose in diabetic patients.

**PROCHLORPERAZINE** *(Compazine, ✦Stemetil)* ▶LK ♀C ▶? $

ADULT - N/V: 5–10 mg PO/IM tid-qid max 40 mg/d; 15–30 mg PO daily or 10 mg PO q12h of sustained release or 15 mg PO qam of sustained release; 25 mg PR q12h; 5–10 mg IV over at least 2 min q3–4h prn max 40 mg/d; 5–10 mg IM q3–4h prn max 40 mg/d.

PEDS - N/V: Age <2 yo or <10 kg: not recommended. >2 yo: 0.4 mg/kg/d PO/PR in 3–4 divided doses; 0.1–0.15 mg/kg/dose IM; IV not recommended.

(cont.)

**PROCHLORPERAZINE** (cont.)

UNAPPROVED ADULT - Migraine: 10 mg IV/IM or 25 mg PR single dose for acute headache.

UNAPPROVED PEDS - N/V during surgery: 5–10 mg IM 1–2 h before anesthesia induction, may repeat in 30 min; 5–10 mg IV 15–30 min before anesthesia induction, may repeat once.

FORMS - Generic/Trade: tabs 5,10,25 mg, supp 25 mg. Trade only: extended-release caps (Compazine Spansules) 10,15,30 mg, supp 2.5,5 mg, liquid 5 mg/5 mL.

NOTES - May cause extrapyramidal reactions (especially in elderly), hypotension (with IV), arrhythmias, sedation, seizures, hyperprolactinemia, gynecomastia, dry mouth, constipation, urinary retention, leukopenia, thrombocytopenia. Elderly more prone to adverse effects.

**PROMETHAZINE** (*Phenergan*) ▶LK ♀C ▶- $

WARNING - Contraindicated if <2 yo due to risk of fatal respiratory depression; caution in older children.

ADULT - Nausea/vomiting: 12.5–25 mg q4–6h PO/IM/PR prn. Motion sickness: 25 mg PO/PR 30–60 min prior to departure and q12h prn. Hypersensitivity reactions: 25 mg IM/IV, may repeat in 2 h. Allergic conditions: 12.5 mg PO/PR/IM/IV qid or 25 mg PO/PR qhs.

PEDS - Nausea/vomiting, ≥2 yo: 0.25–1 mg/kg/dose PO/IM/PR q4–6h prn. Motion sickness: 0.5 mg/kg PO 30–60 min prior to departure and q12h prn. Max 25 mg/dose. Hypersensitivity reactions, >2 yo: 6.25–12.5 mg PO/PR/IM/IV q6h prn.

UNAPPROVED ADULT - Nausea/vomiting: 12.5–25 mg IV q4h prn.

UNAPPROVED PEDS - Nausea/vomiting, ≥2 yo: 0.25–0.5 mg/kg/dose IV q4h prn.

FORMS - Generic/Trade: tab/supp 12.5, 25, 50 mg. Generic only: syrup 6.25 mg/5ml.

NOTES - May cause sedation, extrapyramidal reactions (esp. with high IV doses), hypotension with rapid IV administration, anticholinergic side effects, eg, dry mouth, blurred vision.

**SCOPOLAMINE** (*Transderm-Scop, Scopace, ✦Transderm-V*) ▶L ♀C ▶+ $$

ADULT - Motion sickness: 1 disc behind ear at least 4h before travel and q3 d prn or 0.4–0.8 mg PO 1 h before travel and q8h prn. Prevention of post-op N/V: Apply patch behind ear 4 h before surgery, remove 24 h after surgery. Spastic states, postencephalitic parkinsonism: 0.4–0.8 mg PO q8h prn.

PEDS - Not approved in children <12 yo.

UNAPPROVED PEDS - Pre-op and antiemetic: 6 mcg/kg/dose IM/IV/SC (max dose 0.3 mg/dose). May repeat q6–8h. Has been used in severe drooling.

FORMS - Trade only: topical disc 1.5 mg/72h, box of 4. Oral tab 0.4 mg.

NOTES - Dry mouth common. Also causes drowsiness, blurred vision.

**THIETHYLPERAZINE** (*Torecan*) ▶L ♀? ▶? $

ADULT - N/V: 10 mg PO/IM 1–3 times/d.

PEDS - Not approved in children.

FORMS - Trade only: tab 10 mg.

**TRIMETHOBENZAMIDE** (*Tigan*) ▶LK ♀C but + ▶? $

ADULT - N/V: 250 mg PO q6–8h, 200 mg PR/IM q6–8h.

PEDS - N/V: Children <13.6kg (except neonates): 100 mg PR q6–8h. Children 13.6–40.9 kg: 100–200 mg PO/PR q6–8h.

FORMS - Generic/Trade: Caps 300 mg. Generic only: Caps 250 mg.

NOTES - Not for IV use. May cause sedation. Reduce starting dose in the elderly or if reduced renal function to minimize risk of adverse effects.

## GASTROENTEROLOGY: Anti-Ulcer—Antacids

***ALKA-SELTZER*** (aspirin + citrate + bicarbonate) ▶LK ♀? (- 3rd trimester) ▶? $

ADULT - Relief of upset stomach: 2 regular strength tabs in 4 oz water q4h PO prn, max 8 tabs (<60 yo) or 4 tabs (>60 yo) in 24h or 2 extra-strength tabs in 4 oz water q6h PO prn, max 7 tabs (<60 yo) or 4 tabs (>60 yo) in 24h.

PEDS - Not approved in children.

FORMS - OTC Trade only: regular strength, original: ASA 325 mg + citric acid 1000 mg + sodium bicarbonate 1916 mg. Regular strength lemon lime and cherry: 325 mg + 1000 mg + 1700 mg. Extra-strength: 500 mg + 1000 mg + 1985 mg. Not all forms of Alka Seltzer contain aspirin (eg, Alka Seltzer Heartburn Relief).

NOTES - Avoid ASA-containing forms in children and teenagers due to risk of Reye's syndrome.

**ALUMINUM HYDROXIDE** (*Alternagel, Amphojel, Alu-Tab, Alu-Cap, ✦Basalgel, Mucaine*) ▶K ♀+ (? 1st trimester) ▶? $

ADULT - Hyperphosphatemia in chronic renal failure (short term treatment only to avoid aluminum accumulation): 30–60 mL PO with meals. Upset stomach, indigestion: 5–10 mL or 1–2 tabs PO 6 times/d, between meals and qhs and prn.

PEDS - Not approved in children.

UNAPPROVED ADULT - Hyperphosphatemia in chronic renal failure (short term treatment only to avoid aluminum accumulation): 30–60 mL PO with meals. Symptomatic reflux: 15–30 mL PO q30–60 min. For long-term management of reflux disease: 15–30 mL PO 1 and 3 h after meals and qhs prn. Peptic ulcer disease: 15–45 mL or 1–3 tab PO 1 and 3h after meals and qhs. Prophylaxis against GI bleeding (titrate dose to maintain gastric pH >3.5): 30–60 mL or 2–4 tab PO q1–2h.

UNAPPROVED PEDS - Peptic ulcer disease: 5–15 mL PO 1 and 3h after meals and qhs. Prophylaxis against GI bleeding (titrate dose to maintain gastric pH >3.5): Neonates 0.5–1 mL/kg/dose PO q4h. Infants 2–5 mL PO q1–2h. Child: 5–15 mL PO q1–2h.

FORMS - OTC Generic/Trade: cap 475 mg, susp 320 & 600 mg/5 mL. Trade only: cap 400 mg (Alu-Cap)

NOTES - For concentrated suspensions, use ½ the recommended dose. May cause constipation.

**ALUMINUM HYDROXIDE** (*cont.*)

Avoid administration with tetracyclines, digoxin, iron, isoniazid, buffered/enteric aspirin, diazepam, fluoroquinolones.

***CITROCARBONATE*** (**bicarbonate + citrate**) ▶K ♀? ▶? $

ADULT - 1–2 teaspoonfuls in cold water PO 15 min to 2 h after meals prn.

PEDS - 6–12 yo: ¼-1/2 teaspoonful in cold water PO after meals prn.

FORMS - OTC Trade only: sodium bicarbonate 0.78 g + sodium citrate anhydrous 1.82 g in each 1 teaspoonful dissolved in water, 150, 300g.

NOTES - Chronic use may cause metabolic alkalosis. Contains sodium.

***GAVISCON*** (**aluminum hydroxide + magnesium carbonate**) ▶K ♀? ▶? $

ADULT - 2–4 tabs or 15–30 mL (regular strength) or 10 mL (extra strength) PO qid prn.

PEDS - Not approved in children.

UNAPPROVED PEDS - Peptic ulcer disease: 5–15 mL PO after meals and qhs.

FORMS - OTC Trade only: Tab: regular strength (Al hydroxide 80 mg + Mg trisilicate 20 mg), extra strength (Al hydroxide 160 mg + Mg carbonate 105 mg). Liquid: regular strength (Al hydroxide 95 mg + Mg carbonate 358 mg per 15 mL), extra strength (Al hydroxide 508 mg + Mg carbonate 475 mg per 30 mL )

NOTES - Contains alginic acid or sodium alginate which is considered an "inactive" ingredient. Alginic acid forms foam barrier which floats in stomach to minimize esophageal contact with acid. Chronic use may cause metabolic alkalosis. Contains sodium.

***MAALOX*** (**aluminum hydroxide + magnesium hydroxide**) ▶K ♀ + (? 1st trimester) ▶? $

ADULT - Heartburn/indigestion: 10–20 mL or 1–4 tab PO qid, after meals and qhs and prn.

PEDS - Not approved in children.

UNAPPROVED ADULT - Peptic ulcer disease: 15–45 mL PO 1 & 3h after meals & qhs. Symptomatic reflux: 15–30 mL PO q30–60 min. For long-term management of reflux disease: 15–30 mL PO 1 and 3 h after meals & qhs prn. Prophylaxis against GI bleeding (titrate dose to maintain gastric pH >3.5): 30–60 mL PO q1–2h.

UNAPPROVED PEDS - Peptic ulcer disease: 5–15 mL PO 1 and 3h after meals and qhs. Prophylaxis against GI bleeding (titrate dose to maintain gastric pH >3.5): Neonates 1 mL/kg/dose PO q4h. Infants 2–5 mL PO q1–2h. Child: 5–15 mL PO q1–2h.

FORMS - OTC Generic/Trade: regular strength chew tab (Al hydroxide + Mg hydroxide 200/200 mg), susp (225/200 mg per 5 mL).

NOTES - Maalox Extra Strength and Maalox TC are more concentrated than Maalox. Maalox Plus has added simethicone. May cause constipation or diarrhea. Avoid concomitant administration with tetracyclines, digoxin, iron, isoniazid, buffered/enteric aspirin, diazepam, fluoroquinolones. Avoid chronic use in patients with renal dysfunction due to potential for magnesium accumulation.

***MAGALDRATE*** (*Riopan*) ▶K ♀ + (? 1st trimester) ▶? $

ADULT - Relief of upset stomach: 5–10 mL between meals and qhs and prn.

PEDS - Not approved in children.

UNAPPROVED PEDS - Peptic ulcer disease: 5–10 mL PO 1 and 3h after meals and qhs.

FORMS - OTC Trade only: susp 540 mg/5 mL. Riopan Plus (with simethicone) available as susp 540/20 mg/5 mL, chew tab 540/20 mg.

NOTES - Riopan Plus has added simethicone. Avoid concomitant administration with tetracyclines, fluoroquinolones, digoxin, iron, isoniazid, buffered/enteric aspirin, diazepam. Avoid chronic use in patients with renal failure.

***MYLANTA*** (**aluminum hydroxide + magnesium hydroxide + simethicone**) ▶K ♀ + (? 1st trimester) ▶? $

ADULT - Heartburn/indigestion: 10–45 mL or 2–4 tab PO qid, after meals and qhs and prn.

PEDS - Safe dosing has not been established.

UNAPPROVED ADULT - Peptic ulcer disease: 15–45 mL PO 1 and 3h after meals and qhs. Symptomatic reflux: 15–30 mL PO q30–60 min. For long-term management of reflux: 15–30 mL PO 1 and 3 h postprandially and qhs prn.

UNAPPROVED PEDS - Peptic ulcer disease: 5–15 mL PO 1 and 3h after meals and qhs.

FORMS - OTC Generic/Trade: Liquid, double strength liquid, tab, double strength tab. Trade only: tab sodium + sugar + dye free.

NOTES - Mylanta Gelcaps contain calcium carbonate and magnesium hydroxide. May cause constipation or diarrhea. Avoid concomitant administration with tetracyclines, fluoroquinolones, digoxin, iron, isoniazid, buffered/enteric aspirin, diazepam. Avoid chronic use in renal dysfunction.

***ROLAIDS*** (**calcium carbonate + magnesium hydroxide**) ▶K ♀? ▶? $

ADULT - 2–4 tabs PO q1h prn, max 12 tabs/d (regular strength) or 10 tabs/d (extra-strength).

PEDS - Not approved in children.

FORMS - OTC Trade only: Tab: regular strength (Ca carbonate 550 mg, Mg hydroxide 110 mg), extra-strength (Ca carbonate 675 mg, Mg hydroxide 135 mg).

NOTES - Chronic use may cause metabolic alkalosis.

## GASTROENTEROLOGY: Anti-Ulcer—H2 Antagonists

**CIMETIDINE** (*Tagamet, Tagamet HB*) ▶LK ♀B ▶+ $$$

ADULT - Treatment of duodenal or gastric ulcer: 800 mg qhs or 300 mg PO qid with meals and qhs or 400 mg PO bid. Prevention of duodenal ulcer: 400 mg PO qhs. Erosive esophagitis: 800 mg PO

bid or 400 mg PO qid. Prevention or treatment of heartburn (OTC product only approved for this indication): 200 mg PO prn max 400 mg/d for up to 14 d. Hypersecretory conditions: 300 mg PO qid with meals and qhs. Patients unable to take oral

(cont.)

**CIMETIDINE** (*cont.*)
medications: 300 mg IV/IM q6–8h or 37.5 mg/h continuous IV infusion. Prevention of upper GI bleeding in critically ill patients: 50 mg/h continuous infusion.

PEDS - Not approved in children.

UNAPPROVED ADULT - Prevention of aspiration pneumonitis during surgery: 400–600 mg PO or 300 mg IV 60–90 min prior to anesthesia. Has been used as adjunctive therapy with H1 antagonist for severe allergic reactions.

UNAPPROVED PEDS - Treatment of duodenal or gastric ulcers, erosive esophagitis, hypersecretory conditions: Neonates: 5–10 mg/kg/d PO/IV/IM divided q 8–12h. Infants: 10–20 mg/kg/d PO/IV/ IM divided q6h. Children: 20–40 mg/kg/d PO/IV/ IM divided q6h. Chronic viral warts in children: 25–40 mg/kg/d PO in divided doses.

FORMS - Rx Generic/Trade: tab 200, 300, 400, 800 mg. Rx Generic liquid 300 mg/5 mL. OTC Generic/ Trade: tab 200 mg.

NOTES - May cause dizziness, drowsiness, headache, diarrhea, nausea. Decreased absorption of ketoconazole, itraconazole. Increased levels of carbamazepine, cyclosporine, diazepam, labetalol, lidocaine, theophylline, phenytoin, procainamide, quinidine, propranolol, tricyclic antidepressants, valproic acid, warfarin. Stagger doses of cimetidine and antacids. Decrease dose with CrCl <30 mL/min.

**FAMOTIDINE** (*Pepcid, Pepcid AC, Maximum Strength Pepcid AC*) ▶LK ♀B ▶? $$
ADULT - Treatment of duodenal ulcer: 40 mg PO qhs or 20 mg PO bid. Maintenance of duodenal ulcer: 20 mg PO qhs. Treatment of gastric ulcer: 40 mg PO qhs. GERD: 20 mg PO bid. Treatment or prevention of heartburn: (OTC product only approved for this indication) 10–20 mg PO prn. Hypersecretory conditions: 20 mg PO q6h. Patients unable to take oral medications: 20 mg IV q12h.

PEDS - Not approved in children.

UNAPPROVED ADULT - Prevention of aspiration pneumonitis during surgery: 40 mg PO/IM prior to anesthesia. Upper GI bleeding: 20 mg IV q12h. Has been used as adjunctive therapy with H1 antagonist for severe allergic reactions.

UNAPPROVED PEDS - Treatment of duodenal or gastric ulcers, GERD, hypersecretory conditions: 0.6–0.8 mg/kg/d IV in 2–3 divided doses or 1–1.2 mg/kg/d PO in 2–3 divided doses, max 40 mg/d. GERD: <3 mo: 0.5 mg/kg PO daily; 3–12 mo: 0.5 mg/kg PO bid; 1–16 yo:1 mg/kg/d PO divided bid.

FORMS - Generic/Trade: tab 10 mg (OTC, Pepcid AC Acid Controller), 20 (Rx and OTC, Max Strength Pepcid AC), 30, 40 mg. Rx Trade only: susp.40 mg/5 mL.

NOTES - May cause dizziness, headache, constipation, diarrhea. Decreased absorption of ketoconazole, itraconazole. Adjust dose in patients with CrCl <60 mL/min.

**NIZATIDINE** (*Axid, Axid AR*) ▶K ♀B ▶? $$$$
ADULT - Treatment of duodenal or gastric ulcer: 300 mg PO qhs or 150 mg PO bid. Maintenance of

duodenal ulcer: 150 mg PO qhs. GERD: 150 mg PO bid. Treatment or prevention of heartburn: (OTC product only approved for this indication) 75 mg PO prn, max 150 mg/d.

PEDS - Age ≥12 yo: Esophagitis, GERD: 150 mg PO bid.

UNAPPROVED ADULT - Has been used as adjunctive therapy with H1 antagonist for severe allergic reactions.

UNAPPROVED PEDS - 6 mo-11 yo (limited data): 6–10 mg/kg/d PO in 2 divided doses.

FORMS - OTC Trade only (Axid AR): tabs 75 mg Rx Trade only: oral solution 15 mg/mL (120, 480 mL). Rx Generic/Trade: cap 150, 300 mg.

NOTES - May cause dizziness, headache, constipation, diarrhea. Decrease absorption of ketoconazole, itraconazole. Adjust dose if CrCl <80 mL/min.

**PEPCID COMPLETE** (*famotidine + calcium carbonate + magnesium hydroxide*) ▶LK ♀B ▶? $
ADULT - Treatment of heartburn: 1 tab PO prn. Max 2 tabs/d.

PEDS - Not approved in children.

FORMS - OTC: Trade only: chew tab famotidine 10 mg with calcium carbonate 800 mg & magnesium hydroxide 165 mg.

**RANITIDINE** (*Zantac, Zantac 25, Zantac 75, Zantac 150, Peptic Relief*) ▶K ♀B ▶? $$$
ADULT - Treatment of duodenal ulcer: 150 mg PO bid or 300 mg qhs. Treatment of gastric ulcer or GERD: 150 mg PO bid. Maintenance of duodenal or gastric ulcer: 150 mg PO qhs. Treatment of erosive esophagitis: 150 mg PO qid. Treatment of erosive esophagitis: 150 mg PO bid. Prevention/treatment of heartburn: (OTC product only approved for this indication) 75–150 mg PO prn, max 300 mg/d. Hypersecretory conditions: 150 mg PO bid. Patients unable to take oral meds: 50 mg IV/IM q6–8h or 6.25 mg/h continuous IV infusion.

PEDS - Children 1 mo - 16 yr: Treatment of duodenal or gastric ulcers: 2–4 mg/kg/24h PO divided bid (max 300 mg) or 2–4 mg/kg/d IV divided q6–8h. GERD, erosive esophagitis: 5–10 mg/kg/24h PO divided bid or 2–4 mg/kg/d IV divided q6–8h. Maintenance of duodenal or gastric ulcers: 2–4 mg/kg/24h PO daily (max 150 mg).

UNAPPROVED ADULT - Prevention of upper GI bleeding in critically ill patients: 6.25 mg/h continuous IV infusion (150 mg/d). Has been used as adjunctive therapy with H1 antagonist for severe allergic reactions.

UNAPPROVED PEDS - Treatment of duodenal or gastric ulcers, GERD, hypersecretory conditions: Neonates: 2–4 mg/kg/24h PO divided q12h or 2 mg/kg/24h IV divided q12h. Infants and children: 2–4 mg/kg/24h IV/IM divided q12h or 0.1–0.2 mg/kg/h continuous IV infusion. Premature and term infants <2 wk of age: 2 mg/kg/d PO divided q12h. 1.5 mg/kg IV x1 then 12 h later 1.5–2 mg/ kg/d IV divided q12h. Continuous infusion 1.5 mg/kg x1 then 0.04–0.08 mg/kg/h infusion.

**RANITIDINE** (*cont.*)
FORMS - Generic/Trade: tabs 75 mg (OTC, Zantac 75, Zantac 150), 150,300 mg, syrup 75 mg/5 mL. Rx Trade only: effervescent tab 25,150 mg. Rx Generic only: caps 150,300 mg.
NOTES - May cause dizziness, sedation, headache, drowsiness, rash, nausea, constipation, diarrhea.

Variable effects on warfarin, decreased absorption of ketoconazole, itraconazole. Dissolve granules and effervescent tabs in water. Stagger doses of ranitidine and antacids. Adjust dose in patients with CrCl <50 mL/min.

### HELICOBACTER PYLORI THERAPY

Triple therapy PO × 7-14 d: clarithromycin 500 mg bid + amoxicillin 1 g bid (or metronidazole 500 mg bid) + a proton pump inhibitor

Quadruple therapy PO × 14 d: bismuth subsalicylate 525 mg (or 30 mL) tid-qid + metronidazole 500 mg tid-qid + tetracycline 500 mg tid-qid + a proton pump inhibitor or a H2 blocker

PPI's: esomeprazole 40 mg qd, lansoprazole 30 mg bid, omeprazole 20 mg bid, pantoprazole 40 mg bid, rabeprazole 20 mg bid.

H2 blockers: cimetidine 400 mg bid, famotidine 20 mg bid, nizatidine 150 mg bid, ranitidine 150 mg bid.
Adapted from *The Medical Letter Treatment Guidelines* 2004:10.

## GASTROENTEROLOGY: Anti-Ulcer—*Helicobacter pylori* Treatment

***HELIDAC*** (**bismuth subsalicylate + metronidazole + tetracycline**) ▶LK ♀D ▶- $$$$
ADULT - Active duodenal ulcer associated with Helicobacter pylori: 1 dose (2 bismuth subsalicylate chewable tabs, 1 metronidazole tab and 1 tetracycline cap) PO qid, at meals and qhs for 2 wk with an H2 antagonist.
PEDS - Not approved in children.
UNAPPROVED ADULT - Active duodenal ulcer associated with Helicobacter pylori: Same dose as in "adult", but substitute proton pump inhibitor for H2 antagonist.
FORMS - Trade only: Each dose: bismuth subsalicylate 524 (2x262 mg) chewable tab + metronidazole 250 mg tab + tetracycline 500 mg cap.
NOTES - See components.

***PREVPAC*** (**lansoprazole + amoxicillin + clarithromycin, ◆HP-Pac**) ▶LK ♀C ▶? $$$$$
ADULT - Active duodenal ulcer associated with Helicobacter pylori: 1 dose PO bid × 10–14 d.
PEDS - Not approved in children.
FORMS - Trade only: lansoprazole 30 mg × 2 + amoxicillin 1 g (2x500 mg) × 2, clarithromycin 500 mg × 2.
NOTES - See components.
***PYLERA*** (**biskalcitrate + metronidazole + tetracycline**) ▶LK ♀D ▶- $$$$$
ADULT - Duodenal ulcer associated with H. pylori: 3 caps PO qid (after meals and at bedtime) × 10 d. To be given with omeprazole 20 mg PO bid.
PEDS - Not approved in children.
FORMS - Trade only: Each cap: biskalcitrate 140 mg + metronidazole 125 mg + tetracycline 125 mg.
NOTES - See components.

## GASTROENTEROLOGY: Anti-Ulcer—Proton Pump Inhibitors

**ESOMEPRAZOLE** (*Nexium*) ▶L ♀B ▶? $$$$
ADULT - Erosive esophagitis: 20–40 mg PO daily × 4–8 wk. Maintenance of erosive esophagitis: 20 mg PO daily. Zollinger-Ellison: 40 mg PO bid × 4–8 wk, may repeat for additional 4–8 wk. GERD: 20 mg PO daily × 4 wk. GERD with esophagitis: 20–40 mg IV daily × 10 d until taking PO. Prevention of NSAID-associated gastric ulcer: 20–40 mg PO daily × up to 6 mo. H pylori eradication: 40 mg PO daily with amoxicillin 1000 mg PO bid & clarithromycin 500 mg PO bid × 10 d.
PEDS - 1–11 yo: GERD: 10–20 mg daily for up to 8 wk. 12–17 yo: GERD: 20–40 mg daily for up to 8 wk.
FORMS - Trade only: Delayed release cap 20, 40 mg. Delayed release granules for oral susp 10, 20, 40 mg per packet.
NOTES - May decrease absorption of ketoconazole, itraconazole, digoxin, iron, and ampicillin. Concomitant administration with voriconazole, an

inhibitor of CYP2C19 and CYP3A4 may lead to a more than doubling of esomeprazole exposure.
**LANSOPRAZOLE** (*Prevacid, Prevacid NapraPac*) ▶L ♀B ▶? $$$$
ADULT - Erosive esophagitis: 30 mg PO daily or 30 mg IV daily × 7 d or until taking PO. Maintenance therapy following healing of erosive esophagitis: 15 mg PO daily. NSAID-induced gastric ulcer: 30 mg PO daily × 8 wk (treatment), 15 mg PO daily for up to 12 wk (prevention). GERD: 15 mg PO daily. Duodenal ulcer treatment and maintenance: 15 mg PO daily. Gastric ulcer: 30 mg PO daily. Part of a multidrug regimen for H. pylori eradication: 30 mg PO bid with amoxicillin 1000 mg PO bid & clarithromycin 500 mg PO bid × 10–14 d (see table) or 30 mg PO tid with amoxicillin 1000 mg PO tid × 14 d. Hypersecretory conditions: 60 mg PO daily.
PEDS - Erosive esophagitis and GERD (1–11 yo) ≤30 kg: 15 mg PO daily × up to 12 wk. >30 kg:

**(cont.)**

**LANSOPRAZOLE** (*cont.*)

30 mg PO daily × up to 12 wk. Non-erosive GERD (12–17 yo): 15 mg PO daily × up to 8 wk. GERD with erosive esophagitis (12–17 yo): 30 mg PO daily × up to 8 wk.

FORMS - Trade only: Cap 15, 30 mg. Susp 15, 30 mg packets. Orally disintegrating tab 15, 30 mg. Prevacid NapraPac: 7 lansoprazole 15 mg caps packaged with 14 naproxen tabs 375 mg or 500 mg.

NOTES - Take before meals. Avoid concomitant administration with sucralfate. May decrease absorption of atazanavir, ketoconazole, itraconazole, ampicillin, digoxin and iron. Orally disintegrating tabs can be dissolved water (15 mg tab in 4 mL, 30 mg tab in 10 mL) and administered via an oral syringe or nasogastric tube ≥8 French.

**OMEPRAZOLE** (*Prilosec*, *◆Losec*) ▶L ♀C ▶? OTC $, Rx $$$$

ADULT - GERD, duodenal ulcer, erosive esophagitis: 20 mg PO daily. Heartburn (OTC): 20 mg PO daily × 14 d. Gastric ulcer: 40 mg PO daily. Hypersecretory conditions: 60 mg PO daily. Part of a multidrug regimen for H pylori eradication: 20 mg PO bid with amoxicillin 1000 mg PO bid & clarithromycin 500 mg PO bid × 10 d, with additional 18 d of omeprazole 20 mg PO daily if ulcer present (see table). Or 40 mg PO daily with clarithromycin 500 mg PO tid × 14 d, with additional 14 d of omeprazole 20 mg PO daily if ulcer present.

PEDS - GERD (1–16 yo) 5 to <10 kg: 5 mg PO daily, 10 to <20 kg: 10 mg PO daily. ≥20 kg: 20 mg PO daily.

UNAPPROVED ADULT - Upper GI bleeding: 80 mg IV, then infusion 8 mg/h until endoscopy.

UNAPPROVED PEDS - Gastric or duodenal ulcers, hypersecretory states: 0.7–3.3 mg/kg/dose PO daily. GERD: 1 mg/kg/d PO daily or bid.

FORMS - Rx Generic/Trade: Cap 10, 20 mg. Trade only: Cap 40 mg, granules for susp 2.5 mg, 10 mg. OTC: Cap 20 mg.

NOTES - Take before meals. Caps contain enteric-coated granules; do not chew. Caps may be opened and administered in acidic liquid (eg, apple juice). May increase levels of diazepam, warfarin, and phenytoin. May decrease absorption of ketoconazole, itraconazole, iron, ampicillin, and digoxin. Reduces plasma levels of atazanavir. Concomitant administration with voriconazole, an inhibitor of CYP2C19 and CYP3A4 may lead to a more than doubling of omeprazole exposure. Avoid administration with sucralfate.

**PANTOPRAZOLE** (*Protonix*, *◆Pantoloc*) ▶L ♀B ▶? $$$$

ADULT - 40 mg PO daily for 8–16 wk. Maintenance therapy following healing of erosive esophagitis:

40 mg PO daily. Zollinger-Ellison syndrome: 80 mg IV q8–12h × 6 d until taking PO. GERD associated with a history of erosive esophagitis: 40 mg IV daily × 7–10 d until taking PO.

PEDS - Not approved in children.

UNAPPROVED ADULT - Has been studied as part of various multidrug regimens for H. pylori eradication. Decreases peptic ulcer rebleeding after hemostasis: 80 mg IV bolus, then 8 mg/h continuous IV infusion × 3 d, followed by oral therapy (or 40 mg IV q12h for 4–7 d if unable to tolerate PO).

UNAPPROVED PEDS - GERD associated with a history of erosive esophagitis: 0.5–1 mg/kg/d (max 40 mg/d).

FORMS - Generic/Trade: Tabs 20, 40 mg. Trade only: Granules for susp 40 mg/packet.

NOTES - May decrease absorption of ketoconazole, itraconazole, digoxin, iron, and ampicillin. Reduces atazanavir concentrations (avoid together). Can increase INR when used with warfarin.

**RABEPRAZOLE** (*AcipHex*, *◆Pariet*) ▶L ♀B ▶? $$$$

ADULT - GERD: 20 mg PO daily × 4–16 wk. Duodenal ulcers: 20 mg PO daily × 4 wk. Zollinger-Ellison syndrome: 60 mg PO daily, may increase up to 100 mg daily or 60 mg bid. Part of a multidrug regimen for H. pylori eradication: 20 mg PO bid, with amoxicillin 1000 mg PO bid & clarithromycin 500 mg PO bid × 7 d.

PEDS - Children ≥12 yo: : 20 mg PO daily for up to 8 wk.

FORMS - Generic/Trade: Tab 20 mg.

NOTES - May decrease absorption of ketoconazole, itraconazole, digoxin, iron, and ampicillin.

**ZEGERID** (omeprazole + bicarbonate) ▶L ♀C ▶? $$$$

ADULT - Duodenal ulcer, GERD, erosive esophagitis: 20 mg PO daily × 4–8 wk. Gastric ulcer: 40 mg PO once daily × 4–8 wk. Reduction of risk of upper GI bleed in critically ill (susp only): 40 mg PO, then 40 mg 6–8 h later, then 40 mg once daily thereafter × 14 d.

PEDS - Not approved in children.

FORMS - Trade only: Caps 20/1100 & 40/1100 mg omeprazole/sodium bicarbonate, powder packets for susp 20/1680 & 40/1680 mg.

NOTES - Do not combine two 20 mg doses for a 40 mg dose, since the dose of sodium bicarbonate is the same in both dose strengths. May increase levels of diazepam, warfarin, and phenytoin. May decrease absorption of ketoconazole, itraconazole, iron, ampicillin, and digoxin. Reduces plasma levels of atazanavir. Avoid administration with sucralfate.

---

## GASTROENTEROLOGY: Anti-Ulcer—Other

**BELLERGAL-S** (phenobarbital + belladonna + ergotamine, *◆Bellergal Spacetabs*) ▶LK ♀X ▶- $

WARNING - Serious or life-threatening peripheral ischemia has been noted with ergotamine component when used with cytochrome P450 3A4

inhibitors such as ritonavir, nelfinavir, indinavir, erythromycin, clarithromycin, ketoconazole, and itraconazole.

ADULT - Hypermotility/hypersecretion: 1 tab PO bid.

PEDS - Not approved in children.

**BELLERGAL-S (cont.)**
FORMS - Generic/Trade: Tab phenobarbital 40 mg, ergotamine 0.6 mg, belladonna 0.2 mg.
NOTES - May decrease INR in patients receiving warfarin. Variable effect on phenytoin levels. May cause sedation especially with alcohol, phenothiazines, opioids, or tricyclic antidepressants. Additive anticholinergic effects with tricyclic antidepressants.

**DICYCLOMINE (*Bentyl, Bentylol, Antispas, ✦Formulex, Protylol, Lomine*)** ▶LK ♀B ▶- $
ADULT - Treatment of functional bowel/irritable bowel syndrome (irritable colon, spastic colon, mucous colon): Initiate with 20 mg PO qid and increase to 40 mg PO qid, if tolerated. Patients who are unable to take oral medications: 20 mg IM q6h.
PEDS - Not approved in children.
UNAPPROVED PEDS - Treatment of functional/irritable bowel syndrome: Infants >6 mo: 5 mg PO tid-qid. Children: 10 mg PO tid-qid.
FORMS - Generic/Trade: Tab 20 mg, cap 10 mg, syrup 10 mg/5 mL. Generic only: Cap 20 mg.
NOTES - Although some use lower doses (ie, 10–20 mg PO qid), the only adult oral dose proven to be effective is 160 mg/d.

**DONNATAL (phenobarbital + atropine + hyoscyamine + scopolamine)** ▶LK ♀C ▶- $
ADULT - Adjunctive therapy of irritable bowel syndrome or adjunctive treatment of duodenal ulcers: 1–2 tabs/caps or 5–10 mL PO tid-qid or 1 extended release tab PO q8–12h.
PEDS - Adjunctive therapy of irritable bowel syndrome: 0.1 mL/kg/dose PO q4h, max dose 5 mL. Adjunctive treatment of duodenal ulcers: 0.1 mL/kg/dose q4h. Alternative dosing regimen: Weight 4.5kg: 0.5 mL PO q4h or 0.75 mL PO q6h; 9.1kg: 1 mL PO q4h or 1.5 mL PO q6h; 13.6kg: 1.5 mL PO q4h or 2 mL PO q6h; 22.7kg: 2.5 mL PO q4h or 3.75 mL PO q6h; 34kg: 3.75 mL PO q4h or 5 mL PO q6h; ≥45.5kg: 5 mL PO q4h or 7.5 mL PO q6h.
FORMS - Generic/Trade: Phenobarbital 16.2 mg + hyoscyamine 0.1 mg + atropine 0.02 mg + scopolamine 6.5 mcg in each tab, cap or 5 mL. Extended-release tab 48.6 + 0.3111 + 0.0582 + 0.0195 mg.
NOTES - The FDA has classified Donnatal as "possibly effective" for treatment of irritable bowel syndrome and duodenal ulcer. Heat stroke may occur in hot weather. Can cause anticholinergic side effects; use caution in narrow-angle glaucoma, BPH, etc.

**GI COCKTAIL (*Green Goddess*)** ▶LK ♀See individual ▶See individual $
ADULT - See components
PEDS - Not approved in children.
UNAPPROVED ADULT - Acute GI upset: mixture of Maalox/Mylanta 30 mL + viscous lidocaine (2%) 10 mL + Donnatal 10 mL administered PO in a single dose.
NOTES - Avoid repeat dosing due to risk of lidocaine toxicity.

**HYOSCINE (✦*BUCOSPAN*)** ▶LK ♀C ▶? ?
ADULT - Canada: GI or bladder spasm: 10–20 mg PO/IV up to 60 mg daily (PO) or 100 mg daily (IV).

PEDS - Not approved in children.
FORMS - Canada: Trade: Tab 10 mg.
NOTES - May cause dizziness, drowsiness, blurred vision, dry mouth, N/V, urinary retention. Contraindicated in glaucoma, obstructive conditions (eg, pyloric, duodenal or other intestinal obstructive lesions, ileus, and obstructive uropathies), and myasthenia gravis.

**HYOSCYAMINE (*Anaspaz, A-spaz, Cystospaz, ED Spaz, Hyosol, Hyospaz, Levbid, Levsin, Levsinex, Medispaz, NuLev, Spacol, Spasdel, Symax*)** ▶LK ♀C ▶- $
ADULT - Bladder spasm, control gastric secretion, GI hypermotility, irritable bowel syndrome: 0.125–0.25 mg PO q4h or prn. 0.375–0.75 mg PO q12h (extended release). Max 1.5 mg/d.
PEDS - Bladder spasm >12 yo: Adult dosing. Control gastric secretion, GI hypermotility, irritable bowel syndrome, and others: Initial oral dose by weight for children <2 yo: 12.5 mcg (2.3 kg), 16.7 mcg (3.4 kg), 20.8 mcg (5 kg), 25 mcg (7 kg), 31.3–33.3 mcg (10 kg), and 45.8 mcg (15 kg). Alternatively, if <2 yo: 3 drops (2.3 kg), 4 drops (3.4 kg), 5 drops (5 kg), 6 drops (7 kg), 8 drops (10 kg), 11 drops (15 kg). Doses can be repeated q4h prn, but max daily dose is six times initial dose. Initial oral dose by weight for children 2–12 yo: 31.3–33.3 mcg (10kg), 62.5 mcg (20kg), 93.8 mcg (40kg), and 125 mcg (50kg). Doses may be repeated q4h, but max daily dose should not exceed 750 mcg.
FORMS - Generic/Trade: Tab 0.125. Sublingual Tab 0.125 mg. Extended release Tab 0.375 mg. Extended release Cap 0.375 mg. Elixir 0.125 mg/5 mL. Drops 0.125 mg/1 mL. Trade: Tab 0.15 mg (Hyospaz, Cystospaz). Tab, orally disintegrating 0.125 (NuLev).
NOTES - May cause dizziness, drowsiness, blurred vision, dry mouth, N/V, urinary retention. Contraindicated in glaucoma, obstructive conditions (eg, pyloric, duodenal or other intestinal obstructive lesions, ileus, achalasia, GI hemorrhage, and obstructive uropathies), unstable cardiovascular status, and myasthenia gravis.

**MEPENZOLATE (*Cantil*)** ▶LK ♀B ▶? $$$$$
ADULT - Adjunctive therapy in peptic ulcer disease: 25–50 mg PO tid-qid, with meals and qhs.
PEDS - Not approved in children.
FORMS - Trade only: Tab 25 mg.
NOTES - Contraindicated in glaucoma, obstructive uropathy, paralytic ileus, toxic megacolon, myasthenia gravis.

**METHSCOPOLAMINE (*Pamine, Pamine Forte*)** ▶LK ♀C ▶? $$$$
ADULT - Adjunctive therapy in peptic ulcer disease: 2.5–5 mg PO 30 min ac & qhs.
PEDS - Not approved in children.
FORMS - Generic/Trade: Tab 2.5 mg (Pamine), 5 mg (Pamine Forte).
NOTES - Has not been shown to be effective in treating peptic ulcer disease.

**MISOPROSTOL (*PGE1, Cytotec*)** ▶LK ♀X ▶- $
WARNING - Contraindicated in desired early or preterm pregnancy due to its abortifacient property.
**(cont.)**

**MISOPROSTOL** (cont.)

Pregnant women should avoid contact/exposure to the tabs. Uterine rupture reported with use for labor induction & medical abortion.

ADULT - Prevention of NSAID-induced gastric ulcers: 200 mcg PO qid. If not tolerated, use 100 mcg PO qid.

PEDS - Not approved in children.

UNAPPROVED ADULT - Cervical ripening and labor induction: 25 mcg intravaginally q3–6h (or 50 mcg q6h). First-trimester pregnancy failure: 800 mcg intravaginally, repeat on d 3 if expulsion incomplete. Medical abortion ≤49 d gestation: w/ mifepristone, see mifepristone; w/ methotrexate: 800 mcg intravaginally 5–7 d after 50 mg/m² PO or IM methotrexate. Preop cervical ripening: 400 mcg intravaginally 3–4h before mechanical cervical dilation. Post-partum hemorrhage: 800 mcg PR × 1. Oral dosing has been used but is controversial. Treatment of duodenal ulcers: 100 mcg PO qid.

UNAPPROVED PEDS - Improvement in fat absorption in cystic fibrosis in children 8 - 16 yo: 100 mcg PO qid.

FORMS - Generic/Trade: Oral tabs 100 & 200 mcg.

NOTES - Contraindicated with prior C-section. Oral tabs can be inserted into the vagina for labor induction/cervical ripening. Monitor for uterine hyperstimulation & abnormal fetal heart rate. Risk factors for uterine rupture: prior uterine surgery & ≥5 previous pregnancies.

**PROPANTHELINE** (*Pro-Banthine*, ✦*Propanthel*) ▶LK ♀C ▶- $$$

ADULT - Adjunctive therapy in peptic ulcer disease: 7.5–15 mg PO 30 min before meals and qhs.

PEDS - Not approved in children.

UNAPPROVED ADULT - Irritable bowel, pancreatitis, urinary bladder spasms: 7.5–15 mg PO qid.

UNAPPROVED PEDS - Antisecretory effects: 1.5 mg/kg/d PO in 3–4 divided doses. Antispasmodic effects: 2–3 mg/kg/d PO divided q4–6h and qhs.

FORMS - Generic/Trade: Tab 15 mg. Trade only: Tab 7.5 mg.

NOTES - For elderly adults and those with small stature use 7.5 mg dose. May cause constipation, dry mucous membranes.

**SIMETHICONE** (*Mylicon, Gas-X, Phazyme, ✦Ovol*) ▶Not absorbed ♀C but + ▶? $

ADULT - Excessive gas in GI tract: 40–160 mg PO after meals and qhs prn, max 500 mg/d.

PEDS - Excessive gas in GI tract: <2 yo: 20 mg PO qid prn, max of 240 mg/d. Children 2–12 yo: 40 mg PO qid prn.

UNAPPROVED PEDS - Although used to treat infant colic (in approved dose for gas), several studies suggest no benefit.

FORMS - OTC: Generic/Trade: Tab 60,95 mg, chew tab 40,80,125 mg, cap 125 mg, drops 40 mg/0.6 mL.

NOTES - For administration to infants, may mix dose in 30 mL of liquid. Chew tabs should be chewed thoroughly.

**SUCRALFATE** (*Carafate, ✦Sulcrate*) ▶Not absorbed ♀B ▶? $$$

ADULT - Duodenal ulcer: 1g PO qid, 1h before meals and qhs. Maintenance therapy of duodenal ulcer: 1g PO bid.

PEDS - Not approved in children.

UNAPPROVED ADULT - Gastric ulcer, reflux esophagitis, NSAID-induced GI symptoms, stress ulcer prophylaxis: 1g PO qid 1h before meals & qhs. Oral and esophageal ulcers due to radiation/chemo/sclerotherapy: (susp only) 5–10 mL swish and spit /swallow qid.

UNAPPROVED PEDS - Reflux esophagitis, gastric or duodenal ulcer, stress ulcer prophylaxis: 40–80 mg/kg/d PO divided q6h. Alternative dosing: children <6 yo: 500 mg 1/2 tab qid, children >6 yo: 1g PO qid.

FORMS - Generic/Trade: Tab 1 g, susp 1g/10 mL.

NOTES - May cause constipation. May reduce the absorption of cimetidine, ciprofloxacin, digoxin, ketoconazole, itraconazole, norfloxacin, phenytoin, ranitidine, tetracycline, theophylline and warfarin; separate doses by at least 2 h. Antacids should be separated by at least 30 min.

## GASTROENTEROLOGY: Laxatives—Bulk-Forming

**METHYLCELLULOSE** (*Citrucel*) ▶Not absorbed ♀+ ▶? $

ADULT - Laxative: 1 heaping tablespoon in 8 ounces cold water PO daily-tid.

PEDS - Laxative: Age 6–12 yo: 1½ heaping teaspoons in 4 ounces cold water daily-tid PO prn.

FORMS - OTC Trade only: regular & sugar-free packets and multiple use canisters, clear-mix solution, caplets 500 mg.

NOTES - Must be taken with water to avoid esophageal obstruction or choking.

**POLYCARBOPHIL** (*FiberCon, Fiberall, Konsyl Fiber, Equalactin*) ▶Not absorbed ♀+ ▶? $

ADULT - Laxative: 1 g PO qid prn.

PEDS - Laxative: Children 3–5 yo: 500 mg PO daily-bid prn. ≥6 yo: 500 mg PO daily-tid prn.

UNAPPROVED ADULT - Diarrhea: 1 g PO q30min prn. Max daily dose 6 g.

UNAPPROVED PEDS - Diarrhea: Children 3–5 yo: 500 mg PO q30min prn. Max daily dose 1.5 g. >6 yo: 500 mg PO daily-tid or prn. Max daily dose 3 g.

FORMS - OTC Generic/Trade: Tab 500,625 mg, chew tab 500,1000 mg.

NOTES - When used as a laxative, take dose with at least 8 ounces of fluid. Do not administer concomitantly with tetracycline; separate by at least 2 h.

**PSYLLIUM** (*Metamucil, Fiberall, Konsyl, Hydrocil, ✦Prodium Plain*) ▶Not absorbed ♀+ ▶? $

ADULT - Laxative: 1 rounded tsp in liquid, 1 packet in liquid or 1 wafer with liquid PO daily-tid.

PEDS - Laxative (children 6–11yo): ½-1 rounded tsp in liquid, ½-1 packet in liquid or 1 wafer with liquid PO daily-tid.

UNAPPROVED ADULT - Reduction in cholesterol: 1 rounded tsp in liquid, 1 packet in liquid or 1–2

**PSYLLIUM** (*cont.*)
wafers with liquid PO tid. Prevention of GI side effects with orlistat: 6 g in liquid with each orlistat dose or 12 g in liquid qhs.
FORMS - OTC: Generic/Trade: regular and sugar-free powder, granules, caps, wafers, including various flavors and various amounts of psyllium.

NOTES - Powders and granules must be mixed with liquid prior to ingestion. Start with 1 dose/d and gradually increase to minimize gas and bloating. Can bind with warfarin, digoxin, potassium-sparing diuretics, salicylates, tetracycline and nitrofurantoin; space at least 3 h apart.

## GASTROENTEROLOGY: Laxatives—Osmotic

**GLYCERIN** (*Fleet*) ▶Not absorbed ♀C ▶? $
ADULT - Constipation: 1 adult supp PR prn.
PEDS - Constipation: Neonates: 0.5 mL/kg/dose PR prn. Children <6 yo: 1 infant supp or 2–5 mL rectal solution as an enema PR prn. Children ≥6 yo: 1 adult supp or 5–15 mL of rectal solution as enema PR prn.
FORMS - OTC Generic/Trade: supp infant & adult, solution (Fleet Babylax) 4 mL/applicator.

**LACTULOSE** (*Chronulac, Cephulac, Kristalose*) ▶Not absorbed ♀B ▶? $$
ADULT - Constipation: 15–30 mL (syrup) or 10–20 g (powder for oral solution) PO daily. Evacuation of barium following barium procedures: 5–10 mL (syrup) PO bid. Acute hepatic encephalopathy: 30–45 mL syrup/dose PO q1h until laxative effect observed or 300 mL in 700 mL water or saline PR as a retention enema q4–6h. Prevention of encephalopathy: 30–45 mL syrup PO tid-qid.
PEDS - Prevention or treatment of encephalopathy: Infants: 2.5–10 mL/d (syrup) PO in 3–4 divided doses. Children/adolescents: 40–90 mL/d (syrup) PO in 3–4 divided doses.
UNAPPROVED ADULT - Restoration of bowel movements in hemorrhoidectomy patients: 15 mL syrup PO bid on d before surgery and for 5 d following surgery.
UNAPPROVED PEDS - Constipation: 7.5 mL syrup PO daily, after breakfast.
FORMS - Generic/Trade: syrup 10 g/15 mL. Trade only (Kristalose): 10, 20 g packets for oral solution.
NOTES - May be mixed in water, juice or milk to improve palatability. Packets for oral solution should be mixed in 4 oz of water. Titrate dose to produce 2–3 soft stools/d.

**MAGNESIUM CITRATE**, ◆*CITRO-MAG* ▶K ♀+ ▶? $
ADULT - Evacuate bowel prior to procedure: 150–300 mL PO divided daily-bid.
PEDS - Evacuate bowel prior to procedure: Children <6 yo: 2–4 mL/kg/24h PO divided daily-bid. Children 6–12 yo: 100–150 mL/24h PO divided daily-bid.
FORMS - OTC Generic only: solution 300 mL/bottle. Low sodium & sugar-free available.
NOTES - Use caution with impaired renal function. May decrease absorption of phenytoin, ciprofloxacin, benzodiazepines, and glyburide. May cause additive CNS depression with CNS depressants. Chill to improve palatability.

**MAGNESIUM HYDROXIDE** (*Milk of Magnesia*) ▶K ♀+ ▶? $
ADULT - Laxative: 30–60 mL PO as a single dose or divided doses. Antacid: 5–15 mL/dose PO qid prn or 622–1244 mg PO qid prn.
PEDS - Laxative: Age <2 yo: 0.5 mL/kg PO as a single dose. 2–5 yo: 5–15 mL/d PO as a single dose or in divided doses. 6–11 yo: 15–30 mL PO in a single dose or in divided doses. Antacid (children >12yo): 2.5–5 mL/dose PO qid prn.
FORMS - OTC Generic/Trade: susp 400 mg/5ml. Trade only: chew tab 311 mg. Generic only: susp (concentrated) 1200 mg/5 mL, sugar-free 400 mg/5 mL.
NOTES - Milk of magnesia concentrated liquid contains 800 mg/5 mL, so use half of the dose. Use caution with impaired renal function.

**POLYETHYLENE GLYCOL** (*MiraLax, GlycoLax*) ▶Not absorbed ♀C ▶? $
ADULT - Constipation: 17 g (1 heaping tablespoon) in 4–8 oz water, juice, soda, coffee, or tea PO daily.
PEDS - Not approved in children.
UNAPPROVED PEDS - Constipation: 0.8 g/kg/d PO in 2 divided doses.
FORMS - OTC Generic/Trade: powder for oral solution 17g/scoop. Rx Trade only: 17 g packets for oral solution.
NOTES - Takes 2–4 d to produce bowel movement. Indicated for up to 14 d.

**POLYETHYLENE GLYCOL WITH ELECTROLYTES** (*GoLytely, Colyte, TriLyte, NuLytely, Moviprep, HalfLytely and Bisacodyl Tablet Kit, ◆Klean-Prep, Electropeg, Peg-Lyte*) ▶Not absorbed ♀C ▶? $
ADULT - Bowel cleansing prior to GI examination: 240 mL PO every 10 min or 20–30 mL/min NG until 4L are consumed or rectal effluent is clear. Moviprep: 240 mL q15 min × 4 (over 1 h) the night before plus 16 additional ounces of clear liquid and 240 mL q15 min × (over 1 h) plus 16 additional ounces of clear liquid on the morning of the colonoscopy. Alternatively, 240 mL q15 min × 4 (over 1 h) at 6pm on the evening before the colonoscopy and then 1.5 h later, 240 mL q15 min × 4 (over 1h) plus 32 additional ounces of clear liquid on the evening before the colonoscopy (Moviprep only).
PEDS - Bowel prep, >6 mo (NuLYTELY, TriLyte): 25 mL/kg/h PO/NG, until rectal effluent clear, max 4L.
UNAPPROVED ADULT - Chronic constipation: 125–500 mL/d PO daily-bid.
UNAPPROVED PEDS - Bowel cleansing prior to GI examination: 25–40 mL/kg/h PO/NG for 4–10 h or until rectal effluent is clear or 20–30 mL/
(cont.)

**POLYETHYLENE GLYCOL** (*cont.*)
min NG until 4L are consumed or rectal effluent is clear. Acute iron overdoses: children <3 yo: 0.5 L/h.
FORMS - Generic/Trade: powder for oral solution in disposable jug 4L or 2L (Moviprep). Also, as a kit of 2L bottle of polyethylene glycol with electrolytes and 2 or 4 bisacodyl tabs 5 mg (HalfLytely and Bisacodyl Tablet Kit). Trade only (GoLytely): packet for oral solution to make 3.785 L.
NOTES - Solid food should not be given within 2 h of solution. Effects should occur within 1–2 h. Chilling improves palatability.

**SODIUM PHOSPHATE** (*Fleet enema, Fleet Phospho-Soda, Accu-Prep, Visicol, +Enemol, Phoslax*) ▶Not absorbed ♀C ▶? $
WARNING - Phosphate-containing bowel cleansing regimens have been rarely reported to cause acute phosphate nephropathy. Risk factors include advanced age, kidney disease or decreased intravascular volume, and medications that affect renal perfusion or function such as diuretics, ACE inhibitors, ARBs, and maybe NSAIDs.
ADULT - 1 adult or pediatric enema PR or 20–30 mL of oral soln PO prn (max 45 mL/24 h). Visicol: Evening before colonoscopy: 3 tabs with 8 oz clear liquid q15 min until 20 tabs are consumed. Day of colonoscopy: starting 3–5 h before procedure, 3 tabs with 8 oz clear liquid q15 min until 20 tabs are consumed.

PEDS - Laxative: 1 pediatric enema (67.5 mL) PR prn or 5–9 yo: 5 mL of oral solution PO prn. 10–12 yo: 10 mL of oral solution PO prn.
UNAPPROVED ADULT - Visicol: Evening before colonoscopy: 3 tabs with 8 oz clear liquid q15 min until 20 tabs are consumed. Day of colonoscopy: starting 3–5 h before procedure, 3 tabs with 8 oz clear liquid q15 min until 8–12 tabs are consumed.
FORMS - OTC Trade only: pediatric & adult enema, oral solution. Rx Trade only: Visicol tab (trade $$$): 1.5 g.
NOTES - Taking the last 2 doses of Visicol with ginger ale appears to minimize residue. Excessive doses (>45 mL/24 h) of oral products may lead to serious electrolyte disturbances. Use with caution in severe renal impairment.

**SORBITOL** ▶Not absorbed ♀+ ▶? $
ADULT - Laxative: 30–150 mL (of 70% solution) PO or 120 mL (of 25–30% solution) PR. Cathartic: 1–2 mL/kg PO.
PEDS - Laxative: Children 2–11 yo: 2 mL/kg (of 70% solution) PO or 30–60 mL (of 25–30% solution) PR.
UNAPPROVED PEDS - Cathartic: 4.3 mL/kg of 35% soln (diluted from 70% soln) PO × 1.
FORMS - Generic only: solution 70%.
NOTES - When used as a cathartic, can be given with activated charcoal to improve taste and decrease gastric transit time of charcoal. May precipitate electrolyte changes.

## GASTROENTEROLOGY: Laxatives—Stimulant

**BISACODYL** (*Correctol, Dulcolax, Feen-a-Mint*) ▶L ♀+ ▶? $
ADULT - Constipation/colonic evacuation prior to a procedure: 10–15 mg PO daily prn, 10 mg PR daily prn.
PEDS - Constipation/colonic evacuation prior to a procedure: 0.3 mg/kg/d PO daily prn. Children <2 yo: 5 mg PR prn. 2–11 yo: 5–10 mg PR prn. >11 yo: 10 mg PR prn.
FORMS - OTC Generic/Trade: tab 5 mg, supp 10 mg.
NOTES - Oral tab has onset of action of 6–10 h. Onset of action of susp is approximately 15–60 min. Do not chew tabs, swallow whole. Do not give within 1h of antacids or dairy products. Chronic use of stimulant laxatives may be habit forming.

**CASCARA** ▶L ♀C ▶+ $
ADULT - Constipation: 325 mg PO qhs prn or 5 mL/d of aromatic fluid extract PO qhs prn.
PEDS - Constipation: Infants: 1.25 mL/d of aromatic fluid extract PO daily prn. Children 2–11 yo: 2.5 mL/d of aromatic fluid extract PO daily prn.
FORMS - OTC Generic only: tab 325 mg, liquid aromatic fluid extract.
NOTES - Cascara sagrada fluid extract is 5 times more potent than cascara sagrada aromatic fluid extract. Chronic use of stimulant laxatives may be habit forming.

**CASTOR OIL** (*Purge, Fleet Flavored Castor Oil*) ▶Not absorbed ♀- ▶? $
ADULT - Constipation: 15 mL PO daily prn. Colonic evacuation prior to procedure: 15–30 mL of castor oil or 30–60 mL emulsified castor oil PO as a single dose 16h prior to procedure.
PEDS - Colonic evacuation prior to procedure: Children <2 yo: 1–5 mL of castor oil or 5–15 mL emulsified castor oil PO as a single dose 16h prior to procedure. 2–11 yo: 5–15 mL of castor oil or 7.5–30 mL of emulsified castor oil PO as a single dose 16h prior to procedure.
FORMS - OTC Generic/Trade: liquid 30,60,120,480 mL, emulsified susp 45,60,90,120 mL.
NOTES - Emulsions somewhat mask bad taste. Onset of action approx. 2–6h. Do not give at bedtime. Chill or administer with juice to improve taste.

**SENNA** (*Senokot, SenokotXTRA, Ex-Lax, Fletcher's Castoria, +Glysennid*) ▶L ♀C ▶+ $
ADULT - Laxative or evacuation of the colon for bowel or rectal examinations: 1 tsp granules in water or 10–15 mL or 2 tabs PO qhs. Max daily dose 4 tsp of granules, 30 mL of syrup, 8 tabs or 2 supp.
PEDS - Laxative: 10–20 mg/kg/dose PO qhs. Alternative regimen: 1 mo–2 yo: 1.25–2.5 mL syrup PO qhs, max 5 mL/d; 2–5yo: 2.5–3.75 mL syrup PO qhs, max 7.5 mL/d; 6–12 yo: 5–7.5 mL syrup PO qhs, max 15 mL/d.
FORMS - OTC Generic/Trade (All dosing is based on sennosides content; 1 mg sennosides = 21.7

**SENNA (cont.)**

mg standardized senna concentrate): granules 15 mg/tsp, syrup 8.8 mg/5 mL, liquid 3 mg/mL (Fletcher's Castoria), tab 8.6, 15, 17, 25 mg, chewable tab 15 mg.

NOTES - Effects occur 6–24 h after oral administration. Use caution in renal dysfunction. Chronic use of stimulant laxatives may be habit forming.

## GASTROENTEROLOGY: Laxatives—Stool Softener

**DOCUSATE** (*Colace, Surfak, Kaopectate Stool Softener*) ▶L ♀+ ▶? $

ADULT - Constipation. Docusate calcium: 240 mg PO daily. Docusate sodium: 50–500 mg/d PO in 1–4 divided doses.

PEDS - Constipation, docusate sodium: Children <3 yo: 10–40 mg/d PO in 1–4 divided doses. 3–6 yo: 20–60 mg/d PO in 1–4 divided doses. 6–12 yo: 40–150 mg/d PO in 1–4 divided doses.

UNAPPROVED ADULT - Docusate sodium, constipation: Can be given as a retention enema: Mix 50–100 mg docusate liquid with saline or oil retention enema for rectal use. Cerumen removal:

Instill 1 mL liquid (not syrup) in affected ear; allow to remain for 10–15 min, then irrigate with 50 mL lukewarm NS if necessary.

UNAPPROVED PEDS - Docusate sodium: Cerumen removal: Instill 1 mL liquid (not syrup) in affected ear; allow to remain for 10–15 min, then irrigate with 50 mL lukewarm NS if necessary.

FORMS - Docusate calcium OTC Generic/Trade: cap 240 mg. Docusate sodium OTC Generic/Trade: cap 50,100, 250 mg, tab 50,100 mg, liquid 10 & 50 mg/5 mL, syrup 16.75 & 20 mg/5 mL.

NOTES - Takes 1–3 d to notably soften stools.

## GASTROENTEROLOGY: Laxatives—Other or Combinations

**LUBIPROSTONE** (*Amitiza*) ▶Gut ♀C ▶? $$$$$

WARNING - Avoid if symptoms or history of mechanical gastrointestinal obstruction.

ADULT - Chronic idiopathic constipation: 24 mcg PO bid with meals. Irritable bowel syndrome with constipation in women >18 yo: 8 mcg PO bid.

PEDS - Not approved in children.

FORMS - Trade only: 8, 24 mcg caps.

**MINERAL OIL** (*Kondremul, Fleet Mineral Oil Enema, ✦Lansoyl*) ▶Not absorbed ♀C ▶? $

ADULT - Laxative: 15–45 mL PO in a single dose or in divided doses, 60–150 mL PR.

PEDS - Laxative: Children 6–11 yo: 5–15 mL PO in a single dose or in divided doses. Children 2–11 yo: 30–60 mL PR.

FORMS - OTC Generic/Trade: plain mineral oil, mineral oil emulsion (Kondremul).

NOTES - Use with caution in young children due to concerns for aspiration pneumonitis. Although usual directions for plain mineral oil are to administer at bedtime, this increases risk of

lipid pneumonitis. Mineral oil emulsions may be administered with meals.

**PERI-COLACE** (docusate + sennosides) ▶L ♀C ▶? $

ADULT - Constipation: 2–4 tabs PO once daily or in divided doses prn.

PEDS - Constipation 6–12 yo: 1–2 tabs PO daily prn. 2–6 yo: up to 1 tab PO daily prn.

FORMS - OTC Generic/Trade: tab 50 mg docusate + 8.6 mg sennosides

NOTES - Dilute syrup in 6–8 oz of juice, milk or infant formula to prevent throat irritation. Chronic use of stimulant laxatives (casanthranol) may be habit forming.

**SENOKOT-S** (senna + docusate) ▶L ♀C ▶+ $

ADULT - 2 tabs PO daily, max 4 tabs bid.

PEDS - 6–12 yo: 1 tab PO daily, max 2 tabs bid. 2–6 yo: ½ tab PO daily, max 1 tab bid.

FORMS - OTC Generic/Trade: tab 8.6 mg senna concentrate/50 mg docusate.

NOTES - Effects occur 6–24 h after oral administration. Use caution in renal dysfunction. Chronic use of stimulant laxatives may be habit forming.

## GASTROENTEROLOGY: Ulcerative Colitis

**BALSALAZIDE** (*Colazal*) ▶Minimal absorption ♀B ▶? $$$$$

ADULT - Ulcerative colitis: 2.25 g PO tid × 8–12 wk.

PEDS - 5–17 yo: Mild to moderately ulcerative colitis: 2.25 g PO tid × 8 wk or 750 mg PO tid × 8 wk.

FORMS - Generic/Trade: cap 750 mg.

NOTES - Contraindicated in salicylate allergy. Caution with renal insufficiency.

**MESALAMINE** (*5-aminosalicylic acid, 5-ASA, Asacol, Lialda, Pentasa, Canasa, Rowasa, ✦Mesasal, Salofalk*) ▶Gut ♀B ▶? $$$$$

ADULT - Ulcerative colitis: Tab: 800–1600 mg PO tid.

Pentasa: 1 g PO qid. Lialda: 2.4–4.8 g PO daily with a meal × 8 wk. Susp: 4 g (60 mL) PR retained for 8h qhs. Maintenance of ulcerative colitis: 1600 mg/d PO in divided doses. Ulcerative proctitis: Canasa supp: 500 mg PR bid-tid or 1000 mg PR qhs.

PEDS - Not approved in children.

UNAPPROVED ADULT - Active Crohn's: 0.4–4.8 g/d PO in divided doses. Maintenance of remission of Crohn's: 2.4 g/d in divided doses.

UNAPPROVED PEDS - Tab: 50 mg/kg/d PO divided q6–12h. Cap: 50 mg/kg/d PO divided q8–12h.

(cont.)

**MESALAMINE** *(cont.)*
FORMS - Trade only: delayed-release tab 400 mg (Asacol), controlled-release cap 250 & 500 mg (Pentasa), delayed-release tab 1200 mg (Lialda), rectal supp 1000 mg (Canasa). Generic/Trade: rectal susp 4 g/60 mL (Rowasa).
NOTES - Avoid in salicylate sensitivity or hepatic dysfunction. May decrease digoxin levels. May discolor urine yellow-brown. Most common adverse effects include headache, abdominal pain, fever, rash.

**OLSALAZINE** *(Dipentum)* ▶L ♀C ▶- $$$$
ADULT - Maintenance of remission of ulcerative colitis in patients intolerant to sulfasalazine: 500 mg PO bid.
PEDS - Not approved in children.
UNAPPROVED ADULT - Crohn's: 1.5–3 g/d PO in divided doses.
FORMS - Trade only: cap 250 mg.
NOTES - Diarrhea in up to 17%. Avoid in salicylate sensitivity.

**SULFASALAZINE** *(Azulfidine, Azulfidine EN-tabs, ✦Salazopyrin En-tabs, S.A.S.)* ▶L ♀B ▶- $$
WARNING - Beware of hypersensitivity, marrow suppression, renal & liver damage, irreversible neuromuscular & CNS changes, fibrosing alveolitis.

ADULT - Colitis: Initially 500–1000 mg PO qid. Maintenance: 500 mg PO qid. RA: 500 mg PO daily-bid after meals to start. Increase to 1g PO bid.
PEDS - JRA: ≥6 yo: 30–50 mg/kg/d (EN-Tabs) PO divided bid to max of 2 g/d. Colitis, >2 yo: Initially 30–60 mg/kg/d PO divided into 3–6 doses. Max 75 mg/kg/d. Maintenance: 30 mg/kg/d PO divided qid.
UNAPPROVED ADULT - Ankylosing spondylitis: 1–1.5 g PO bid. Psoriasis: 1.5–2g PO bid. Psoriatic arthritis: 1g PO bid.
FORMS - Generic/Trade: Tabs 500 mg, scored. Enteric coated, Delayed-release (EN-Tabs) 500 mg.
NOTES - Contraindicated in children <2 yo. Avoid with hepatic or renal dysfunction, intestinal or urinary obstruction, porphyria, sulfonamide or salicylate sensitivity. Monitor CBC q 2–4 wk for 3 mo, then q 3 mo. Monitor LFTs & renal function. Oligospermia & infertility, and photosensitivity may occur. May decrease folic acid, digoxin, cyclosporine & iron levels. May turn body fluids, contact lenses, or skin orange-yellow. Enteric coated (Azulfidine EN, Salazopyrin EN) tabs may cause fewer GI adverse effects.

## GASTROENTEROLOGY: Other GI Agents

**ALOSETRON** *(Lotronex)* ▶L ♀B ▶? $$$$$
WARNING - Can cause severe constipation & ischemic colitis. Concomitant use with fluvoxamine, a potent CYP1A2 inhibitor, is contraindicated. Use caution with moderate CYP1A2 inhibitors such as quinolone antibiotics and cimetidine. Use caution with strong inhibitors of CYP3A4 such as ketoconazole, clarithromycin, telithromycin, protease inhibitors, voriconazole and itraconazole. Can be prescribed only by drug company authorized clinicians using special sticker and written informed consent.
ADULT - Diarrhea-predominant irritable bowel syndrome in women who have failed conventional therapy: 0.5 mg PO twice daily for 4 wk; in patients who become constipated, decrease to 0.5 mg PO once daily. If well tolerated after 4 wk, may increase to 1 mg PO bid. Discontinue if symptoms not controlled in 4 wk on 1 mg PO bid.
PEDS - Not approved in children.
FORMS - Trade only: tab 0.5, 1 mg.
NOTES - Specific medication guide must be distributed with prescriptions.

**ALPHA-GALACTOSIDASE** *(Beano)* ▶Minimal absorption ♀? ▶? $
ADULT - 5 drops per ½ cup gassy food, 3 tabs PO (chew, swallow or crumble) or 15 drops per typical meal.
PEDS - Not approved in children <12 yo.
FORMS - OTC Trade only: drops 150 GalU/5 drops, tab 150 GalU.
NOTES - Beano produces 2–6 grams of carbohydrates for every 100 grams of food treated by Beano; may increase glucose levels.

**ALVIMOPAN** *(Entereg)* ▶Intestinal flora ♀B ▶? ?
ADULT - Short-term (up to 15 doses) in hospitalized patients undergoing partial large or small bowel resection surgery with primary anastomosis: 12 mg PO 30 min prior to surgery, then 12 mg bid for up to 7 d.
PEDS - Not approved in children.
FORMS - Trade only: Cap: 12 mg.
NOTES - Only available to hospitals who are authorized to use the medication.

**BUDESONIDE** *(Entocort EC)* ▶L ♀C ▶? $$$$$
ADULT - Mild-moderate Crohn's, induction of remission 9 mg PO daily × 8 wk. May repeat 8 wk course for recurring episodes. Maintenance: 6 mg PO daily × 3 mo.
PEDS - Not approved in children.
UNAPPROVED PEDS - Mild-moderate Crohn's and ≥9 yo: 0.45 mg/kg up to 9 mg PO daily × 8–12 wk.
FORMS - Trade only: cap 3 mg.
NOTES - May taper dose to 6 mg for 2 wk prior to discontinuation.

**CERTOLIZUMAB** *(Cimzia)* ▶Plasma, K ♀B ▶? $$$$$
ADULT - Crohn's: 400 mg SQ at 0, 2, and 4 wk. If response occurs, then 400 mg SQ every 4 wk.
PEDS - Not approved in children.
FORMS - Trade: 400 mg kit.
NOTES - Monitor patients for TB infections.

*CHLORDIAZEPOXIDE-CLIDINIUM* ▶K ♀D ▶- $
ADULT - Irritable bowel syndrome: 1 cap PO tid-qid.
PEDS - Not approved in children.
FORMS - Generic only: cap clidinium 2.5 mg + chlordiazepoxide 5 mg.

**CHLORDIAZEPOXIDE-CLIDINIUM** (*cont.*)
NOTES - May cause drowsiness. After prolonged use, gradually taper to avoid withdrawal symptoms. Contains ingredients formerly contained in Librax.

**CISAPRIDE** (*Propulsid*) ▶LK ♀C ▶? from manufacturer only
WARNING - Available only through limited-access protocol through manufacturer. Can cause potentially fatal cardiac arrhythmias. Many drug and disease interactions.
ADULT - 10 mg PO qid, at least 15 min before meals and qhs. Some patients may require 20 mg PO qid. Max 80 mg/d.
PEDS - Not approved in children.
UNAPPROVED PEDS - Gastroesophageal reflux disease: 0.2–0.3 mg/kg/dose PO tid-qid.
FORMS - Trade only: Tab 10,20 mg, susp 1 mg/1 mL.

**GLYCOPYRROLATE** (*Robinul, Robinul Forte*) ▶K ♀B ▶? $$$$
ADULT - Drooling: 0.1 mg/kg PO bid-tid, max 8 mg/d. Pre-op/intraoperative respiratory antisecretory: 0.1 mg IV/IM prn.
PEDS - Not approved in children <16 yo.
UNAPPROVED PEDS - Drooling: 0.04–0.1 mg/kg PO tid-qid, max 8 mg/d. Pre-op/intraoperative respiratory antisecretory: 0.004–0.01 mg/kg IV/IM prn, max 0.2 mg/dose or 0.8 mg/24h.
FORMS - Generic/Trade: Tab 1, 2 mg.
NOTES - Contraindicated in glaucoma, obstructive uropathy, paralytic ileus or GI obstruction, myasthenia gravis, severe ulcerative colitis, toxic megacolon and unstable cardiovascular status in acute hemorrhage.

**LACTASE** (*Lactaid*) ▶Not absorbed ♀+ ▶+ $
ADULT - Swallow or chew 3 caplets (Original strength), 2 caplets (Extra strength), 1 caplet (Ultra) with first bite of dairy foods. Adjust dose based on response.
PEDS - Titrate dose based on response.
FORMS - OTC Generic/Trade: caplets, chew tab.

**LIBRAX** (**chlordiazepoxide + methscopolamine**) ▶K ♀D ▶- $$$$$
ADULT - Irritable bowel syndrome: 1 cap PO tid-qid.
PEDS - Not approved in children.
FORMS - Trade only: cap methscopolamine 2.5 mg + chlordiazepoxide 5 mg.
NOTES - May cause drowsiness. After prolonged use, gradually taper to avoid withdrawal symptoms.

**METHYLNALTREXONE** (*Relistor*) ▶unchanged ♀B ▶? ?
ADULT - Opioid-induced constipation in patients with advanced illness who are receiving palliative care and when response to laxative therapy has not been sufficient: 38 to <62 kg: 8 mg SC qod, 62 to 114 kg: 12 mg SC qod. All others: 0.15 mg/kg SC qod.
PEDS - Not approved in children.
FORMS - Injectable solution 12 mg/0.6 mL.
NOTES - Do not use with GI obstruction. Usual dose every other d, but no more frequently than once daily.

**NEOMYCIN - ORAL** (*Mycifradin, Neo-Fradin*) ▶Minimally absorbed ♀D ▶? $$$
ADULT - Suppression of intestinal bacteria (given with erythromycin): 1 g PO at 19h, 18h and 9h prior to procedure (ie, 1 pm, 2 pm, 11 pm on prior d). Alternative regimen 1 g PO q1h for 4 doses then 1 g PO q4h for 5 doses. Hepatic encephalopathy: 4–12 g/d PO divided q6h. Diarrhea caused by enteropathogenic E. coli: 3 g/d PO divided q6h.
PEDS - Suppression of intestinal bacteria (given with erythromycin): 25 mg/kg PO at 19h, 18h and 9h prior to procedure (ie, 1 pm, 2 pm, 11 pm on prior d). Alternative regimen 90 mg/kg/d PO divided q4h for 2–3 d. Hepatic encephalopathy: 50–100 mg/kg/d PO divided q6–8h. Diarrhea caused by enteropathogenic E. coli: 50 mg/kg/d PO divided q6h.
FORMS - Generic only: tab 350, 500 mg. Trade only (Neo-Fradin): solution 125 mg/5 mL.
NOTES - Increased INR with warfarin, decreased levels of digoxin, methotrexate.

**OCTREOTIDE** (*Sandostatin, Sandostatin LAR*) ▶LK ♀B ▶? $$$$$
ADULT - Diarrhea associated with carcinoid tumors: 100–600 mcg/d SC/IV in 2–4 divided doses or 20 mg IM (Sandostatin LAR) q4 wk × 2 mo. Adjust dose based on response. Diarrhea associated with vasoactive intestinal peptide-secreting tumors: 200–300 mcg/d SC/IV in 2–4 divided doses or 20 mg IM (Sandostatin LAR) q4 wk × 2 mo. Adjust dose based on response.
PEDS - Not approved in children.
UNAPPROVED ADULT - Variceal bleeding: Bolus 50–100 mcg IV followed by 25–50 mcg/h continuous IV infusion. AIDS diarrhea: 100–500 mcg SC tid. Irritable bowel syndrome: 100 mcg as a single dose to 125 mcg SC bid. GI and pancreatic fistulas: 50–200 mcg SC/IV q8h.
UNAPPROVED PEDS - Diarrhea: initially 1–10 mcg/kg SC/IV q12h. Congenital hyperinsulinism 1 to 40 mcg/kg SC daily. Hypothalamic obesity in children 6 to 17 yr: 40 mg IM every 4 wk (Sandostatin LAR) or 5–15 mcg/kg SC daily.
FORMS - Generic/Trade: injection vials 0.05, 0.1, 0.2, 0.5, 1 mg. Trade only: long-acting injectable susp (Sandostatin LAR) 10,20,30 mg.
NOTES - For treatment of variceal bleeding, most studies treat for 3–5 d. Individualize dose based on response. Dosage reduction often necessary in elderly. May cause hypoglycemia, hyperglycemia; caution especially in diabetes. May cause hypothyroidism, cardiac arrhythmias. Increases bioavailability of bromocriptine. Sandostatin LAR only indicated for patients stabilized on Sandostatin.

**ORLISTAT** (*Alli, Xenical*) ▶Gut ♀B ▶? $$$$$
ADULT - Weight loss and weight management: 120 mg PO tid with meals or up to 1 h after meals.
PEDS - Children 12–16 yo: 120 mg PO tid with meals. Not approved in children <12 yo.
FORMS - Trade only: Caps 60 (OTC), 120 (Rx) mg.
NOTES - May cause fatty stools, fecal urgency, flatus with discharge and oily spotting in >20% of

**(cont.)**

**ORLISTAT** (*cont.*)

patients. GI adverse effects greater when taken with high fat diet.

**PANCREATIN** (*Creon, Donnazyme, Ku-Zyme, ✦Entozyme*) ▶Gut ♀C ▶? $$$

ADULT - Enzyme replacement (initial dose): 8,000–24,000 units lipase (1–2 cap/tab) PO with meals and snacks.

PEDS - Enzyme replacement (initial dose): <1 yo: 2,000 units lipase PO with meals. 1–6 yo: 4,000–8,000 units lipase PO with meals, 4,000 units lipase with snacks. 7–12 yo: 4,000–12,000 units lipase PO with meals and snacks.

FORMS - Tab, cap with varying amounts of pancreatin, lipase, amylase and protease.

NOTES - Titrate dose to stool fat content. Products are not interchangeable. Avoid concomitant calcium carbonate and magnesium hydroxide since these may affect the enteric coating. Do not crush/chew microspheres or tabs. Possible association of colonic strictures and high doses of lipase (>16,000 units/kg/meal) in pediatric patients.

**PANCRELIPASE** (*Viokase, Pancrease, Pancrecarb, Cotazym, Ku-Zyme HP*) ▶Gut ♀C ▶? $$$

ADULT - Enzyme replacement (initial dose): 4,000–33,000 units lipase (1–3 cap/tab) PO with meals and snacks.

PEDS - Enzyme replacement (initial dose): 6 mo -1 yo: 2,000 units lipase or 1/8 tsp PO with feedings. 1–6 yo: 4,000–8,000 units lipase PO with meals, 4,000 units lipase with snacks. 7–12 yo: 4,000–12,000 units lipase PO w/ meals/snacks.

FORMS - Tab, cap, powder with varying amounts of lipase, amylase and protease.

NOTES - Titrate dose to stool fat content. Products are not interchangeable. Avoid concomitant calcium carbonate and magnesium hydroxide since these may affect the enteric coating. Do not crush/chew microspheres or tabs. Possible association of colonic strictures and high doses of lipase (>16,000 units/kg/meal) in pediatric patients.

**PINAVERIUM,** ✦*DICETEL*▶? ♀C ▶- $$$

ADULT - Canada only. Irritable bowel syndrome: 50 mg PO tid, may increase to max of 100 mg tid.

PEDS - Not for children.

FORMS - Trade only: tabs 50, 100 mg.

NOTES - Take with a full glass of water during meal or snack.

**SECRETIN** (*SecreMax*) ▶Serum ♀C ▶? $$$$$

ADULT - Stimulation of pancreatic secretions, to aid in diagnosis of exocrine pancreas dysfunction: Test dose 0.2 mcg IV. If tolerated, 0.2 mcg/kg IV over 1 min. Stimulation of gastrin to aid in diagnosis of gastrinoma: Test dose 0.2 mcg IV. If tolerated, 0.4 mcg/kg IV over 1 min. Identification of ampulla of Vater and accessory papilla during ERCP: 0.2 mcg/kg IV over 1 min.

PEDS - Not approved in children.

NOTES - Previously known as Secreflo. Contraindicated in acute pancreatitis.

**TEGASEROD** (*Zelnorm*) ▶stomach/L ♀B ▶? free (investigational)

WARNING - Restricted (investigational) use; contact manufacturer to obtain. Severe diarrhea leading to hypovolemia, hypotension and syncope has been reported, as has ischemic colitis and other forms of intestinal ischemia; discontinue immediately if symptoms occur.

ADULT - Constipation-predominant irritable bowel syndrome in women <55 yo: 6 mg PO bid before meals for 4–6 wk. May repeat for an additional 4–6 wk.

PEDS - Not approved in children.

FORMS - Restricted use only. Trade only: tab 2, 6 mg.

**URSODIOL** (*Actigall, Ursofalk, URSO, URSO Forte*) ▶Bile ♀B ▶? $$$$

ADULT - Radiolucent gallstone dissolution (Actigall): 8–10 mg/kg/d PO divided in 2–3 doses. Prevention of gallstones associated with rapid weight loss (Actigall): 300 mg PO bid. Primary biliary cirrhosis (URSO): 13–15 mg/kg/d PO divided in 2–4 doses.

PEDS - Not approved in children.

UNAPPROVED ADULT - Cholestasis of pregnancy: 300–600 mg PO bid.

UNAPPROVED PEDS - Biliary atresia: 10–15 mg/kg/d PO divided tid. Cystic fibrosis with liver disease: 30 mg/kg/d PO divided bid. TPN-induced cholestasis: 30 mg/kg/d PO divided tid.

FORMS - Generic/Trade: cap 300 mg. Trade only: tab 250 (URSO), 500 mg scored (URSO Forte).

NOTES - Gallstone dissolution requires mo of therapy. Complete dissolution does not occur in all patients and 5-yr recurrence up to 50%. Does not dissolve calcified cholesterol stones, radiopaque stones or radiolucent bile pigment stones. Avoid concomitant antacids, cholestyramine, colestipol, estrogen, oral contraceptives.

## HEMATOLOGY: Anticoagulants—Heparin, LMW Heparins, & Fondaparinux

**NOTE:** See cardiovascular section for antiplatelet drugs & thrombolytics. Contraindicated in active major bleeding. High risk of spinal/epidural hematoma if spinal puncture or neuraxial anesthesia before/during treatment (see: http://www.asra.com/consensus-statements/2.html). Risk of bleeding increased by oral anticoagulants, ASA, dipyridamole, dextran, glycoprotein IIb/IIIA inhibitors, NSAIDs (including ketorolac), ticlopidine, clopidogrel, and thrombolytics. Monitor platelets, Hb, stool for occult blood.

**DALTEPARIN** (*Fragmin*) ▶KL ♀B ▶+ $$$$$

ADULT - DVT prophylaxis, acute medical illness with restricted mobility: 5000 units SC daily × 12–14 d.

DVT prophylaxis, abdominal surgery: 2,500 units SC 1–2 h preop and daily postop × 5–10 d. DVT prophylaxis, abdominal surgery in patients with

**DALTEPARIN** (cont.)

malignancy: 5,000 units SC evening before surgery and daily postop × 5–10 d. Alternatively, 2,500 units SC 1–2 h preop and 12 h later, then 5,000 units SC daily × 5–10 d. DVT prophylaxis, hip replacement: Give SC for up to 14 d. Preop start regimens: 2,500 units 2 h preop and 4–8h postop, then 5,000 units daily starting ≥6h after 2nd dose. Alternatively, 5,000 units 10–14 h preop, 4–8h postop, then daily (approximately 24h between doses). Postop start regimen: 2,500 units 4–8h postop, then 5,000 units daily starting ≥6h after first dose. Treatment of DVT/PE in cancer: 200 units/kg SC daily × 1 mo, then 150 units/kg SC daily × 5 mo. Max 18,000 units/d, round to nearest commercially available syringe dose. Unstable angina or non-Q-wave MI: 120 units/kg up to 10000 units SC q12h with aspirin (75–165 mg/d PO) until clinically stable.

PEDS - Not approved in children.

UNAPPROVED ADULT - Therapeutic anticoagulation: 200 units/kg SC daily or 100–120 units/kg SC bid. Venous thromboembolism in pregnancy. Prevention: 5,000 units SC daily. Treatment: 100 units/kg SC q12h or 200 units/kg SC daily. To avoid unwanted anticoagulation during delivery, stop LMWH 24 h before elective induction of labor.

FORMS - Trade only: Single-dose syringes 2,500 & 5,000 anti-Xa units/0.2 mL, 7500 Anti-Xa/0.3 mL, 10,000 anti-Xa units/1 mL, 12,500 anti-Xa units/0.5 mL, 15000 anti-Xa units/0.6 mL, 18,000 anti-Xa units/0.72 mL; multi-dose vial 10,000 units/mL, 9.5 mL and 25,000 units/mL, 3.8 mL.

NOTES - Longer prophylaxis may be warranted based on individual thromboembolic risk. ACCP recommendations suggest that patients with total hip or knee replacement or hip fracture surgery receive prophylaxis for ≥10 d; consider extended prophylaxis (28–35 d) in hip replacement or hip fracture surgery. Contraindicated in heparin or pork allergy, history of heparin-induced thrombocytopenia. Use caution and consider monitoring anti-Xa levels if morbidly obese, underweight, pregnant, or renal/liver failure. Drug effect can be reversed with protamine.

**ENOXAPARIN** (*Lovenox*) ▶KL ♀B ▶+ $$$$$

ADULT - DVT prophylaxis, acute medical illness with restricted mobility: 40 mg SC daily for ≤14 d (CrCl <30 mL/min: 30 mg SC daily). DVT prophylaxis, hip/knee replacement: 30 mg SC q12h starting 12–24 h postop for ≤14 d (CrCl <30 mL/min: 30 mg SC daily). Alternative for hip replacement: 40 mg SC daily starting 12 h preop. After hip replacement may continue 40 mg SC daily × 3 wk. DVT prophylaxis, abdominal surgery: 40 mg SC daily starting 2 h preop for ≤12 d (CrCl <30 mL/min: 30 mg SC daily). Outpatient treatment of DVT without pulmonary embolus: 1 mg/kg SC q12h. Inpatient treatment of DVT with/without pulmonary embolus: 1 mg/kg SC q12h or

1.5 mg/kg SC q24h (CrCl <30 mL/min: 1 mg/kg SC daily). Give at the same time each d. Continue enoxaparin for ≥5 d and until therapeutic oral anticoagulation established. Unstable angina or non-Q-wave MI (NSTEMI): 1 mg/kg SC q12h with aspirin (100–325 mg PO daily) for ≥2 d and until clinically stable (CrCl <30 mL/min: 1 mg/kg SC daily). Acute ST-elevation MI: if ≤75 yo: 30 mg IV bolus followed 15 min later by 1 mg/kg SC dose then 1 mg/kg (max 100 mg/dose for the first two doses) SC q12 h (CrCl <30 mL/min: 30 mg IV bolus followed 15 min later by 1 mg/kg SC dose then 1 mg/kg SC daily); if >75 yo: 0.75 mg/kg (max 75 mg/dose for the first two doses, no bolus) SC q12 h (CrCl <30 mL/min: 1 mg/kg SC daily, no bolus). Given with aspirin (75–325 mg PO daily) until hospital discharge or for ≥8 d.

PEDS - Not approved in children.

UNAPPROVED ADULT - Prevention of venous thromboembolism. After major trauma: 30 mg SC q12h starting 12–36 h postinjury if hemostasis achieved. Acute spinal cord injury: 30 mg SC q12h. Venous thromboembolism in pregnancy: Prevention: 40 mg SC daily. Treatment: 1 mg/kg SC q12h. To avoid unwanted anticoagulation during delivery, stop LMWH 24 h before elective induction of labor.

UNAPPROVED PEDS - Therapeutic anticoagulation: Age <2 mo: 1.5 mg/kg/dose SC q12h titrated to anti-Xa level of 0.5–1 units/mL. Age >2 mo: 1 mg/kg/dose SC q12h titrated to anti-Xa level of 0.5–1.0 units/mL. DVT prophylaxis: Age <2 mo: 0.75 mg/kg/dose q12h. Age >2 mo: 0.5 mg/kg/dose q12h.

FORMS - Trade only: Multi-dose vial 300 mg; Syringes 30,40 mg; graduated syringes 60,80,100,120,150 mg. Concentration is 100 mg/mL except for 120,150 mg which are 150 mg/mL.

NOTES - Longer prophylaxis may be warranted based on individual thromboembolic risk. ACCP recommendations suggest that patients with total hip or knee replacement or hip fracture surgery receive prophylaxis for ≥10 d; consider extended prophylaxis (28–35 d) in hip replacement or hip fracture surgery. Dosage adjustments for CrCl <30 mL/min. Use caution and consider monitoring anti-Xa levels if renal dysfunction, pregnancy, morbidly obese, underweight, or abnormal coagulation/bleeding. In unstable angina or NSTEMI, can give 30 mg IV bolus 15 min before first SC dose. In acute ST-elevation MI, if administered with thrombolytic give between 15 min before or 30 min after start of thrombolytic therapy. In PCI, if last enoxaparin administration was >8h before balloon inflation, give 0.3 mg/kg IV bolus. Contraindicated in patients with heparin or pork allergy, history of heparin-induced thrombocytopenia. Use caution in mechanical heart valves, especially in pregnancy; reports of valve thrombosis (maternal & fetal deaths reported). Congenital anomalies linked to enoxaparin use

(cont.)

**ENOXAPARIN** *(cont.)*

during pregnancy; causality unclear. Multidose formulation contains benzyl alcohol, which can cause hypersensitivity and cross placenta in pregnancy. Drug effect can be reversed with protamine.

**FONDAPARINUX** *(Arixtra)* ▶K ♀B ▶? $$$$$

ADULT - DVT prophylaxis, hip/knee replacement or hip fracture surgery, abdominal surgery: 2.5 mg SC daily starting 6–8 h postop (giving earlier increases risk of bleeding). Usual duration is 5–9 d; extend prophylaxis up to 24 additional d (max 32 d) in hip fracture surgery. DVT/PE treatment based on weight: 5 mg (if <50 kg), 7.5 mg (if 50–100 kg), 10 mg (if >100 kg) SC daily for ≥5 d & therapeutic oral anticoagulation.

PEDS - Not approved in children.

UNAPPROVED ADULT - Unstable angina or non-ST elevation MI: 2.5 mg SC daily until hospital discharge or for up to 8 d. ST-elevation MI and creatinine <3 mg/dL: 2.5 mg IV loading dose, then 2.5 mg SC daily until hospital discharge or for up to 8 d.

FORMS - Trade only: Pre-filled syringes 2.5 mg/0.5 mL, 5 mg/0.4 mL, 7.5 mg/0.6 mL, 10 mg/0.8 mL.

NOTES - May cause thrombocytopenia, however, lacks in vitro cross-reactivity with heparin-induced thrombocytopenia antibodies. Risk of major bleeding increased in elderly. Contraindicated if CrCl <30 mL/min due to increased bleeding risk. Caution advised if CrCl 30–50 mL/min. Monitor renal function in all patients; discontinue if severely impaired or labile. In DVT prophylaxis, contraindicated if body weight <50 kg. Protamine ineffective for reversing anticoagulant effect. Factor VIIa partially reverses anticoagulant effect in small studies. Risk of catheter thrombosis in PCI; use in conjunction with anticoagulant with anti-IIa activity. Store at room temperature.

**HEPARIN,** *✦HEPALEAN* (▶ *Reticuloendothelial system)* ♀C but + ▶+ $

ADULT - Venous thrombosis/pulmonary embolus treatment: Load 80 units/kg IV, then initiate infusion at 18 units/kg/h. Adjust based on coagulation testing (PTT). DVT prophylaxis: 5000 units SC q8–12h. Low-dose for prevention of thromboembolism in pregnancy: 5,000–10,000 units SC q12h. Treatment of thromboembolism in pregnancy: 80 units/kg IV load, then infuse 18 units/kg/h with dose titrated to achieve full anticoagulation for ≥5 d. Then continue via SC route with ≥10,000 units SC q8–12h adjusted to achieve PTT of 1.5–2.5 × control. To avoid unwanted anticoagulation during delivery, stop SC heparin 24 h before elective induction of labor.

PEDS - Venous thrombosis/pulmonary embolus treatment: Load 50 units/kg IV, then 25 units/kg/h infusion.

UNAPPROVED ADULT - Venous thrombosis/pulmonary embolus treatment: Load 333 units/kg SC, then 250 units/kg SC q12h based on max 100 kg weight. Adjust to achieve goal PTT 1.5–2 × control (approximately 50–70 sec). Anticoagulation for acute MI not treated with thrombolytics: 75 units/kg IV load, then initiate infusion at 1,000–1,200 units/h adjusted to achieve PTT of 1.5–2.5 × control. Unstable angina/non ST-elevation MI: 60–70 units/kg IV load (max 5000 units), then initiate infusion at 12–15 units/kg/h (max 1000 units) and adjust to achieve goal PTT 1.5–2.5 × control. Adjunct to thrombolytics for acute MI. For use with alteplase, reteplase, or tenecteplase: 60 units/kg IV load (max 4,000 units), then initial infusion 12 units/kg/h (max 1,000 units/h) adjusted to achieve PTT 1.5–2 × control (approximately 50–70 sec). Maintain for ≥48 h, duration based on concomitant therapy and patient thromboembolic risk. For use with streptokinase: start ≥4 h after start of streptokinase and PTT <70 sec; 12,500 units SC q12h. IV heparin only for patients receiving streptokinase who are at high risk for systemic/ venous thromboembolism, duration based on concomitant therapy and patient thromboembolic risk.

UNAPPROVED PEDS - Venous thrombosis/pulmonary embolus treatment: Load 75 units/kg IV over 10 min, then 28 units/kg/h if age <1 yo, 20 units/kg/h if age >1 yo.

FORMS - Generic only: 1000, 2500, 5000, 7500, 10,000, 20,000 units/mL in various vial and syringe sizes.

NOTES - Beware of heparin-induced thrombocytopenia (HIT; immune-mediated thrombocytopenia associated with thrombotic events), elevated LFTs, hyperkalemia/ hypoaldosteronism. HIT can occur up to several wk after heparin discontinued. Osteoporosis with long-term use. Bleeding risk increased by high dose; concomitant thrombolytic or platelet GPIIb/IIIa receptor inhibitor; recent surgery, trauma, or invasive procedure; concomitant hemostatic defect. Monitor platelets, hemoglobin, stool for occult blood. Anti-Xa is an alternative to PTT for monitoring. Drug effect can be reversed with protamine.

**TINZAPARIN** *(Innohep)* ▶K ♀B ▶+ $$$$$

ADULT - DVT with/without pulmonary embolus: 175 units/kg SC daily for ≥6 d & until adequate anticoagulation with warfarin.

PEDS - Not approved in children.

UNAPPROVED ADULT - Treatment of venous thromboembolism in pregnancy: 175 units/kg SC daily.

FORMS - Trade only: 20,000 anti-Xa units/mL, 2 mL multi-dose vial.

NOTES - Contraindicated if history of heparin-induced thrombocytopenia, or allergy to heparin, pork, sulfites, or benzyl alcohol. Can cause thrombocytopenia, priapism (rare), increased AST/ALT. Tinzaparin may slightly prolong PT; draw blood for INR just before giving tinzaparin. Use caution and consider monitoring anti-Xa levels if morbidly obese, underweight, pregnant, or renal dysfunction. Drug effect can be reversed with protamine.

| WEIGHT-BASED HEPARIN DOSING FOR DVT/PE* |
|---|
| Initial dose: 80 units/kg IV bolus, then 18 units/kg/h. Check PTT in 6 h. |
| PTT <35 sec (<1.2 × control): 80 units/kg IV bolus, then ↑ infusion rate by 4 units/kg/h. |
| PTT 35–45 sec (1.2–1.5 × control): 40 units/kg IV bolus, then ↑ infusion by 2 units/kg/h. |
| PTT 46–70 sec (1.5–2.3 × control): No change. |
| PTT 71–90 sec (2.3–3 × control): ↑ infusion rate by 2 units/kg/h. |
| PTT >90 sec (>3 × control): Hold infusion for 1 h, then ↑ infusion rate by 3 units/kg/h. |

*PTT = Activated partial thromboplastin time. Reagent-specific target PTT may differ; use institutional nomogram when available. Consider establishing a max bolus dose/max initial infusion rate or use an adjusted body weight in obesity. Monitor PTT 6 h after heparin initiation and 6 h after each dosage adjustment. When PTT is stable within therapeutic range, monitor every morning. Therapeutic PTT range corresponds to anti-factor Xa activity of 0.3-0.7 units/mL. Check platelets between d 3 and 5. Can begin warfarin on 1st d of heparin; continue heparin for ≥4 to 5 d of combined therapy. Adapted from *Ann Intern Med* 1993;119:874; *Chest* 2008:133:463S-464S, *Circulation* 2001; 103:2994.

## HEMATOLOGY: Anticoagulants—Other

**ARGATROBAN ▶L ♀B ▶- $$$$$**
ADULT - Prevention/treatment of thrombosis in heparin-induced thrombocytopenia: Start 2 mcg/kg/min IV infusion. Get PTT at baseline and 2 h after starting infusion. Adjust dose (up to 10 mcg/kg/min) until PTT is 1.5–3 times baseline (but not >100 sec). Percutaneous coronary intervention in those with or at risk for heparin-induced thrombocytopenia: Bolus 350 mcg/kg IV over 3 to 5 min then 25 mcg/kg/min infusion. Target activated clotting time (ACT: 300–450 sec). If ACT<300 sec, give 150 mcg/kg bolus and increase infusion rate to 30 mcg/kg/min. If ACT >450 sec, reduce infusion rate to 15 mcg/kg/min. Maintain ACT 300–450 sec for the duration of the procedure.
PEDS - Not approved in children.
NOTES - Argatroban prolongs INR with warfarin; discontinue when INR >4 on combined therapy, recheck INR in 4–6 h and restart argatroban if INR subtherapeutic. Dosage reduction recommended in liver dysfunction.

**BIVALIRUDIN (*Angiomax*) ▶proteolysis/K ♀B ▶? $$$$$**
ADULT - Anticoagulation in patients undergoing PCI (including patients with or at risk of heparin-induced thrombocytopenia or heparin-induced thrombocytopenia and thrombosis syndrome): 0.75 mg/kg IV bolus prior to intervention, then 1.75 mg/kg/h for duration of procedure (with provisional Gp IIb/IIIa inhibition) and optionally up to 4 h post-procedure. For CrCl <30 mL/min, reduce infusion dose to 1 mg/kg/h after bolus. For patients on dialysis, reduce infusion dose to 0.25 mg/kg/h. Use with aspirin 300–325 mg PO daily. Additional bolus of 0.3 mg/kg if activated clotting time <225 sec. Can additionally infuse 0.2 mg/kg/h for up to 20 h more.
PEDS - Not approved in children.
UNAPPROVED ADULT - Anticoagulation with streptokinase thrombolysis in ST elevation MI & known heparin-induced thrombocytopenia, start 3 min before streptokinase: 0.25 mg/kg bolus followed by 0.5 mg/kg/h for first 12 h, then 0.25 mg/kg/h for subsequent 36 h (consider dose reduction if PTT >75 sec within first 12 h). Acute coronary syndrome (with or without Gp IIb/IIIa inhibition): 0.1 mg/kg bolus followed by 0.25 mg/kg/h. If PCI, then additional bolus 0.5 mg/kg then 1.75 mg/kg/h. Use with aspirin.
NOTES - Contraindicated in active major bleeding. Monitor activated clotting time. Former trade name Hirulog.

| THERAPEUTIC GOALS FOR ANTICOAGULATION | |
|---|---|
| INR Range* | Indication |
| 2.0–3.0 | Atrial fibrillation, deep venous thrombosis†, pulmonary embolism†, bioprosthetic heart valve, mechanical prosthetic heart valve (aortic position, bileaflet or tilting disk with normal sinus rhythm and normal left atrium) |
| 2.5–3.5 | Mechanical prosthetic heart valve: (1) mitral position, (2) aortic position with atrial fibrillation, (3) caged ball or caged disk |

*Aim for an INR in the middle of the INR range (eg, 2.5 for range of 2–3 and 3.0 for range of 2.5–3.5). Adapted from: *Chest* 2008; 133: 456-7S, 459S, 547S, 594-5S; see this manuscript for additional information and other indications.
†For first-event unprovoked DVT/PE, after 3 mo of therapy at goal INR 2-3, may consider low-intensity therapy (INR range 1.5-2.0) in patients with strong preference for less frequent INR testing.

## WARFARIN—SELECTED DRUG INTERACTIONS

Assume possible interactions with any new medication. When starting/stopping a medication, the INR should be checked at least weekly for ≥2-3 wk and dose adjusted accordingly. For further information regarding mechanism or management, refer to the Tarascon Pocket Pharmacopoeia drug interactions database (PDA edition). Similarly monitor if significant change in diet (including supplements) or illness resulting in decreased oral intake.

### Increased anticoagulant effect of warfarin/Increased risk of bleeding

*Monitor INR when agents below started, stopped, or dosage changed. Consider alternative agent.*
acetaminophen ≥2 g/day for ≥3-4 days, allopurinol, amiodarone*, amprenavir, **anabolic steroids**, aspirin¶, cefixime, cefoperazone, celecoxib, chloramphenicol, cimetidine†, **corticosteroids**, danazol, danshen, delavirdine, disulfiram, dong quai , erlotinib, etravirine, **fibrates**, fish oil, fluconazole, **fluoroquinolones**, fluorouracil, fluvoxamine, fosphenytoin (acute), garlic supplements, gemcitabine, gemfibrozil, glucosamine-chondroitin, ginkgo, ifosfamide, imatinib, isoniazid, itraconazole, ketoconazole, leflunomide, lepirudin, levothyroxine#, **macrolides**‡, metronidazole, miconazole (intravaginal), neomycin (PO for >1–2 days), **NSAIDs**¶, olsalazine, omeprazole, paroxetine, penicillin (high-dose IV), pentoxifylline, phenytoin (acute), propafenone, propoxyphene, quinidine, quinine, **statins**§, sulfinpyrazone (with later inhibition), **sulfonamides**, tamoxifen, **testosterones**, **tetracyclines**, tramadol, tigecycline, tipranavir, tricyclic ≥, valproate, voriconazole, vorinostat, vitamin A (high-dose), vitamin E, zafirlukast, zileuton

### Decreased anticoagulant effect of warfarin/Increased risk of thrombosis

*Monitor INR when agents below started, stopped, or dosage changed. Consider alternative agent.*
Aminoglutethimide, aprepitant, azathioprine, barbiturates, bosentan, carbamazepine, coenzyme Q-10, dicloxacillin, fosphenytoin (chronic), ginseng (American), griseofulvin, mercaptopurine, mesalamine, methimazole#, mitotane, nafcillin, oral contraceptives**, phenytoin (chronic), primidone, propylthiouracil#, raloxifene, ribavirin, rifabutin, rifampin, rifapentine, ritonavir, St John's wort, vitamin C (high-dose).
*Use alternative to agents below. Or give at different times of day and monitor INR when agent started, stopped, or dose/dosing schedule changed*
cholestyramine, colestipol††, sucralfate

*Interaction may be delayed; monitor INR for several wk after starting & several mo after stopping amiodarone. May need to decrease warfarin dose by 33–50%.
† Famotidine, nizatidine or ranitidine are alternatives.
‡ Azithromycin appears to have lower risk of interaction than clarithromycin or erythromycin.
§ Pravastatin appears to have lower risk of interaction.
# Hyperthyroidism/thyroid replacement increases metabolism of clotting factors, increasing response to warfarin therapy and increased bleed risk (typically requires lowering warfarin dose).
¶ Does not necessarily increase INR, but increases bleeding risk. Check INR frequently and monitor for GI bleeding.
**Do not necessarily ↓ INR, but may induce hypercoagulability.
†† Likely lower risk than cholestyramine
Adapted from: Coumadin® product information; *Am Fam Phys* 1999;59:635; *Chest* 2004; 126: 204S; Hansten and Horn's Drug Interactions Analysis and Management; *Ann Intern Med* 2004;141:23; *Arch Intern Med* 2005;165:1095. *Tarascon Pocket Pharmacopoeia drug interactions database (PDA edition).*

**LEPIRUDIN (*Refludan*)** ▶K ♀B ▶? $$$$$
ADULT - Anticoagulation in heparin-induced thrombocytopenia (HIT) and associated thromboembolic disease: Bolus 0.4 mg/kg up to 44 mg IV over 15–20 sec, then infuse 0.15 mg/kg/h up to 16.5 mg/h × 2–10 d. Adjust dose to maintain APTT ratio of 1.5–2.5.
PEDS - Not approved in children.
UNAPPROVED ADULT - Adjunct to thrombolytics for acute MI in patients with HIT: 0.1 mg/kg IV bolus, then infuse 0.15 mg/h.
NOTES - May increase INR. Dosage adjustment for renal impairment: Bolus 0.2 mg/kg IV followed by 0.075 mg/kg/h for CrCl 45–60 mL/min, 0.045 mg/kg/h for CrCl 30–44 mL/min, 0.0225 mg/kg/h for CrCl 15–29 mL/min. Hemodialysis/CrCl <15 mL/

min: Bolus 0.1 mg/kg IV qod if APTT ratio <1.5. Severe anaphylactic reactions resulting in death have been reported upon initial or re-exposure.
**WARFARIN (*Coumadin, Jantoven*)** ▶L ♀X ▶+ $
WARNING - Many important drug interactions that increase/decrease INR, see table.
ADULT - Oral anticoagulation for prophylaxis/treatment of DVT/PE, thromboembolic complications associated with A-fib, mechanical and bioprosthetic heart valves: Start 2–5 mg PO daily × 3–4 d, then adjust dose to maintain therapeutic PT/INR. Consider initial dose <5 mg if elderly, malnourished, liver disease, or high bleeding risk. Target INR of 2–3 for most indications, 2.5–3.5 for mechanical heart valves. See table for specific target INR and duration of anticoagulation.

**WARFARIN** (*cont.*)

PEDS - Not approved in children.

UNAPPROVED ADULT - Oral anticoagulation treatment of acute DVT/PE: Start 5–10 mg PO daily (with ≥5 d of LMWH/heparin) until target INR (2.0 to 3.0) reached. See table for target INR and duration of anticoagulation for specific indications.

FORMS - Generic/Trade: Tabs 1, 2, 2.5, 3, 4, 5, 6, 7.5, 10 mg.

NOTES - ACCP guidelines suggest initial dose of 2–10 mg, with lower doses if high risk of bleeding, elderly,

malnourished or congestive heart failure. Consider lower initial dose if genetic variation in CYP2C9 and VKORC1 enzymes. Tissue necrosis in protein C or S deficiency. Many important drug interactions that increase/decrease INR, see table for significant drug interactions. Warfarin onset of action is within 24 h, peak effect delayed by 3–4 d. Most patients can begin warfarin at the same time as heparin/LMWH. Continue heparin/LMWH treatment for thrombosis until the INR has been in the therapeutic range for ≥2 d. See phytonadione (vitamin K) entry for management of abnormally high INR.

## HEMATOLOGY: Antihemophilic Agents

**ANTI-INHIBITOR COAGULANT COMPLEX** (*Feiba VH, ✦Feiba VH Immuno*) ▶L ♀C ▶? $$$$$

ADULT - Hemophilia A or B with factor VIII inhibitors, XI and XII (if surgery or active bleeding): 50–100 units/kg IV; specific dose and frequency based on site of bleeding, max 200 units/kg/d.

PEDS - Not approved in children.

NOTES - Contraindicated if normal coagulation. Human plasma product, thus risk of infectious agent transmission. Avoid in active or impending disseminated intravascular coagulation (DIC).

**FACTOR IX** (*Benefix, Mononine, ✦Immunine VH*) ▶L ♀C ▶? $$$$$

ADULT - Hemophilia B: individualize factor IX dose.

PEDS - Hemophilia B: individualize factor IX dose.

FORMS - Specific formulation usually chosen by specialist in Hemophilia Treatment Center.

NOTES - Risk of HIV/hepatitis transmission varies by product. Products that contain factors II, VII, & X may cause thrombosis in at-risk patients. Stop infusion if signs of DIC.

**FACTOR VIIA** (*NovoSeven, NovoSeven RT, ✦Niastase*) ▶L ♀C ▶? $$$$$

ADULT - Hemophilia A or B: individualize factor VIIa dose.

PEDS - Hemophilia A or B: individualize factor VIIa dose.

UNAPPROVED ADULT - Reversal of excessive warfarin anticoagulation (INR >10): 15–20 mcg/kg IV over 3–5 min. Intracerebral hemorrhage (within 4 h of symptom onset): 40–160 mcg/kg IV over

1 to 2 min. Perioperative blood loss in retropubic prostatectomy: 20 or 40 mcg/kg IV bolus.

FORMS - Trade only: 1200, 2400, 4800 mcg/vial.

NOTES - Contraindicated with hypersensitivity to mouse, hamster or bovine proteins. Patients with DIC, advanced atherosclerotic disease, crush injury or septicemia may be at increase thrombotic risk. If DIC or thrombosis confirmed, reduce dose or stop treatment depending on symptoms.

**FACTOR VIII** (*Advate, Alphanate, Helixate, Hemofil M, Humate P, Koate, Kogenate, Monoclate P, Monarc-M, Recombinate, ReFacto, Xyntha*) ▶L ♀C ▶? $$$$$

ADULT - Hemophilia A: individualize factor VIII dose. Surgical procedures in patients with von Willebrand disease (Alphanate, Humate P): individualized dosing. Bleeding in patients with von Willebrand disease (Humate P): individualized dosing.

PEDS - Hemophilia A: individualize factor VIII dose.

FORMS - Specific formulation usually chosen by specialist in Hemophilia Treatment Center. Recombinant formulations: Advate, Helixate, Kogenate, Recombinate, ReFacto, Xyntha. Human plasma-derived formulations: Alphanate, Hemofil M, Humate P, Koate, Monoclate P, Monarc-M.

NOTES - Risk of HIV/hepatitis transmission varies by product; no such risk with recombinant product. Reduced response with development of factor VIII inhibitors. Hemolysis with large/repeated doses in patients with A, B, AB blood type.

## HEMATOLOGY: Colony Stimulating Factors

**DARBEPOETIN** (*Aranesp, NESP*) ▶cellular sialidases, L ♀C ▶? $$$$$

WARNING - Increased risk of death and serious cardiovascular events, including arterial and venous thrombotic events; may shorten time to tumor progression in cancer patients. To minimize risks, use lowest dose to minimum level to avoid blood transfusion; individualize dosing to maintain Hb 10–12 g/dL; risks have not been excluded with targeted Hb <12 g/dL. Consider antithrombotic

DVT prophylaxis. Not approved for use in cancer patients with anemia not due to concurrent myelosuppressive chemotherapy; discontinue when chemotherapy completed. Not for patients receiving myelosuppressive chemotherapy in whom anticipated outcome is cure.

ADULT - Anemia of chronic renal failure: 0.45 mcg/kg IV/SC q weekly, or SC q 2 wk for some patients. Maintenance dose may be lower in predialysis patients than dialysis patients. Adjust

**(cont.)**

**DARBEPOETIN** (cont.)

dose based on Hb to maintain Hg 10–12 g/dL. Anemia in cancer chemo patients: initially 2.25 mcg/kg SC q wk, or 500 mcg SC every 3 wk. For weekly administration, max 4.5 mcg/kg/dose. Adjust dose based on Hb to maintain lowest level to avoid transfusion. Weekly dose conversion to darbepoetin (D) from erythropoietin (E): 6.25 mcg D for <2,500 units E; 12.5 mcg D for 2,500–4,999 units E; 25 mcg D for 5,000–10,999 units E; 40 mcg D for 11,000–17,999 units E; 60 mcg D for 18,000–33,999 units E; 100 mcg D for 34,000–89,999 units E; 200 mcg D for ≥90,000 units E. Give D once weekly for patients taking E 2–3 times weekly; give D once every 2 wk for patients taking E once weekly. Monitor Hb weekly until stable, then at least monthly.

PEDS - Not approved in children.

UNAPPROVED ADULT - Chemotherapy-induced anemia: 3 mcg/kg or 200 mcg SC q2 wk.

FORMS - Trade only: All forms are available with or without albumin. Single-dose vials 25, 40, 60, 100, 200, 300, 500 mcg/1 mL, and 150 mcg/0.75 mL. Single-dose prefilled syringes or autoinjectors - 25 mcg/0.42 mL, 40 mcg/0.4 mL, 60 mcg/0.3 mL, 100 mcg/0.5 mL, 150 mcg/0.3 mL, 200 mcg/0.4 mL, 300 mcg/0.6 mL, 500 mcg/1 mL.

NOTES - May exacerbate HTN; contraindicated if uncontrolled HTN. Not for immediate correction of anemia. Evaluate iron stores before and during treatment; most patients eventually require iron supplements. Consider other causes of anemia if no response. Use only one dose per vial/syringe; discard any unused portion. Do not shake. Protect from light.

**EPOETIN ALFA (Epogen, Procrit, erythropoietin alpha, ✦Eprex)** ▶L ♀C ▶? $$$$$

WARNING - Increased risk of death and serious cardiovascular events, including arterial and venous thrombotic events; may shorten time to tumor progression in cancer patients. To minimize risks, use lowest dose to minimum level to avoid blood transfusion; individualize dosing to maintain Hb 10–12 g/dL; risks have not been excluded with targeted Hb <12 g/dL. Consider antithrombotic DVT prophylaxis. Not approved for use in cancer patients with anemia not due to concurrent myelosuppressive chemotherapy; discontinue when chemotherapy completed. Not for patients receiving myelosuppressive chemotherapy in whom anticipated outcome is cure.

ADULT - Anemia of chronic renal failure: Initial dose 50–100 units/kg IV/SC 3 times/wk. Adjust dose based on Hb to maintain Hg 10–12 g/dL. Zidovudine-induced anemia in HIV-infected patients: 100–300 units/kg IV/SC 3 times/wk. Anemia in cancer chemo patients: 150–300 units/kg SC 3 times/wk or 40,000 units SC once/wk. Monitor Hb weekly until stable, then at least monthly. Adjust dose based on Hb to maintain lowest level to avoid transfusion. Reduction of allogeneic blood transfusion in surgical patients: 300 units/kg/d SC × 10 d preop, on the d of surgery, and 4 d postop. Or 600 units/kg SC

once weekly starting 21 d preop and ending on d of surgery (4 doses).

PEDS - Not approved in children.

UNAPPROVED PEDS - Anemia of chronic renal failure: Initial dose 50–100 units/kg IV/SC 3 times/wk. Zidovudine-induced anemia in HIV-infected patients: 100 units/kg SC 3 times/wk; max of 300 units/kg/dose.

FORMS - Trade only: Single-dose 1 mL vials 2,000, 3,000, 4,000, 10,000, 40,000 units/mL. Multi-dose vials 10,000 units/mL 2 mL & 20,000 units/mL 1 mL.

NOTES - May exacerbate HTN; contraindicated if uncontrolled HTN. Not for immediate correction of anemia. Evaluate iron stores before and during treatment; most patients eventually require iron supplements. Consider other causes of anemia if no response. Single-dose vials contain no preservatives. Use one dose per vial; do not re-enter vial. Discard unused portion.

**EPOETIN BETA (Mircera, erythropoietin beta)** ▶L ♀C ▶? $$$$$

WARNING - Increased risk of death and serious cardiovascular events, including arterial and venous thrombotic events; may shorten time to tumor progression in cancer patients. To minimize risks, use lowest dose to minimum Hb level to avoid blood transfusion; individualize dosing to maintain Hb 10–12 g/dL; risks have not been excluded with targeted Hb <12 g/dL. Consider antithrombotic DVT prophylaxis. Not indicated for treatment of anemia due to cancer chemotherapy.

ADULT - Approved, but not yet available in US. Anemia in chronic renal failure: 0.6 mcg/kg IV/SC q2 wk; may be given q mo in some patients. Adjust dose based on Hb. Monitor Hb q2 wk until stable, then at least monthly. Target Hb not to exceed 12 g/dL. Reduce dose by 25% if Hb is increasing and approaches 12 g/dL or if Hb increases by 1 g/dL per 2 wk time period. Increase or decrease dose by approximately 25% to maintain desired Hb.

PEDS - Not approved in children.

FORMS - Trade only: Single-dose 1 mL vials 50, 100, 200, 300, 400, 600 or 1000 mcg/mL. Single-use pre-filled syringes: 50, 75, 100, 150, 200, 250 mcg/0.3 mL; 400, 600, 800 mcg/0.6mL.

NOTES - Approved, but not yet available in US. See PI for conversion doses from other erythropoiesis-stimulating agents. May exacerbate HTN; contraindicated if uncontrolled HTN. Monitor for seizures and premonitory neurologic symptoms. Discontinue if pure red cell aplasia suspected. Not for immediate correction of anemia. Evaluate iron stores before and during treatment; most patients eventually require iron supplements. Consider other causes of anemia if no response. Contains no preservatives; discard unused portion.

**FILGRASTIM (G-CSF, Neupogen)** ▶L ♀C ▶? $$$$$

ADULT - Reduction of febrile neutropenia after chemo for non-myeloid malignancies: 5 mcg/kg/d SC/IV for ≤2 wk until post-nadir ANC is ≥10,000/mm³. Can increase by 5 mcg/kg/d with each cycle prn.

**FILGRASTIM** (cont.)
PEDS - Reduction of febrile neutropenia after che-motherapy for non-myeloid malignancies: 5 mcg/kg/d SC/IV.
UNAPPROVED ADULT - AIDS: 0.3–3.6 mcg/kg/d.
FORMS - Trade only: Single-dose vials 300 mcg/1 mL, 480 mcg/1.6 mL. Single-dose syringes 300 mcg/0.5 mL, 480 mcg/0.8 mL.
NOTES - Allergic-type reactions, bone pain, cutane-ous vasculitis. Do not give within 24 h before/after cytotoxic chemotherapy. Store in refrigerator; use within 24 h when kept at room temperature.

**OPRELVEKIN** (*Neumega*) ▶K ♀C ▶? $$$$$
WARNING - Risk of allergic reactions and anaphylaxis.
ADULT - Prevention of severe thrombocytopenia after chemo for nonmyeloid malignancies: 50 mcg/kg SC daily starting 6–24 h after chemo and continuing until post-nadir platelet count is ≥50,000 cells/mcL.
PEDS - Not approved in children. Safe and effective dose not established. Papilledema with 100 mcg/kg; 50 mcg/kg ineffective.

FORMS - Trade only: 5 mg single-dose vials with diluent.
NOTES - Fluid retention - monitor fluid and electro-lyte balance. Transient atrial arrhythmias, visual blurring, papilledema.

**PEGFILGRASTIM** (*Neulasta*) ▶Plasma ♀C ▶? $$$$$
WARNING - Do not use if <45 kg.
ADULT - To reduce febrile neutropenia after chemo for non-myeloid malignancies: 6 mg SC once each chemo cycle.
PEDS - Not approved in children.
FORMS - Trade only: Single-dose syringes 6 mg/0.6 mL.
NOTES - Bone pain common. Do not give <14 d before or 24 h after cytotoxic chemo. Store in refrigerator. Stable at room temperature for ≤48 h. Protect from light

**SARGRAMOSTIM** (*GM-CSF, Leukine*) ▶L ♀C ▶? $$$$$
ADULT - Specialized dosing for leukemia, bone mar-row transplantation.
PEDS - Not approved in children.

## HEMATOLOGY: Other Hematological Agents

**NOTE:** See endocrine section for vitamins and minerals.

**AMINOCAPROIC ACID** (*Amicar*) ▶K ♀D ▶? $$
ADULT - To improve hemostasis when fibrinolysis contributes to bleeding: 4–5 g IV/PO over 1h, then 1 g/h for 8 h or until bleeding controlled.
PEDS - Not approved in children.
UNAPPROVED ADULT - Prevention of recurrent sub-arachnoid hemorrhage: 6 g IV/PO q4h (6 doses/d). Reduction of postop bleeding after cardiopulmo-nary bypass: 5 g IV, then 1 g/h × 6–8 h.
UNAPPROVED PEDS - To improve hemostasis when fibrinolysis contributes to bleeding: 100 mg/kg or 3 g/m² IV infusion during first h, then continuous infusion of 33.3 mg/kg/h or 1 g/m²/h. Max dose of 18 g/m²/d. IV prep contains benzyl alcohol - do not use in newborns.
FORMS - Generic/Trade: Syrup or oral soln 250 mg/mL, tabs 500 mg.
NOTES - Contraindicated in active intravascu-lar clotting. Do not use in DIC without heparin. Can cause intrarenal thrombosis, hyperkalemia. Skeletal muscle weakness, necrosis with pro-longed use - monitor CPK. Use with estrogen/oral contraceptives can cause hypercoagulability. Rapid IV administration can cause hypotension, bradycardia, arrhythmia.

**ANAGRELIDE** (*Agrylin*) ▶LK ♀C ▶? $$$$$
ADULT - Thrombocythemia due to myeloproliferative disorders (including essential thrombocythemia): Start 0.5 mg PO qid or 1 mg PO bid, then after 1 wk adjust to lowest effective dose that main-tains the platelet count <600,000/mcL. Max of 10 mg/d or 2.5 mg as a single dose. Usual dose 1.5 to 3 mg/d.
PEDS - Limited data. Thrombocythemia due to myeloproliferative disorders (including essential

thrombocythemia): Start 0.5 mg PO daily, then after 1 wk adjust to lowest effective dose that maintains platelet count <600,000/mcL. Max 10 mg/d or 2.5 mg as a single dose. Usual dose 1.5 to 3 mg/d.
FORMS - Generic/Trade: Caps, 0.5, 1 mg.
NOTES - Caution in patients with heart disease—may cause vasodilation, tachycardia, palpitations, heart failure. Contraindicated in severe hepatic impairment, use with caution in mild to moderate hepatic impairment. Dosage should be increased by not more than 0.5 mg/d in any one wk.

**ECULIZUMAB** (*Soliris*) ▶Serum ♀C ▶? $$$$$
ADULT - Reduction of hemolysis in paroxysmal noc-turnal hemoglobinuria: 600 mg IV infusion q7d × 4 wk, then increase to 900 mg for fifth dose 7d later, then 900 mg q14d. Administer infusion over 35 min.
PEDS - Not approved in children.
NOTES - Contraindicated if there is active menin-gococcal infection or without current meningo-coccal vaccination. Administer meningococcal vaccine ≥2 wk prior to therapy and revaccinate according to current guidelines. Caution if sys-temic infection. Dose may be given within 2 d of scheduled dosing date. Monitor LDH for response. Need to monitor hemolysis for ≥8 wk after discontinuation.

**HYDROXYUREA** (*Hydrea, Droxia*) ▶LK ♀D ▶- $ varies by therapy
WARNING - Mutagenic and clastogenic; may cause secondary leukemia. Instruct patients to report promptly fever, sore throat, signs of local infec-tion, bleeding from any site, or symptoms sugges-tive of anemia. Cutaneous vasculitic toxicities,
**(cont.)**

**HYDROXYUREA (cont.)**

including vasculitic ulcerations and gangrene, have been reported most often in patients on interferon therapy.

ADULT - Sickle cell anemia (Droxia): Start 15 mg/kg PO daily while monitoring CBC q 2 wk. If WBC ≥ 2500/mm³, Plt ≥ 95,000/mm³, Hb > 5.3 g/dl, then increase dose q 12 wk by 5 mg/kg/d (max 35 mg/kg/d). Give concomitant folic acid 1 mg/d. Chemotherapy: doses will vary by indication, eg, melanoma, CML, recurrent, metastatic or inoperable carcinoma of the ovary, squamous cell carcinoma of the head and neck, acute leukemia.

PEDS - Not approved in children.

UNAPPROVED ADULT - Essential thrombocythemia at high risk for thrombosis: 0.5–1 g PO daily adjusted to keep platelets <400/mm³. Also has been used for HIV, psoriasis, polycythemia vera.

UNAPPROVED PEDS - Sickle cell anemia.

FORMS - Generic/Trade: Cap 500 mg. Trade only: (Droxia) Caps 200, 300, 400 mg.

NOTES - Reliable contraception is recommended. Monitor CBC & renal function. Elderly may need lower doses. Minimize exposure to the drug by wearing gloves during handling.

**PROTAMINE** ▶PLASMA ♀C ▶? $

ADULT - Heparin overdose: 1 mg antagonizes ~100 units heparin. Give IV over 10 min in doses of not >50 mg.

PEDS - Not approved in children.

UNAPPROVED ADULT - Reversal of low molecular weight heparin: 1 mg protamine per 100 anti-Xa units of dalteparin or tinzaparin. Give additional 0.5 mg protamine per 100 anti-Xa units of tinzaparin if PTT remains prolonged 2–4 h after first infusion of protamine. 1 mg protamine per 1 mg enoxaparin.

UNAPPROVED PEDS - Heparin overdose: if <30 min since last heparin dose, give 1 mg protamine per 100 units of heparin received; if 30–60 min since last heparin dose, give 0.5–0.75 mg protamine per 100 units of heparin received; if 60–120 min since last heparin dose, give 0.375–0.5 mg protamine per 100 units of heparin; if >120 min since last heparin dose, give 0.25–0.375 mg protamine per 100 units of heparin.

NOTES - Severe hypotension/anaphylactoid reaction with too rapid administration. Allergic reactions in patients with fish allergy, previous exposure to protamine (including insulin). Risk of allergy unclear in infertile/vasectomized men with anti-protamine antibodies. Additional doses of protamine may be required in some situations (neutralization of SC heparin, heparin rebound after cardiac surgery). Monitor APTT to confirm heparin neutralization.

**PROTEIN C CONCENTRATE (Ceprotin)** ▶Serum ♀C ▶? $$$$$

ADULT - Severe congenital protein C deficiency (prevention and treatment of venous thrombosis and purpura fulminans): Individualized dosing.

PEDS - Severe congenital protein C deficiency (prevention and treatment of venous thrombosis and purpura fulminans): Individualized dosing.

NOTES - Product contains heparin; do not use if history of heparin induced thrombocytopenia. Check platelets and discontinue if heparin induced thrombocytopenia suspected. Product contains sodium. Made from pooled human plasma, may transmit infectious agents.

**THROMBIN - TOPICAL (Evithrom, Recothrom, Thrombin-JMI)** ▶? ♀C ▶? $$$

WARNING - The bovine form (Thrombin-JMI) has been associated with rare but potentially fatal abnormalities in hemostasis ranging from asymptomatic alterations in PT and/or aPTT to severe bleeding or thrombosis. Hemostatic abnormalities are likely due to antibody formation, may cause factor V deficiency, and are more likely with repeated applications. Consult hematologist if abnormal coagulation, bleeding or thrombosis after topical thrombin use.

ADULT - Hemostatic aid for minor bleeding: Apply topically to site of bleeding; dose depends on area to be treated.

PEDS - Hemostatic aid for minor bleeding (Evithrom): Apply topically to site of bleeding; dose depends on area to be treated. Recothrom/Thrombin-JMI not approved in children.

NOTES - Do not inject; drug for topical use only. Do not use for severe or brisk arterial bleeding. Thaw Evithrom prior to use. Reconstitute Recothrom and Thrombin-JMI prior to use. Evithrom is human-derived and carries the risk of viral transmission. Recothrom is a recombinant product; risk of allergic reaction with known hypersensitivity to snake proteins; contraindicated with hypersensitivity to hamster proteins. Thrombin-JMI is a bovine origin product; contraindicated with hypersensitivity to products of bovine origin.

**TRANEXAMIC ACID (Cyklokapron)** ▶K ♀B ▶- $$$

ADULT - Prophylaxis/reduction of bleeding during tooth extraction in hemophilia patients: 10 mg/kg IV immediately before surgery, then 25 mg/kg PO 3–4 times/d for 2–8 d post surgery. Additional regimens: 10 mg/kg IV 3–4 times/d if intolerant of oral therapies or 25 mg/kg PO 3–4 times/d beginning the day before surgery.

PEDS - Not approved in children.

NOTES - Dose adjustment in renal impairment-Creat 1.36–2.83 mg/dL: 10 mg/kg IV bid or 15 mg/kg PO bid. Creat 2.83–5.66 mg/dL: 10 mg/kg IV daily or 15 mg/kg PO daily. Creat >5.66 mg/dL: 10 mg/kg IV q48h or 5 mg/kg IV q24h; 15 mg/kg PO q48h or 7.5 mg/kg PO q24h.

## HERBAL & ALTERNATIVE THERAPIES

**NOTE:** In the US, herbal and alternative therapy products are regulated as dietary supplements, not drugs. Premarketing evaluation and FDA approval are not required unless specific therapeutic claims are made. Since these products are not required to demonstrate efficacy, it is unclear whether many of them have health benefits. In addition, there may be considerable variability in content from lot to lot or between products. See www.tarascon.com/herbals for the evidence-based efficacy ratings used by Tarascon editorial staff.

**ALOE VERA (*acemannan, burn plant*)** ▶LK ♀oral- topical +? ▶oral- topical +? $
UNAPPROVED ADULT - Topical: Efficacy unclear for seborrheic dermatitis, psoriasis, genital herpes, partial-thickness skin burns. Gel possibly effective for oral lichen planus. Does not prevent radiation-induced skin injury. Do not apply to surgical incisions; impaired healing reported. Oral: Mild to moderate active ulcerative colitis (possibly effective): 100 mL PO bid. Efficacy unclear for type 2 diabetes.
UNAPPROVED PEDS - Not for use in children.
FORMS - Not by prescription.
NOTES - OTC laxatives containing aloe were removed from the US market in 2002 due to concerns about increased risk of colon cancer. International Aloe Science Council seal may help ensure aloe content.

**ANDROSTENEDIONE (*andro*)** ▶L, peripheral conversion to estrogens & androgens ♀- ▶- $
UNAPPROVED ADULT - Marketed as anabolic steroid to enhance athletic performance. Advise patients against use because of potential for androgenic and estrogenic side effects.
UNAPPROVED PEDS - Not for use in children.
FORMS - Not by prescription.
NOTES - In 2004 FDA warned manufacturers to stop marketing. Also banned by many athletic associations. In theory, chronic use may increase risk of hormone-related cancers (prostate, breast, ovarian). Increase in androgen levels could exacerbate hyperlipidemia.

**ARISTOLOCHIC ACID (*Aristolochia, Asarum, Bragantia*)** ▶? ♀- ▶- $
UNAPPROVED ADULT - Do not use. Was promoted for weight loss.
UNAPPROVED PEDS - Do not use.
FORMS - Not by prescription.
NOTES - Banned by FDA due to risk of nephrotoxicity and cancer. May be present as an adulterant in other Chinese herbal products like Akebia, Clematis, Stephania, and others. Rule out aristolochic acid nephrotoxicity in cases of unexplained renal failure.

**ARNICA (*Arnica montana, leopard's bane, wolf's bane*)** ▶? ♀- ▶- $
UNAPPROVED ADULT - Toxic if taken by mouth. Topical preparations promoted for treatment of skin wounds, bruises, aches, and sprains; but insufficient data to assess efficacy. Do not use on open wounds.

UNAPPROVED PEDS - Not for use in children.
FORMS - Not by prescription.
NOTES - Repeated topical application can cause skin reactions.

**ARTICHOKE LEAF EXTRACT (*Cynara-SL, Cynara scolymus*)** ▶? ♀? ▶? $
UNAPPROVED ADULT - May reduce total cholesterol, but clinical significance is unclear. Cynara-SL is promoted as digestive aid (possibly effective for dyspepsia) at a dose of 1–2 caps PO daily. Does not appear to prevent alcohol-induced hangover.
UNAPPROVED PEDS - Not for use in children.
FORMS - Not by prescription.
NOTES - Advise against use by patients with bile duct obstruction or gallstones. Artichoke leaf is an ingredient in CholesTame and Digestive Formula.

**ASTRAGALUS (*Astragalus membranaceus, huang qi, vetch*)** ▶? ♀? ▶? $
UNAPPROVED ADULT - Used in combination with other herbs in traditional Chinese medicine, but efficacy unclear for CHD, CHF, chronic kidney disease, viral infections, upper respiratory tract infections. Astragalus-based Chinese herbal medicine may improve survival, tumor response, and performance status of patients receiving platinum-based chemotherapy for non-small cell lung cancer.
UNAPPROVED PEDS - Not for use in children.
FORMS - Not by prescription.
NOTES - Not used for >3 wk without close follow-up in traditional Chinese medicine. In theory, may enhance activity of drugs for diabetes, hypertension, and anticoagulation.

**BILBERRY (*Vaccinium myrtillus, huckleberry, Tegens, VMA extract*)** ▶Bile, K ♀- ▶- $
UNAPPROVED ADULT - Cataracts (efficacy unclear): 80–160 mg PO bid-tid of 25% anthocyanosides extract. Insufficient data to evaluate efficacy for macular degeneration. Does not appear effective for improving night vision.
UNAPPROVED PEDS - Not for use in children.
FORMS - Not by prescription.
NOTES - High doses may impair platelet aggregation, affect clotting time, and cause GI distress.

**BITTER MELON (*Momordica charantia, ampalaya, karela*)** ▶? ♀- ▶- $$
UNAPPROVED ADULT - Efficacy unclear for type 2 diabetes. Dose unclear; juice may be more potent than dried fruit powder.

(cont.)

**BITTER MELON** (*cont.*)

UNAPPROVED PEDS - Not for use in children. Two cases of hypoglycemic coma in children ingesting bitter melon tea.

FORMS - Not by prescription.

**BITTER ORANGE** (*Citrus aurantium, Seville orange, Acutrim Natural AM, Dexatrim Natural Ephedrine Free*) ▶ K ♀ - ▶ - $

UNAPPROVED ADULT - Marketed as substitute for ephedra in weight-loss dietary supplements; safety and efficacy not established.

UNAPPROVED PEDS - Not for use in children.

FORMS - Not by prescription.

NOTES - Contains sympathomimetics including synephrine and octopamine. Synephrine banned by some sports organizations. Case reports of stroke and MI in patients taking bitter orange with caffeine. Do not use within 14 d of an MAOI. Juice may inhibit CYP 3A4 metabolism of felodipine and midazolam.

**BLACK COHOSH** (*Cimicifuga racemosa, Remifemin, Menofem*) ▶? ♀ - ▶ - $

UNAPPROVED ADULT - Ineffective for relief of menopausal symptoms.

UNAPPROVED PEDS - Not for use in children.

FORMS - Not by prescription.

NOTES - Do not alter vaginal epithelium, endometrium, or estradiol levels in postmenopausal women.

**BUTTERBUR** (*Petesites hybridus, Petadolex, Petaforce, Tesalin, ZE 339*) ▶? ♀ - ▶ - $

UNAPPROVED ADULT - Migraine prophylaxis (possibly effective): Petadolex 50–75 mg PO bid. Allergic rhinitis prophylaxis (possibly effective): Petadolex 50 mg PO bid or Tesalin (ZE 339; 8 mg petasin/tab) 1 tab PO qid or 2 tabs tid. Efficacy unclear for asthma.

UNAPPROVED PEDS - Not for children.

FORMS - Not by prescription. Standardized pyrrolizidine-free extracts: Petadolex (7.5 mg of petasin & isopetasin/50 mg tab). Tesalin (ZE 339; 8 mg petasin/tab).

NOTES - Do not use raw butterbur; it may contain hepatotoxic pyrrolizidine alkaloids which are removed by processing. Butterbur is related to Asteraceae and Compositae; consider the potential for cross-allergenicity between plants in these families.

**CHAMOMILE** (*Matricaria recutita - German chamomile, Anthemis nobilis - Roman chamomile*) ▶? ♀ - ▶? $

UNAPPROVED ADULT - Promoted as a sedative or anxiolytic, to relieve GI distress, for skin infections or inflammation, many other indications. Efficacy unclear for any indication. Does not appear to reduce mucositis caused by 5-fluorouracil or radiation.

UNAPPROVED PEDS - Supplements not for use in children. Efficacy and safety unclear for treatment of infant colic with multi-ingredient teas/extracts of chamomile, fennel, and lemon balm.

FORMS - Not by prescription.

NOTES - Theoretical concern (no clinical evidence) for interactions due to increased sedation, increased risk of bleeding (contains coumarin derivatives), delayed GI absorption of other drugs (due to anti-spasmodic effect). Increased INR with warfarin attributed to chamomile in single case report.

**CHAPARRAL** (*Larrea divaricata, creosote bush*) ▶? ♀ - ▶ - $

UNAPPROVED ADULT - Do not use. Promoted as cancer cure.

UNAPPROVED PEDS - Not for use in children.

FORMS - Not by prescription.

NOTES - Reports of irreversible liver damage in humans.

**CHASTEBERRY** (*Vitex agnus castus fruit extract, Femaprin*) ▶? ♀ - ▶ - $

UNAPPROVED ADULT - Premenstrual syndrome (possibly effective): 20 mg PO daily of extract ZE 440 (ratio 6–12:1; standardized for casticin).

UNAPPROVED PEDS - Not for use in children.

FORMS - Not by prescription.

NOTES - Liquid formulations may contain alcohol. Avoid concomitant dopamine antagonists such as haloperidol or metoclopramide.

**CHONDROITIN** ▶ K ♀? ▶? $

UNAPPROVED ADULT - Does not appear effective for relief of knee osteoarthritis pain, but possibly reduces joint space narrowing. Glucosamine/Chondroitin Arthritis Intervention Trial (GAIT) did not find improvement in pain of knee OA with chondroitin 400 mg PO tid +/- glucosamine. Glucosamine + chondroitin improved pain in subgroup of patients with moderate to severe knee OA.

UNAPPROVED PEDS - Not for use in children.

FORMS - Not by prescription.

NOTES - Chondroitin content not standardized and known to vary. Cosamin DS contains 3 mg manganese/cap; tolerable upper limit of manganese is 11 mg/d. Some products made from bovine cartilage. Case reports of increased INR/bleeding with warfarin in patient taking chondroitin + glucosamine.

**COENZYME Q10** (*CoQ-10, ubiquinone*) ▶ Bile ♀ - ▶ - $

UNAPPROVED ADULT - Heart failure: 100 mg/d PO divided bid-tid (conflicting clinical trials; may reduce hospitalization, dyspnea, edema, but Am Heart Assoc does not recommend). Statin-induced muscle pain: 100–200 mg PO daily (conflicting clinical trials). Parkinson's disease: 1200 mg/d PO divided qid at meals and hs ($$$$; efficacy unclear; might slow progression slightly, but Am Acad Neurol does not recommend). Study for progression of Huntington's disease was inconclusive. Prevention of migraine: 100 mg PO tid (possibly effective). Efficacy unclear for improving athletic performance. Appears ineffective for diabetes, amyotrophic lateral sclerosis.

UNAPPROVED PEDS - Not for use in children.

FORMS - Not by prescription.

NOTES - Case reports of increased INR with warfarin; but a crossover study did not find an interaction.

**COMFREY (Symphytum officinale)** ▶? ♀- ▶- $
UNAPPROVED ADULT - Do not use, even externally (application on broken skin could lead to systemic absorption). Topical use promoted for bruises, burns and sprains.
UNAPPROVED PEDS - Do not use, even externally (application on broken skin could lead to systemic absorption). Topical use promoted for bruises, burns and sprains.
FORMS - Not by prescription.
NOTES - Reports of fatal hepatic veno-occlusive disease in humans. Contains pyrrolizidine alkaloids. FDA banned comfrey products from US market in 2001.

**CRANBERRY (Cranactin, Vaccinium macrocarpon)** ▶? ♀? ▶? $
UNAPPROVED ADULT - Prevention of UTI (possibly effective): 300 mL/d PO cranberry juice cocktail. Usual dose of cranberry juice extract caps/tabs is 300–400 mg PO bid. Insufficient data to assess efficacy for treatment of UTI. Should not be a substitute for antibiotics in acute UTI.
UNAPPROVED PEDS - Insufficient data to assess efficacy for prevention/treatment of UTI. Does not appear to treat or prevent UTI in children with neurogenic bladder. Should not be a substitute for antibiotics in acute UTI.
FORMS - Not by prescription.
NOTES - Warfarin product labeling advises patients to avoid ingestion of cranberry products based on case reports of increased INRs and bleeding. However, new clinical trials did not find an increase in the INR with cranberry. ~100 calories/6 oz of cranberry juice cocktail. Advise diabetics that some products have high sugar content. Not a substitute for antibiotics to treat UTI. Increases urinary oxalate excretion; may increase risk of oxalate kidney stones.

**CREATINE** ▶LK ♀- ▶- $
UNAPPROVED ADULT - Promoted to enhance athletic performance. No benefit for endurance exercise, but modest benefit for intense anaerobic tasks lasting <30 sec. Usually taken as loading dose of 20 g/d PO × 5 d, then 2–5 g/d. A 5-yr phase III NIH trial is evaluating for neuroprotection in Parkinson's disease (http://www.parkinsontrial.ninds.nih.gov). Possibly effective for increasing muscle strength in Duchenne muscular dystrophy, polymyositis/dermatomyositis. Does not appear effective for myotonic dystrophy Type 1, amyotrophic lateral sclerosis, Research ongoing in Huntington's disease.
UNAPPROVED PEDS - Not usually for use in children. Am Acad Peds strongly discourages performance-enhancing substances by athletes. Possibly effective for increasing muscle strength in Duchenne muscular dystrophy.
FORMS - Not by prescription.
NOTES - Caffeine may antagonize the ergogenic effects of creatine. Creatine is metabolized to

creatinine. In young healthy adults, large doses can increase serum creatinine slightly without affecting CrCl. The effect in elderly is unknown.
**DANSHEN (Salvia miltiorrhiza)** ▶? ♀? ▶? $
UNAPPROVED ADULT - Used for treatment of cardiovascular diseases in traditional Chinese medicine.
UNAPPROVED PEDS - Not for use in children.
FORMS - Not by prescription.
NOTES - Case reports of increased INR with warfarin.

**DEHYDROEPIANDROSTERONE (DHEA, Aslera, Fidelin, Prasterone)** ▶Peripheral conversion to estrogens and androgens ♀- ▶- $
UNAPPROVED ADULT - Does not improve cognition, quality of life, or sexual function in elderly. To improve well-being in women with adrenal insufficiency: 50 mg PO daily (possibly effective; conflicting clinical trials). Used by athletes as a substitute for anabolic steroids; but no convincing evidence of enhanced athletic performance or increased muscle mass. Banned by many sports organizations.
UNAPPROVED PEDS - Not for use in children.
FORMS - Not by prescription.
NOTES - In theory, chronic use may increase risk of hormone-related cancers (prostate, breast, ovarian). But analysis of pooled data from epidemiologic studies found no link between sex hormone serum levels and prostate cancer.

**DEVIL'S CLAW (Harpagophytum procumbens, Phyto Joint, Doloteffin, Harpadol)** ▶? ♀- ▶- $
UNAPPROVED ADULT - Osteoarthritis, acute exacerbation of chronic low back pain (possibly effective): 2400 mg extract/d (50–100 mg harpagoside/d) PO divided bid-tid.
UNAPPROVED PEDS - Not for children.
FORMS - Not by prescription. Extracts standardized to harpagoside (iridoid glycoside) content.

**DONG QUAI (Angelica sinensis)** ▶? ♀- ▶- $
UNAPPROVED ADULT - Appears ineffective for postmenopausal symptoms; North American Menopause Society recommends against use. Used with other herbs for treatment and prevention of dysmenorrhea, TIA, stroke, PVD, and cardiovascular conditions in traditional Chinese medicine.
UNAPPROVED PEDS - Not for use in children.
FORMS - Not by prescription.
NOTES - Increased risk of bleeding with warfarin with/without increase in INR; avoid concurrent use.

**ECHINACEA (E. purpurea, E. angustifolia, E. pallida, cone flower, EchinaGuard, Echinacin Madaus)** ▶? ♀- ▶- $
UNAPPROVED ADULT - Promoted as immune stimulant. Conflicting clinical trials for prevention or treatment of upper respiratory infections.
UNAPPROVED PEDS - Not for use in children. Appears ineffective for treatment of upper respiratory tract infections in children. A formulation combining echinacea, vitamin C, and propolis

(cont.)

**ECHINACEA** (*cont.*)

(Chizukit; not available in US) appears effective for preventing respiratory infections.

FORMS - Not by prescription.

NOTES - Single case reports of precipitation of thrombotic thrombocytopenic purpura and exacerbation of pemphigus vulgaris; causality unclear. Rare allergic reactions including anaphylaxis. Cross-hypersensitivity possible with other plants in Compositae family (arnica, chamomile, chrysanthemum, feverfew, ragweed, Artemisia). Photosensitivity is possible. Could interact with immunosuppressants due to immunomodulating effects. Some experts limit use to ≤8 wk and recommend against use in patients with autoimmune disorders. May inhibit CYP 450 1A2.

**ELDERBERRY** (*Sambucus nigra, Rubini, Sambucol, Sinupret*) ▶? ♀- ▶- $

UNAPPROVED ADULT - Efficacy unclear for influenza, sinusitis, and bronchitis.

UNAPPROVED PEDS - Not for use in children.

FORMS - Not by prescription.

NOTES - Sinupret and Sambucol also contain other ingredients. Eating uncooked elderberries may cause nausea or cyanide toxicity.

**EPHEDRA** (*Ephedra sinica, ma huang, Metabolife 356, Biolean, Ripped Fuel, Xenadrine*) ▶K ♀- ▶- $

UNAPPROVED ADULT - Little evidence of efficacy for obesity, other than modest short-term weight loss. Traditional use as bronchodilator. The FDA banned ephedra supplements in 2004.

UNAPPROVED PEDS - Not for use in children.

FORMS - Not by prescription.

NOTES - Linked to CVA, MI, sudden death, HTN, palpitations, tachycardia, seizures. Risk of serious reactions may increase with dose, strenuous exercise, or concomitant use of other stimulants like caffeine (as in Biolean & Dexatrim Results). Metabolife 356 can prolong QT interval and increase systolic BP. Country mallow (Sida cordifolia) contains ephedrine.

**EVENING PRIMROSE OIL** (*Oenothera biennis*) ▶? ♀? ▶? $

UNAPPROVED ADULT - Appears ineffective for premenstrual syndrome, postmenopausal symptoms, atopic dermatitis.

UNAPPROVED PEDS - Not for use in children.

FORMS - Not by prescription.

**FENUGREEK** (*Trigonelle foenum-graecum*) ▶? ♀- ▶- $$

UNAPPROVED ADULT - Efficacy unclear for diabetes or hyperlipidemia. Insufficient data to evaluate efficacy as galactagogue.

UNAPPROVED PEDS - Not for use in children.

FORMS - Not by prescription.

NOTES - Case report of increased INR with warfarin possibly related to fenugreek. Can cause maple syrup-like body odor. Fiber content could decrease GI absorption of some drugs.

**FEVERFEW** (*Chrysanthemum parthenium, MIG-99, Migra-Lief, MigraSpray, Tanacetum parthenium L.*) ▶? ♀- ▶- $

UNAPPROVED ADULT - Prevention of migraine (possibly effective): 50–100 mg extract PO daily; 2–3 fresh leaves PO daily; 50–125 mg freeze-dried leaf PO daily. Take either leaf form with or after meals. Benefit of alcoholic extract questioned. May take 1–2 mo to be effective. Inadequate data to evaluate efficacy for acute migraine.

UNAPPROVED PEDS - Not for use in children.

FORMS - Not by prescription.

NOTES - May cause uterine contractions; avoid with pregnancy. Migra-Lief contains feverfew, riboflavin and magnesium. MigraSpray and Gelstat are homeopathic products unlikely to be beneficial.

**FLAVOCOXID** (*Limbrel, UP446*) ▶? ♀- ▶- $$$

UNAPPROVED ADULT - Osteoarthritis (efficacy unclear): 250–500 mg PO bid. Max 2000 mg/d short-term. Taking 1 h before or after meals may increase absorption.

UNAPPROVED PEDS - Not for use in children.

FORMS - Caps 250,500 mg. Marketed as medical food by prescription only (not all medical foods require a prescription). Medical foods are intended to be given under physician supervision to meet distinctive nutritional needs of a disease, but they do not undergo an approval process to establish safety and efficacy.

NOTES - Be alert for confusion between the brand names, Limbrel and Enbrel, as well misidentification of flavocoxid as a COX-2 inhibitor. Baicalin, a component of Limbrel, may reduce exposure to rosuvastatin in some patients.

**GARCINIA** (*Garcinia cambogia, Citri Lean*) ▶? ♀- ▶- $

UNAPPROVED ADULT - Appears ineffective for weight loss.

UNAPPROVED PEDS - Not for use in children.

FORMS - Not by prescription.

**GARLIC SUPPLEMENTS** (*Allium sativum, Kwai, Kyolic*) ▶LK ♀- ▶- $

UNAPPROVED ADULT - Ineffective for hyperlipidemia, and Am College of Cardiology does not recommend for this indication. Small reduction in BP, but efficacy in HTN unclear. Does not appear effective for diabetes.

UNAPPROVED PEDS - Not for use in children.

FORMS - Not by prescription.

NOTES - Significantly decreases saquinavir levels; may also interact with other protease inhibitors. May increase bleeding risk with warfarin with/without increase in INR. Kyolic (aged garlic extract) did not affect the INR in a clinical study.

**GINGER** (*Zingiber officinale*) ▶? ♀? ▶? $

UNAPPROVED ADULT - Prevention of motion sickness (efficacy unclear): 500–1000 mg powdered rhizome PO single dose 1 h before exposure. American College of Obstetrics and Gynecology

**GINGER** *(cont.)*

considers ginger 250 mg PO qid a nonpharmacologic option for N/V of pregnancy. Some experts advise pregnant women to limit dose to usual dietary amount (≤1 g/d). Does not appear effective for postop N/V. Efficacy unclear for relief of osteoarthritis pain.
UNAPPROVED PEDS - Not for use in children.
FORMS - Not by prescription.
NOTES - Increased INR >10 attributed to ginger in a phenprocoumon-treated patient, but study in healthy volunteers found no effect of ginger on INR or pharmacokinetics of warfarin.

**GINKGO BILOBA** *(EGb 761, Ginkgold, Ginkoba, Quanterra Mental Sharpness)* ▶K ♀- ▶- $
UNAPPROVED ADULT - Dementia (efficacy unclear): 40 mg PO tid of standardized extract containing 24% ginkgo flavone glycosides and 6% terpene lactones. It may take up to 4 wk to be effective. Am Psychiatric Assn finds evidence too weak to support use for Alzheimers or other dementias. Does not appear to improve memory or prevent dementia in elderly with normal cognitive function. Does not improve cognition in healthy younger people. Does not appear effective for prevention of acute altitude sickness. Limited benefit in intermittent claudication. Am College of Cardiology found insufficient evidence for treatment of peripheral vascular disease. ArginMax (also contains L-arginine and other ingredients) promoted for SSRI-induced sexual dysfunction.
UNAPPROVED PEDS - Not for use in children.
FORMS - Not by prescription.
NOTES - Case reports of intracerebral, subdural, and ocular bleeding. Does not appear to increase INR with warfarin, but monitoring for bleeding is advised. Ginkgo seeds contain a neurotoxin. A few reports attributing exacerbation or precipitation of seizures to ginkgo supplements has raised concern about possible contamination with the neurotoxin. Some experts advise caution or avoidance of ginkgo by those with seizures or taking drugs that lower the seizure threshold.

**GINSENG - AMERICAN** *(Panax quinquefolius L.)* ▶K ♀- ▶- $
UNAPPROVED ADULT - Reduction of postprandial glucose in type 2 diabetes (possibly effective): 3 g ground root caps PO taken with or up to 2h before meal.
UNAPPROVED PEDS - Not for use in children.
FORMS - Not by prescription.
NOTES - Ginseng content varies widely and some products are mislabeled or adulterated with caffeine. American, Asian, and Siberian ginseng are often misidentified. Decreased INR with warfarin.

**GINSENG - ASIAN** *(Panax ginseng, Ginsana, Ginsai, G115, Korean red ginseng)* ▶? ♀- ▶- $
UNAPPROVED ADULT - Promoted to improve vitality and well-being: 200 mg PO daily. Ginsana: 2 caps PO daily or 1 cap PO bid. Ginsana Sport: 1 cap PO

daily. Efficacy unclear for improving physical or psychomotor performance, diabetes, herpes simplex infections, cognitive or immune function. American College of Obstetrics and Gynecologists and North American Menopause Society recommend against use for postmenopausal hot flashes.
UNAPPROVED PEDS - Not for use in children.
FORMS - Not by prescription.
NOTES - Some formulations may contain up to 34% alcohol. Ginsana Gold also contains vitamins and minerals. Reports of an interaction with the MAOI, phenelzine. Decreased INR with warfarin. Ginseng content varies widely and some products are mislabeled or adulterated with caffeine. American, Asian, and Siberian ginseng are often misidentified. May interfere with FPIA and MEIA digoxin assays.

**GINSENG - SIBERIAN** *(Eleutherococcus senticosus, Ci-wu-jia)* ▶? ♀- ▶- $
UNAPPROVED ADULT - Does not appear to improve athletic endurance. Did not appear effective in single clinical trial for chronic fatigue syndrome.
UNAPPROVED PEDS - Not for use in children.
FORMS - Not by prescription.
NOTES - May interfere with FPIA and MEIA digoxin assays. A case report of thalamic stroke attributed to Siberian ginseng plus caffeine.

**GLUCOSAMINE** *(Aflexa, Cosamin DS, Dona, Flextend, Promotion)* ▶L ♀- ▶- $
UNAPPROVED ADULT - Osteoarthritis: Glucosamine HCl 500 mg PO tid. Glucosamine sulfate (Dona) 1500 mg PO once daily (a packet dissolved in glass of water or caplet). Efficacy for OA is unclear (conflicting data). Glucosamine/Chondroitin Arthritis Intervention Trial (GAIT) did not find improvement in pain of knee OA with glucosamine HCl 500 mg +/- chondroitin 400 mg both PO tid. Glucosamine + chondroitin did improve pain in subgroup of patients with moderate to severe OA. Some earlier studies reported improved pain with glucosamine sulfate, a different salt (Dona 1500 mg PO once daily). Glucosamine sulfate 1500 mg/d (not Dona brand) was ineffective for hip OA in GOAL study.
UNAPPROVED PEDS - Not for use in children.
FORMS - Not by prescription.
NOTES - Use cautiously or avoid in patients with shellfish allergy. Case reports of increased INR/bleeding with warfarin in patient taking chondroitin + glucosamine.

**GOLDENSEAL** *(Hydrastis canadensis)* ▶? ♀- ▶- $
UNAPPROVED ADULT - Often used in attempts to achieve false-negative urine test for illicit drug use (efficacy unclear). Often combined with echinacea in cold remedies; but insufficient data to assess efficacy of goldenseal for the common cold or URIs.
UNAPPROVED PEDS - Not for use in children.
FORMS - Not by prescription.
NOTES - Alkaloids in goldenseal with antibacterial activity not well-absorbed orally. Oral use contraindicated in pregnancy (may cause uterine *(cont.)*

**GOLDENSEAL** *(cont.)*

contractions), newborns (may cause kernicterus), and hypertension (high doses may cause peripheral vasoconstriction). Adding goldenseal directly to urine turns it brown. May inhibit CYP 2D6 and 3A4. Berberine, a component of goldenseal, may increase cyclosporine levels.

**GRAPE SEED EXTRACT** (*Vitis vinifera L., procyanidolic oligomers, PCO*) ▶? ♀? ▶? $

UNAPPROVED ADULT - Small clinical trials suggest benefit in chronic venous insufficiency. No benefit demonstrated in single study of seasonal allergic rhinitis.

UNAPPROVED PEDS - Not for use in children.

FORMS - Not by prescription.

NOTES - Pine bark (pycnogenol) and grape seed extract are often confused; they both contain oligomeric proanthocyanidins.

**GREEN TEA** (*Camellia sinensis*) ▶? ♀+ in moderate amount in food, - in supplements ▶+ in moderate amount in food, - in supplements $

PEDS - Not for children.

UNAPPROVED ADULT - Some population studies suggest a reduction in adenomatous polyps and chronic atrophic gastritis in green tea drinkers. Efficacy unclear for cancer prevention, weight loss, hypercholesterolemia. Phase I studies of green tea extract in advanced lung and prostate cancer did not suggest antineoplastic activity. Currently under evaluation for prevention of prostate cancer in men with high-grade prostate intraepithelial neoplasia.

FORMS - Not available by prescription. Green tea extract available in caps standardized to polyphenol content.

NOTES - Case report of decreased INR with warfarin attributed to drinking large amounts of green tea (due to vitamin K content). The vitamin K content of green tea is low with usual consumption.

**GUARANA** (*Paullinia cupana*) ▶? ♀+ in food, - in supplements ▶+ in food, - in supplements $

UNAPPROVED ADULT - Marketed as an ingredient in weight-loss dietary supplements. Seeds contain caffeine. Use of guarana in weight loss dietary supplements may provide high doses of caffeine.

UNAPPROVED PEDS - Not for children.

FORMS - Not by prescription.

**GUGGULIPID** (*Commiphora mukul extract, guggul*) ▶? ♀- ▶- $$

UNAPPROVED ADULT - Does not appear effective for hyperlipidemia. A randomized controlled trial conducted in US with 1000 mg or 2000 mg PO tid reported no change in total cholesterol, triglycerides, or HDL, and a small increase in LDL. Earlier studies of weaker design reported reductions in total cholesterol of up to 27%.

UNAPPROVED PEDS - Not for use in children.

FORMS - Not by prescription.

NOTES - May decrease levels of propranolol and diltiazem.

**HAWTHORN** (*Crataegus laevigata, monogyna, oxyacantha, standardized extract WS 1442 - Crataegutt novo, HeartCare*) ▶? ♀- ▶- $

UNAPPROVED ADULT - Symptomatic improvement of mild CHF (NYHA I-II; possibly effective): 80 mg PO bid to 160 mg PO tid of standardized extract (19% oligomeric procyanidins; WS 1442; HeartCare 80 mg tabs); doses as high as 900–1800 mg/d have been studied. Initial presentation of SPICE study found no benefit for primary outcome (composite of cardiac death/ hospitalization), but possible reduction of sudden cardiac death for LVEF 25–35%. Am College of Cardiology found evidence insufficient to recommend for mild heart failure. Does not appear effective for hypertension.

UNAPPROVED PEDS - Not for use in children.

FORMS - Not by prescription.

NOTES - Unclear whether hawthorn and digoxin should be used together; mechanisms of action may be similar.

**HONEY** (*Medihoney*) ▶? ♀+ ▶+ $ for PO $$$ for Medihoney

UNAPPROVED ADULT - Topical for burn/wound care (including diabetic foot, leg statis ulcers, pressure ulcers, 1st and 2nd degree partial thickness burns, donor sites, surgical/traumatic wounds): Apply Medihoney to wound for 12–24 h/d. Oral. Constipation (efficacy unclear): 1–2 tbsp (30–60 g) in glass of water. Topical. Efficacy unclear for prevention of dialysis catheter infections.

UNAPPROVED PEDS - Topical for burn/wound care (including diabetic foot, leg statis ulcers, pressure ulcers, 1st and 2nd degree partial thickness burns, donor sites, surgical/traumatic wounds): Apply Medihoney to wound for 12–24 h/d. Do not feed honey to children <1 yo due to risk of infant botulism. Nocturnal cough due to upper RTI (efficacy unclear): Give honey 30 min before sleep. Give ½ tsp for 2–5 yo, 1 tsp for 6–11 yo, 2 tsp for 12–18 yo. WHO considers honey a cheap, popular, and safe demulcent for children.

FORMS - Mostly not by prescription. Medihoney is FDA approved product.

NOTES - Honey may contain trace amounts of antimicrobials used to treat infection in honeybee hives. Medihoney sterile dressings contain Leptospermum (Manuka) honey that is irradiated to inactivate C botulinum spores.

**HORSE CHESTNUT SEED EXTRACT** (*Aesculus hippocastanum, HCE50, Venastat*) ▶? ♀- ▶- $

UNAPPROVED ADULT - Chronic venous insufficiency (effective): 1 cap Venastat PO bid with water before meals. Response within 1 mo. Venastat is 16% aescin in standardized extract. Am College of Cardiology found evidence insufficient to recommend for peripheral vascular disease.

UNAPPROVED PEDS - Not for use in children.

FORMS - Not by prescription.

NOTES - Venastat does not contain aesculin, a toxin in horse chestnuts.

**KAVA (*Piper methysticum, One-a-d Bedtime & Rest, Sleep-Tite*)** ▶K ♀- ▶- $
UNAPPROVED ADULT - Promoted as anxiolytic (possibly effective) or sedative; recommend against use due to hepatotoxicity.
UNAPPROVED PEDS - Not for use in children.
FORMS - Not by prescription.
NOTES - Reports of severe hepatotoxicity leading to liver transplantation. May potentiate CNS effects of benzodiazepines and other sedatives, including alcohol. Reversible yellow skin discoloration with long-term use.

**KOMBUCHA TEA (*Manchurian or Kargasok tea*)** ▶? ♀- ▶- $
UNAPPROVED ADULT - Promoted for many indications, but no scientific evidence to support benefit for any condition. FDA advises caution due to a case of fatal acidosis.
UNAPPROVED PEDS - Not for use in children.
FORMS - Not by prescription.
NOTES - Culture of bacteria and yeast that is very acidic after preparation. Tea is made by steeping mushroom culture in tea and sugar for ~1 wk. Tea may contain alcohol, ethyl acetate, acetic acid, and lactate.

**LICORICE (*Cankermelt, Glycyrrhiza glabra, Glycyrrhiza uralensis*)** ▶Bile ♀- ▶- $
UNAPPROVED ADULT - Insufficient data to assess efficacy for postmenopausal vasomotor symptoms. Cankermelt (dissolving oral patch): Efficacy unclear for pain relief and healing of aphthous stomatitis. Apply patch to ulcer for 16 h/d until ulcer is healed.
UNAPPROVED PEDS - Not for use in children.
FORMS - Not by prescription.
NOTES - Diuretics or stimulant laxatives could potentiate licorice-induced hypokalemia. In the US, "licorice" candy usually does not contain licorice. Deglycyrrhizinated licorice does not have mineralocorticoid effects.

**MELATONIN (*N-acetyl-5-methoxytryptamine*)** ▶L ♀- ▶- $
UNAPPROVED ADULT - To reduce jet lag after flights across >5 time zones (possibly effective; especially when traveling East; may also help when crossing 2–4 time zones): 0.5–5 mg PO qhs (10 pm to midnight) × 3–6 nights starting on d of arrival. Faster onset and better sleep quality with 5 mg over 0.5 mg, but no greater benefit with >5 mg. No benefit with use before departure or with slow-release formulations. Do not take earlier in day (may cause drowsiness and delay adaptation to local time). To promote daytime sleep in night shift workers: 1.8–3 mg PO prior to daytime sleep. Delayed sleep phase disorder: 0.3–5 mg PO 1.5–6 h before habitual bedtime. Orphan drug for treatment of circadian rhythm-related sleep disorders in blind patients with no light perception. Possibly effective for difficulty falling asleep, but not for staying asleep.

UNAPPROVED PEDS - Not usually used in children. Sleep-onset insomnia in ADHD, ≥6 yo (possibly effective): 3–6 mg PO qhs. Orphan drug treatment of circadian rhythm-related sleep disorders in blind patients with no light perception.
FORMS - Not by prescription.
NOTES - High melatonin levels linked to nocturnal asthma; some experts advise patients with nocturnal asthma to avoid melatonin supplements until more data available.

**METHYLSULFONYLMETHANE (*MSM, dimethyl sulfone, crystalline DMSO2*)** ▶? ♀- ▶- $
UNAPPROVED ADULT - Insufficient data to assess efficacy of oral and topical MSM for arthritis pain.
UNAPPROVED PEDS - Not for use in children.
FORMS - Not by prescription.
NOTES - Can cause nausea, diarrhea, headache. DMSO metabolite promoted as a source of sulfur without odor.

**MILK THISTLE (*Silybum marianum, Legalon, silymarin, Thisylin*)** ▶LK ♀- ▶- $
UNAPPROVED ADULT - Hepatic cirrhosis (possibly effective): 100–200 mg PO tid of standardized extract with 70–80% silymarin. Hepatitis C: May decrease serum transaminase levels, but does not appear to improve viral load or liver histology; American Gastroenterology Assoc recommends against use. Used in Europe to treat Amanita mushroom poisoning.
UNAPPROVED PEDS - Not for use in children.
FORMS - Not by prescription.
NOTES - May inhibit cytochrome P450 2C9 and 3A4; but no effect on pharmacokinetics of indinavir in human studies. May decrease blood glucose in patients with cirrhosis and diabetes.

**NETTLE ROOT (*stinging nettle, Urtica dioica radix*)** ▶? ♀- ▶- $
UNAPPROVED ADULT - Efficacy unclear for treatment of BPH.
UNAPPROVED PEDS - Not for use in children.
FORMS - Not by prescription.
NOTES - Lead contamination led to recall of some lots of Nature's Way nettle caps.

**NONI (*Morinda citrifolia*)** ▶? ♀- ▶- $$$
UNAPPROVED ADULT - Promoted for many medical disorders; but insufficient data to assess efficacy.
UNAPPROVED PEDS - Not for use in children.
FORMS - Not by prescription.
NOTES - Potassium concentration comparable to orange juice. Hyperkalemia reported in a patient with chronic renal failure. Case reports of hepatotoxicity.

**POLICOSANOL (*One-A-Day Cholesterol Plus, CholeRx, Cholest Response, Cholesstor, Cholestin*)** ▶? ♀- ▶- $
UNAPPROVED ADULT - Ineffective for hyperlipidemia. A Cuban formulation (unavailable in US) reduced LDL cholesterol in studies by a single **(cont.)**

**POLICOSANOL** (*cont.*)

group of researchers, but studies by other groups found no benefit. Clinical study of a US formulation (Cholesstor) also found no benefit.

UNAPPROVED PEDS - Not for use in children.

FORMS - Not by prescription.

NOTES - An old formulation of Cholestin contained red yeast rice; the current formulation contains policosanol.

**PROBIOTICS** (*Acidophilus, Align, Bifantis, Bifidobacteria, Lactobacillus, Bacid, Culturelle, Florastor, IntestiFlora, Lactinex, LiveBac, Power-Dophilus, Primadophilus, Probiotica, Saccharomyces boulardii, VSL#3*) ▶? ♀+ ▶+ $

ADULT - VSL#3 approved as medical food. Ulcerative colitis (possibly effective): 1–2 packets or 4–8 caps/d. Active ulcerative colitis: 4–8 packets or 16–32 caps/d. Pouchitis (effective): 2–4 packets or 6–18 caps/d. Irritable bowel syndrome (may relieve gas and bloating): ½ -1 packet PO daily or 2–4 caps daily. Mix powder from packets with ≥4 oz of cold water before taking.

PEDS - VSL#3 approved as medical food for ulcerative colitis (possibly effective) or pouchitis (effective), age ≥3 mo: Dose based on weight and number of bowel movements/d. See http://www.vsl3.com/VSL3/about-take-vsl.asp. Use adult dose for ≥15 yo. Mix powder with ≥4 oz of cold water before taking.

UNAPPROVED ADULT - Antibiotic-associated diarrhea (effective): Saccharomyces boulardii 500 mg PO bid (Florastor 2 caps PO bid). Give 2 h before/after antibiotic so culture isn't killed. Probiotics may reduce GI side effects of H pylori eradication regimens. May improve abdominal pain and bloating in irritable bowel syndrome (eg, Align 1 cap PO once daily). Efficacy of probiotics unclear for travelers' diarrhea (conflicting evidence), Crohn's disease, H pylori, radiation enteritis. Lactobacillus GG appears ineffective for prevention of post-antibiotic vulvovaginitis. Safety and efficacy of probiotics unclear for prevention of recurrent C difficile diarrhea.

UNAPPROVED PEDS - Prevention of antibiotic-associated diarrhea (effective): Lactobacillus GG 10–20 billion cells/d PO (Culturelle 1 cap PO once daily or bid) or S boulardii 250 mg PO bid (Floraster 1 cap PO bid). Rotavirus gastroenteritis: Lactobacillus GG ≥10 billion cells/d PO started early in illness. Efficacy of probiotics unclear for travelers' diarrhea (conflicting evidence), radiation enteritis, irritable bowel syndrome. Lactobacillus GG does not appear effective for Crohn's disease in children. Research ongoing for prevention and treatment of atopic dermatitis.

FORMS - Not by prescription. Culturelle contains Lactobacillus GG 10 billion cells/cap. Florastor contains Saccharomyces boulardii 5 billion cells/250 mg cap. Probiotica contains Lactobacillus reuteri 100 million cells/chew tab. VSL#3 contains 450 billion cells/packet,

225 billion cells/2 caps (Bifidobacterium breve, longum, infantis; Lactobacillus acidophilus, plantarum, casei, bulgaricus; Streptococcus thermophilus). Align contains Bifidobacterium infantis 35624, 1 billion cells/cap. VSL#3 is marketed as non-prescription medical food. Medical foods are intended to be given under physician supervision to meet distinctive nutritional needs of a disease, but they do not undergo an approval process to establish safety and efficacy.

NOTES - Do not use probiotics in patients with acute pancreatitis; increased mortality and bowel ischemia reported in clinical trial. Use cautiously in immunosuppressed patients; acquired infection possible. Lactobacillus sepsis and Saccharomyces fungemia reported rarely in probiotic-treated patients; possible central venous access port contamination in some cases. Microbial type and content varies by product. Pick yogurt products labeled "Live and active cultures". Refrigerate packets of VSL#3; can store at room temp for 1 wk.

**PYCNOGENOL** (*French maritime pine tree bark*) ▶L ♀? ▶? $

UNAPPROVED ADULT - Promoted for many medical disorders, but efficacy unclear for chronic venous insufficiency, sperm dysfunction, melasma, osteoarthrits, hypertension, type 2 diabetes, diabetic retinopathy, and ADHD.

UNAPPROVED PEDS - Not for use in children.

FORMS - Not by prescription.

NOTES - Pine bark (pycnogenol) and grape seed extract are often confused; they both contain oligomeric proanthocyanidins.

**PYGEUM AFRICANUM** (*African plum tree, Prostata, Prostatonin, Provol*) ▶? ♀- ▶- $

UNAPPROVED ADULT - Benign prostatic hypertrophy (may have modest efficacy): 50–100 mg PO bid or 100 mg PO daily of standardized extract containing 14% triterpenes. Prostatonin (also contains Urtica dioica): 1 cap PO bid with meals; up to 6 wk for full response. Prostata also contains saw palmetto and other ingredients.

UNAPPROVED PEDS - Not for use in children.

FORMS - Not by prescription.

NOTES - Appears well-tolerated. Self-treatment could delay diagnosis of prostate cancer.

**RED CLOVER ISOFLAVONE EXTRACT** (*Trifolium pratense, trefoil, Promensil, Rimostil, Supplifem, Trinovin*) ▶Gut, L, K ♀- ▶- $$

UNAPPROVED ADULT - Promensil (1 tab PO daily-bid with meals) marketed for menopausal symptoms; Rimostil (1 tab PO daily) for bone & cholesterol health, and to promote health & well-being after menopause; Trinovin (1 tab PO daily) for maintaining prostate health & urinary function in men. Conflicting evidence of efficacy for postmenopausal vasomotor symptoms. Does not appear effective overall, but may have modest benefit for severe symptoms. Efficacy unclear for prevention of osteoporosis & treatment of hyperlipidemia in postmenopausal women, and for BPH symptoms in men.

**RED CLOVER ISOFLAVONE EXTRACT** (cont.)

UNAPPROVED PEDS - Not for use in children.

FORMS - Not by prescription. Isoflavone content (genistein, daidzein, biochanin, formononetin) is 40 mg/tab in Promensil and Trinovin, 57 mg/tab in Rimostil.

NOTES - Does not appear to stimulate endometrium. Effect on breast cancer risk is unclear; some experts recommend against use of isoflavone supplements by women with breast cancer. No effect on breast density in women with Wolfe P2 or DY mammographic breast density patterns. H2 blockers, proton pump inhibitors, and antibiotics may decrease metabolic activation of isoflavones in GI tract. Ingesting large amounts of red clover can cause bleeding in cattle; bleeding risk of supplements in humans is theoretical. Supplifem contains soy and red clover extract (51 mg isoflavones/caplet).

**RED WINE** ▶L ♀- ▶- $

ADULT - Red wine, alcoholic beverage.

PEDS - Not appropriate for children.

FORMS - Not by prescription.

**RED YEAST RICE** (*Monascus purpureus, Xuezhikang, Zhibituo, Hypocol, Lipolysar*) ▶L ♀- ▶- $$

UNAPPROVED ADULT - Efficacy of currently available US products for hyperlipidemia is unclear. Some products were removed from the US market because they contained up to 10 mg/d of lovastatin. Others, such as Cholestin, were reformulated with policosanol (ineffective for hyperlipidemia). Xuezhikang (reduces LDL by 10–33%) was effective for secondary prevention of CHD events in Chinese trial. Xuezihang 2 caps PO bid or Zhibituo 3 tabs PO tid provides ~ 10 mg lovastatin/d.

UNAPPROVED PEDS - Not for use in children.

FORMS - Not by prescription. Xuezhikang marketed in Asia, Norway (HypoCol), Italy (Lipolysar).

NOTES - In 1997, a red yeast rice product called Cholestin was marketed in the US as a cholesterol-lowering supplement. It was removed from the market in 2001 after a judge ruled it an unapproved drug because it contained lovastatin (5–7 mg/d at usual doses). Cholestin later returned to the market; it now contains policosanol (ineffective for hyperlipidemia). Current red yeast rice products should not contain more than trace amounts of statins. In 2007, the FDA warned consumers that 3 products promoted on the internet contained illegal amounts of lovastatin (5–10 mg/d). Cases of myopathy have been reported with red yeast rice supplements.

**S-ADENOSYLMETHIONINE** (*SAM-e, sammy*) ▶L ♀? ▶? $$$

UNAPPROVED ADULT - Depression (possibly effective): 400–1600 mg/d PO. Osteoarthritis (possibly effective): 400–1200 mg/d PO. Onset of response in OA in 2–4 wk. Efficacy unclear for alcoholic liver disease.

UNAPPROVED PEDS - Not for use in children.

FORMS - Not by prescription.

NOTES - Serotonin syndrome possible with SSRIs. Do not use within 2 wk of an MAOI or in bipolar disorder.

**SAINT JOHN'S WORT** (*Alterra, Hypericum perforatum, Kira, Movana, One-a-Day Tension & Mood, LI-160, St John's wort*) ▶L ♀- ▶- $

UNAPPROVED ADULT - Short-term treatment of mild depression (effective): 300 mg PO tid of standardized extract (0.3% hypericin). Conflicting clinical trials for moderate major depression.

UNAPPROVED PEDS - Not for use in children. Does not appear effective for attention-deficit/hyperactivity disorder.

FORMS - Not by prescription.

NOTES - Photosensitivity possible with >1800 mg/d. Inducer of hepatic cytochrome P450 3A4, 2C9, 2C19, and P-glycoprotein. May decrease efficacy of drugs with hepatic metabolism including alprazolam, cyclosporine, methadone, non-nucleoside reverse transcriptase inhibitors, omeprazole, oral contraceptives, protease inhibitors, statins, voriconazole. May need increased dose of digoxin, theophylline, tricyclic antidepressants. Decreased INR with warfarin. Administration with SSRIs, nefazodone, triptans may cause serotonin syndrome. Do not use within 14 d of monoamine oxidase inhibitors.

**SAW PALMETTO** (*Serenoa repens, One-a-Day Prostate Health, Quanterra*) ▶? ♀- ▶- $

UNAPPROVED ADULT - BPH (possibly effective for mild to moderate; appears ineffective for moderate to severe): 160 mg PO bid or 320 mg PO daily of standardized liposterolic extract. Take with food. Brewed teas may not be effective.

UNAPPROVED PEDS - Not for use in children.

FORMS - Not by prescription.

NOTES - Not for use by women of child-bearing potential. Does not interfere with PSA test. Self-treatment could delay diagnosis of prostate cancer.

**SHARK CARTILAGE** (*BeneFin, Cancenex, Cartilade*) ▶? ♀- ▶- $$$$$

UNAPPROVED ADULT - Appears ineffective for palliative care of advanced cancer. Neovastat (AE-941), a derivative of shark cartilage was ineffective in phase III clinical trial for non-small cell lung cancer.

UNAPPROVED PEDS - Not for use in children.

FORMS - Not by prescription.

NOTES - Contamination with salmonella was reported in some shark cartilage caps.

**SILVER - COLLOIDAL** (*mild & strong silver protein, silver ion*) ▶? ♀- ▶- $

UNAPPROVED ADULT - The FDA does not recognize OTC colloidal silver products as safe or effective for any use.

UNAPPROVED PEDS - Not for use in children.

FORMS - Not by prescription. May come as silver chloride, cyanide, iodide, oxide, or phosphate.

NOTES - Silver accumulates in skin (leads to grey tint), conjunctiva, and internal organs with chronic use.

**SOY (*Genisoy, Healthy Woman, Novasoy, Phytosoya, Supro*)** ▶Gut, L, K ♀+ for food, ? for supplements ▶+ for food, ? for supplements $
UNAPPROVED ADULT - Cardiovascular risk reduction: ≥25 g/d soy protein (50 mg/d isoflavones) PO. Hypercholesterolemia: ~50 g/d soy protein PO reduces LDL cholesterol by ~3%; effects on HDL, triglycerides, BP appear insignificant. No apparent benefit for isoflavone supplements. Postmenopausal vasomotor symptoms (modest benefit if any): 20–60 g/d soy protein PO (40–80 mg/d isoflavones). Conflicting clinical trials for reducing postmenopausal bone loss. American Heart Assn recommends against isoflavone supplements for treatment or prevention of hyperlipidemia, or breast, endometrial, or prostate cancer.
UNAPPROVED PEDS - Soy foods are regarded as safe for children.
FORMS - Not by prescription.
NOTES - Effect on breast cancer risk is unclear; some experts recommend against use of isoflavone or phytoestrogen supplements by women with endometrial or breast cancer (esp. estrogen receptor-positive tumor or receiving tamoxifen). Case report of decreased INR with ingestion of soy milk by patient taking warfarin. Report of decreased levothyroxine absorption with soy protein.

**STEVIA (*Stevia rebaudiana*)** ▶L ♀- ▶? $
UNAPPROVED ADULT - Leaves traditionally used as a sweetener, but not enough safety data for FDA approval as such. Per Health Canada, acceptable daily intake for stevioside is 1 mg/kg/d up to 70 mg; stevia leaf powder max of 280 mg/d for adults. Efficacy unclear for treatment of type 2 diabetes or hypertension.
UNAPPROVED PEDS - Not for use in children.
FORMS - Not by prescription.
NOTES - Stevia available as dietary supplement, but not approved by the FDA as food sweetener in the US. Canadian labeling advises against use by pregnant women, children, or those with low BP.

**TEA TREE OIL (*melaleuca oil, Melaleuca alternifolia*)** ▶? ♀- ▶- $
UNAPPROVED ADULT - Not for oral use; CNS toxicity reported. Efficacy is unclear for onychomycosis, tinea pedis, acne vulgaris, dandruff, and pediculosis.
UNAPPROVED PEDS - Not for use in children.
FORMS - Not by prescription.

**VALERIAN (*Valeriana officinalis, Alluna, One-a-d Bedtime & Rest, Sleep-Tite*)** ▶? ♀- ▶- $
UNAPPROVED ADULT - Insomnia (possibly effective; conflicting clinical trials): 400–900 mg of standardized extract PO 30 min before bedtime. Response reported in 2–4 wk. Alluna (valerian + hops): 2 tabs PO 1 h before bedtime. Some products have unpleasant smell.
UNAPPROVED PEDS - Not for use in children.
FORMS - Not by prescription.
NOTES - Do not combine with CNS depressants. Withdrawal symptoms reported after long-term use. Valerian does not appear to inhibit CYP 1A2, 2D6, 2E1, or 3A4.

**WILD YAM (*Dioscorea villosa*)** ▶L ♀? ▶? $
UNAPPROVED ADULT - Ineffective as topical "natural progestin".
UNAPPROVED PEDS - Not for use in children.
FORMS - Not by prescription.

**WILLOW BARK EXTRACT (*Salix alba, Salicis cortex, Assalix, salicin*)** ▶K ♀- ▶- $
UNAPPROVED ADULT - Osteoarthritis, low back pain (possibly effective): 60 to 240 mg/d salicin PO divided bid-tid. Onset of pain relief is about 2 h. It is often included in multi-ingredient weight-loss supplements based on preliminary research suggesting that aspirin increases thermogenesis.
UNAPPROVED PEDS - Not for use in children. Do not give to febrile children who could develop Reye's syndrome.
FORMS - Not by prescription. Some products standardized to 15% salicin content.
NOTES - Contraindicated in third trimester of pregnancy, and also in patients with intolerance or with allergy to aspirin or other NSAIDs. Consider contraindications and precautions that apply to other salicylates. Avoid concomitant use of NSAIDs.

**YOHIMBE (*Corynanthe yohimbe, Pausinystalia yohimbe, Potent V*)** ▶L ♀- ▶- $
UNAPPROVED ADULT - Nonprescription yohimbe promoted for impotence and as aphrodisiac, but these products rarely contain much yohimbine (active constituent). FDA considers yohimbe bark in herbal remedies an unsafe herb. Yohimbine HCl is available in US as a prescription drug, but Am Urological Assoc does not recommend for erectile dysfunction.
UNAPPROVED PEDS - Not for use in children.
FORMS - Yohimbine is the primary alkaloid in the bark of the yohimbe tree. Yohimbine HCl is a prescription drug in the US; yohimbe bark is available without prescription. Yohimbe bark (not by prescription) and prescription yohimbine HCl are not interchangeable.
NOTES - Can cause CNS stimulation. High doses of yohimbine have MAOI activity and can increase BP. Avoid in patients with hypotension, diabetes, heart, liver or kidney disease. Reports of renal failure, seizures, death in patients taking products containing yohimbe.

## IMMUNOLOGY: Immunizations

**NOTE:** For vaccine info see CDC website (www.cdc.gov).

**AVIAN INFLUENZA VACCINE H5N1 - INACTIVATED INJECTION ▶IMMUNE SYSTEM ♀C ▶? ?**
ADULT - 18–64 yo: 1 mL IM × 2 doses, separated by 21–35 d.
PEDS - Not approved for use in children.
NOTES - Caution if hypersensitivity to chicken or egg proteins. The immunocompromised may have a blunted immune response.

**BCG VACCINE (*Tice BCG, ✦Oncotice, Immucyst*)** ▶Immune system ♀C ▶? $$$$
ADULT - 0.2–0.3 mL percutaneously (using 1 mL sterile water for reconstitution).
PEDS - Age >1 mo: use adult dose. Age <1 mo: Decrease concentration by 50% using 2 mL sterile water for reconstitution, then 0.2–0.3 mL percutaneously. May revaccinate with full dose (adult dose) after 1 yo if necessary.

**COMVAX (haemophilus B vaccine + hepatitis B vaccine)** ▶Immune system ♀C ▶? $$$
ADULT - Do not use in adults.
PEDS - Infants born of HBsAg (-) mothers: 0.5 mL IM × 3 doses at 2, 4, and 12–15 mo of age.
NOTES - Combination is made of PedvaxHIB (Haemophilus b vaccine) + Recombivax HB (hepatitis B vaccine). For infants >8 wk of age.

**DIPHTHERIA TETANUS AND ACELLULAR PERTUSSIS VACCINE (*DTaP, Tdap, Tripedia, Infanrix, Daptacel, Boostrix, Adacel, ✦Tripacel*)** ▶Immune system ♀C ▶- $$
ADULT - 0.5 mL IM in deltoid as a single dose, 2 to 5 yr since last tetanus dose (Adacel).
PEDS - Check immunization history: DTaP is preferred for all DTP doses. Give first dose of 0.5 mL IM at approximately 2 mo, 2nd dose at 4 mo, third dose at 6 mo, fourth dose at 15–18 mo, and fifth dose (booster) at 4–6 yo. Use Boostrix only if adolescents 10–18 yo, and ≥2–5 yr after the last

childhood dose of DTP. Use Adacel only in adolescents ≥11 yo and at least 2 to 5 yr after last childhood dose of DTP or Td.
NOTES - When feasible, use the same brand for first 3 doses. Do not give drug if prior DTP vaccination caused anaphylaxis or encephalopathy within 7 d. Avoid Tripedia in patients with thimerosal allergy. Do not use Boostrix or Adacel for primary childhood vaccination series, if prior DTP vaccination caused anaphylaxis or encephalopathy, or if progressive neurologic disorders (eg, encephalopathy) or uncontrolled epilepsy. Adacel is only DTaP vaccine approved for use in adults up to age 64 yo. For adolescents and adults, only one dose should be given, at least 2–5 yr after last tetanus dose. No information currently available on repeat doses in adolescents or adults.

**DIPHTHERIA-TETANUS TOXOID (*Td, DT, ✦D2T5*)** ▶Immune system ♀C ▶? $
ADULT - Age ≥7 yo: 0.5 mL IM, 2nd dose 4–8 wk later, and third dose 6–12 mo later. Give 0.5 mL booster dose at 10 yr intervals. Use the adult formulation (Td) for adults and children ≥7 yr of age.
PEDS - Age 6 wk- 6 yo: 0.5 mL IM , 2nd dose 4–8 wk later, and third dose 6–12 mo later using DT for pediatric use. If immunization of infants begins in the first yr of life using DT rather than DTP (ie, pertussis is contraindicated), give three 0.5 mL doses 4–8 wk apart, followed by a fourth dose 6- 12 mo later.
FORMS - Injection DT (pediatric: 6 wk- 6 yo). Td (adult and children: ≥7 yr).
NOTES - DTaP is preferred for most children <7 yr of age. Td is preferred for adults and children ≥7 yo. Avoid in thimerosal allergy.

| TETANUS WOUND CARE (www.cdc.gov) | | |
|---|---|---|
| | Uncertain or <3 prior tetanus immunizations | ≥3 prior tetanus immunizations |
| Non tetanus-prone wound (e.g., clean and minor) | Td (DT if <7 yo) | Td if >10 yr since last dose |
| Tetanus-prone wound (e.g., dirt, contamination, punctures, crush components) | Td (DT if <7 yo) and tetanus immune globulin 250 units IM at site other than dT | Td if >5 yr since last dose |

**HAEMOPHILUS B VACCINE (*ActHIB, HibTITER, Pedvax HIB*)** ▶Immune system ♀C ▶? $$
PEDS - Doses vary depending on formulation used and age at first dose. ActHIB/OmniHIB/HibTITER: 2- 6 mo- 0.5 mL IM × 3 doses at two mo intervals. 7- 11 mo- 0.5 mL IM × 2 doses at two mo intervals. 12- 14 mo- 0.5 mL IM × 1 dose. A single 0.5 mL IM (booster) dose is given to children ≥15 mo old, and at least 2 mo after the previous injection. 15- 60 mo: 0.5 mL IM × 1 dose (no booster). PedvaxHIB: 2- 14 mo- 0.5 mL IM × 2 doses at two mo intervals. If the 2 doses are given before 12 mo of age, a third 0.5 mL IM (booster) dose is given at least 2 mo after the 2nd dose. 15- 60 mo- 0.5 mL IM × 1 dose (no booster).
UNAPPROVED ADULT - Asplenia, ≥14 d prior to elective splenectomy, or immunodeficiency: 0.5 mL IM × 1 dose of any Hib conjugate vaccine.
UNAPPROVED PEDS - Asplenia, ≥14 d prior to elective splenectomy, or immunodeficiency age ≥5 yo: 0.5 mL IM × 1 dose of any Hib vaccine.
NOTES - Not for IV use. No data on interchangeability between brands; AAP & ACIP recommend use of any product in children ≥12- 15 mo of age.

**HEPATITIS A VACCINE (*Havrix, Vaqta, ◆Avaxim, Epaxal*)** ▶Immune system ♀C ▶+ $$$
ADULT - Havrix ≥18 yo: 1 mL (1440 ELU) IM, then 1 mL (1440 ELU) IM booster dose 6- 12 mo later. Vaqta ≥18 yo: 1 mL (50 U) IM, then 1 mL (50 U) IM booster 6-18 mo later.
PEDS - Havrix 1–18 yo: 0.5 mL (720 ELU) IM × 1 dose, then 0.5 mL (720 ELU) IM booster 6–12 mo after first dose. Vaqta 1–18 yo: 0.5 mL (25 U) IM × 1 dose, then 0.5 mL (25 U) IM booster 6–18 mo later.
FORMS - Single dose vial (specify pediatric or adult).
NOTES - Do not inject IV, SC, or ID. Brands may be used interchangeably. Need for boosters is unclear. Post-exposure prophylaxis with hepatitis A vaccine alone is not recommended. Should be given 4 wk prior to travel to endemic area. May be given at the same time as immune globulin, but preferably at different site.

**HEPATITIS B VACCINE (*Engerix-B, Recombivax HB*)** ▶Immune system ♀C ▶+ $$$
ADULT - Engerix-B ≥20 yo: 1 mL (20 mcg) IM, repeat in 1 and 6 mo. Hemodialysis: Give 2.0 mL (40 mcg) IM, repeat in 1, 2, & 6 mo. Give 2.0 mL (40 mcg) IM booster when antibody levels <10 mIU/mL. Recombivax HB: 1 mL (10 mcg) IM, repeat in 1 and 6 mo. Hemodialysis: 1 mL (40 mcg) IM, repeat in 1 & 6 mo. Give 1 mL (40 mcg) IM booster when antibody levels <10 mIU/mL.
PEDS - Specialized dosing based on age and maternal HBsAg status. Infants of hepatitis B negative and positive mothers, children, adolescents <20 yr: Engerix-B 10 mcg (0.5 mL) IM 0, 1, 6 mo. Recombivax 5 mcg (0.5 mL) IM 0, 1, 6 mo. In adolescents 11–15 yr, a 2-dose schedule can be used (Recombivax HB 10 mcg (1.0 mL) IM 0, 4–6 mo).
NOTES - Infants born to hepatitis B positive mothers should also receive hepatitis B immune globulin

and hepatitis B vaccine within 12 h of birth. Not for IV or ID use. May interchange products. Recombivax HB Dialysis Formulation is intended for adults only. Avoid if yeast allergy. Adult formulations contain thimerosal; avoid if allergy.

**HUMAN PAPILLOMAVIRUS RECOMBINANT VACCINE (*Gardasil*)** ▶Immune system ♀B ▶? $$$$$
ADULT - Females up to age 26 yr: 0.5 mL IM at time 0, 2 and 6 mo.
PEDS - Females 9 yr or older: 0.5 mL IM at time 0, 2 and 6 mo.
NOTES - Includes types 6, 11, 16, 18. Patients must be counseled to continue to use condoms. Immunosuppression may reduce response. Fainting and falling may occur after vaccination; observe patient for 15 min after vaccination.

**INFLUENZA VACCINE - INACTIVATED INJECTION (*Afluria, Fluarix, FluLaval, Fluzone, Fluvirin, ◆Fluviral, Vaxigrip*)** ▶Immune system ♀C ▶+ $
ADULT - 0.5 mL IM single dose once yearly.
PEDS - Fluarix and FluLaval are not indicated if <18 yo, Fluvirin not indicated if <4 yo. Age 6- 35 mo: 0.25 mL IM, repeat dose ≥4 wk if previously unvaccinated. Age 3- 8 yo: 0.5 mL IM, repeat dose ≥4 wk if previously unvaccinated. Age 9–12 yo: 0.5 mL IM once yearly.
NOTES - Avoid in Guillain-Barre Syndrome, chicken egg allergy, ASA therapy in children (Reye's risk), thimerosal allergy. Optimal administration October to November.

**INFLUENZA VACCINE - LIVE INTRANASAL (*FluMist*)** ▶Immune system ♀C ▶+ $
ADULT - Healthy adults ages 18–49 yo: 1 dose (0.2 mL) intranasally once yearly.
PEDS - Healthy children 2–17 yo: 1 dose (0.2 mL) intranasally, repeat dose ≥4 wk if previously unvaccinated and 2–8 yo.
NOTES - Avoid in Guillain-Barre Syndrome, chicken egg allergy, ASA therapy in children (Reye's risk), recurrent wheezing and <5 yo. Optimal administration October to November. Since FluMist is a live vaccine, do not use with immune deficiencies (eg, HIV, malignancy, etc.) or altered immune status (eg, taking systemic corticosteroids, chemotherapy, radiation, etc.)

**JAPANESE ENCEPHALITIS VACCINE (*JE-Vax*)** ▶Immune system ♀C ▶? $$$$
ADULT - 1 mL SC × 3 doses on d 0, 7, and 30.
PEDS - Age ≥3 yo: 1.0 mL SC × 3 doses on d 0, 7, and 30. Age 1–3 yo: 0.5 mL SC × 3 doses on d 0, 7, and 30.
NOTES - Give at least 10 d before travel to endemic areas. An abbreviated schedule on d 0, 7, and 14 can be given if time limits. A booster dose may be given after 2 yr. Avoid in thimerosal allergy.

**MEASLES MUMPS & RUBELLA VACCINE (*M-M-R II, ◆Priorix*)** ▶Immune system ♀C ▶+ $$$
ADULT - 0.5 mL (1 vial) SC.
PEDS - 12–15 mo of age: 0.5 mL (1 vial) SC. Revaccinate prior to elementary and/or middle school according to local health guidelines. If

**MEASLES MUMPS & RUBELLA VACCINE (cont.)**

measles outbreak, may immunize infants 6–12 mo old with 0.5 mL SC; then start 2 dose regimen between 12–15 mo of age.

NOTES - Do not inject IV. Contraindicated in pregnancy. Advise women to avoid pregnancy for 4 wk following vaccination. Live virus, contraindicated in immunocompromised patients. Avoid if allergic to neomycin or gelatin; caution in egg allergy.

**MEASLES VACCINE (Attenuvax)** ▶Immune system ♀C ▶+ $

ADULT - 0.5 mL (1 vial) SC.

PEDS - 12–15 mo of age: 0.5 mL (1 vial) SC. Revaccinate prior to elementary school. If measles outbreak, may immunize infants 6–12 mo old with 0.5 mL SC; then start 2 dose regimen (usually with MMR) between 12–15 mo of age.

NOTES - Do not inject IV. Contraindicated in pregnancy. Advise women to avoid pregnancy for 4 wk following vaccination. Live virus, contraindicated in immunocompromised patients. Avoid if allergic to neomycin or gelatin; caution in patients with egg allergies.

**MENINGOCOCCAL VACCINE (Menomune-A/C/Y/W-135, Menactra, ◆Menjugate)** ▶Immune system ♀C ▶? $$$$

WARNING - Reports of associated Guillain-Barre Syndrome; avoid if prior history of this condition.

ADULT - 0.5 mL SC (Menomune) or IM (Menactra).

PEDS - Age ≥2 yo: 0.5 mL SC.

UNAPPROVED PEDS - Age 3–18 mo: 0.5 mL SC × 2 doses separated by 3 mo.

NOTES - Give 2 wk before elective splenectomy or before travel to endemic areas. May consider revaccination q3–5 yr in high risk patients. Do not inject IV. Contraindicated in pregnancy. Consider vaccinating 11–12 yo and first-yr college students living in dormitories. Avoid in thimerosal allergy.

**MUMPS VACCINE (Mumpsvax)** ▶Immune system ♀C ▶+ $$

ADULT - 0.5 mL (1 vial) SC.

PEDS - 12–15 mo of age: 0.5 mL (1 vial) SC. Revaccinate prior to elementary school.

NOTES - Do not inject IV. Contraindicated in pregnancy. Advise women to avoid pregnancy for 4 wk following vaccination. Live virus, contraindicated in immunocompromised patients. Avoid if allergic to neomycin or gelatin; caution in patients with egg allergies.

**PEDIARIX (diphtheria tetanus and acellular pertussis vaccine + hepatitis B vaccine + polio vaccine)** ▶Immune system ♀C ▶? $$$

PEDS - 0.5 mL at 2, 4, 6 mo IM.

NOTES - Do not administer before 6 wk of age.

**PLAGUE VACCINE ▶IMMUNE SYSTEM** ♀C ▶+ $

ADULT - Age 18–61 yo: 1 mL IM × 1 dose, then 0.2 mL IM 1–3 mo after the 1st injection, then 0.2 mL IM 5–6 mo after the 2nd injection.

PEDS - Not approved in children.

NOTES - Up to 3 booster doses (0.2 mL) may be administered at 6 mo intervals in high risk patients. Jet injector gun may be used for IM administration.

**PNEUMOCOCCAL 23-VALENT VACCINE (Pneumovax, ◆Pneumo 23)** ▶Immune system ♀C ▶+ $$

ADULT - All adults 65 yr or older: 0.5 mL IM/SCx1. Vaccination also recommended for high-risk individuals < 65 yo. Routine revaccination in immunocompetent patients is not recommended. Consider revaccination once in patients ≥65 yo (if <65 yo at initial vaccination) or patients at high risk of developing serious pneumococcal infection if >5 yr from initial vaccine.

PEDS - ≥2 yo: 0.5 mL IM/SC. Consider revaccination once in patients at high risk of developing serious pneumococcal infection after 3–5 yo from initial vaccine in patients that would be ≤10 yo at revaccination.

NOTES - Do not give IV or ID. May be given in conjunction with influenza virus vaccine at different site. OK for high risk children ≥2 yo who received Prevnar series already to provide additional serotype coverage. Avoid in thimerosal allergy.

**PNEUMOCOCCAL 7-VALENT CONJUGATE VACCINE (Prevnar)** ▶Immune system ♀C ▶? $$$

ADULT - Not approved in adults.

PEDS - 0.5 mL IM × 3 doses 6–8 wk apart starting at 2–6 mo of age, followed by a 4th dose of 0.5 mL IM at 12–15 mo. For previously unvaccinated older infants and children age 7–11 mo: 0.5 mL × 2 doses 6–8 wk apart, followed by a 3rd dose of 0.5 mL at 12–15 mo. Age 12–23 mo: 0.5 mL × 2 doses 6–8 wk apart. Age 2–9 yo: 0.5 mL × 1 dose; give 2nd dose 4 wk later in immunocompromised or chronically ill children.

NOTES - For IM use only; do not inject IV. Shake susp vigorously prior to administration.

**POLIO VACCINE (IPOL)** ▶Immune system ♀C ▶? $$

ADULT - Not generally recommended. Previously unvaccinated adults at increased risk of exposure should receive a complete primary immunization series of 3 doses (two doses at intervals of 4–8 wk; a third dose at 6–12 mo after the 2nd dose). Accelerated schedules are available. Travelers to endemic areas who have received primary immunization should receive a single booster in adulthood.

PEDS - 0.5 mL IM or SC at 2 mo of age, with 2nd dose at 4 mo, 3rd dose at 6–18 mo, and 4th dose at 4–6 yo.

NOTES - Oral polio vaccine no longer available.

**PROQUAD (measles mumps & rubella vaccine + varicella vaccine, MMRV)** ▶Immune system ♀C ▶? $$$$

ADULT - Not indicated in adults.

PEDS - 12 mo - 12 yo: 0.5 mL (1 vial) SC.

NOTES - Give ≥1 mo after a MMR-containing vaccine and ≥3 mo after a varicella-containing vaccine. Do not inject IV. Contraindicated in pregnancy. Following vaccination avoid pregnancy for 3 mo and ASA/salicylates for 6 wk. Live virus, contraindicated in immunocompromise or untreated TB. Avoid if allergic to neomycin; caution with egg allergies.

**RABIES VACCINE (*RabAvert, Imovax Rabies, BioRab, Rabies Vaccine Adsorbed*)** ►Immune system ♀C ▶? $$$$$
ADULT - Post-exposure prophylaxis: Give rabies immune globulin (20 IU/kg) immediately after exposure, then give rabies vaccine 1 mL IM in deltoid region on d 0, 3, 7, 14, and 28. If patients have received pre-exposure immunization, give 1 mL IM rabies vaccine on d 0 and 3 only without rabies immune globulin. Pre-exposure immunization: 1 mL IM rabies vaccine on d 0, 7, and between d 21–28. Or 0.1 mL ID on d 0, 7, and between d 21–28. (Imovax Rabies I.D. vaccine formula only). Repeat q2–5 yr based on antibody titer.
PEDS - Same as adults.
NOTES - Do not use ID preparation for post-exposure prophylaxis.

**ROTAVIRUS VACCINE (*RotaTeq, Rotarix*)** ►Immune system ♀ ▶? $$$$$
ADULT - Not recommended.
PEDS - RotaTeq: Give the first dose (2 mL PO) between 6–12 wk of age, and then the 2nd & 3rd doses at 4–10 wk intervals thereafter (last dose no later than 32 wk). Rotarix: Give first dose (1 mL) at 6 wk of age, and 2nd dose (1 mL) at least 4 wk later, and prior to 24 wk of age.
FORMS - Trade only: Oral susp 2 mL (RotaTeq), 1 mL (Rotarix).
NOTES - Live vaccine so potential for transmission, especially to immunodeficient close contacts. Safety unclear in immunocompromised infants.

**RUBELLA VACCINE (*Meruvax II*)** ►Immune system ♀C ▶+ $
ADULT - 0.5 mL (1 vial) SC.
PEDS - 12–15 mo of age: 0.5 mL (1 vial) SC. Revaccinate prior to elementary school according to local health guidelines.
NOTES - Do not inject IV. Contraindicated in pregnancy. Advise women to avoid pregnancy for 4 wk following vaccination. Live virus, contraindicated in immunocompromised patients. Avoid if allergic to neomycin or gelatin.

**SMALLPOX VACCINE (*ACAM 2000, vaccinia vaccine*)** ►Immune system ♀C ▶- Not available to civilians
ADULT - Prevention of smallpox or monkeypox: Specialized administration using bifurcated needle SC × 1.
PEDS - >1 yo: Specialized administration using bifurcated needle SC × 1.
NOTES - Caution in polymyxin, neomycin, tetracycline, or streptomycin allergy. Avoid in those (or household contacts of those) with eczema or a history of eczema, those with a rash due to other causes (eg, burns, zoster, impetigo, psoriasis), immunocompromise, or pregnancy. Persons with known cardiac disease or ≥3 risk factors for cardiac disease should not be vaccinated as response team members in the pre-event smallpox vaccination program.

**TETANUS TOXOID ►IMMUNE SYSTEM ♀C ▶+ $**
WARNING - Td is preferred in adults and children ≥7 yo. DTP is preferred in children <7 yo. Use fluid tetanus toxoid in assessing cell-mediated immunity only.
ADULT - 0.5 mL IM (adsorbed) × 2 doses 4–8 wk apart. Give third dose 6–12 mo after 2nd injection. Give booster q10 yr. Assess cell-mediated immunity: 0.1 mL of 1:100 diluted skin-test reagent or 0.02 mL of 1: 10 diluted skin-test reagent injected intradermally.
PEDS - 0.5 mL IM (adsorbed) × 2 doses 4–8 wk apart. Give third dose 6–12 mo after 2nd injection. Give booster q10 yr.
NOTES - May use tetanus toxoid fluid for active immunization in patients hypersensitive to the aluminum adjuvant of the adsorbed formulation: 0.5 mL IM or SC × 3 doses at 4- 8 wk intervals. Give fourth dose 6- 12 mo after third injection. Give booster dose q10 yr. Avoid in thimerosal allergy

*TRIHIBIT*(**haemophilus B vaccine + diphtheria tetanus and acellular pertussis vaccine**) ►Immune system ♀C ▶- $$$
PEDS - For 4th dose only, 15–18 mo: 0.5 mL IM.
NOTES - Tripedia (DTaP) is used to reconstitute ActHIB (Haemophilus b) to make TriHIBit and will appear whitish in color. Use within 30 min. Avoid in thimerosal allergy.

**TWINRIX (hepatitis A vaccine + hepatitis B vaccine)** ►Immune system ♀C ▶? $$$
ADULT - ≥18 yo: 1 mL IM in deltoid only, repeat in 1 & 6 mo. Accelerated dosing schedule: 0, 7, 21–30 d and booster dose at 12 mo.
PEDS - Not approved in children.
NOTES - Not for IV or ID use. 1 mL = 720 ELU inactivated hepatitis A + 20 mcg hepatitis B surface antigen.

**TYPHOID VACCINE - INACTIVATED INJECTION (*Typhim Vi, ✦Typherix*)** ►Immune system ♀C ▶? $$
ADULT - 0.5 mL IM × 1 dose given at least 2 wk prior to potential exposure. May consider revaccination q2 yr in high risk patients.
PEDS - Age ≥2 yo: same as adult dose.
NOTES - Recommended for travel to endemic areas.

**TYPHOID VACCINE - LIVE ORAL (*Vivotif Berna*)** ►Immune system ♀C ▶? $$
ADULT - 1 cap 1 h before a meal with cold or lukewarm drink qod × 4 doses to be completed at least 1 wk prior to potential exposure. May consider revaccination q5 yr in high risk patients.
PEDS - Age ≥6 yo: same as adult dose.
FORMS - Trade only: Caps
NOTES - Recommended for travel to endemic areas. Oral vaccine may be inactivated by antibiotics, including antimalarials.

**VARICELLA VACCINE (*Varivax, ✦Varilrix*)** ►Immune system ♀C ▶+ $$$
ADULT - 0.5 mL SC. Repeat 4- 8 wk later.
PEDS - age 1- 12 yo: 0.5 mL SC × 1 dose. Age ≥13 yo: same as adult dose. Not recommended for infants <1 yo.
UNAPPROVED PEDS - Postexposure prophylaxis: 0.5 mL SC within 3–5 d of exposure.

| CHILDHOOD IMMUNIZATION SCHEDULE* | | | | | | Months | | | Years | | |
|---|---|---|---|---|---|---|---|---|---|---|---|
| Age | Birth | 1 | 2 | 4 | 6 | 12 | 15 | 18 | 2 | 4-6 | 11-12 |
| Hepatitis B | HB | HB | | | | HB | | | | | |
| Rotavirus | | | Rota | Rota | Rota | | | | | | |
| DTP | | | DTaP | DTaP | DTaP | | DTaP | | | DTaP | DTaP |
| H influenza b | | | Hib | Hib | Hib | Hib | | | | | |
| Pneumococci | | | PCV | PCV | PCV | PCV | | | | | |
| Polio | | | IPV | IPV | | IPV | | | | IPV | |
| Influenza† | | | | | | Influenza (yearly)† | | | | | |
| MMR | | | | | | MMR | | | | | MMR |
| Varicella | | | | | | Varicella | | | | | Vari |
| Hepatitis A¶ | | | | | | Hep A × 2¶ | | | | | |
| Papillomavirus§ | | | | | | | | | | | HPV × 3§ |
| Meningococcal | | | | | | | | | | | MCV |

*2007 schedule from the CDC, ACIP, AAP, & AAFP, see CDC website (www.cdc.gov).
†If ≥5 yo and healthy can use intransal form. If <9 yo receiving for first time, should get 2 doses ≥4 weeks apart for injected form and ≥6 weeks apart for intranasal.
¶Two doses at least 6 months apart.
§Second and third doses 2 and 6 months after first dose.

## VARICELLA VACCINE (cont.)

NOTES - Do not inject IV. Following vaccination avoid pregnancy for 3 mo and ASA/salicylates for 6 wk. The need for booster doses is currently not defined. This live vaccine is contraindicated in immunocompromised. Vaccine is stored in freezer; thawed vaccine must be used within 30 min.

## YELLOW FEVER VACCINE (YF-Vax) ▶Immune system ♀C ▶+ $$$
ADULT - 0.5 mL SC.
PEDS - 0.5 mL SC into the thigh (6 mo - 3 yo) or deltoid region (≥3 yo).
NOTES - Approval by state and/or federal authorities required to obtain vaccine. A booster dose (0.5 mL) may be administered q10 yr.

## ZOSTER VACCINE - LIVE (Zostavax) ▶Immune system ♀C ▶? $$$$
ADULT - Adults ≥60 yr: 0.65 mL SC × 1.
PEDS - Not approved in children.
NOTES - Avoid if there is history of anaphylactic/anaphylactoid reaction to gelatin or neomycin, if primary or acquired immunodeficiency states, or if taking immunosuppressives. Do not administer if active untreated tuberculosis or in possible pregnancy. Theoretically possible to transmit to pregnant household contact who has not had varicella infection or immunocompromised contact. Do not substitute for Varivax in children.

## IMMUNOLOGY: Immunoglobulins

NOTE: Adult IM injections should be given in the deltoid region; injection in the gluteal region may result in suboptimal response.

## ANTIVENIN - CROTALIDAE IMMUNE FAB OVINE POLYVALENT (CroFab) ▶? ♀C ▶? $$$$$
ADULT - Rattlesnake envenomation: Give 4–6 vials IV infusion over 60 min, within 6 h of bite if possible. Administer 4–6 additional vials if no initial control of envenomation syndrome, then 2 vials q6h for up to 18 h (3 doses) after initial control has been established.

PEDS - Same as adults, although specific studies in children have not been conducted.
NOTES - Contraindicated with allergy to papaya or to papain. Start IV infusion slowly over the first 10 min at 25–50 mL/h and observe for allergic reaction, then increase to full rate of 250 mL/h.

| ADULT IMMUNIZATION SCHEDULE* | |
|---|---|
| Hepatitis A | For all ages with clotting factor disorders, chronic liver disease, or exposure risk (travel to endemic areas, IV drug use, men having sex with men), 2 doses (0, 6–12 mo). |
| Hepatitis B | For all ages with medical (hemodialysis, clotting factor recipients), occupational (healthcare or public safety workers with blood exposure), behavioral (IV drug use, multiple sex partners, recent sexually transmitted disease, men having sex with men) or other (household/sex contacts of those with chronic HBV infections, clients/staff of developmentally disabled, >6 mo travel to high risk areas, inmates of correctional facilitites) indications , 3 doses (0, 1–2, 4–6 mo). |
| Herpes zoster | Consider single dose of vaccine in individuals 60 yr of age or older. |
| Human papillomavirus | Consider HPV vaccine in women 9–26 yr at 0, 2, and 6 mo. |
| Influenza | 1 yearly dose if ≥65 yo. If <65 yr, then 1 yearly dose if healthcare worker, chronic underlying illness, or household contact of person with chronic underlying illness. Intranasal vaccine indicated for healthy adults <50 yr. |
| Measles, mumps, rubella (MMR) | If <50 yo and immunity in doubt, see www.cdc.gov. |
| Meningococcal (polysaccharide) | For all ages if medical (complement deficiency, anatomic or functional asplenia) or other (travel to endemic regions, consider for college dormitory residents) indications, 1 dose. Consider revaccination in 3–5 yr if high-risk. |
| Pertussis | Consider single dose of pertussis in adults as part of DTaP (Adacel), at least 10 yr since last tetanus dose. |
| Pneumococcal (polysaccharide) | 1 dose if ≥65 yo. If <65 yr, consider immunizing if chronic underlying illness, nursing home resident, or Native American. Consider revaccination 5 yr later if high risk or if ≥65 yr and received primary dose before age 65. |
| Tetanus, diphtheria (Td) | For all ages, 1 dose booster every 10 yr. |
| Varicella | For all ages if immunity in doubt, if ≥13 yr, 2 doses separated by 4–8 wk, see www.cdc.gov |

*2005 schedule from the CDC, ACIP, & AAFP, see CDC website (www.cdc.gov).

**ANTIVENIN - CROTALIDAE POLYVALENT** ▶L ♀C ▶? $$$$$
ADULT - Pit viper envenomation: minimal envenomation: 20- 40 mL (2- 4 vials) IV infusion; moderate envenomation: 50- 90 mL (5- 9 vials) IV infusion; severe envenomation: ≥100- 150 mL (10- 15 vials) IV infusion. Administer within 4 h of bite, less effective after 8 h, and of questionable value after 12 h. May give additional 10- 50 mL (1- 5 vials) IV infusion based on clinical assessment and response to initial dose.
PEDS - Larger relative doses of antivenin are needed in children and small adults because of small volume of body fluid to dilute the venom. The dose is not based on weight.
NOTES - Test first for sensitivity to horse serum. Serum sickness may occur 5–24 d after dose. IV route is preferred. May give IM.

**ANTIVENIN - LATRODECTUS MACTANS** ▶L ♀C ▶? $$
ADULT - Specialized dosing for black widow spider toxicity; consult poison center.
PEDS - Specialized dosing for black widow spider toxicity; consult poison center.
NOTES - Test first for horse serum sensitivity. Serum sickness may occur 5–24 d after dose.

**BOTULISM IMMUNE GLOBULIN (BabyBIG)** ▶L ♀? ▶? $$$$$
ADULT - Not approved in >1 yo.
PEDS - Infant botulism <1 yo: 1 mL (50 mg)/kg IV.

**CYTOMEGALOVIRUS IMMUNE GLOBULIN HUMAN (Cytogam)** ▶L ♀C ▶? $$$$$
ADULT - Specialized dosing based on indication and time since transplant.
PEDS - Specialized dosing based on indication and time since transplant.

**HEPATITIS B IMMUNE GLOBULIN (H-BIG, HyperHep B, HepaGam B, NABI-HB)** ▶L ♀C ▶? $$$
ADULT - Post-exposure prophylaxis for needlestick, ocular, mucosal exposure: 0.06 mL/kg IM (usual dose 3- 5 mL) within 24 h of exposure. Initiate hepatitis B vaccine series within 7 d. Consider a 2nd dose of hepatitis B immune globulin (HBIG) one mo later if patient refuses hepatitis B vaccine series. Post-exposure prophylaxis for sexual exposure: 0.06 mL/kg IM within 14d of sexual contact. Initiate hepatitis B vaccine series. Prevention of hepatitis B recurrence following liver transplantation in HBsAg-positive (HepaGam B): first dose given during transplantation surgery. Subsequent doses daily for 7 d, then biweekly up to 3 mo and

**HEPATITIS B IMMUNE GLOBULIN** *(cont.)*

monthly thereafter. Doses adjusted based on regular monitoring of HBsAg, HBV-DNA, HBeAg and anti-HBs antibody levels.

PEDS - Prophylaxis of infants born to HBsAg (+) mothers: 0.5 mL IM within 12 h of birth. Initiate hepatitis B vaccine series within 7 d. If hepatitis B vaccine series is refused, repeat HBIG dose at 3 and 6 mo. Household exposure <12 mo of age: 0.5 mL IM within 14d of exposure. Initiate hep B vaccine series.

NOTES - HBIG may be administered at the same time or up to 1 mo prior to hepatitis B vaccine without impairing the active immune response from hepatitis B vaccine.

**IMMUNE GLOBULIN - INTRAMUSCULAR** *(Baygam, ◆Gamastan)* ▶L ♀C ▶? $$$$
ADULT - Hepatitis A post-exposure prophylaxis for household or institutional contacts): 0.02 mL/kg IM within 2 wk of exposure. Hepatitis A pre-exposure prophylaxis (ie, travel to endemic area): <3 mo length of stay = 0.02 mL/kg IM. >3 mo length of stay = 0.06 mL/kg IM and repeat q4–6 mo. Measles: 0.2–0.25 mL/kg IM within 6 d of exposure, max 15 mL. Varicella zoster (if VariZIG unavailable): 0.6–1.2 mL/kg IM. Rubella exposure in pregnant, susceptible women: 0.55 mL/kg IM. Immunoglobulin deficiency: 0.66 mL/kg IM every 3–4 wk.

PEDS - Not approved in children.

UNAPPROVED PEDS - Measles: 0.2–0.25 mL/kg IM within 6 d of exposure. In susceptible immunocompromised children use 0.5 mL/kg IM (max 15 mL) immediately after exposure. Varicella zoster (if VariZIG unavailable): 0.6–1.2 mL/kg IM.

NOTES - Human derived product, increased infection risk. Hepatitis A vaccine preferred over immune globulin for persons >2 yo who plan to travel to high risk areas repeatedly or for long periods of time.

**IMMUNE GLOBULIN - INTRAVENOUS** *(Carimune, Polygam, Panglobulin, Octagam, Flebogamma, Gammagard, Gamunex, Iveegam, Privigen, Venoglobulin)* ▶L ♀C ▶? $$$$$
ADULT - Idiopathic thrombocytopenic purpura (induction): 400 mg/kg IV daily × 5 d (or 1 g/kg IV daily for 1–2 d). Bone marrow transplant (>20 yo): 500 mg/kg IV daily, given 7 and 2 d before transplant, and then weekly until 90 d post transplant. Primary humoral immunodeficiency: 200–300 mg/kg IV each mo; increase as needed to max 400–800 mg/kg/mo. B-cell chronic lymphocytic leukemia: specialized dosing.

PEDS - Pediatric HIV: 400 mg/kg IV q28 d. Idiopathic thrombocytopenic purpura (induction): 400 mg/kg IV daily × 5 d (or 1 g/kg IV daily for 1–2 d). Kawasaki Syndrome (acute): 400 mg/kg IV daily × 4 d (or 2 g/kg IV × 1 over 10 h). Primary humoral immunodeficiency: 200–300 mg/kg IV each mo; increase as needed to max 400–800 mg/kg/mo.

UNAPPROVED ADULT - First-line therapy in severe Guillain-Barré syndrome, chronic inflammatory demyelinating polyneuropathy, multifocal motor neuropathy, severe post-transfusion purpura, inclusion body myositis, fetomaternal alloimmune thrombocytopenia; sec-line therapy in stiff-person syndrome, dermatomyositis, myasthenia gravis, and Lambert-Eaton myasthenic syndrome: Various dosing regimens have been used; a common one is myasthenia gravis (induction): 400 mg/kg IV daily × 5 d (total 2 g/kg). Has been used in multiple sclerosis and inflammatory myositis (polymyositis & dermatomyositis), renal transplant rejection, systemic lupus erythematosus, toxic epidermal necrolysis and Stevens-Johnson syndrome, Clostridium difficile colitis, Graves' ophthalmopathy, pemphigus, Wegener's granulomatosis, Churg-Strauss syndrome and Duchenne muscular dystrophy

UNAPPROVED PEDS - Myasthenia gravis (induction): 400 mg/kg IV daily × 5 d. Other dosing regimens have been used.

NOTES - Indications and doses vary by product. Follow LFTs, renal function, vital signs, and urine output closely. Contraindicated in IgA deficiency. Use caution (and lower infusion rates) if risk factors for thrombosis, heart failure, or renal insufficiency. Use slower infusion rates for initial doses. Consider pretreatment with acetaminophen and/or diphenhydramine to minimize some infusion-related adverse effects. Human-derived product; although donors are carefully screened there is risk of transmission of infectious agents.

**IMMUNE GLOBULIN - SUBCUTANEOUS** *(Vivaglobulin)* ▶L ♀C ▶? $$$$$
ADULT - Primary immune deficiency: 100–200 mg/kg SC weekly. In patients already receiving IV immune globulin: SC dose = (previous IV dose × 1.37) divided by frequency of IV regimen in wk.

PEDS - Limited information. Dosing appears to be same as in adults.

NOTES - Do not administer IV. Contraindicated in IgA deficiency. Human-derived product, increased infection risk.

**LYMPHOCYTE IMMUNE GLOBULIN** *(Atgam)* ▶L ♀C ▶? $$$$$
ADULT - Renal allograft recipients: 10–30 mg/kg IV daily. Delaying onset of allograft rejection: 15 mg/kg IV daily × 14 d, then qod × 14 d. Treatment of renal transplant rejection: 10–15 mg/kg IV × 14 d. Aplastic anemia: 10–20 mg/kg IV daily × 8–14 d, then qod, as needed, up to 21 total doses.

PEDS - Limited experience. Has been safely administered to a limited number of children with renal transplant and aplastic anemia at doses comparable to adults.

NOTES - Equine product. Doses should be administered over ≥4 h.

**RABIES IMMUNE GLOBULIN HUMAN** *(Imogam Rabies-HT, HyperRAB S/D)* ▶L ♀C ▶? $$$$$
ADULT - Post-exposure prophylaxis: 20 units/kg (0.133 mL/kg), with as much as possible infiltrated around the bite and the rest given IM. Give as soon

(cont.)

**RABIES IMMUNE GLOBULIN HUMAN** (*cont.*)
as possible after exposure. Administer with the first dose of vaccine, but in a different extremity.
PEDS - Not approved in children.
UNAPPROVED PEDS - Use adult dosing.
NOTES - Do not repeat dose once rabies vaccine series begins. Do not give to patients who have been completely immunized with rabies vaccine. Do not administer IV.

**RSV IMMUNE GLOBULIN** (*RespiGam*) ▶Plasma ♀C ▶? $$$$$
PEDS - RSV prophylaxis in children <24 mo: 1.5 mL/kg/h × 15 min. Increase rate as clinical condition permits to 3 mL/kg/h × 15 min, then to a max rate of 6 mL/kg/h. Max total dose/mo is 750 mg/kg.
NOTES - May cause fluid overload; monitor vital signs frequently during IV infusion. RSV season is typically November-April.

**TETANUS IMMUNE GLOBULIN** (*BayTet*, *✦Hypertet*) ▶L ♀C ▶? $$$$
ADULT - See tetanus wound management table.

Post-exposure prophylaxis in tetanus prone wounds in patients ≥7 yr of age: if <3 doses of tetanus vaccine have been administered or if history is uncertain, give 250 units IM × 1 dose along with dT. If ≥3 doses of tetanus vaccine have been administered in the past, do not give tetanus immune globulin. Tetanus treatment: 3000–6000 units IM in combination with other therapies.
PEDS - <7 yo: 4 units/kg IM or 250 units IM. Initiate tetanus toxoid vaccine (DTP or DT).
NOTES - Do not give tetanus immune globulin for clean, minor wounds. May be given at the same time as tetanus toxoid active immunization. Do not inject IV.

**VARICELLA-ZOSTER IMMUNE GLOBULIN** (*VariZIG, VZIG*) ▶L ♀C ▶? $$$$$
ADULT - Specialized dosing for post-exposure prophylaxis.
PEDS - Specialized dosing for post-exposure prophylaxis.

---

## IMMUNOLOGY: Immunosuppression

**BASILIXIMAB** (*Simulect*) ▶Plasma ♀B ▶? $$$$$
ADULT - Specialized dosing for organ transplantation.
PEDS - Specialized dosing for organ transplantation.

**CYCLOSPORINE** (*Sandimmune, Neoral, Gengraf*) ▶L ♀C ▶- $$$$$
ADULT - Specialized dosing for organ transplantation, RA, and psoriasis.
PEDS - Not approved in children.
UNAPPROVED ADULT - Specialized dosing for autoimmune eye disorders, vasculitis, inflammatory myopathies, Behcet's disease, psoriatic arthritis, chronic refractory idiopathic thrombocytopenia.
UNAPPROVED PEDS - Specialized dosing for organ transplantation, chronic refractory idiopathic thrombocytopenia.
FORMS - Generic/Trade: microemulsion Caps 25, 100 mg. Generic/Trade: Caps (Sandimmune) 25, 100 mg, solution (Sandimmune) 100 mg/mL, microemulsion solution (Neoral, Gengraf) 100 mg/mL.
NOTES - Monitor cyclosporine blood concentrations closely. Many drug interactions including atorvastatin, azithromycin, lovastatin, oral contraceptives, rosuvastatin, simvastatin, sirolimus, terbinafine, voriconazole. Use caution when combining with methotrexate or potassium sparing drugs such as ACE inhibitors. Reduce dose in renal dysfunction. Monitor BP and renal function closely. Avoid excess UV light exposure. Monitor patients closely when switching from Sandimmune to microemulsion formulations.

**DACLIZUMAB** (*Zenapax*) ▶L ♀C ▶? $$$$$
ADULT - Specialized dosing for organ transplantation.
PEDS - Not approved in children.
UNAPPROVED PEDS - Specialized dosing for organ transplantation.

**MYCOPHENOLATE MOFETIL** (*Cellcept, Myfortic*) ▶? ♀D ▶? $$$$$
ADULT - Specialized dosing for organ transplantation.
PEDS - Not approved in children.
UNAPPROVED ADULT - Lupus nephritis: 1000 mg PO bid. Has been used in pemphigus, bullous pemphigoid, and refractory uveitis.
UNAPPROVED PEDS - Specialized dosing for organ transplantation.
FORMS - Trade only (CellCept): caps 250 mg, tabs 500 mg, oral susp 200 mg/mL. Trade (Myfortic): tab, extended-release: 180, 360 mg.
NOTES - Increased risk of first trimester pregnancy loss and increased risk of congenital malformations, especially external ear and facial abnormalities.

**SIROLIMUS** (*Rapamune*) ▶L ♀C ▶- $$$$$
WARNING - Increased risk of infection and lymphoma. Combination of sirolimus plus cyclosporine or tacrolimus is associated with hepatic artery thrombosis in liver transplant patients. Combination with tacrolimus and corticosteroids in lung transplant patients may cause bronchial anastomotic dehiscence. Can cause hypersensitivity reactions including anaphylactic and/or anaphylactoid reactions, angioedema, vasculitis. Avoid with strong inhibitors of CYP3A4 and/or P-glycoprotein (ketoconazole, voriconazole, itraconazole, erythromycin, telithromycin, clarithromycin) or strong inducers CYP3A4 and/or P-glycoprotein (rifampin, rifabutin). Monitor level if cyclosporine is discontinued or has dose markedly changed.
ADULT - Specialized dosing for organ transplantation.
PEDS - Not approved in children.
UNAPPROVED PEDS - Specialized dosing for organ transplantation.

**SIROLIMUS** (*cont.*)
FORMS - Trade only: oral solution 1 mg/mL (60 mL). Tab 1, 2 mg.
NOTES - Wear protective clothing and sunscreen when exposed to sunlight to reduce the risk of skin cancer. Adjust dose by 1/3 to 1/2 in liver dysfunction. Monitor trough levels—particularly in patients likely to have altered drug metabolism, ≥13 yo who weigh <40 kg, hepatic impairment, when changing doses or with interacting medications . Do not adjust dose more frequently than q1–2 wk. Oral solution & tabs are clinically equivalent from a dosing standpoint at the 2 mg level; however this is unknown at higher doses.

**TACROLIMUS** (*Prograf, FK 506*) ▶L ♀C ▶- $$$$$
ADULT - Specialized dosing for organ transplantation.
PEDS - Specialized dosing for organ transplantation.
UNAPPROVED ADULT - RA (approved in Canada), active vasculitis, systemic lupus erythematosus nephritis & vasculitis.
FORMS - Trade only: Caps 0.5, 1, 5 mg.
NOTES - Reduce dose in renal dysfunction. Monitor BP and renal function closely. Many drug interactions.

## IMMUNOLOGY: Other

**HYMENOPTERA VENOM ▶SERUM ♀C ▶? $$$$**
ADULT - Specialized desensitization dosing protocol.
PEDS - Specialized desensitization dosing protocol.
NOTES - Venom products available: honey bee (Apis mellifera) and yellow jacket (Vespula sp.), yellow hornet (Dolichovespula arenaria), white-faced hornet (Dolichovespula maculata) and wasp (Polistes sp.). Mixed vespid venom protein (yellow jacket, yellow hornet and white-faced hornet) is also available.

**RILONACEPT** (*Arcalyst*) ▶? ♀? ▶? $$$$$
ADULT - Familial cold auto-inflammatory syndrome (FCAS) and Muckle-Wells syndrome (MWS): Begin therapy with a loading dose of 320 mg (160 mg SC on the same d at two different sites), then 160 mg SC once weekly.
PEDS - Familial cold auto-inflammatory syndrome (FCAS) and Muckle-Wells syndrome (MWS): Begin therapy with a loading dose of 4.4 mg/kg (to a max of 320 mg) SC in one or two doses, then 2.2 mg/kg (to a max of 160 mg) SC once weekly.
NOTES - Increased risk of infections.

**TUBERCULIN PPD** (*Aplisol, Tubersol, Mantoux, PPD*) ▶L ♀C ▶+ $
ADULT - 5 TU (0.1 mL) intradermally.
PEDS - Same as adult dose. AAP recommends screening at 12 mo, 4- 6 yo, and 14- 16 yo.
NOTES - Avoid SC injection. Read 48- 72 h after intradermal injection. Repeat testing in patients with known prior positive PPD may cause scarring at injection site.

## NEUROLOGY: Alzheimer's Disease—Cholinesterase Inhibitors

**NOTE:** Avoid concurrent use of anticholinergic agents. Use caution in asthma/COPD. May be co-administered with memantine.

**DONEPEZIL** (*Aricept*) ▶LK ♀C ▶? $$$$
ADULT - Alzheimer's disease: Start 5 mg PO qhs. May increase to 10 mg PO qhs in 4–6 wk. For severe disease (MMSE ≤10), the recommended dose is 10 mg/d.
PEDS - Not approved in children.
UNAPPROVED ADULT - Dementia in Parkinson's disease: 5–10 mg/d.
FORMS - Generic/Trade: Tabs 5,10 mg. Trade only: Orally disintegrating tabs 5,10 mg.
NOTES - Some clinicians start with 5 mg PO qod to minimize GI side effects.

**GALANTAMINE** (*Razadyne, Razadyne ER, ◆Reminyl*) ▶LK ♀B ▶? $$$$
ADULT - Alzheimer's disease: Extended release: Start 8 mg PO q am with food; increase to 16 mg q am after 4 wk. May increase to 24 mg q am after another 4 wk. Immediate release: Start 4 mg PO bid with food; increase to 8 mg bid after 4 wk. May increase to 12 mg PO bid after another 4 wk.
PEDS - Not approved in children.
UNAPPROVED ADULT - Dementia in Parkinson's disease: 4–8 mg PO bid (immediate release).
FORMS - Trade only: Tabs (Razadyne) 4, 8, 12 mg; oral solution 4 mg/mL. Extended release caps (Razadyne ER) 8, 16, 24 mg. Prior to April 2005 was called Reminyl.
NOTES - Do not exceed 16 mg/d with renal or hepatic impairment. Use caution with CYP3A4 and CYP2D6 inhibitors (eg, cimetidine, ranitidine, ketoconazole, erythromycin, paroxetine). Avoid abrupt discontinuation. If therapy has been interrupted for several d or more, then restart at the lowest dose.

**RIVASTIGMINE** (*Exelon, Exelon Patch*) ▶K ♀B ▶? $$$$$
ADULT - Alzheimer's disease: Start 1.5 mg PO bid with food. Increase to 3 mg bid after 2 wk. Usual effective dose is 6–12 mg/d. Max 12 mg/d. Patch: Start 4.6 mg/24h once daily; may increase after ≥1 mo to max 9.5 mg/24h. Dementia associated with Parkinson's disease: Start 1.5 mg PO bid with food. Increase by 3 mg/d at intervals >4 wk to max 12 mg/d. Patch: Start 4.6 mg/24h once daily; may increase after ≥1 mo to max 9.5 mg/24h.
PEDS - Not approved in children.
FORMS - Generic/Trade: Caps 1.5, 3, 4.5, 6 mg. Trade only: Oral solution 2 mg/mL (120 mL). Transdermal patch: 4.6 mg/24h (9 mg/patch), 9.5 mg/24h (18 mg/patch).

(cont.)

**RIVASTIGMINE** (*cont.*)

NOTES - Restart treatment with the lowest daily dose (ie, 1.5 mg PO bid) if discontinued for several d to reduce the risk of severe vomiting. Use solution if difficulty swallowing. When changing from PO to patch, patients taking <6 mg/d can be placed on 4.6 mg/24h patch. For those taking 6–12 mg/d, may start with 9.5 mg/24h patch. Have patient start the d after stopping oral dosing. Rotate application sites and do not apply to same spot for 14 d.

**TACRINE** (*Cognex*) ▶L ♀C ▶? $$$$$

ADULT - Alzheimer's disease (not first line): Start 10 mg PO qid for 4 wk, then increase to 20 mg qid. Titrate to higher doses q4 wk as tolerated. Max 160 mg/d.

PEDS - Not approved in children.

FORMS - Trade only: Caps 10, 20, 30, 40 mg.

NOTES - Hepatotoxicity may occur. Monitor LFTs q2 wk × 16 wk, then q3 mo.

## NEUROLOGY: Alzheimer's Disease—NMDA Receptor Antagonists

**MEMANTINE** (*Namenda*, ✦*Ebixa*) ▶KL ♀B ▶? $$$$

ADULT - Alzheimer's disease (moderate to severe): Start 5 mg PO daily. Increase by 5 mg/d at weekly intervals to max 20 mg/d. Doses >5 mg/d should be divided bid.

PEDS - Not approved in children.

FORMS - Trade only: Tabs 5, 10 mg. Oral soln 2 mg/mL.

NOTES - May be used in combination with acetylcholinesterase inhibitors. Reduce target dose to 5 mg PO bid in severe renal impairment (CrCl 5–29 mL/min). No dosage adjustment needed for mild-moderate renal impairment.

## NEUROLOGY: Anticonvulsants

**NOTE:** Avoid rapid discontinuation of anticonvulsants, since this can precipitate seizures or other withdrawal symptoms. Recent data suggest an increased risk of suicidal ideation or behaviors with antiepileptic drugs. Monitor closely for signs of depression, anxiety, hostility, hypomania/mania, or suicidality. Symptoms may develop within one wk of initiation, and risk continues for at least 24 wk.

**CARBAMAZEPINE** (*Tegretol, Tegretol XR, Carbatrol, Epitol, Equetro*) ▶L ♀D ▶+ $$

WARNING - Risk of aplastic anemia and agranulocytosis; contraindicated if prior marrow depression. Monitor CBC at baseline and periodically.

ADULT - Epilepsy: Start 200 mg PO bid. Increase by 200 mg/d at weekly intervals, divided tid-qid (regular release), bid (extended-release), or qid (susp) to max 1,600 mg/d. Trigeminal neuralgia: Start 100 mg PO bid or 50 mg PO qid (susp); increase by 200 mg/d until pain relief. Max 1,200 mg/d. Bipolar disorder, acute manic/mixed episodes (Equetro): Start 200 mg PO bid; increase by 200 mg/d to max 1,600 mg/d. See "unapproved adult" section for alternative bipolar dosing.

PEDS - Epilepsy, age >12 yo: Start 200 mg PO bid or 100 mg PO qid (susp); increase by 200 mg/d at weekly intervals, divided tid-qid (regular release), bid (extended-release), or qid (susp) to max 1,000 mg/d (age 12–15 yo) or 1,200 mg/d (age >15 yo). Epilepsy, age 6–12 yo: Start 100 mg PO bid or 50 mg PO qid (susp); increase by 100 mg/d at weekly intervals divided tid-qid (regular release), bid (extended-release), or qid (susp) to max 1,000 mg/d. Epilepsy, age <6 yo: Start 10–20 mg/kg/d PO divided bid-tid or qid (susp). Increase weekly prn. Max 35 mg/kg/d.

UNAPPROVED ADULT - Neuropathic pain: Start 100 mg PO bid; usual effective dose is 200 mg PO bid-qid. Max 1,200 mg/d. Mania (American Psychiatric Association guidelines): Start 200–600 mg/d divided tid-qid (standard release) or bid (extended-release), then increase by 200 mg/d q2–4 d. Mean effective dose is 1,000 mg/d. Max 1,600 mg/d.

UNAPPROVED PEDS - Bipolar disorder (manic or mixed phase): Start 100–200 mg PO daily or bid; titrate to usual effective dose of 200–600 mg/d for children and up to 1,200 mg/d for adolescents.

FORMS - Generic/Trade: Tabs 200 mg, chew tabs 100 mg, susp 100 mg/5 mL. Generic Only: Tabs 100,300,400 mg, chew tabs 200 mg. Trade only: Extended-release tabs (Tegretol XR): 100, 200, 400 mg. Extended-release caps (Carbatrol & Equetro): 100, 200, 300 mg.

NOTES - Usual therapeutic level is 4–12 mcg/mL. Stevens-Johnson Syndrome, hepatitis, aplastic anemia, and hyponatremia may occur. Monitor CBC and LFTs. Many drug interactions. Should not be used for absence or atypical absence seizures. Dangerous and possibly fatal skin reactions are more common with the HLA-B*1502 allele most common in people of Asian and Indian ancestry; screen new patients for this allele prior to starting therapy.

**CLOBAZAM** (✦*FRISIUM*) ▶L ♀X (first trimester) D (2nd/3rd trimesters) ▶- $

WARNING - Caution in the elderly; may accumulate and cause side effects such as psychomotor impairment.

ADULT - Canada only. Epilepsy, adjunctive: Start 5–15 mg PO daily. Gradually increase prn to max 80 mg/d.

PEDS - Canada only. Epilepsy, adjunctive, <2 yo: Start 0.5–1 mg/kg PO daily. 2–16 yo: Start 5 mg PO daily; may increase prn to max 40 mg/d.

FORMS - Generic/Trade: Tabs 10 mg.

NOTES - Reduce dose in hepatic or renal dysfunction. Drug interactions with enzyme-inducing

**CLOBAZAM** (*cont.*)

anticonvulsants such as carbamazepine and phenytoin; may need to adjust dose.

**ETHOSUXIMIDE** (*Zarontin*) ▶LK ♀C ▶+ $$$$

ADULT - Absence seizures: Start 500 mg PO given once daily or divided bid. Increase by 250 mg/d q4–7 d prn. Max 1.5 g/d.

PEDS - Absence seizures, 3–6 yo: Start 250 mg PO daily or divided bid. Max 500 mg/d. Age >6 yo: use adult dosing.

UNAPPROVED PEDS - Absence seizures, age <3 yo: start 15 mg/kg/d PO divided bid. Increase q4–7 d prn. Usual effective dose is 15–40 mg/kg/d divided bid. Max 500 mg/d.

FORMS - Generic/Trade: Caps 250 mg. Syrup 250 mg/5 mL.

NOTES - Usual therapeutic level is 40–100 mcg/mL. Monitor CBC for blood dyscrasias. Use caution in hepatic and renal impairment. May increase the risk of grand mal seizures in some patients.

**ETHOTOIN** (*Peganone*) ▶L ♀C ▶+ $$$$

ADULT - Generalized tonic/clonic or complex partial seizures: Start ≤1 g/d given in 4–6 divided doses. Usual effective dose is 2–3 g/d.

PEDS - Generalized tonic/clonic or complex partial seizures: Start ≤750 mg/d in 4–6 divided doses. Usual effective dose is 0.5–1 g/d. Max 2–3 g/d.

FORMS - Trade only: Tabs 250 mg.

NOTES - Usual therapeutic level is 15–50 mcg/mL. Doses <2 g/d are usually ineffective in adults. Give after food to reduce GI side effects.

**FELBAMATE** (*Felbatol*) ▶KL ♀C ▶- $$$$$

WARNING - Aplastic anemia and fatal hepatic failure have occurred.

ADULT - Severe, refractory epilepsy: Start 400 mg PO tid. Increase by 600 mg/d q2 wk to max 3,600 mg/d.

PEDS - Lennox-Gastaut syndrome, adjunctive therapy, age 2–14 yo: Start 15 mg/kg/d PO in 3–4 divided doses. Increase by 15 mg/kg/d at weekly intervals to max 45 mg/kg/d.

FORMS - Trade only: Tabs 400, 600 mg. Susp 600 mg/5 mL.

NOTES - Use only after discussing the risks and obtaining written informed consent. Many drug interactions.

**FOSPHENYTOIN** (*Cerebyx*) ▶L ♀D ▶+ $$$$$

ADULT - Status epilepticus: Load 15–20 mg "phenytoin equivalents" (PE) per kg IV no faster than 100–150 mg PE/min. Non-emergent loading dose: 10–20 mg PE/kg IM/IV at rate ≤150 mg/min. Maintenance: 4–6 mg PE/kg/d.

PEDS - Not approved in children.

UNAPPROVED PEDS - Status epilepticus: 15–20 mg PE/kg IV at a rate <2 mg PE/kg/min. Nonemergent use >7 yo: 4–6 mg PE/kg/24 h IV/IM no faster than 100–150 mg PE/min.

NOTES - Fosphenytoin is dosed in "phenytoin equivalents" (PE). Use beyond 5 d has not been systematically studied. Monitor ECG & vital signs continuously during and after infusion. Contraindicated in cardiac conduction block.

Many drug interactions. Usual therapeutic level is 10–20 mcg/mL in normal hepatorenal function. Renal/hepatic disease may change protein binding and levels. Low albumin levels may increase free fraction.

**GABAPENTIN** (*Neurontin*) ▶K ♀C ▶? $$$$

ADULT - Partial seizures, adjunctive therapy: Start 300 mg PO qhs. Increase gradually to usual effective dose of 300–600 mg PO tid. Max 3,600 mg/d. Postherpetic neuralgia: Start 300 mg PO on d 1. Increase to 300 mg bid on d 2, and to 300 mg tid on d 3. Max 1,800 mg/d divided tid.

PEDS - Partial seizures, adjunctive therapy, 3–12 yo: Start 10–15 mg/kg/d PO divided tid. Titrate over 3 d to usual effective dose of 25–40 mg/kg/d divided tid. Max 50 mg/kg/d. Age >12 yo: Use adult dosing.

UNAPPROVED ADULT - Partial seizures, initial monotherapy: Titrate as above. Usual effective dose is 900–1,800 mg/d. Neuropathic pain: 300 mg PO tid, max 3,600 mg/d in 3–4 divided doses. Migraine prophylaxis: Start 300 mg PO daily, then gradually increase to 1,200–2,400 mg/d in 3–4 divided doses. Restless legs syndrome: Start 300 mg PO qhs. Max 3,600 mg/d divided tid. Hot flashes: 300 mg PO tid.

UNAPPROVED PEDS - Neuropathic pain: Start 5 mg/kg PO at bedtime. Increase to 5 mg/kg bid on d 2 and 5 mg/kg tid on d 3. Titrate to usual effective level of 8–35 mg/kg/24 h.

FORMS - Generic only: Tabs 100, 300, 400 mg. Generic/Trade: Caps 100, 300, 400 mg. Tabs (scored) 600, 800 mg. Soln 50 mg/mL.

NOTES - Decrease dose in renal impairment (CrCl <60 mL/min); table in package insert. Discontinue gradually over ≥1 wk.

**LAMOTRIGINE** (*Lamictal, Lamictal CD*) ▶LK ♀C (see notes) ▶- $$$$

WARNING - Potentially life-threatening rashes (eg, Stevens-Johnson Syndrome) have been reported in 0.3% of adults and 0.8% of children, usually within 2–8 wk of initiation; discontinue at first sign of rash. Drug interaction with valproate – see adjusted dosing guidelines.

ADULT - Partial seizures, Lennox Gastaut syndrome, or generalized tonic-clonic seizures, adjunctive therapy with an enzyme-inducing anticonvulsant (age >12 yo): Start 50 mg PO daily × 2 wk, then 50 mg PO bid × 2 wk. Increase by 100 mg/d q1–2 wk to usual maintenance dose of 150–250 mg PO bid. Partial seizures, conversion to monotherapy from adjunctive therapy with a single enzyme-inducing anticonvulsant (age ≥16 yo): Use above guidelines to gradually increase the dose to 250 mg PO bid; then taper the enzyme-inducing anticonvulsant by 20% a wk over 4 wk. Partial seizures, Lennox-Gastaut syndrome, or generalized tonic-clonic seizures, adjunctive therapy with valproate (age >12 yo): Start 25 mg PO qod × 2 wk, then 25 mg PO daily × 2 wk. Increase by 25–50 mg/d q1–2 wk to usual maintenance dose

(cont.)

**LAMOTRIGINE** *(cont.)*

of 100–400 mg/d (when used with valproate + other anticonvulsants) or 100–200 mg/d (when used with valproate alone) given once daily or divided bid. Partial seizures, conversion to monotherapy from adjunctive therapy with valproate (age ≥16 yo): Use above guidelines to gradually increase the dose to 200 mg/d PO given daily or divided bid; then decrease valproate weekly by ≤500 mg/d to an initial goal of 500 mg/d. After 1 wk at these doses, increase lamotrigine to 300 mg/d and decrease valproate to 250 mg/d divided bid. A wk later, discontinue valproate; then increase lamotrigine weekly by 100 mg/d to usual maintenance dose of 500 mg/d. Partial seizures, Lennox-Gastaut syndrome, or generalized tonic-clonic seizures, adjunctive therapy with other anticonvulsants (not valproate or enzyme inducers) (>12 yo): Start 25 mg PO daily × 2 wk, the 50 mg PO daily × 2 wk. Increase by 50 mg/d q1–2 wk to usual maintenance dose of 225–375 mg/d divided bid. See psychiatry section for bipolar disorder dosing.

PEDS – Partial seizures, Lennox-Gastaut syndrome or generalized tonic-clonic seizures, adjunctive therapy with an enzyme-inducing anticonvulsant, age 2–12 yo: Start 0.6 mg/kg/d PO divided bid × 2 wk, then 1.2 mg/kg/d PO divided bid × 2 wk. Increase q1–2 wk by 1.2 mg/kg/d (rounded down to the nearest whole tab) to usual maintenance dose of 5–15 mg/kg/d. Max 400 mg/d. Partial seizures, Lennox-Gastaut syndrome, or generalized tonic-clonic seizures, adjunctive therapy with valproate, age 2–12 yo: Start 0.15 mg/kg/d PO (given daily or divided bid) × 2 wk, then 0.3 mg/kg/d PO (given daily or divided bid) × 2 wk. Increase q1–2 wk by 0.3 mg/kg/d (rounded down to nearest whole tab) to usual maintenance dose of 1–5 mg/kg/d (lamotrigine + valproate and other anticonvulsants) or 1–3 mg/kg/d if used with valproate alone. Max 200 mg/d. Partial seizures, Lennox-Gastaut syndrome, or generalized tonic-clonic seizures, adjunctive therapy with other anticonvulsants (not valproate or enzyme inducers), age 2–12 yo: Start 0.3 mg/kg/d (given daily or divided bid) × 2 wk, then 0.6 mg/kg/d × 2 wk. Increase q1–2 wk by 0.6 mg/kg/d (rounded down to nearest whole tab) to usual maintenance dose of 4.5–7.5 mg/kg/d. Max 300 mg/d. Age >12 yo: use adult dosing for all of the above indications.

UNAPPROVED ADULT – Initial monotherapy for partial seizures: Start 25 mg PO daily. Usual maintenance dose is 100–300 mg/d divided bid. Max 500 mg/d.

UNAPPROVED PEDS - Initial monotherapy for partial seizures: Start 0.5 mg/kg/d given daily or divided bid. Max 10 mg/kg/d. Newly-diagnosed absence seizures: Titrate as above. Usual effective dose is 2–15 mg/kg/d.

FORMS – Generic/Trade: Chewable dispersible tabs 5, 25 mg. Trade only: Tabs 25, 100, 150, 200 mg. Chewable dispersible tabs (Lamictal CD) 2 mg not available in pharmacies; obtain through manufacturer representative, or by calling 1-888-825-5249.

NOTES – Drug interactions with valproate and enzyme-inducing antiepileptic drugs (ie, carbamazepine, phenobarbital, phenytoin, primidone); may need to adjust dose. May increase carbamazepine toxicity. Women taking estrogen-containing oral contraceptives without an enzyme-inducing anticonvulsant will generally require an increase of the lamotrigine maintenance dose by up to 2-fold. Consider increasing the lamotrigine dose when the contraceptive is started. Taper lamotrigine by ≤25% of daily dose q wk over a 2-wk period if the contraceptive is stopped. Preliminary evidence suggests that exposure during the first trimester of pregnancy is associated with a risk of cleft palate and/or cleft lip. Please report all fetal exposure to the Lamotrigine Pregnancy Registry (800-336-2176) and the North American Antiepileptic Drug Pregnancy Registry (888-233-2334).

**LEVETIRACETAM** *(Keppra)* ▶K ♀C ▶? $$$$$

ADULT – Partial seizures, juvenile myoclonic epilepsy (JME), or primary generalized tonic-clonic seizures (GTC), adjunctive therapy: Start 500 mg PO/IV bid ; increase by 1,000 mg/d q2 wk prn to max 3,000 mg/d (partial seizures) or to target dose of 3,000 mg/d (JME or GTC).

PEDS – Partial seizures, adjunctive therapy, age >4 yo: Start 20 mg/kg/d PO (or IV if ≥16 yo) divided bid. Increase q2 wk as tolerated to target dose of 60 mg/kg/d. Juvenile myoclonic epilepsy, adjunctive therapy, age ≥12 yo: See adult dosing (IV approved for ≥16 yo only). Primary generalized tonic-clonic seizures (GTC), adjunctive therapy, 6–15 yo: Start 20 mg/kg/d PO (or IV if ≥16 yo) divided bid. Increase by 20 mg/kg/d q2 wk to target dose of 60 mg/kg/d. GTC, adjunctive therapy, >16 yo: Use adult dosing.

UNAPPROVED ADULT – Myoclonus: Start 500–1,000 mg/d in divided doses. May increase to max 1,500–3,000 mg/d or 50 mg/kg/d.

FORMS – Trade only: Tabs 250, 500, 750, 1,000 mg. Oral solution 100 mg/mL.

NOTES – Drug interactions unlikely. Decrease dose in renal dysfunction (CrCl <80 mL/min). Emotional lability, hostility, and depression may occur. Use same dose when switching between IV and PO forms.

**METHSUXIMIDE** *(Celontin)* ▶L ♀C ▶? $$$

ADULT – Refractory absence seizures: Start 300 mg PO daily; increase weekly by 300 mg/d. Max 1,200 mg/d.

PEDS – Refractory absence seizures: Start 10–15 mg/kg/d PO in 3–4 divided doses; increase weekly prn. Max 30 mg/kg/d.

FORMS – Trade only: Caps 150, 300 mg.

NOTES – Monitor CBC, UA, and LFTs.

**OXCARBAZEPINE (Trileptal)** ▶LK ♀C ▶- $$$$$
WARNING - Serious multi-organ hypersensitivity reactions and life-threatening rashes (eg, Stevens-Johnson Syndrome, toxic epidermal necrolysis) have occurred, with some fatalities. Consider discontinuation if skin reactions occur.
ADULT - Partial seizures, monotherapy: Start 300 mg PO bid. Increase by 300 mg/d q3 d to usual effective dose of 1,200 mg/d. Max 2,400 mg/d. Partial seizures, adjunctive: Start 300 mg PO bid. Increase by ≤600 mg/d at weekly intervals to usual effective dose of 1,200 mg/d. Max 2,400 mg/d.
PEDS - Partial seizures, adjunctive, age 2–16 yo: Start 8–10 mg/kg/d PO divided bid (max starting dose 600 mg/d). Titrate to max 60 mg/kg/d (age 2 to <4 yo), or to target dose of 900 mg/d (20–29 kg), 1,200 mg/d (29.1–39 kg), or 1,800 mg/d (>39 kg). Consider using a starting dose of 16–20 mg/kg for children aged 2 to <4 yo who weigh <20 kg to account for higher clearance. Partial seizures, initial monotherapy, 4–16 yo: Start 8–10 mg/kg/d divided bid. Increase by 5 mg/kg/d q3 d to recommended dose (in mg/d) of: 600–900 if ~20 kg, 900–1,200 if ~25–30 kg, 900–1,500 if ~35–40 kg, 1,200–1,500 if ~45 kg, 1,200–1,800 if ~50–55 kg, 1,200–2,100 if ~60–65 kg, 1,500–2,100 if ~70 kg. Partial seizures, conversion to monotherapy, age 4–16 yo: Start 8–10 mg/kg/d divided bid. Increase at weekly intervals by ≤10 mg/kg/d to target dose listed for initial monotherapy.
FORMS - Generic/Trade: Tabs (scored) 150, 300, 600 mg. Trade only: Oral susp 300 mg/5 mL.
NOTES - Monitor serum sodium. Decrease initial dose by one-half in renal dysfunction (CrCl <30 mL/min). Inhibits CYP 2C19 and induces CYP 3A4/5. Interactions with other antiepileptic drugs, oral contraceptives, and dihydropyridine calcium channel blockers.

**PHENOBARBITAL (Luminal)** ▶L ♀D ▶- ©IV $
ADULT - Epilepsy: 100–300 mg/d PO divided dailytid. Status epilepticus: 20 mg/kg IV at rate ≤60 mg/min.
PEDS - Epilepsy: 3–5 mg/kg/d PO divided bid-tid. Status epilepticus: 20 mg/kg IV at rate ≤60 mg/min.
UNAPPROVED ADULT - Status epilepticus: may give up to a total dose of 30 mg/kg IV.
UNAPPROVED PEDS - Status epilepticus: 15–20 mg/kg IV load; may give additional 5 mg/kg doses q15–30 min to max total dose of 30 mg/kg. Epilepsy: 3–5 mg/kg/d given once daily or divided bid (neonates), 5–6 mg/kg/d given once daily or divided bid (infants), 6–8 mg/kg/d given once daily or divided bid (age 1–5 yo), 4–6 mg/kg/d given once daily or divided bid (age 6–12 yo), or 1–3 mg/kg/d given once daily or divided bid (age >12 yo).
FORMS - Generic only: Tabs 15, 16.2, 30, 32.4, 60, 100 mg. Elixir 20 mg/5 mL.
NOTES - Usual therapeutic level is 15- 40 mcg/

mL. Monitor cardiopulmonary function closely when administering IV. Decrease dose in renal or hepatic dysfunction. Many drug interactions.
**PHENYTOIN (Dilantin, Phenytek)** ▶L ♀D ▶+ $$
ADULT - Status epilepticus: 10–15 mg/kg IV at rate ≤50 mg/min, then 100 mg IV/PO q6–8h. Epilepsy, oral loading dose: 400 mg PO initially, then 300 mg in 2 h and 4 h. Epilepsy, maintenance dose: 300 mg/d PO given once daily (extended release) or divided tid (standard release) and titrated to a therapeutic level.
PEDS - Epilepsy, age >6 yo: 5 mg/kg/d PO divided bid-tid, to max 300 mg/d. Status epilepticus: 15–20 mg/kg IV at a rate ≤1 mg/kg/min.
FORMS - Generic/Trade: Extended-release caps 30, 100 mg (Dilantin). Susp 125 mg/5 mL. Trade only: Extended-release caps 200, 300 mg (Phenytek). Chew tabs 50 mg (Dilantin Infatabs).
NOTES - Usual therapeutic level is 10–20 mcg/mL. Monitor ECG and vital signs when administering IV. Many drug interactions. Monitor serum levels closely when switching between forms (free acid vs. sodium salt). The free fraction may be increased in patients with low albumin levels. IV loading doses of 15–20 mg/kg have also been recommended. May need to reduce loading dose if patient is already on phenytoin.
**PREGABALIN (Lyrica)** ▶K ♀C ▶? ©V $$$$$
ADULT - Painful diabetic peripheral neuropathy: Start 50 mg PO tid; may increase within 1 wk to max 100 mg PO tid. Postherpetic neuralgia: Start 150 mg/d PO divided bid-tid; may increase within 1 wk to 300 mg/d divided bid-tid; max 600 mg/d. Partial seizures (adjunctive): Start 150 mg/d PO divided bid-tid; may increase prn to max 600 mg/d divided bid-tid. Fibromyalgia: Start 75 mg PO bid; may increase to 150 mg bid within 1 wk; max 225 mg bid.
PEDS - Not approved in children.
FORMS - Trade only: Caps 25, 50, 75, 100, 150, 200, 225, 300 mg.
NOTES - Adjust dose if CrCl <60 mL/min; refer to package insert. Warn patients to report changes in visual acuity and muscle pain. May increase creatine kinase. Must taper if discontinuing to avoid withdrawal symptoms. Increased risk of peripheral edema when used in conjunction with thiazolidinedione antidiabetic agents.
**PRIMIDONE (Mysoline)** ▶LK ♀D ▶- $$$$
ADULT - Epilepsy: Start 100–125 mg PO qhs. Increase over 10 d to usual maintenance dose of 250 mg PO tid-qid. Max 2 g/d.
PEDS - Epilepsy <8 yo: Start 50 mg PO qhs. Increase over 10 d to usual maintenance dose of 125–250 mg PO tid or 10- 25 mg/kg/d.
UNAPPROVED ADULT - Essential tremor: Start 12.5–25 mg PO qhs. May increase weekly prn by 50 mg/d to 250 mg/d given once daily or in divided doses. Max 750 mg/d.
FORMS - Generic/Trade: Tabs 50, 250 mg.
NOTES - Usual therapeutic level = 5–12 mcg/mL. Metabolized to phenobarbital.

**TIAGABINE (*Gabitril*)** ▶L ♀C ▶? $$$$$

WARNING - New onset-seizures and status epilepticus may occur when used in patients without epilepsy, particularly when combined with other medications that lower the seizure threshold. Avoid off-label use.

ADULT - Partial seizures, adjunctive therapy with an enzyme-inducing anticonvulsant: Start 4 mg PO daily. Increase by 4–8 mg/d prn at weekly intervals to max 56 mg/d divided bid-qid.

PEDS - Partial seizures, adjunctive therapy with an enzyme-inducing anticonvulsant, age 12–18 yo: Start 4 mg PO daily. Increase by 4 mg/d prn q1–2 wk to max 32 mg/d divided bid-qid.

FORMS - Trade only: Tabs 2, 4, 12, 16 mg.

NOTES - Take with food. Dosing is for patients on enzyme-inducing anticonvulsants such as carbamazepine, phenobarbital, phenytoin, or primidone. Reduce dosage in patients who are not taking enzyme-inducing medications, and in those with liver dysfunction.

**TOPIRAMATE (*Topamax*)** ▶K ♀C ▶? $$$$$

ADULT - Partial seizures or primary generalized tonic-clonic seizures, monotherapy: Start 25 mg PO bid (wk 1), 50 mg bid (wk 2), 75 mg bid (wk 3), 100 mg bid (wk 4), 150 mg bid (wk 5), then 200 mg bid as tolerated. Partial seizures, primary generalized tonic-clonic seizures, or Lennox Gastaut Syndrome, adjunctive therapy: Start 25–50 mg PO qhs. Increase weekly by 25–50 mg/d to usual effective dose of 200 mg PO bid. Doses >400 mg/d not shown to be more effective. Migraine prophylaxis: Start 25 mg PO qhs (wk 1), then 25 mg bid (wk 2), 25 mg q am and 50 mg q pm (wk 3), then 50 mg bid (wk 4 and thereafter).

PEDS - Partial seizures or primary generalized tonic-clonic seizures, monotherapy (age >10 yo): Use adult dosing. Partial seizures, primary generalized tonic-clonic seizures, or Lennox-Gastaut Syndrome, adjunctive therapy, 2–16 yo: Start 1–3 mg/kg (max 25 mg) PO qhs. Increase by 1–3 mg/kg/d q 1–2 wk to usual effective dose of 5–9 mg/kg/d divided bid.

UNAPPROVED ADULT - Essential tremor: Start 25 mg PO daily. Increase by 25 mg/d at weekly intervals to 100 mg/d; max 400 mg/d. Bipolar disorder: Start 25–50 mg PO daily. Titrate prn to max 400 mg/d. Alcohol dependence: Start 25 mg PO qd; increase by 25 mg/d at weekly intervals as tolerated to 300 mg/d for up to 14 wk total.

FORMS - Trade only: Tabs 25, 50, 100, 200 mg. Sprinkle Caps 15, 25 mg.

NOTES - Give ½ usual adult dose in renal impairment (CrCl <70 mL/min). Confusion, nephrolithiasis, glaucoma, and weight loss may occur. Risk of oligohidrosis and hyperthermia, particularly in children; use caution in warm ambient temperatures and/or with vigorous physical activity. Hyperchloremic, non-anion gap metabolic acidosis may occur; monitor serum bicarbonate and either reduce dose or taper off entirely if this occurs. Max dose tested was 1,600 mg/d.

**VALPROIC ACID (*Depakene, Depakote, Depakote ER, Depacon, Stavzor, divalproex, sodium valproate, ✦Epival, Deproic*)** ▶L ♀D ▶+ $$$$

HEPATOTOXICITY, DRUG INTERACTIONS, REDUCE DOSE IN ELDERLY.

WARNING - Fatal hepatic failure has occurred; monitor LFTs during first 6 mo of treatment. Life-threatening pancreatitis has been reported after initial or prolonged use. Evaluate for abdominal pain, N/V, and/or anorexia. Discontinue if pancreatitis occurs. May be more teratogenic than other anticonvulsants (eg, carbamazepine, lamotrigine, and phenytoin). Hepatic failure and clotting disorders have occurred when used during pregnancy.

ADULT - Epilepsy: 10–15 mg/kg/d (absence start 15 mg/kg/d) PO or IV infusion over 60 min (≤20 mg/min) divided bid to qid (standard release, delayed release, or IV) or given once daily (Depakote ER). Increase dose by 5–10 mg/kg/d at weekly intervals to max 60 mg/kg/d. Migraine prophylaxis: Start 250 mg PO bid (Depakote or Stavzor) or 500 mg PO daily (Depakote ER) × 1 wk, then increase to max 1,000 mg/d PO divided bid (Depakote or Stavzor) or given once daily (Depakote ER).

PEDS - Seizures >2 yo: 10–15 mg/kg/d PO or IV infusion over 60 min (rate ≤20 mg/min). Increase dose by 5–10 mg/kg/d at weekly intervals to max 60 mg/kg/d. Divide doses >250 mg/d into bid-qid; may give once daily (Depakote ER) if >10 yo. For complex partial seizures Stavzor is for ages ≥ 10 yo.

UNAPPROVED ADULT - Status epilepticus (not first-line): Load 20–40 mg/kg IV (rate ≤6 mg/kg/min), then continue 4–8 mg/kg IV tid to achieve therapeutic level. May use lower loading dose if already on valproate.

UNAPPROVED PEDS - Status epilepticus, age >2 yo (not first-line): Load 20–40 mg/kg IV over 1–5 min, then 5 mg/kg/h adjusted to achieve therapeutic level. May use lower loading dose if already on valproate.

FORMS - Generic/Trade: Immediate release caps 250 mg (Depakene), syrup (Depakene, valproic acid) 250 mg/5 mL. Trade only (Depakote): Delayed release sprinkle caps 125 mg, delayed release tabs 125, 250, 500 mg; extended release tabs (Depakote ER) 250, 500mg. Trade only (Stavzor): Delayed release caps 125, 250, 500mg.

NOTES - Contraindicated in urea cycle disorders or hepatic dysfunction. Usual therapeutic trough level is 50–100 mcg/mL. Depakote and Depakote ER are not interchangeable. Depakote ER is ~10% less bioavailable than Depakote. Depakote releases divalproex sodium over 8–12h (daily-qid dosing); Depakote ER releases divalproex sodium over 18–24h (daily dosing). Many drug interactions. Patients receiving other anticonvulsants

| DERMATOMES | |
|---|---|
| **MOTOR FUNCTION BY NERVE ROOTS** | |
| *Level* | *Motor Function* |
| C3/C4/C5 | Diaphragm |
| C5/C6 | Deltoid/biceps |
| C7/C8 | Triceps |
| C8/T1 | Finger flexion/intrinsics |
| T1–T12 | Intercostal/abd muscles |
| L2/L3 | Hip flexion |
| L2/L3/L4 | Hip adduction/quads |
| L4/L5 | Ankle dorsiflexion |
| S1/S2 | Ankle plantarflexion |
| S2/S3/S4 | Rectal tone |

| | *Root* | *Motor* | *Sensory* | *Reflex* |
|---|---|---|---|---|
| **LUMBOSACRAL** | L4 | quadriceps | medial foot | knee-jerk |
| **NERVE ROOT** | L5 | dorsiflexors | dorsum of foot | medial hamstring |
| **COMPRESSION** | S1 | plantarflexors | lateral foot | ankle-jerk |

| GLASGOW COMA SCALE | | *Motor Activity* |
|---|---|---|
| | *Verbal Activity* | 6. Obeys commands |
| *Eye Opening* | 5. Oriented | 5. Localizes pain |
| 4. Spontaneous | 4. Confused | 4. Withdraws to pain |
| 3. To command | 3. Inappropriate | 3. Flexion to pain |
| 2. To pain | 2. Incomprehensible | 2. Extension to pain |
| 1. None | 1. None | 1. None |

**VALPROIC ACID** (*cont.*)

may require higher doses of valproic acid. Reduce dose in the elderly. Hyperammonemia, GI irritation, or thrombocytopenia may occur.

**VIGABATRIN, ✦SABRIL** ▶K ♀C ▶- $$$$

WARNING - Ophthalmologic abnormalities have been reported. Visual field testing should be performed prior to treatment and q3 mo thereafter. Given the limitations of visual field testing in children <9 yo, vigabatrin should be used in this age group only if clearly indicated. Do not use with other retinotoxic drugs.

ADULT - Canada only. Epilepsy (adjunct treatment): Start: 1 g/d in divided doses. Maintenance: 2–3 g/d in divided doses.

PEDS - Canada only. Epilepsy (adjunct treatment) or infantile spasms (monotherapy): Start: 40 mg/kg/d, maintenance: 50–100 mg/kg/d in divided doses.

FORMS - Trade only: Tabs 500 mg. Oral powder 500 mg/sachet.

**ZONISAMIDE (*Zonegran*)** ▶LK ♀C ▶? $$$$

ADULT - Partial seizures, adjunctive: Start 100 mg PO daily × 2 wk, then increase to 200 mg PO daily. May increase prn q2 wk to 300–400 mg/d, given once daily or divided bid. Max 600 mg/d.

PEDS - Not approved in children.

FORMS - Generic/Trade: Caps 25, 50, 100 mg.

NOTES - This is a sulfonamide; contraindicated in sulfa allergy. Fatalities and severe reactions including Stevens-Johnson syndrome, toxic epidermal necrolysis, fulminant hepatic necrosis, and blood dyscrasias have occurred with sulfonamides. Clearance is affected by CYP3A4 inhibitors or inducers such as phenytoin, carbamazepine, phenobarbital, and valproic acid. Nephrolithiasis may occur. Oligohidrosis and hyperthermia may occur, and are more common in children. Patients with renal disease may require slower titration.

## NEUROLOGY: Migraine Therapy—Triptans (5-HT1 Receptor Agonists)

**NOTE:** May cause vasospasm. Avoid in ischemic or vasospastic heart disease, cerebrovascular syndromes, peripheral arterial disease, uncontrolled HTN, and hemiplegic or basilar migraine. Do not use within 24 h of ergots or other triptans. Risk of serotonin syndrome if used with SSRIs or MAOIs.

**ALMOTRIPTAN (*Axert*)** ▶LK ♀C ? $$
ADULT - Migraine treatment: 6.25–12.5 mg PO. May repeat in 2 h prn. Max 25 mg/d.
PEDS - Not approved in children.
FORMS - Trade only: Tabs 6.25, 12.5 mg.
NOTES - MAOIs inhibit almotriptan metabolism; use together only with extreme caution. Use lower doses (6.25 mg) in renal and/or hepatic dysfunction.

**ELETRIPTAN (*Relpax*)** ▶LK ♀C ? $$
ADULT - Migraine treatment: 20–40 mg PO at onset. May repeat in >2 h prn. Max 40 mg/dose or 80 mg/d.
PEDS - Not approved in children.
FORMS - Trade only: Tabs 20, 40 mg.
NOTES - Do not use within 72 h of potent CYP3A4 inhibitors such as ketoconazole, itraconazole, nefazodone, troleandomycin, clarithromycin, ritonavir, or nelfinavir.

**FROVATRIPTAN (*Frova*)** ▶LK ♀C ? $
ADULT - Migraine treatment: 2.5 mg PO. May repeat in 2 h prn. Max 7.5 mg/24 h.
PEDS - Not approved in children.
FORMS - Trade only: Tabs 2.5 mg.

**NARATRIPTAN (*Amerge*)** ▶KL ♀C ? $$$
ADULT - Migraine treatment: 1–2.5 mg PO. May repeat in 4 h prn. Max 5 mg/24 h.
PEDS - Not approved in children.
FORMS - Trade only: Tabs 1, 2.5 mg.
NOTES - Contraindicated in severe renal or hepatic impairment.

**RIZATRIPTAN (*Maxalt, Maxalt MLT*)** ▶LK ♀C ? $$
ADULT - Migraine treatment: 5–10 mg PO; May repeat in 2 h prn. Max 30 mg/24 h.
PEDS - Not approved in children.
FORMS - Trade only: Tabs 5, 10 mg. Orally disintegrating tabs (MLT) 5, 10 mg.
NOTES - Should not be combined with MAOIs. MLT form dissolves on tongue without liquids.

**SUMATRIPTAN (*Imitrex*)** ▶LK ♀C ? + $$
ADULT - Migraine treatment: 4–6 mg SC. May repeat in 1 h prn. Max 12 mg/24 h. Tablets: 25–100 mg PO (50 mg most common). May repeat q2h prn with 25–100 mg doses. Max 200 mg/24 h. Intranasal spray: 5–20 mg. May repeat q2h prn. Max 40 mg/24 h. Cluster headache treatment: 6 mg SC. May repeat in >1h prn. Max 12 mg/24 h. Initial oral dose of 50 mg appears to be more

effective than 25 mg. If HA returns after initial SC injection, then tabs may be used q2h prn, max 100 mg/24 h.
PEDS - Not approved in children.
UNAPPROVED PEDS - Acute migraine, intranasal spray, 8–17 yo: 20 mg (if ≥40 kg) or 10 mg (if 20–39 kg) intranasally at headache onset. May repeat after 2 h prn.
FORMS - Trade only: Tabs 25, 50, 100 mg. Nasal spray 5, 20 mg/spray. Injection (single-dose vial) 6 mg/0.5 mL. Injection (STATdose System) 4, 6 mg prefilled cartridges.
NOTES - Should not be combined with MAOIs. Avoid IM/IV route.

**TREXIMET (sumatriptan + naproxen)** ▶LK ♀C ▶- $$$$
WARNING - May cause vasospasm. Avoid in ischemic or vasospastic heart disease, cerebrovascular syndromes, peripheral arterial disease, uncontrolled HTN, and hemiplegic or basilar migraine. Do not use within 24 h of ergots or other triptans. Risk of serotonin syndrome if used with SSRIs or MAOIs. There is a risk of gastrointestinal bleeding and perforation. Do not use ergots within 24 h of Treximet.
ADULT - Migraine treatment: 1 tab PO at onset; may repeat in ≥2 h. Max 2 tabs/24 h.
PEDS - Not approved in children.
FORMS - Trade only: Tabs 85 mg sumatriptan + 500 mg naproxen sodium.
NOTES - Avoid if CrCl <30 mL/min, hepatic impairment, cerebrovascular, cardiovascular, or peripheral vascular disease, uncontrolled HTN. Contraindicated with MAOIs.

**ZOLMITRIPTAN (*Zomig, Zomig ZMT*)** ▶L ♀C ? $$
ADULT - Migraine treatment: Tabs: 1.25–2.5 mg PO q2h. Max 10 mg/24 h. Orally disintegrating tabs (ZMT): 2.5 mg PO. May repeat in 2 h prn. Max 10 mg/24 h. Nasal spray: 5 mg (1 spray) in one nostril. May repeat in 2 h prn. Max 10 mg/24 h.
PEDS - Not approved in children.
FORMS - Trade only: Tabs 2.5, 5 mg. Orally disintegrating tabs $$$ (ZMT) 2.5, 5 mg. Nasal spray 5 mg/spray.
NOTES - Risk of vasospastic complications. Should not be combined with MAOIs. Use lower doses (<2.5 mg) in hepatic dysfunction. May break 2.5 mg tabs in half.

## NEUROLOGY: Migraine Therapy—Other

*CAFERGOT* (ergotamine + caffeine) ▶L ♀X ▶- $
WARNING - Contraindicated with concomitant use of potent CYP 3A4 inhibitors (eg, macrolides, protease inhibitors) due to risk of serious/life-threatening peripheral ischemia. Ergots have

been associated with potentially life-threatening fibrotic complications.
ADULT - Migraine and cluster headache treatment: 2 tabs PO at onset, then 1 tab q30 min prn to max 6 tabs/attack or 10 tabs/wk.

*CAFERGOT* (cont.)
PEDS - Not approved in children.
UNAPPROVED PEDS - Migraine treatment: 1 tab PO at onset, then 1 tab q 30 min prn to max 3 tabs/attack.
FORMS - Trade only: Tabs 1/100 mg ergotamine/caffeine.
NOTES - Contraindicated in sepsis, CAD, peripheral arterial disease, HTN, impaired hepatic or renal function, malnutrition, or severe pruritus.

**DIHYDROERGOTAMINE (*D.H.E. 45, Migranal*)** ▶L ♀X ▶- $$
WARNING - Contraindicated with concomitant use of potent CYP 3A4 inhibitors (eg, macrolides, protease inhibitors) due to risk of serious/life-threatening peripheral ischemia. Ergots have been associated with potentially life-threatening fibrotic complications.
ADULT - Migraine treatment: Solution (DHE 45): 1 mg IV/IM/SC; may repeat q1h prn to max 2 mg (IV) or 3 mg (IM/SC) per 24 h. Nasal spray (Migranal): 1 spray (0.5 mg) in each nostril; may repeat in 15 min prn to max 6 sprays (3 mg)/24 h or 8 sprays (4 mg)/wk.
PEDS - Not approved in children.
FORMS - Trade only: Nasal spray 0.5 mg/spray (Migranal). Self-injecting solution (D.H.E 45): 1 mg/mL.
NOTES - Contraindicated in basilar or hemiplegic migraine, sepsis, ischemic or vasospastic cardiac disease, peripheral vascular disease, vascular surgery, impaired hepatic or renal function, or uncontrolled HTN. Avoid concurrent ergotamine, methysergide, or triptan use.

**ERGOTAMINE (*Ergomar*)** ▶L ♀X ▶- $$
ADULT - Vascular headache: Start 2 mg SL; may repeat q30 min to max 6 mg/24 h. Drug interactions. Fibrotic complications.

PEDS - Not approved in children.
FORMS - Trade only: Sublingual tabs (ergotamine tartrate) 2 mg.
NOTES - Avoid use with potent CYP3A4 inhibitors (eg, ritonavir, nelfinavir, indinavir, erythromycin, clarithromycin, troleandomycin); severe peripheral vasoconstriction may result.

**FLUNARIZINE, ✦*SIBELIUM*** ▶L ♀C ▶- $$
ADULT - Canada only. Migraine prophylaxis: 10 mg PO qhs; if side effects occur, then reduce dose to 5 mg qhs. Safety of long-term use (>4 mo) has not been established.
PEDS - Not approved in children.
FORMS - Generic/Trade: Caps 5 mg
NOTES - Gradual onset of benefit, over 6–8 wk. Not for acute therapy. Contraindicated if history of depression or extrapyramidal disorders.

***MIDRIN* (isometheptene + dichloralphenazone + acetaminophen, Amidrine, Durdrin, Migquin, Migratine, Migrazone, Va-Zone)** ▶L ♀? ▶?
©IV $
ADULT - Tension and vascular headache treatment: 1–2 caps PO q4h, to max of 8 caps/d. Migraine treatment: 2 caps PO × 1, then 1 cap q1h prn to max 5 caps/12 h.
PEDS - Not approved in children.
FORMS - Generic only: Caps (isometheptene/dichloralphenazone/acetaminophen) 65/100/325 mg.
NOTES - Midrin brand no longer available; generics only. FDA has classified as possibly effective for migraine treatment. Contraindicated in glaucoma, severe renal disease, heart disease, hepatic disease, or concurrent MAOI use. Use caution in HTN, peripheral arterial disease, or recent MI.

## NEUROLOGY: Multiple sclerosis

**GLATIRAMER (*Copaxone*)** ▶Serum ♀B ▶? $$$$$
ADULT - Multiple sclerosis (relapsing-remitting): 20 mg SC daily.
PEDS - Not approved in children.
FORMS - Trade only: Injection 20 mg single dose vial.
NOTES - Do not inject IV.

**INTERFERON BETA-1A (*Avonex, Rebif*)** ▶L ♀C ▶? $$$$$
WARNING - Risk of severe hepatic injury and failure, possibly greater when used with other hepatotoxic drugs. Monitor LFTs. Suicidality risk; use caution in depression.
ADULT - Multiple sclerosis (relapsing forms): Avonex- 30 mcg (6 million units) IM q wk. Rebif- start 8.8 mcg SC three times weekly; titrate over 4 wk to maintenance dose of 44 mcg three times weekly.
PEDS - Not approved in children.
FORMS - Trade only: Avonex: Injection 30 mcg single dose vial with & without albumin. Pre-filled syringe 30 mcg. Rebif: Starter kit 20 mcg pre-filled syringe. Pre-filled syringe 22, 44 mcg.

NOTES - Use caution in patients with depression, seizure disorders, or cardiac disease. Follow LFTs and CBC. Avonex: indicated for the first attack of MS. Rebif: give same dose 3 d each wk, with at least 48 h between doses.

**INTERFERON BETA-1B (*Betaseron*)** ▶L ♀C ▶? $$$$$
ADULT - Multiple sclerosis (relapsing-remitting): Start 0.0625 mg SC qod; titrate over six wk to 0.25 mg (8 million units) SC qod.
PEDS - Not approved in children.
FORMS - Trade only: Injection 0.3 mg (9.6 million units) single dose vial.
NOTES - Suicidality risk; use caution in depression. Check LFTs after 1, 3, and 6 mo and then periodically. Product can be stored at room temp until reconstituted; then refrigerate and use within 3 h.

**NATALIZUMAB (*Tysabri*)** ▶Serum ♀C ▶? $$$$$
WARNING - May cause progressive multifocal leukoencephalopathy; avoid concomitant use of other immunomodulators. Risk of severe hepatotoxicity; discontinue if jaundice or evidence of liver injury. Risk of anaphylaxis or other hypersensitivity reactions; permanently discontinue if they occur.

**(cont.)**

**NATALIZUMAB** *(cont.)*
ADULT - Refractory, relapsing multiple sclerosis (monotherapy) and Crohn's disease: 300 mg IV infusion over 1 h q4 wk.
PEDS - Not approved in children.
NOTES - Not first line - recommended only when there has been an inadequate response or failure to tolerate other therapies. Available only through the MS-TOUCH or CD-TOUCH prescribing programs at 1-800-456-2255. Observe closely for infusion reactions. Avoid other immunosuppressants when using for Crohn's disease; discontinue if no response by 12 wk. For patients on steroids, taper them as soon as a benefit is noted and discontinue natalizumab if steroids cannot be tapered off within 6 mo. Consider stopping natalizumab in patients who require steroids more than 3 mo per yr. Severe hepatotoxicity has been reported; discontinue if jaundice or evidence of liver injury.

## NEUROLOGY: Myasthenia Gravis

**AMBENONIUM** *(Mytelase)* ▶L ♀C ▶? $$$$$
ADULT - Myasthenia gravis: Start 5 mg PO tid-qid. Adjust q1–2 d to usual effective dose of 5–25 mg tid-qid. Usual max 200 mg/d. Narrow therapeutic window. Doses >200 mg/d require close supervision.
PEDS - Not approved in children.
FORMS - Trade only: Tabs 10 mg
NOTES - Avoid concomitant use of atropine, ganglionic blocking agents, or other cholinergic drugs. Narrow therapeutic window and variable individual dose requirements, so titrate slowly. Extended or high-dose (>200 mg/d) therapy requires close supervision. Cholinergic crisis may be treated by discontinuing the drug and giving atropine 0.5 to 1.0 mg IV plus supportive care.

**EDROPHONIUM** *(Tensilon)* ▶Plasma ♀C ▶? $
ADULT - Evaluation for myasthenia gravis: 2 mg IV over 15–30 sec (test dose) while on cardiac monitor, then 8 mg IV after 45 sec. Reversal of neuromuscular blockade: 10 mg IV over 30–45 sec; repeat prn to max 40 mg.
PEDS - Evaluation for myasthenia gravis, weight ≤34 kg: 1 mg IV (test dose), then 1 mg IV q30–45 sec to max 5 mg. Weight >34 kg: 2 mg IV (test dose), then 2 mg IV q30- 45 sec to max 10 mg.
UNAPPROVED ADULT - Reversal of non-depolarizing neuromuscular blockade: 0.5–1.0 mg/kg IV together with atropine 0.007–0.014 mg/kg.
NOTES - Not for maintenance therapy of myasthenia gravis because of short duration of action (5–10 min). May give IM. Monitor cardiac function. Atropine should be readily available in case of cholinergic reaction. Contraindicated in mechanical urinary or intestinal obstruction.

**NEOSTIGMINE** *(Prostigmin)* ▶L ♀C ▶? $$$
ADULT - Myasthenia gravis: 15–375 mg/d PO in divided doses, or 0.5 mg IM/SC when oral therapy is not possible. Reversal of non-depolarizing neuromuscular blocking agents: 0.5–2.0 mg slow IV (preceded by atropine 0.6–1.2 mg or glycopyrrolate 0.2–0.6 mg); repeat prn to max 5 mg.
PEDS - Not approved in children.
UNAPPROVED PEDS - Myasthenia gravis: 7.5–15 mg PO tid-qid; or 0.03 mg/kg IM q2–4h. Reversal of non-depolarizing neuromuscular blocking agents: 0.025–0.08 mg/kg/dose slow IV, preceded by either atropine (0.4 mg for each mg of neostigmine) or glycopyrrolate (0.2 mg for each mg of neostigmine).
FORMS - Trade only: Tabs 15 mg.
NOTES - Oral route preferred when possible.

**PYRIDOSTIGMINE** *(Mestinon, Mestinon Timespan, Regonal)* ▶Plasma, K ♀C ▶+ $$
ADULT - Myasthenia gravis, standard release tabs: Start 60 mg PO tid; gradually increase to usual therapeutic dose of 200 mg PO tid. Extended release tabs: Start 180 mg PO daily or divided bid. Max 1,500 mg/d. May give 2 mg IM or slow IV injection q2–3h.
PEDS - Not approved in children.
UNAPPROVED PEDS - Myasthenia gravis, neonates: 5 mg PO q4–6h or 0.05- 0.15 mg/kg IM/IV q4–6h. Myasthenia gravis, children: 7 mg/kg/d PO in 5–6 divided doses, or 0.05–0.15 mg/kg/dose IM/IV q4–6h. Max 10 mg IM/IV single dose.
FORMS - Generic/Trade: Tabs 60 mg. Trade only: Extended release tabs 180 mg. Syrup 60 mg/5 mL.
NOTES - Give injection at 1/30th of oral dose when oral therapy is not possible.

## NEUROLOGY: Parkinsonian Agents—Anticholinergics

**NOTE:** Anticholinergic medications may cause memory loss, delirium, or psychosis, particularly in elderly patients or those with baseline cognitive impairment.

**BENZTROPINE MESYLATE** *(Cogentin)* ▶LK ♀C ▶? $
ADULT - Parkinsonism: Start 0.5–2 mg/d PO/IM/IV. Increase in 0.5 mg increments at weekly intervals to max 6 mg/d. May divide doses daily-qid. Drug-induced extrapyramidal disorders: 1–4 mg PO/IM/IV given once daily or divided bid.
PEDS - Not approved in children.
UNAPPROVED PEDS - Parkinsonism (>3 yo): 0.02–0.05 mg/kg/dose given once daily or divided bid. Use caution; potential for undesired anticholinergic effects.
FORMS - Generic only: Tabs 0.5, 1, 2 mg.
NOTES - Contraindicated in narrow-angle glaucoma. Avoid concomitant use of donepezil, rivastigmine, galantamine, or tacrine.

**BIPERIDEN (*Akineton*)** ▶LK ♀C ▶? $$$
ADULT - Parkinsonism: 2 mg PO tid-qid. Titrate to max 16 mg/d. Drug-induced extrapyramidal disorders: 2 mg PO daily-tid to max 8 mg/24 h.
PEDS - Not approved in children.
FORMS - Trade only: Tabs 2 mg
NOTES - Contraindicated in narrow-angle glaucoma, bowel obstruction, and megacolon.

**TRIHEXYPHENIDYL (*Artane*)** ▶LK ♀C ▶? $
ADULT - Parkinsonism: 1 mg PO daily. Increase by 2 mg/d at 3–5 d intervals to usual therapeutic dose of 6–10 mg/d divided tid with meals. Max 15 mg/d.
PEDS - Not approved in children.
FORMS - Generic only: Tabs 2, 5 mg. Elixir 2 mg/ 5 mL.

## NEUROLOGY: Parkinsonian Agents—COMT Inhibitors

**ENTACAPONE (*Comtan*)** ▶L ♀C ▶? $$$$$
ADULT - Parkinson's disease, adjunctive: Start 200 mg PO with each dose of carbidopa/levodopa. Max 8 tabs (1,600 mg)/d.
PEDS - Not approved in children.
FORMS - Trade only: Tabs 200 mg.
NOTES - Adjunct to carbidopa/levodopa in patients who have end-of-dose "wearing off." Has no antiparkinsonian effect on its own. Avoid concomitant use of non-selective MAOIs. Use caution in hepatobiliary dysfunction. Avoid rapid withdrawal, which may precipitate neuroleptic malignant syndrome.

**TOLCAPONE (*Tasmar*)** ▶LK ♀C ▶? $$$$$
WARNING - Fatal hepatic failure has occurred. Use only in patients on carbidopa/levodopa who fail alternative therapies and provide written informed consent. Monitor LFTs at baseline, q2–4 wk × 6 mo, and then periodically. Discontinue if

LFT elevation >2 times upper limit of normal or if there is no clinical benefit after 3 wk of therapy.
ADULT - Parkinson's disease, adjunctive (not first line): Start 100 mg PO tid. Increase to 200 mg PO tid only if expected benefit justifies the risk. Max 600 mg/d. Only effective when used in combination with carbidopa/levodopa.
PEDS - Not approved in children.
FORMS - Trade only: Tabs 100, 200 mg.
NOTES - Adjunct to carbidopa-levodopa in patients who have refractory end-of-dose "wearing off." Has no antiparkinsonian effect on its own. Contraindicated in hepatic dysfunction. Monitor LFTs. Avoid concomitant use of non-selective MAOIs. Avoid rapid withdrawal, which may precipitate neuroleptic malignant syndrome. Informed consent forms are available from the manufacturer (www.tasmar.com).

## NEUROLOGY: Parkinsonian Agents—Dopaminergic Agents & Combinations

**NOTE:** Dopaminergic medications may cause hallucinations, particularly when used in combination. They have also been associated with sudden-onset episodes of sleep without warning ("sleep attacks"), and with the development of impulse control disorders such as compulsive gambling, hypersexuality, and hyperphagia. Avoid rapid discontinuation, which may precipitate neuroleptic malignant syndrome.

**APOMORPHINE (*Apokyn*)** ▶L ♀C ▶? $$$$$
WARNING - Never administer IV due to risk of severe adverse effects including pulmonary embolism.
ADULT - Acute, intermittent treatment of hypomobility ("off episodes") in Parkinson's disease: Start 0.2 mL SC test dose in the presence of medical personnel. May increase dose by 0.1 mL every few d as tolerated. Max 0.6 mL/dose or 2 mL/d. Monitor for orthostatic hypotension after initial dose and with dose escalation. Potent emetic - pretreat with trimethobenzamide 300 mg PO tid (or domperidone 20 mg PO tid) starting three d prior to use, and continue for ≥2 mo before weaning.
PEDS - Not approved in children.
FORMS - Trade only: Cartridges (for injector pen, 10 mg/mL) 3 mL. Ampules (10 mg/mL) 2 mL.
NOTES - Write doses exclusively in mL rather than mg to avoid errors. Most effective when administered at (or just prior to) the onset of an "off" episode. Avoid concomitant use of 5HT3 antagonists (eg, ondansetron, granisetron, dolasetron, palonosetron, alosetron), which can precipitate severe hypotension and loss of consciousness. Inform patients that the dosing pen is labeled

in mL (not mg), and that it is possible to dial in a dose of medication even if the cartridge does not contain sufficient drug. Rotate injection sites. Restart at 0.2 mL/d if treatment is interrupted for ≥1 wk. Adjust dosing in hepatic impairment. Reduce starting dose to 0.1 mL in patients with mild or moderate renal failure. Contains sulfites.

**CARBIDOPA (*Lodosyn*)** ▶LK ♀C ▶? $$$
ADULT - Parkinson's Disease, adjunct to carbidopa/ levodopa: start 25 mg PO daily with first daily dose of carbidopa/levodopa. May give an additional 12.5–25 mg with each dose of carbidopa/ levodopa as needed. Max 200 mg/d.
PEDS - Not approved in children.
FORMS - Trade only: Tabs 25 mg.
NOTES - Adjunct to carbidopa/levodopa to reduce peripheral side-effects such as nausea. Also increases the CNS availability of levodopa. Monitor for CNS side-effects such as dyskinesias and hallucinations when initiating therapy, and reduce the dose of levodopa as necessary.

**CARBIDOPA-LEVODOPA (*Sinemet, Sinemet CR, Parcopa*)** ▶L ♀C ▶- $$$$
ADULT - Parkinsonism: Standard release and orally disintegrating tab: start 1 tab (25/100 mg) PO

**(cont.)**

**CARBIDOPA-LEVODOPA** (cont.)
tid. Increase by 1 tab/d q 1–2 d prn. Use 1 tab (25/250 mg) PO tid-qid when higher levodopa doses are needed. Sustained release: Start 1 tab (50/200 mg) PO bid; separate doses by ≥4 h. Increase as needed at intervals ≥3 d. Typical max dose is 1,600–2,000 mg/d of levodopa, but higher doses have been used.
PEDS - Not approved in children.
UNAPPROVED ADULT - Restless legs syndrome: start 1/2 tab (25/100 mg) PO qhs; increase q3–4d to max 50/200 mg (two 25/100 tabs) qhs. If symptoms recur during the night, then a combination of standard release (25/100 mg, 1–2 tabs qhs) and sustained release (25/100 or 50/200 mg qhs) tabs may be used.
FORMS - Generic/Trade: Tabs (carbidopa/levodopa) 10/100, 25/100, 25/250 mg. Tabs, sustained release (Sinemet CR, carbidopa-levodopa ER) 25/100, 50/200 mg. Trade only: orally disintegrating tab (Parcopa) 10/100, 25/100, 25/250.
NOTES - Motor fluctuations and dyskinesias may occur. The 25/100 mg tabs are preferred as initial therapy, since most patients require at least 70–100 mg/d of carbidopa to reduce the risk of N/V. The 10/100 mg tabs have limited clinical utility. Extended-release formulations have a lower bioavailability than conventional preparations. Do not use within two wk of a nonselective MAOI. When used for restless legs syndrome, may precipitate rebound (recurrence of symptoms during the night) or augmentation (earlier daily onset of symptoms). Orally disintegrating tab is placed on top of the tongue and does not require water or swallowing, but is absorbed through the GI tract (not sublingually). Use caution in patients with undiagnosed skin lesions or a history of melanoma.

**PRAMIPEXOLE** (*Mirapex*) ▶K ♀C ▶? $$$$$
ADULT - Parkinson's disease: Start 0.125 mg PO tid × 1 wk, then 0.25 mg × 1 wk; after that, increase by 0.75 mg/wk divided tid. Usual effective dose is 0.5–1.5 mg PO tid. Restless legs syndrome: Start 0.125 mg PO 2–3 h prior to bedtime. May increase q4–7 d to 0.25 mg then 0.5 mg if needed.
PEDS - Not approved in children.
FORMS - Generic/Trade: Tabs 0.125, 0.25, 0.5, 1, 1.5 mg. Trade only: Tabs 0.75 mg.
NOTES - Decrease dose in renal impairment. Sleep attacks, syncope, and/or orthostatic hypotension may occur. Titrate slowly.

**ROPINIROLE** (*Requip, Requip XL*) ▶L ♀C ▶? $$$$$
ADULT - Parkinson's disease: Start 0.25 mg PO tid. Increase by 0.25 mg/dose at weekly intervals to 1 mg PO tid. Extended-release: Start 2 mg PO daily,

then gradually titrate dose at ≥ weekly intervals. Max 24 mg/d. Restless legs syndrome: Start 0.25 mg PO 1–3 h before sleep for 2 d, then increase to 0.5 mg/d on d 3–7. Increase by 0.5 mg/d at weekly intervals prn to max 4 mg/d given 1–3 h before sleep.
PEDS - Not approved in children.
FORMS - Generic/Trade: Tabs 0.25, 0.5, 1, 2, 3, 4 mg. Trade only: Tabs 5 mg, Extended-release caps 2, 3, 4, 8 mg.
NOTES - Sleep attacks, impulse control disorders, syncope, and/or orthostatic hypotension may occur. Titrate slowly. Retitrate if significant interruption of therapy occurs.

**ROTIGOTINE** (*Neupro*) ▶L ♀C ▶? $$$$$
ADULT - Product being discontinued altogether spring 2008. Parkinson's disease: Start 2 mg/24 h patch daily × 1 wk, then increase to lowest effective dose of 4 mg/24 h. May increase prn in ≥1 wk to max 6 mg/24 h.
PEDS - Not approved in children.
FORMS - Trade only: Transdermal patch 2, 4, 6 mg/24 h.
NOTES - Contains sulfites. Remove prior to MRI or cardioversion to avoid burns. Apply to clean, dry, intact skin of the abdomen, thigh, flank, shoulder, or upper arm, and hold in place for 20–30 sec. Rotate application sites daily, and wash skin after removal. Taper by 2 mg/24 h every other d when discontinuing.

***STALEVO*** (carbidopa + levodopa + entacapone) ▶L ♀C ▶- $$$$$
ADULT - Parkinson's disease (conversion from carbidopa-levodopa +/- entacapone): Start Stalevo tab that contains the same amount of carbidopa-levodopa as the patient was previously taking, and titrate to desired response. May need to lower the dose of levodopa in patients not already taking entacapone. Max 1,600 mg/d of entacapone or 1,600–2,000 mg/d of levodopa.
PEDS - Not approved in children.
FORMS - Trade only: Tabs (carbidopa/levodopa/entacapone): Stalevo 50 (12.5/50/200 mg), Stalevo 100 (25/100/200 mg), Stalevo 150 (37.5/150/200 mg), Stalevo 200 (50/200/200 mg).
NOTES - Patients who are not currently taking entacapone may benefit from titration of the individual components of this medication before conversion to this fixed-dose preparation. Avoid concomitant use of non-selective MAOIs. Use caution in hepatobiliary dysfunction. Motor fluctuations and dyskinesias may occur. Should not be used in patients with undiagnosed skin lesions or a history of melanoma.

## NEUROLOGY: Parkinsonian Agents—Monoamine Oxidase Inhibitors (MAOIs)

**RASAGILINE** (*Azilect*) ▶L ♀C ▶? $$$$$
ADULT - Parkinson's disease, monotherapy: 1 mg PO qam. Parkinson's disease, adjunctive: 0.5 mg PO qam. Max 1 mg/d.
PEDS - Not approved in children.

FORMS - Trade only: Tabs 0.5, 1 mg.
NOTES - Requires an MAOI diet. Contraindicated (risk of hypertensive crisis) with meperidine, methadone, tramadol, propoxyphene, dextromethorphan, sympathomimetic amines (eg, pseudoephedrine,

RASAGILINE (cont.)

phenylephrine, ephedrine), antidepressants, other MAOIs, cyclobenzaprine, and general anesthesia. Discontinue ≥14 d before liberalizing diet, starting one of these medications, or proceeding with elective surgery that requires general anesthesia. May need to reduce levodopa dose when used in combination. Reduce dose to 0.5 mg when used with CYP1A2 inhibitors (eg, ciprofloxacin) and in mild hepatic impairment. Do not use in moderate or severe liver disease.

**SELEGILINE (Eldepryl, Zelapar)** ▶LK ♀C ▶? $$$$
ADULT - Parkinsonism (adjunct to levodopa): 5 mg PO q am and q noon; max 10 mg/d. Zelapar ODT:

Start 1.25 mg sublingual q am for >6 wk, then increase prn to max 2.5 mg q am.
PEDS - Not approved in children.
UNAPPROVED ADULT - Parkinsonism (monotherapy): 5 mg PO q am and q noon; max 10 mg/d.
FORMS - Generic/Trade: Caps 5 mg. Tabs 5 mg. Trade only: Oral disintegrating tabs (Zelapar ODT) 1.25 mg.
NOTES - Should not be combined with meperidine or other opioids. Do not exceed max recommended dose; risk of non-selective MAO inhibition. Zelapar should be taken in the morning before food and without water.

## NEUROLOGY: Other Agents

**BETAHISTINE (*SERC)** ▶LK ♀? ▶? $
ADULT - Canada only. Vertigo of Meniere's disease: 8–16 mg PO tid.
PEDS - Not approved in children.
FORMS - Trade only: Tabs 8, 16 mg.
NOTES - Contraindicated in peptic ulcer disease and pheochromocytoma; use caution in asthmatics.

**BOTULINUM TOXIN TYPE A (Botox, Botox Cosmetic)** ▶Not absorbed ♀C ▶? $$$$$
WARNING - Symptoms of systemic botulism have been reported, particularly in children treated for spasticity due to cerebral palsy.
ADULT - Moderate to severe glabellar lines in patients ≤65 yo: inject 0.1 mL into each of 5 sites. Blepharospasm: 1.25–5 units IM into each of several sites in the orbicularis oculi of upper and lower lids q 3 mo; use lower doses at initial visit. Strabismus: 1.25–5.0 units depending on diagnosis, injected into extraocular muscles. Cervical dystonia: 15–100 units IM (with or without EMG guidance) into affected muscles q 3 mo (eg, splenius capitis/cervicis, sternocleidomastoid, levator scapulae, trapezius, semispinalis, scalene, longissimus); usual total dose is 200–300 units/treatment. Primary axillary hyperhidrosis: 50 units/axilla intradermally, divided over 10–15 sites.
PEDS - Not approved in children <12 yo (for blepharospasm), <16 yo (for cervical dystonia), or <18 yo (for hyperhidrosis).
UNAPPROVED ADULT - Hemifacial spasm: 1.25–2.5 units IM into affected muscles q 3–4 mo (eg, corrugator, orbicularis oculi, zygomaticus major, buccinator, depressor anguli oris, platysma); usual total dose is 10–34 units/treatment.
FORMS - Trade only: 100 unit single-use vials.
NOTES - Clinical benefit occurs in ≤2 wk (2–3 d for facial injections), peaks at 1–6 wk, and wears off in about 3 mo. Contraindicated in peripheral motor neuropathic disease (eg, ALS, motor neuropathy) or neuromuscular junction disease (eg, myasthenia gravis, Lambert-Eaton syndrome). The use of lower doses and longer dosing intervals may decrease the risk of producing neutralizing

antibodies. Increased risk of dysphagia when >100 units are injected into the sternocleidomastoid or with bilateral sternocleidomastoid injections.

**BOTULINUM TOXIN TYPE B (Myobloc)** ▶Not significantly absorbed ♀+ ▶? $$$$$
WARNING - Symptoms of systemic botulism have been reported, particularly in children treated for spasticity due to cerebral palsy.
ADULT - Cervical dystonia: Start 2,500–5,000 units IM in affected muscles. Use lower initial dose if no prior history of botulinum toxin therapy. Benefits usually last for 12–16 wk when a total dose of 5,000–10,000 units has been administered. Titrate to effective dose. Give treatments ≥3 mo apart to decrease the risk of producing neutralizing antibodies.
PEDS - Not approved in children.
NOTES - Low systemic concentrations are expected with IM injection; monitor closely for dysphagia. Use caution in peripheral motor neuropathic disease (eg, ALS, motor neuropathy) or neuromuscular junction disease (eg, myasthenia gravis, Lambert-Eaton syndrome due to an increased risk of systemic effects) and with other drugs that block neuromuscular function (eg, aminoglycosides, curare-like compounds).

**MANNITOL (Osmitrol, Resectisol)** ▶K ♀C ▶? $$
ADULT - Intracranial HTN: 0.25–2 g/kg IV over 30–60 min as a 15%, 20%, or 25% solution.
PEDS - Not approved in children.
UNAPPROVED ADULT - Increased ICP/Head trauma: 0.25–1 g/kg IV push over 20 min. Repeat q4–6h prn.
UNAPPROVED PEDS - Increased ICP/Cerebral edema: 0.25–1 g/kg/dose IV push over 20–30 min, then 0.25–0.5 g/kg/dose IV q4–6h prn.
NOTES - Monitor fluid and electrolyte balance and cardiac function. Filter IV solutions with concentrations ≥20%; crystals may be present.

**NIMODIPINE (Nimotop)** ▶L ♀C ▶- $$$$$
ADULT - Subarachnoid hemorrhage: 60 mg PO q4h for 21 d.
PEDS - Not approved in children.
FORMS - Generic/Trade: Caps 30 mg.

(cont.)

**RASAGILINE** (*cont.*)
NOTES - Begin therapy within 96 h. Give 1 h before or 2 h after meals. May give cap contents SL or via NG tube. Reduce dose in hepatic dysfunction.

**OXYBATE** (*Xyrem, GHB, gamma hydroxybutyrate*) ▶L ♀B ▶? ©Ⅲ $$$$$
WARNING - CNS depressant with abuse potential; avoid concurrent alcohol or sedative use.
ADULT - Narcolepsy-associated cataplexy or excessive daytime sleepiness: 2.25 g PO qhs. Repeat in 2.5–4 h. May increase by 1.5 g/d at >2 wk intervals to max 9 g/d. Dilute each dose in 60 mL water.
PEDS - Not approved in children.
FORMS - Trade only: Solution 180 mL (500 mg/mL) supplied with measuring device and child-proof dosing cups.
NOTES - Available only through the Xyrem Success Program centralized pharmacy (1-866-997-3688). Adjust dose in hepatic dysfunction. Prepare doses just prior to bedtime, and use within 24 h. May need an alarm to signal 2nd dose.

**RILUZOLE** (*Rilutek*) ▶LK ♀C ▶- $$$$$
ADULT - Amyotrophic lateral sclerosis: 50 mg PO q12h.
PEDS - Not approved in children.
FORMS - Trade only: Tabs 50 mg.
NOTES - Take 1 h before or 2 h after meals. Monitor LFTs.

**TETRABENAZINE** (✦*NITOMAN*) ▶L ♀? ▶- $$$$
WARNING - Contraindicated if history of depression or suicidality; monitor closely and discontinue at the first signs thereof.
ADULT - Hyperkinetic movement disorders (Canada only): Start 12.5 mg PO bid-tid. May increase by 12.5 mg/d q3–5 d to usual dose of 25 mg PO tid. Max 200 mg/d, but most patients do not tolerate more than 75 mg/d. Discontinue if there is no benefit after 7 d of treatment at max tolerated dose.
PEDS - Not approved in children.
UNAPPROVED PEDS - Limited data suggest that ½ of the adult dose may be used and titrated as tolerated.
FORMS - Trade only: Tabs 25 mg.
NOTES - Used for the treatment of Huntington's chorea, hemiballismus, senile chorea, tic disorders (including Tourette's syndrome), and tardive dyskinesia. May cause or exacerbate parkinsonism, depression, and/or suicidality. Contraindicated in Parkinson's disease or depression. Don't use with MAOIs; use caution when combined with antipsychotics and other dopamine receptor blocking agents. May attenuate the effects of levodopa and antidepressants.

## OB/GYN: Contraceptives—Oral Biphasic

**NOTE:** Not recommended in women >35 yo who smoke. Increased risk of thromboembolism, stroke, MI, hepatic neoplasia & gallbladder disease. Nausea, breast tenderness, & breakthrough bleeding are common transient side effects. Nighttime dosing may minimize nausea. Effectiveness is reduced by hepatic enzyme-inducing drugs such as certain anticonvulsants and barbiturates, rifampin, rifabutin, griseofulvin & protease inhibitors. Additionally, products that contain St John's wort may decrease efficacy. Vomiting or diarrhea may also increase the risk of contraceptive failure. An additional form of birth control may be advisable. Advise patients to take at the same time every d. See PI for instructions on missing doses. Most available in 21 and 28 d packs. Although not approved by the FDA, combined OCPs are used for dysfunctional uterine bleeding, dysmenorrhea, pelvic pain, and hirsutism (with spironolactone): 1 tab PO daily. Wait 6 wk postpartum to initiate combination OCPs to decrease the risk of thromboembolism and to support lactation.

**NECON 10/11** (ethinyl estradiol + norethindrone) ▶L ♀X ▶- $$
ADULT - Contraception: 1 tab PO daily.
PEDS - Not approved in children.
FORMS - Trade only: Tabs 35 mcg ethinyl estradiol/0.5 mg norethindrone (10) & 35 mcg ethinyl estradiol/1 mg norethindrone (11).
NOTES - Same as Ortho-Novum 10/11.

**ORTHO NOVUM 10/11** (ethinyl estradiol + norethindrone) ▶L ♀X ▶- $$$
ADULT - Contraception: 1 tab PO daily.
PEDS - Not approved in children.
FORMS - Trade only: Tabs 35 mcg ethinyl estradiol/0.5 mg norethindrone (10) & 35 mcg ethinyl estradiol/1 mg norethindrone (11).

## OB/GYN: Contraceptives—Oral Monophasic

**NOTE:** Not recommended in women >35 yo who smoke. Increased risk of thromboembolism, stroke, MI, hepatic neoplasia & gallbladder disease. Nausea, breast tenderness, and breakthrough bleeding are common transient side effects. Nighttime dosing may minimize nausea. Effectiveness is reduced by hepatic enzyme-inducing drugs such as certain anticonvulsants and barbiturates, rifampin, rifabutin, griseofulvin & protease inhibitors. Additionally, products that contain St John's wort may decrease efficacy. Vomiting or diarrhea may also increase the risk of contraceptive failure. An additional form of birth control may be advisable. Advise patients to take at the same time every d. See product insert for instructions on missing doses. Most available in 21 and 28 d packs. Although not approved by the FDA, combined OCPs are used for dysfunctional uterine bleeding, emergency contraception, dysmenorrhea, pelvic pain, and hirsutism (with spironolactone): 1 tab PO daily. Wait 6 wk postpartum to initiate combination OCPs to decrease the risk of thromboembolism and to support lactation.

*ALESSE* (ethinyl estradiol + levonorgestrel) ▶L ♀X ▶- $$
ADULT - Contraception: 1 tab PO daily.
PEDS - Not approved in children.
UNAPPROVED ADULT - Postcoital contraception: see table.
FORMS - Trade only: Tabs 20 mcg ethinyl estradiol/0.1 mg levonorgestrel.
NOTES - May cause less nausea & breast tenderness and may increase breakthrough bleeding due to lower estrogen content.

*APRI* (ethinyl estradiol + desogestrel) (♦*Marvelon*) ▶L ♀X ▶- $$
ADULT - Contraception: 1 tab PO daily.
PEDS - Not approved in children.
FORMS - Trade only: Tabs 30 mcg ethinyl estradiol/0.15 mg desogestrel.
NOTES - Same as Desogen.

*AVIANE* (ethinyl estradiol + levonorgestrel) ▶L ♀X ▶- $$
ADULT - Contraception: 1 tab PO daily.
PEDS - Not approved in children.
UNAPPROVED ADULT - Postcoital contraception: see table.
FORMS - Trade only: Tabs 20 mcg ethinyl estradiol/0.1 mg levonorgestrel.
NOTES - May cause less nausea & breast tenderness & may increase breakthrough bleeding due to lower estrogen content. Same as Alesse.

*BALZIVA* (ethinyl estradiol + norethindrone) ▶L ♀X ▶- $$
ADULT - Contraception: 1 tab PO daily.
PEDS - Not approved in children.
FORMS - Trade only: Tabs 35 mcg ethinyl estradiol/0.4 mg norethindrone.
NOTES - Same as Ovcon-35.

*BREVICON* (ethinyl estradiol + norethindrone) ▶L ♀X ▶- $$$
ADULT - Contraception: 1 tab PO daily.
PEDS - Not approved in children.
FORMS - Trade only: Tabs 35 mcg ethinyl estradiol/0.5 mg norethindrone.

*CRYSELLE* (ethinyl estradiol + norgestrel) ▶L ♀X ▶- $$
ADULT - Contraception: 1 tab PO daily.
PEDS - Not approved in children.
UNAPPROVED ADULT - Postcoital contraception: see table.
FORMS - Trade only: Tabs: 30 mcg ethinyl estradiol/0.3 mg norgestrel.
NOTES - Same as Lo/Ovral

*DEMULEN* (ethinyl estradiol + ethynodiol) ▶L ♀X ▶- $$
WARNING - Multiple strengths; see FORMS & write specific product on Rx.
ADULT - Contraception: 1 tab PO daily.
PEDS - Not approved in children.
FORMS - Trade only: Tabs 35 mcg ethinyl estradiol/1 mg ethynodiol (Demulen 1/35); 50 mcg ethinyl estradiol/1 mg ethynodiol (Demulen 1/50).
NOTES - 50 mcg estrogen component rarely necessary.

*DESOGEN* (ethinyl estradiol + desogestrel) (♦*Marvelon*) ▶L ♀X ▶- $$
ADULT - Contraception: 1 tab PO daily.
PEDS - Not approved in children.
FORMS - Trade only: Tabs 30 mcg ethinyl estradiol/0.15 mg desogestrel.

*FEMCON FE* (ethinyl estradiol + norethindrone) ▶L ♀X ▶- $$$
ADULT - Contraception: 1 tab PO daily.
PEDS - Not approved in children.
FORMS - Trade only: Chewable tabs 35 mcg ethinyl estradiol/0.4 mg norethindrone. Placebo tabs are ferrous fumarate 75 mg.
NOTES - Chewable formulation may be swallowed whole or chewed. If chewed, follow with 8 ounces liquid.

*JUNEL* (ethinyl estradiol + norethindrone) ▶L ♀X ▶- $$
WARNING - Multiple strengths; see FORMS & write specific product on Rx.
ADULT - Contraception: 1 tab PO daily.
PEDS - Not approved in children.
FORMS - Trade only: Tabs 1 mg norethindrone/20 mcg ethinyl estradiol (Junel 1/20). 1.5 mg norethindrone/30 mcg ethinyl estradiol (Junel 1.5/30).
NOTES - Junel 1/20 may cause less nausea & breast tenderness and may increase breakthrough bleeding due to lower estrogen content. Same as Loestrin.

*JUNEL FE* (ethinyl estradiol + norethindrone + ferrous fumarate) ▶L ♀X ▶- $$
WARNING - Multiple strengths; see FORMS & write specific product on Rx.
ADULT - Contraception: 1 tab PO daily.
PEDS - Not approved in children.
FORMS - Trade only: Tabs 1 mg norethindrone/20 mcg ethinyl estradiol w/7 d 75 mg ferrous fumarate (Junel Fe 1/20). 1.5 mg norethindrone/30 mcg ethinyl estradiol w/7 d 75 mg ferrous fumarate (1.5/30).
NOTES - Junel Fe 1/20 may cause less nausea & breast tenderness and may increase breakthrough bleeding due to lower estrogen content. Same as Loestrin Fe.

*KARIVA* (ethinyl estradiol + desogestrel) ▶L ♀X ▶- $$$
ADULT - Contraception: 1 tab PO daily.
PEDS - Not approved in children.
FORMS - Trade only: Tabs 0.02 mg ethinyl estradiol/0.15 mg desogestrel (21) & 0.01 mg ethinyl estradiol (5).
NOTES - May have less breakthrough bleeding. All 28 tabs must be taken. Same as Mircette.

*KELNOR* (ethinyl estradiol + ethynodiol) ▶L ♀X ▶- $$
ADULT - Contraception: 1 tab PO daily.
PEDS - Not approved in children.
FORMS - Generic/Trade: Tabs 35 mcg ethinyl estradiol + 1 mg ethynodiol.
NOTES - Same as Demulen

***LESSINA*** (ethinyl estradiol + levonorgestrel) ▶L ♀X ▶- $$
ADULT - Contraception: 1 tab PO daily.
PEDS - Not approved in children.
UNAPPROVED ADULT - Postcoital contraception: see table.
FORMS - Generic/Trade: Tabs 20 mcg ethinyl estradiol/0.1 mg levonorgestrel.
NOTES - May cause less nausea & breast tenderness and may increase breakthrough bleeding due to lower estrogen content. Same as Levlite.

***LEVLEN*** (ethinyl estradiol + levonorgestrel) (✦*Min-Ovral*) ▶L ♀X ▶- $$
ADULT - Contraception: 1 tab PO daily.
PEDS - Not approved in children.
UNAPPROVED ADULT - Postcoital contraception: see table.
FORMS - Trade only: Tabs 30 mcg ethinyl estradiol/0.15 mg levonorgestrel.
NOTES - Same as Nordette.

***LEVLITE*** (ethinyl estradiol + levonorgestrel) ▶L ♀X ▶- $$
ADULT - Contraception: 1 tab PO daily.
PEDS - Not approved in children.
UNAPPROVED ADULT - Postcoital contraception: see table.
FORMS - Generic/Trade: Tabs 20 mcg ethinyl estradiol/0.1 mg levonorgestrel.
NOTES - May cause less nausea & breast tenderness and may increase breakthrough bleeding due to lower estrogen content. Same as Alesse.

***LEVORA*** (ethinyl estradiol + levonorgestrel) (✦*Min-Ovral*) ▶L ♀X ▶- $$
ADULT - Contraception: 1 tab PO daily.
PEDS - Not approved in children.
UNAPPROVED ADULT - Postcoital contraception: see table.
FORMS - Trade only: Tabs 30 mcg ethinyl estradiol/0.15 mg levonorgestrel.
NOTES - Same as Levlen.

***LO/OVRAL*** (ethinyl estradiol + norgestrel) ▶L ♀X ▶- $$
ADULT - Contraception: 1 tab PO daily.
PEDS - Not approved in children.
UNAPPROVED ADULT - Postcoital contraception: see table.
FORMS - Trade only: Tabs 30 mcg ethinyl estradiol/0.3 mg norgestrel.

***LOESTRIN*** (ethinyl estradiol + norethindrone) (✦*Minestrin 1/20*) ▶L ♀X ▶- $$$
WARNING - Multiple strengths; see FORMS & write specific product on Rx.
ADULT - Contraception: 1 tab PO daily.
PEDS - Not approved in children.
FORMS - Trade only: Tabs 1 mg norethindrone/20 mcg ethinyl estradiol (Loestrin 1/20). 1.5 mg norethindrone/30 mcg ethinyl estradiol (Loestrin 1.5/30).
NOTES - Loestrin 1/20 may cause less nausea & breast tenderness and may increase breakthrough bleeding due to lower estrogen content.

***LOESTRIN 24 FE*** (ethinyl estradiol + norethindrone + ferrous fumarate) ▶L ♀X ▶- $$$
ADULT - Contraception: 1 tab PO daily.
PEDS - Not approved in children.
FORMS - Trade only: Tabs 1 mg norethindrone/20 mcg ethinyl estradiol (24 d) w/4 d 75 mg ferrous fumarate.
NOTES - Loestrin 24 Fe 1/20 may cause less nausea & breast tenderness and may increase breakthrough bleeding due to lower estrogen content.

***LOESTRIN FE*** (ethinyl estradiol + norethindrone + ferrous fumarate) ▶L ♀X ▶- $$$
WARNING - Multiple strengths; see FORMS & write specific product on Rx.
ADULT - Contraception: 1 tab PO daily.
PEDS - Not approved in children.
FORMS - Trade only: Tabs 1 mg norethindrone/20 mcg ethinyl estradiol w/7 d 75 mg ferrous fumarate (Loestrin Fe 1/20); 1.5 mg norethindrone/30 mcg ethinyl estradiol w/7 d 75mg ferrous fumarate (1.5/30).
NOTES - Loestrin Fe 1/20 may cause less nausea & breast tenderness and may increase breakthrough bleeding due to lower estrogen content.

***LOW-OGESTREL*** (ethinyl estradiol + norgestrel) ▶L ♀X ▶- $$
ADULT - Contraception: 1 tab PO daily.
PEDS - Not approved in children.
UNAPPROVED ADULT - Postcoital contraception: see table.
FORMS - Trade only: Tabs: 30 mcg ethinyl estradiol/0.3 mg norgestrel.
NOTES - Same as Lo/Ovral.

***LUTERA*** (ethinyl estradiol + levonorgestrel) ▶L ♀X ▶- $$
ADULT - Contraception: 1 tab PO daily.
PEDS - Not approved in children.
UNAPPROVED ADULT - Postcoital contraception: see table.
FORMS - Trade only: Tabs 20 mcg ethinyl estradiol/0.1 mg levonorgestrel.
NOTES - May cause less nausea & breast tenderness and may increase breakthrough bleeding due to lower estrogen content. Same as Alesse.

***LYBREL*** (ethinyl estradiol + levonorgestrel) ▶L ♀X ▶- $$$
ADULT - Contraception: 1 tab PO daily.
PEDS - Not approved in children.
FORMS - Trade only: Tabs 20 mcg ethinyl estradiol/90 mcg levonorgestrel.
NOTES - Approved for continuous use without a "pill-free" period. May cause breakthrough bleeding.

***MICROGESTIN FE*** (ethinyl estradiol + norethindrone + ferrous fumarate) ▶L ♀X ▶- $$
WARNING - Multiple strengths; see FORMS & write specific product on Rx.
ADULT - Contraception: 1 tab PO daily.
PEDS - Not approved in children.
FORMS - Trade only: Tabs 1 mg norethindrone/20 mcg ethinyl estradiol w/7 d 75 mg ferrous fumarate (Microgestin Fe 1/20). 1.5 mg norethindrone/30

**MICROGESTIN FE** *(cont.)*
    mcg ethinyl estradiol w/7 d 75 mg ferrous fumarate (1.5/30).
    NOTES - Microgestin Fe 1/20 may cause less nausea and breast tenderness and may increase breakthrough bleeding due to lower estrogen content. Same as Loestrin Fe.

**MIRCETTE** (ethinyl estradiol + desogestrel) ▶L ♀X ▶- $$$
    ADULT - Contraception: 1 tab PO daily.
    PEDS - Not approved in children.
    FORMS - Trade only: Tabs 0.02 mg ethinyl estradiol/0.15 mg desogestrel (21) & 0.01 mg ethinyl estradiol (5).
    NOTES - May have less breakthrough bleeding. All 28 tabs must be taken.

**MODICON** (ethinyl estradiol + norethindrone) ▶L ♀X ▶- $$$
    ADULT - Contraception: 1 tab PO daily.
    PEDS - Not approved in children.
    FORMS - Trade only: Tabs 35 mcg ethinyl estradiol/0.5 mg norethindrone.
    NOTES - Same as Brevicon.

**MONONESSA** (ethinyl estradiol + norgestimate) ▶L ♀X ▶- $$
    ADULT - Contraception: 1 tab PO daily.
    PEDS - Not approved in children.
    FORMS - Trade only: Tabs: 35 mcg ethinyl estradiol/0.25 mg norgestimate.
    NOTES - Same as Ortho-Cyclen.

**NECON** (ethinyl estradiol + norethindrone) (✦*Select 1/35, Brevicon 1/35*) ▶L ♀X ▶- $$
    WARNING - Multiple strengths; see FORMS & write specific product on Rx.
    ADULT - Contraception: 1 tab PO daily.
    PEDS - Not approved in children.
    FORMS - Trade only: Tabs 0.5 mg norethindrone/35 mcg ethinyl estradiol (Necon 0.5/35). 1 mg norethindrone/35 mcg ethinyl estradiol (Necon 1/35).
    NOTES - Same as Brevicon (0.5/35), Ortho-Novum 1/35 (1/35).

**NECON 1/50** (mestranol + norethindrone) ▶L ♀X ▶- $$
    ADULT - Contraception: 1 tab PO daily.
    PEDS - Not approved in children.
    FORMS - Trade only: Tabs: 1 mg norethindrone/50 mcg mestranol.
    NOTES - 50 mcg estrogen component rarely necessary. Same as Ortho-Novum 1/50.

**NORDETTE** (ethinyl estradiol + levonorgestrel) (✦*Min-Ovral*) ▶L ♀X ▶- $$$
    ADULT - Contraception: 1 tab PO daily.
    PEDS - Not approved in children.
    UNAPPROVED ADULT - Postcoital contraception: see table.
    FORMS - Trade only: Tabs 30 mcg ethinyl estradiol/0.15 mg levonorgestrel.
    NOTES - Same as Levlen.

**NORINYL 1+35** (ethinyl estradiol + norethindrone) (✦*Select 1/35, Brevicon 1/35*) ▶L ♀X ▶- $$
    ADULT - Contraception: 1 tab PO daily.

    PEDS - Not approved in children.
    FORMS - Trade only: Tabs 1 mg norethindrone/35 mcg ethinyl estradiol.
    NOTES - Same as Ortho-Novum 1/35.

**NORINYL 1+50** (mestranol + norethindrone) ▶L ♀X ▶- $$
    ADULT - Contraception: 1 tab PO daily.
    PEDS - Not approved in children.
    FORMS - Trade only: Tabs 1 mg norethindrone/50 mcg mestranol.
    NOTES - 50 mcg estrogen component rarely necessary. Same as Ortho-Novum 1/50.

**NORTREL** (ethinyl estradiol + norethindrone) ▶L ♀X ▶- $$
    WARNING - Multiple strengths; see FORMS & write specific product on Rx.
    ADULT - Contraception: 1 tab PO daily.
    PEDS - Not approved in children.
    FORMS - Trade only: Tabs 35 mcg ethinyl estradiol/1 mg norethindrone (Nortrel 1/35). 35 mcg ethinyl estradiol/0.5 mg norethindrone (Nortrel 0.5/35).
    NOTES - Same as Brevicon (0.5/35), Ortho-Novum 1/35 (1/35).

**OGESTREL** (ethinyl estradiol + norgestrel) ▶L ♀X ▶- $$
    ADULT - Contraception: 1 tab PO daily.
    PEDS - Not approved in children.
    UNAPPROVED ADULT - Postcoital contraception: see table.
    FORMS - Trade only: Tabs: 50 mcg ethinyl estradiol/0.5 mg norgestrel.
    NOTES - 50 mcg estrogen component rarely necessary. Same as Ovral.

**ORTHO-CEPT** (ethinyl estradiol + desogestrel) (✦*Marvelon*) ▶L ♀X ▶- $$$
    ADULT - Contraception: 1 tab PO daily.
    PEDS - Not approved in children.
    FORMS - Trade only: Tabs 30 mcg ethinyl estradiol/0.15 mg desogestrel.
    NOTES - Same as Desogen.

**ORTHO-CYCLEN** (ethinyl estradiol + norgestimate) (✦*Cyclen*) ▶L ♀X ▶- $$
    ADULT - Contraception: 1 tab PO daily.
    PEDS - Not approved in children.
    FORMS - Generic/Trade: Tabs: 35 mcg ethinyl estradiol/0.25 mg norgestimate.

**ORTHO-NOVUM 1/35** (ethinyl estradiol + norethindrone) ▶L ♀X ▶- $$$
    ADULT - Contraception: 1 tab PO daily.
    PEDS - Not approved in children.
    FORMS - Trade only: Tabs 1 mg norethindrone/35 mcg ethinyl estradiol.

**ORTHO-NOVUM 1/50** (mestranol + norethindrone) ▶L ♀X ▶- $$$
    ADULT - Contraception: 1 tab PO daily.
    PEDS - Not approved in children.
    FORMS - Trade only: Tabs: 1 mg norethindrone/50 mcg mestranol.
    NOTES - 50 mcg estrogen component rarely necessary.

***OVCON-35*** (ethinyl estradiol + norethindrone) ▶L
♀X ▶- $$$
ADULT - Contraception: 1 tab PO daily.
PEDS - Not approved in children.
FORMS - Trade only: Tabs 35 mcg ethinyl estra-
diol/0.4 mg norethindrone.

***OVCON-50*** (ethinyl estradiol + norethindrone) ▶L
♀X ▶- $$$
ADULT - Contraception: 1 tab PO daily.
PEDS - Not approved in children.
FORMS - Trade only: Tabs 50 mcg ethinyl estra-
diol/0.4 mg norethindrone.
NOTES - 50 mcg estrogen component rarely
necessary.

***OVRAL*** (ethinyl estradiol + norgestrel) ▶L ♀X
▶- $$$
ADULT - Contraception: 1 tab PO daily.
PEDS - Not approved in children.
UNAPPROVED ADULT - Postcoital contraception: see
table.
FORMS - Trade only: Tabs 50 mcg ethinyl estra-
diol/0.5 mg norgestrel.
NOTES - 50 mcg estrogen component rarely
necessary.

***PORTIA*** (ethinyl estradiol + levonorgestrel) ▶L ♀X
▶- $$
ADULT - Contraception: 1 tab PO daily.
PEDS - Not approved in children.
UNAPPROVED ADULT - Postcoital contraception: see
table.
FORMS - Trade only: Tabs 30 mcg ethinyl estra-
diol/0.15 mg levonorgestrel.
NOTES - Same as Nordette.

***PREVIFEM*** (ethinyl estradiol + norgestimate) ▶L
♀X ▶- $$
ADULT - Contraception: 1 tab PO daily.
PEDS - Not approved in children.
FORMS - Trade only: Tabs 35 mcg ethinyl estra-
diol/0.25 mg norgestimate.

***QUASENSE*** (ethinyl estradiol + levonorgestrel) ▶L
♀X ▶- $$$
ADULT - Contraception: 1 tab PO daily.
PEDS - Not approved in children.
FORMS - Generic/Trade: Tabs 30 mcg ethinyl estra-
diol/0.15 mg levonorgestrel. 84 white active pills
followed by 7 peach placebo pills.
NOTES - Decreases menstrual periods from q mo
to q 3 mo, however, intermenstrual bleeding and
spotting is more frequent than with 28-d regimens. Same as Seasonale.

***RECLIPSEN*** (ethinyl estradiol + desogestrel) ▶L ♀X
▶- $$
ADULT - Contraception: 1 tab PO daily.
PEDS - Not approved in children.
FORMS - Trade only: Tabs 30 mcg ethinyl estra-
diol/0.15 mg desogestrel.
NOTES - Same as Desogen.

***SEASONALE*** (ethinyl estradiol + levonorgestrel) ▶L
♀X ▶- $$$
ADULT - Contraception: 1 tab PO daily.
PEDS - Not approved in children.

FORMS - Generic/Trade: Tabs 30 mcg ethinyl estra-
diol/0.15 mg levonorgestrel. 84 pink active pills
followed by 7 white placebo pills.
NOTES - Decreases menstrual periods from q mo
to q 3 mo, however, intermenstrual bleeding
and spotting is more frequent than with 28-d
regimens.

***SEASONIQUE*** (ethinyl estradiol + levonorgestrel) ▶L
♀X ▶- $$$
ADULT - Contraception: 1 tab PO daily.
PEDS - Not approved in children.
FORMS - Trade only: Tabs 30 mcg ethinyl estra-
diol/0.15 mg levonorgestrel. 84 light blue-green
active pills followed by 7 yellow pills w/10 mcg
ethinyl estradiol.
NOTES - Decreases menstrual periods from q mo to q
3 mo, however, intermenstrual bleeding and spot-
ting is more frequent than with 28-d regimens.

***SPRINTEC*** (ethinyl estradiol + norgestimate) ▶L ♀X
▶- $$
ADULT - Contraception: 1 tab PO daily.
PEDS - Not approved in children.
FORMS - Trade only: Tabs 35 mcg ethinyl estra-
diol/0.25 mg norgestimate.
NOTES - Same as Ortho-Cyclen.

***YASMIN*** (ethinyl estradiol + drospirenone) ▶L ♀X
▶- $$$
ADULT - Contraception: 1 tab PO daily.
PEDS - Not approved in children.
FORMS - Trade only: Tabs 30 mcg ethinyl estra-
diol/3 mg drospirenone.
NOTES - May cause hyperkalemia due to antimin-
eralocorticoid activity of drospirenone (equal
to 25 mg spironolactone). Monitor potassium
in patients on ACEIs, ARBs, potassium-sparing
diuretics, heparin, aldosterone antagonists, &
NSAIDs.

***YAZ*** (ethinyl estradiol + drospirenone) ▶L ♀X
▶- $$$
ADULT - Contraception, premenstrual dysphoric dis-
order, acne: 1 tab PO daily.
PEDS - Not approved in children.
FORMS - Trade only: Tabs 20 mcg ethinyl estra-
diol/3 mg drospirenone. 24 active pills are followed by 4 inert pills.
NOTES - May cause hyperkalemia due to antimineralocorticoid activity of drospirenone (equal
to 25 mg spironolactone). Monitor potassium
in patients on ACEIs, ARBs, potassium-sparing
diuretics, heparin, aldosterone antagonists, &
NSAIDs.

***ZOVIA*** (ethinyl estradiol + ethynodiol) ▶L ♀X ▶- $$
WARNING - Multiple strengths; see FORMS & write
specific product on Rx.
ADULT - Contraception: 1 tab PO daily.
PEDS - Not approved in children.
FORMS - Trade only: Tabs 1 mg ethynodiol/35 mcg
ethinyl estradiol (Zovia 1/35E). 1 mg ethyno-
diol/50 mcg ethinyl estradiol (Zovia 1/50E).
NOTES - 50 mcg estrogen component rarely neces-
sary. Same as Demulen.

## OB/GYN: Contraceptives—Oral Triphasic

**NOTE:** Not recommended in women >35 yo who smoke. Increased risk of thromboembolism, stroke, MI, hepatic neoplasia & gallbladder disease. Nausea, breast tenderness, & breakthrough bleeding are common transient side effects. Nighttime dosing may minimize nausea. Effectiveness is reduced by hepatic enzyme-inducing drugs such as certain anticonvulsants and barbiturates, rifampin, rifabutin, griseofulvin & protease inhibitors. Additionally, products that contain St John's wort may decrease efficacy. Vomiting or diarrhea may also increase the risk of contraceptive failure. An additional form of birth control may be advisable. Advise patients to take at the same time every d. See PI for instructions on missing doses. Most available in 21 and 28 d packs. Although not approved by the FDA, combined OCPs are used for dysfunctional uterine bleeding, emergency contraception, dysmenorrhea, pelvic pain, and hirsutism (with spironolactone): 1 tab PO daily. Wait 6 wk postpartum to initiate combination OCPs to decrease the risk of thromboembolism and to support lactation.

**ARANELLE (ethinyl estradiol + norethindrone)** ▶L ♀X ▶- $$
ADULT - Contraception: 1 tab PO daily.
PEDS - Not approved in children.
FORMS - Trade only: Tabs 35 mcg ethinyl estradiol/0.5, 1, 0.5 mg norethindrone.
NOTES - Same as Tri-Norinyl.

**CYCLESSA (ethinyl estradiol + desogestrel)** ▶L ♀X ▶- $$
ADULT - Contraception: 1 tab PO daily.
PEDS - Not approved in children.
FORMS - Generic/Trade: Tabs 25 mcg ethinyl estradiol/0.100, 0.125, 0.150 mg desogestrel.

**ENPRESSE (ethinyl estradiol + levonorgestrel) (✦Triquilar)** ▶L ♀X ▶- $$
ADULT - Contraception: 1 tab PO daily.
PEDS - Not approved in children.
UNAPPROVED ADULT - Postcoital contraception: see table.
FORMS - Trade only: Tabs 30, 40, 30 mcg ethinyl estradiol/0.05, 0.075, 0.125 mg levonorgestrel.
NOTES - Same as Triphasil.

**ESTROSTEP FE (ethinyl estradiol + norethindrone + ferrous fumarate)** ▶L ♀X ▶- $$$
ADULT - Contraception: 1 tab PO daily.
PEDS - Not approved in children.
FORMS - Generic/Trade: Tabs 20, 30, 35 mcg ethinyl estradiol/1 mg norethindrone + "placebo" tabs with 75 mg ferrous fumarate. Packs of 28 only.

**LEENA (ethinyl estradiol + norethindrone)** ▶L ♀X ▶- $$
ADULT - Contraception: 1 tab PO daily.
PEDS - Not approved in children.
FORMS - Trade only: Tabs 35 mcg ethinyl estradiol/0.5, 1, 0.5 mg norethindrone.
NOTES - Same as Tri-Norinyl.

**NECON 7/7/7 (ethinyl estradiol + norethindrone)** ▶L ♀X ▶- $$
ADULT - Contraception: 1 tab PO daily.
PEDS - Not approved in children.
FORMS - Trade only: Tabs 35 mcg ethinyl estradiol/0.5, 0.75, 1 mg norethindrone.
NOTES - Same as Ortho-Novum 7/7/7.

**NORTREL 7/7/7 (ethinyl estradiol + norethindrone)** ▶L ♀X ▶- $$
ADULT - Contraception: 1 tab PO daily.
PEDS - Not approved in children.
FORMS - Trade only: Tabs 35 mcg ethinyl estradiol/0.5, 0.75, 1 mg norethindrone.

NOTES - Same as Ortho-Novum 7/7/7.

**ORTHO TRI-CYCLEN (ethinyl estradiol + norgestimate) (✦Tri-Cyclen)** ▶L ♀X ▶- $$
ADULT - Contraception, adult acne: 1 tab PO daily.
PEDS - Not approved in children.
FORMS - Generic/Trade: Tabs 35 mcg ethinyl estradiol/0.18, 0.215, 0.25 mg norgestimate.

**ORTHO TRI-CYCLEN LO (ethinyl estradiol + norgestimate)** ▶L ♀X ▶- $$$
ADULT - Contraception: 1 tab PO daily.
PEDS - Not approved in children.
FORMS - Trade only: Tabs 25 mcg ethinyl estradiol/0.18, 0.215, 0.25 mg norgestimate.

**ORTHO-NOVUM 7/7/7 (ethinyl estradiol + norethindrone)** ▶L ♀X ▶- $$
ADULT - Contraception: 1 tab PO daily.
PEDS - Not approved in children.
FORMS - Trade only: Tabs 35 mcg ethinyl estradiol/0.5, 0.75, 1 mg norethindrone.

**TRI-LEGEST (ethinyl estradiol + norethindrone)** ▶L ♀X ▶- $$$
ADULT - Contraception: 1 tab PO daily.
PEDS - Not approved in children.
FORMS - Trade only: Tabs 20, 30, 35 mcg ethinyl estradiol/1 mg norethindrone.

**TRI-LEGEST FE (ethinyl estradiol + norethindrone + ferrous fumarate)** ▶L ♀X ▶- $$$
ADULT - Contraception: 1 tab PO daily.
PEDS - Not approved in children.
FORMS - Trade only: Tabs 20, 30, 35 mcg ethinyl estradiol/1 mg norethindrone + "placebo" tabs with 75 mg ferrous fumarate.
NOTES - Same as Estrostep Fe.

**TRI-LEVLEN (ethinyl estradiol + levonorgestrel)** ▶L ♀X ▶- $$
ADULT - Contraception: 1 tab PO daily.
PEDS - Not approved in children.
UNAPPROVED ADULT - Postcoital contraception: see table.
FORMS - Trade only: Tabs 30, 40, 30 mcg ethinyl estradiol/0.05, 0.075, 0.125 mg levonorgestrel.
NOTES - Same as Triphasil.

**TRINESSA (ethinyl estradiol + norgestimate)** ▶L ♀X ▶- $$
ADULT - Contraception, adult acne: 1 tab PO daily.
PEDS - Not approved in children.
FORMS - Trade only: Tabs 35 mcg ethinyl estradiol/0.18, 0.215, 0.25 mg norgestimate.
NOTES - Same as Ortho Tri-Cyclen.

*TRI-NORINYL* (ethinyl estradiol + norethindrone) (**Synphasic*) ▶L ♀X ▶- $$
ADULT - Contraception: 1 tab PO daily.
PEDS - Not approved in children.
FORMS - Trade only: Tabs 35 mcg ethinyl estradiol/0.5, 1, 0.5 mg norethindrone.

*TRIPHASIL* (ethinyl estradiol + levonorgestrel) ▶L ♀X ▶- $$
ADULT - Contraception: 1 tab PO daily.
PEDS - Not approved in children.
UNAPPROVED ADULT - Postcoital contraception: see table.
FORMS - Trade only: Tabs 30, 40, 30 mcg ethinyl estradiol/0.05, 0.075, 0.125 mg levonorgestrel.

*TRI-PREVIFEM* (ethinyl estradiol + norgestimate) ▶L ♀X ▶- $$
ADULT - Contraception, adult acne: 1 tab PO daily.
PEDS - Not approved in children.
FORMS - Trade only: Tabs 35 mcg ethinyl estradiol/0.18, 0.215, 0.25 mg norgestimate.
NOTES - Same as Ortho Tri-Cyclen.

*TRI-SPRINTEC* (ethinyl estradiol + norgestimate) ▶L ♀X ▶- $$
ADULT - Contraception, adult acne: 1 tab PO daily.
PEDS - Not approved in children.
FORMS - Trade only: Tabs 35 mcg ethinyl estradiol/0.18, 0.215, 0.25 mg norgestimate.
NOTES - Same as Ortho Tri-Cyclen.

*TRIVORA-28* (ethinyl estradiol + levonorgestrel) ▶L ♀X ▶- $$
ADULT - Contraception: 1 tab PO daily.
PEDS - Not approved in children.
UNAPPROVED ADULT - Postcoital contraception: see table.
FORMS - Trade only: Tabs 30, 40, 30 mcg ethinyl estradiol/0.05, 0.075, 0.125 mg levonorgestrel.
NOTES - Same as Triphasil.

*VELIVET* (ethinyl estradiol + desogestrel) ▶L ♀X ▶- $$
ADULT - Contraception: 1 tab PO daily.
PEDS - Not approved in children.
FORMS - Generic/Trade: Tabs 25 mcg ethinyl estradiol/0.100, 0.125, 0.150 mg desogestrel.
NOTES - Same as Cyclessa.

## OB/GYN: Contraceptives—Other

**ETONOGESTREL** (*Implanon*) ▶L ♀X ▶+ $$$$$
WARNING - Increased risk of thromboembolism & stroke. Effectiveness may be reduced by hepatic enzyme-inducing drugs such as certain anticonvulsants, barbiturates, griseofulvin, rifampin. Additionally, products that contain St John's wort may decrease efficacy; an additional form of birth control may be advisable.
ADULT - Contraception: 1 subdermal implant every three yr.
PEDS - Not approved in children.
FORMS - Trade only: Single rod implant, 68 mg etonogestrel.
NOTES - Not studied in women >130% of ideal body weight; may be less effective if overweight.

**LEVONORGESTREL** (*Plan B*) ▶L ♀X ▶- $$
ADULT - Emergency contraception: 1 tab PO ASAP but within 72h of intercourse. 2nd tab 12h later.
PEDS - Not approved in children.
UNAPPROVED ADULT - 2 tabs (1.5 mg) PO ASAP but within 72h of intercourse (lesser efficacy at up to 120 h).
FORMS - OTC: Trade only: Kit contains 2 tabs 0.75 mg.
NOTES - OTC if ≥ 18 yo; Rx if younger. Nausea uncommon, however, if vomiting occurs within 1h, initial dose must be given again. Consider adding an antiemetic. Patients should be instructed to then contact their healthcare providers. Can be used at any time during the menstrual cycle.

*NUVARING* (ethinyl estradiol vaginal ring + etonogestrel) ▶L ♀X ▶- $$$
WARNING - Not recommended in women >35 yo who smoke. Increased risk of thromboembolism, stroke, MI, hepatic neoplasia & gallbladder disease. Vaginitis, headache, nausea & weight gain are common side effects. Effectiveness is reduced by hepatic enzyme-inducing drugs such as certain anticonvulsants and barbiturates, rifampin, rifabutin, griseofulvin & protease inhibitors. Additionally, products that contain St John's wort may decrease efficacy. An additional form of birth control may be advisable.
ADULT - Contraception: 1 ring intravaginally × 3 wk each mo.
PEDS - Not approved in children.
FORMS - Trade only: Flexible intravaginal ring, 15 mcg ethinyl estradiol/0.120 mg etonogestrel/d. 1 and 3 rings/box.
NOTES - Insert on d 5 of cycle or within 7 d of the last oral contraceptive pill. The ring must remain in place continuously for 3 wk, including during intercourse. Remove for 1 wk, then insert a new ring. May be used continuously for 4 wk & replaced immediately to skip a withdrawal wk. Store at room temperature. In case of accidental removal, reinsert ASAP after rinsing with cool to lukewarm water. If removal >3 h, use back up method until ring in place for ≥7 d. Rare reports of urinary bladder insertion; assess if persistent urinary symptoms & unable to locate the ring.

*ORTHO EVRA* (norelgestromin + ethinyl estradiol transdermal) (**Evra*) ▶L ♀X ▶- $$$
WARNING - Average estrogen concentration 60% higher than common oral contraceptives (ie, 35 mcg ethinyl estradiol), which may further increase the risk of thromboembolism. Not recommended in women >35 yo who smoke. Increased risk of thromboembolism, stroke, MI, hepatic neoplasia & gallbladder disease. Nausea, breast tenderness, & breakthrough bleeding are common transient side effects. Effectiveness is reduced
(cont. on p. 230)

| ORAL CONTRACEPTIVES* ▶L ♀X<br>*Monophasic* | Estrogen<br>(mcg) | Progestin<br>(mg) |
|---|---|---|
| Norinyl 1+50, Ortho-Novum 1/50, Necon 1/50 | 50 mestranol | 1 norethindrone |
| Ovcon-50 | | |
| Demulen 1/50, Zovia 1/50E | 50 ethinyl<br>estradiol | 1 ethynodiol |
| Ovral, Ogestrel | | 0.5 norgestrel |
| Norinyl 1+35, Ortho-Novum 1/35, Necon 1/35, Nortrel 1/35 | | 1 norethindrone |
| Brevicon, Modicon, Necon 0.5/35, Nortrel 0.5/35 | | 0.5 norethindrone |
| Ovcon-35, Femcon Fe, Balziva | 35 ethinyl<br>estradiol | 0.4 norethindrone |
| Previfem | | 0.18 norgestimate |
| Ortho-Cyclen, MonoNessa, Sprintec-28 | | 0.25 norgestimate |
| Demulen 1/35, Zovia 1/35E, Kelnor 1/35 | | 1 ethynodiol |
| Loestrin 21 1.5/30, Loestrin Fe 1.5/30, Junel 1.5/30, Junel 1.5/30 Fe, Microgestin Fe 1.5/30 | | 1.5 norethindrone |
| Cryselle, Lo/Ovral, Low-Ogestrel | 30 ethinyl<br>estradiol | 0.3 norgestrel |
| Apri, Desogen, Ortho-Cept, Reclipsen | | 0.15 desogestrel |
| Levlen, Levora, Nordette, Portia, Seasonale, Seasonique†, Quasense | | 0.15 levonorgestrel |
| Yasmin | | 3 drospirenone |
| Loestrin 21 1/20, Loestrin Fe 1/20,Loestin 24 Fe, Junel 1/20, Junel Fe 1/20, Microgestin Fe 1/20 | | 1 norethindrone |
| Alesse, Aviane, Lessina, Levlite, Lutera | 20 ethinyl<br>estradiol | 0.1 levonorgestrel |
| Lybrel | | 0.09 levonorgestrel |
| Yaz | | 3 drospirenone |
| Kariva, Mircette | 20/10 eth estrad | 0.15 desogestrel |
| **Progestin-only** | | |
| Micronor, Nor-Q.D., Camila, Errin, Jolivette, Nora-BE | none | 0.35 norethindrone |
| **Biphasic** *(estrogen & progestin contents vary)* | | |
| Ortho Novum 10/11, Necon 10/11 | 35 eth estradiol | 0.5/1 norethindrone |
| **Triphasic** *(estrogen & progestin contents vary)* | | |
| Cyclessa, Velivet | 25 ethinyl<br>estradiol | 0.100/0.125/0.150<br>desogestrel |
| Ortho-Novum 7/7/7, Necon 7/7/7, Nortrel 7/7/7 | 35 ethinyl<br>estradiol | 0.5/0.75/1<br>norethindr |
| Tri-Norinyl, Leena, Aranelle | | 0.5/1/0.5 norethindr |
| Enpresse, Tri-Levlen, Triphasil, Trivora-28 | 30/40/30 ethinyl<br>estradiol | 0.5/0.75/0.125<br>levonorgestrel |
| Ortho Tri-Cyclen, Trinessa, Tri-Sprintec, Tri-Previfem | 35 eth<br>estradiol | 0.18/0.215/0.25<br>norgestimate |
| Ortho Tri-Cyclen Lo | 25 eth estradiol | |
| Estrostep Fe, Tri-Legest, Tri-Legest Fe | 20/30/35 eth estr | 1 norethindrone |

*****All**: Not recommended in smokers. Increase risk of thromboembolism, stroke, MI, hepatic neoplasia & gallbladder disease. Nausea, breast tenderness, & breakthrough bleeding are common transient side effects. Effectiveness reduced by hepatic enzyme-inducing drugs such as certain anticonvulsants and barbiturates, rifampin, rifabutin, griseofulvin, & protease inhibitors. Coadministration with St John's wort may decrease efficacy. Vomiting or diarrhea may also increase the risk of contraceptive failure. Consider an additional form of birth control in above circumstances. See product insert for instructions on missing doses. Most available in 21 and 28 d packs. **Progestin only**: Must be taken at the same time every d. Because much of the literature regarding OC adverse effects pertains mainly to estrogen/progestin combinations, the extent to which progestin-only contraceptives cause these effects is unclear. No significant interaction has been found with broad-spectrum antibiotics. The effect of St John's wort is unclear. No placebo days, start new pack immediately after finishing current one. Available in 28 d packs. Readers may find the following website useful: www.managingcontraception.com. †84 light blue-green active pills followed by 7 yellow pills w/ 10 mcg ethinyl estradiol.

**ORTHO EVRA** (cont.)

by hepatic enzyme-inducing drugs such as certain anticonvulsants and barbiturates, rifampin, rifabutin, griseofulvin & protease inhibitors. Additionally, products that contain St John's wort may decrease efficacy. An additional form of birth control may be advisable.
ADULT - Contraception: 1 patch q wk × 3 wk, then 1 wk patch-free.
PEDS - Not approved in children.
FORMS - Trade only: Transdermal patch: 150 mcg norelgestromin + 20 mcg ethinyl estradiol/d. 1 and 3 patches/box.
NOTES - May be less effective in women ≥90 kg (198 lbs). Apply new patch on the same d each wk. Do not exceed 7 d between patches. Rotate application sites, avoid the waistline. Do not use earlier than 4 wk postpartum if not breastfeeding.

**BIEST** (estradiol + estriol) ▶L ♀X ▶- $$$
ADULT - Hormone therapy: Apply topically daily to bid as directed.
PEDS - Not approved in children.
FORMS - Must be compounded by a pharmacist. Gel, cream or troches: 20% estradiol/80% estriol.
NOTES - Although compounded bioidentical hormones have been advocated for hormone therapy, these plant-derived, non-FDA approved formulations lack sufficient evidence to support either effectiveness or safety. Further, in the absence of data otherwise, these products should be considered to have the same safety issues raised by the Women's Health Initiative as those associated with hormone therapy agents that are FDA approved.

---

**EMERGENCY CONTRACEPTION** within 72 h of unprotected sex: Take first dose ASAP, then identical dose 12 h later. *Plan B* kit contains 2 levonorgestrel 0.75 mg tabs. Each dose is 1 pill. The progestin-only method causes less nausea & may be more effective. Alternate regimens: Each dose is either 2 pills of *Ovral or Ogestrel*, 4 pills of *Cryselle, Levlen, Levora, Lo/Ovral, Nordette, Tri-Levlen\*, Triphasil\*, Trivora\*, or Low Ogestrel*, or 5 pills of *Alesse, Aviane, Lessina, or Levlite*. If vomiting occurs within 1 h of taking either dose of medication, consider whether or not to repeat that dose with an antiemetic 1h prior. More info at: www.not-2-late.com.

\*Use 0.125 mg levonorgestrel/30 mcg ethinyl estradiol tabs.

---

## OB/GYN: Estrogens

**NOTE:** See also Hormone Combinations. Unopposed estrogens increase the risk of endometrial cancer in postmenopausal women. Malignancy should be ruled out in cases of persistent or recurrent abnormal vaginal bleeding. In women with an intact uterus, a progestin should be administered daily throughout the mo or for the last 10–12 d of the mo. Do not use during pregnancy. May increase the risk of DVT/PE, gallbladder disease. Interactions with oral anticoagulants, certain anticonvulsants, rifampin, barbiturates, corticosteroids & St John's wort. Estrogens should not be used in the prevention of cardiovascular disease. In the Women's Health Initiative, the use of conjugated estrogens (Premarin) caused an increase in the risk of CVA & PE. Additionally, the combination with medroxyprogesterone increased the risk of breast cancer and MI. Women >65 yo with 4 yr of therapy had an increased risk of dementia. Estrogens should be prescribed at the lowest effective doses and for the shortest durations. Patients should be counseled regarding the risks/benefits of HRT.

**ESTERIFIED ESTROGENS** (*Menest*) ▶L ♀X ▶- $$
ADULT - Moderate to severe menopausal vasomotor symptoms: 1.25 mg PO daily. Atrophic vaginitis: 0.3–1.25 mg PO daily. Female hypogonadism: 2.5 - 7.5 mg PO daily in divided doses for 20 d followed by a 10-d rest period. Repeat until bleeding occurs. Bilateral oophorectomy & ovarian failure: 1.25 mg PO daily. Prevention of postmenopausal osteoporosis: 0.3 - 1.25 mg PO daily.
PEDS - Not approved in children.
FORMS - Trade only: Tabs 0.3, 0.625, 1.25, 2.5 mg.
NOTES - Typical hormone replacement regimen consists of a daily estrogen dose with a progestin added either daily or for the last 10–12 d of the cycle.

**ESTRADIOL** (*Estrace, Gynodiol*) ▶L ♀X ▶- $
ADULT - Moderate to severe menopausal vasomotor symptoms & atrophic vaginitis, female hypogonadism, bilateral oophorectomy & ovarian failure: 1–2 mg PO daily. Prevention of postmenopausal osteoporosis: 0.5 mg PO daily.
PEDS - Not approved in children.
FORMS - Generic/Trade: Tabs, micronized 0.5, 1, 2 mg, scored. Trade only: 1.5 mg (Gynodiol).

NOTES - Typical hormone replacement regimen consists of a daily estrogen dose with a progestin added either daily or for the last 10–12 d of the cycle.

**ESTRADIOL ACETATE** (*Femtrace*) ▶L ♀X ▶- $$
ADULT - Moderate to severe menopausal vasomotor symptoms: 0.45–1.8 mg PO daily.
PEDS - Not approved in children.
FORMS - Trade only: Tabs, 0.45, 0.9, 1.8 mg.
NOTES - Typical hormone replacement regimen consists of a daily estrogen dose with a progestin added either daily or for the last 10–12 d of the cycle.

**ESTRADIOL ACETATE VAGINAL RING** (*Femring*) ▶L ♀X ▶- $$
WARNING - A few cases of toxic shock syndrome have been reported.
ADULT - Menopausal atrophic vaginitis or vasomotor symptoms: insert ring into the vagina and replace after 90 d.
PEDS - Not approved in children.
FORMS - Trade only: 0.05 mg/d and 0.1 mg/d.
NOTES - Should the ring fall out or be removed during the 90 d period, rinse in lukewarm water and re-insert.

**ESTRADIOL CYPIONATE (*Depo-Estradiol*)** ▶L ♀X ▶- $
ADULT - Moderate to severe menopausal vasomotor symptoms: 1–5 mg IM q3–4 wk. Female hypogonadism: 1.5–2 mg IM q mo.
PEDS - Not approved in children.

**ESTRADIOL GEL (*Divigel, Estrogel, Elestrin*)** ▶L ♀X ▶- $$$
ADULT - Moderate to severe menopausal vasomotor symptoms & atrophic vaginitis: Thinly apply contents of one complete pump depression to one entire arm, from wrist to shoulder (Estrogel) or upper arm (Elestrin) or contents of one foil packet to left or right upper thigh on alternating d. Allow to dry completely before dressing. Wash both hands thoroughly after application.
PEDS - Not approved in children.
FORMS - Trade only: Gel 0.06% in non-aerosol, metered-dose pump with #64 or #32 - 1.25 g doses (Estrogel) & #100 - 0.87 g doses (Elestrin). Gel 0.1% in single dose foil packets of 0.25, 0.5 & 1.0 g, carton of 30.
NOTES - Depress the pump twice to prime. Concomitant sunscreen may increase absorption. Typical hormone replacement regimen consists of a daily estrogen dose with a progestin added either daily or for the last 10–12 d of the cycle.

**ESTRADIOL TOPICAL EMULSION (*Estrasorb*)** ▶L ♀X ▶- $$
ADULT - Moderate to severe menopausal vasomotor symptoms: Apply entire contents of one pouch each to left and right legs (spread over thighs & calves) qam. Rub for 3 min until entirely absorbed. Allow to dry completely before dressing. Wash both hands thoroughly after application. Daily dose = two 1.74 g pouches.
PEDS - Not approved in children.
FORMS - Trade only: Topical emulsion, 56 pouches/carton.
NOTES - Typical hormone replacement regimen consists of a daily estrogen dose with a progestin added either daily or for the last 10–12 d of the cycle. Concomitant sunscreen may increase absorption.

**ESTRADIOL TRANSDERMAL PATCH (*Alora, Climara, Esclim, Estraderm, FemPatch, Menostar, Vivelle, Vivelle Dot, ✦Estradot, Oesclim*)** ▶L ♀X ▶- $$
ADULT - Moderate to severe menopausal vasomotor symptoms & atrophic vaginitis, female hypogonadism, bilateral oophorectomy & ovarian failure: initiate with 0.025 - 0.05 mg/d patch once or twice weekly, depending on the product (see FORMS). Prevention of postmenopausal osteoporosis: 0.025–0.1 mg/d patch.
PEDS - Not approved in children.
FORMS - Generic/Trade: Transdermal patches doses in mg/d: Climara (q wk) 0.025, 0.0375, 0.05, 0.06, 0.075, 0.1. Trade only: FemPatch (q wk) 0.025. Esclim (twice/wk) 0.025, 0.0375, 0.05, 0.075, 0.1. Vivelle, Vivelle Dot (twice/wk) 0.025, 0.0375, 0.05, 0.075, 0.1. Estraderm (twice/wk) 0.05, & 0.1. Alora (twice/wk) 0.025, 0.05, 0.075, 0.1.

NOTES - Rotate application sites, avoid the waistline. Transdermal may be preferable for women with high triglycerides & chronic liver disease.

**ESTRADIOL TRANSDERMAL SPRAY (*Evamist*)** ▶L ♀X ▶- $$$
ADULT - Moderate to severe menopausal vasomotor symptoms: Initial: 1 spray daily to adjacent non-overlapping inner surface of the forearm. Allow to dry for 2 min and do not wash for 30 min. Adjust up to 3 sprays daily based on clinical response.
PEDS - Not approved in children.
FORMS - Trade only: Spray: 1.53 mg estradiol per 90 mcL spray, 56 sprays per metered-dose pump.
NOTES - Depress the pump three times with the cover on to prime each new applicator. Hold upright and vertical for spraying; rest the plastic cone against the skin. Typical hormone replacement regimen consists of a daily estrogen dose with a progestin added either daily or for the last 10–12 d of the cycle.

**ESTRADIOL VAGINAL RING (*Estring*)** ▶L ♀X ▶- $$
WARNING - Do not use during pregnancy.
ADULT - Menopausal atrophic vaginitis: insert ring into upper 1/3 of the vaginal vault and replace after 90 d.
PEDS - Not approved in children.
FORMS - Trade only: 2 mg ring single pack.
NOTES - Should the ring fall out or be removed during the 90 d period, rinse in lukewarm water and re-insert. Minimal systemic absorption, probable lower risk of adverse effects than systemic estrogens.

**ESTRADIOL VAGINAL TAB (*Vagifem*)** ▶L ♀X ▶- $-$$
WARNING - Do not use during pregnancy.
ADULT - Menopausal atrophic vaginitis: Begin with 1 tab vaginally daily × 2 wk, maintenance 1 tab vaginally 2x/wk.
PEDS - Not approved in children.
FORMS - Trade only: Vaginal tab: 25 mcg in disposable single-use applicators, 8 & 18/pack.

**ESTRADIOL VALERATE (*Delestrogen*)** ▶L ♀X ▶- $
ADULT - Moderate to severe menopausal vasomotor symptoms & atrophic vaginitis: 10–20 mg IM q4 wk. Female hypogonadism, bilateral oophorectomy & ovarian failure: 10–20 mg IM q4 wk.
PEDS - Not approved in children.

**ESTROGEN VAGINAL CREAM (*Premarin, Estrace*)** ▶L ♀X ▶? $$$$
ADULT - Menopausal atrophic vaginitis: Premarin: 0.5–2 g intravaginally daily. Estrace: 2–4 g intravaginally daily for 1–2 wk. Gradually reduce to a maintenance dose of 1 g 1–3 x/wk.
PEDS - Not approved in children.
FORMS - Trade only: Vaginal cream. Premarin: 0.625 mg conjugated estrogens/g in 42.5 g with or w/o calibrated applicator. Estrace: 0.1 mg estradiol/g in 42.5 g w/calibrated applicator.
NOTES - Possibility of absorption through the vaginal mucosa. Uterine bleeding might be provoked by excessive use in menopausal women. Breast tenderness & vaginal discharge due to mucus

**(cont.)**

**ESTROGEN VAGINAL CREAM** (*cont.*)

hypersecretion may result from excessive estrogenic stimulation. Endometrial withdrawal bleeding may occur if use is discontinued.

**ESTROGENS CONJUGATED** (*Premarin, C.E.S., Congest*) ►L ♀X ►- $$

ADULT - Moderate to severe menopausal vasomotor symptoms, atrophic vaginitis, & urethritis: 0.3–1.25 mg PO daily. Female hypogonadism: 0.3–0.625 mg PO daily for 3 wk with 1 wk off every mo. Bilateral oophorectomy & ovarian failure: 1.25 mg PO daily for 3 wk with 1 wk off every mo. Prevention of postmenopausal osteoporosis: 0.625 mg PO daily. Abnormal uterine bleeding: 25 mg IV/IM. Repeat in 6–12 h if needed.

PEDS - Not approved in children.

UNAPPROVED ADULT - Prevention of postmenopausal osteoporosis: 0.3 mg PO daily. Normalizing bleeding time in patients with AV malformations or underlying renal impairment: 30–70 mg IV/PO daily until bleeding time normalized.

FORMS - Trade only: Tabs 0.3, 0.45, 0.625, 0.9, 1.25 mg.

**ESTROGENS SYNTHETIC CONJUGATED A** (*Cenestin*) ►L ♀X ►- $$$

ADULT - Moderate to severe menopausal vasomotor symptoms: 0.3–1.25 mg PO daily.

PEDS - Not approved in children.

FORMS - Trade only: Tabs 0.3, 0.45, 0.625, 0.9, 1.25 mg.

NOTES - The difference between synthetic conjugated estrogens A and B is the additional component of delta- 8,9-dehydroestrone sulfate in the B preparation. The clinical significance of this is unknown.

**ESTROGENS SYNTHETIC CONJUGATED B** (*Enjuvia*) ►L ♀X ►- $$

ADULT - Moderate to severe menopausal vasomotor symptoms: 0.3–1.25 mg PO daily.

PEDS - Not approved in children.

FORMS - Trade only: Tabs 0.3, 0.45, 0.625, 0.9, 1.25 mg.

NOTES - Typical hormone replacement regimen consists of a daily estrogen dose with a progestin either daily or for the last 10–12 d of the cycle. The difference between synthetic conjugated estrogens A and B is the additional component of delta- 8,9-dehydroestrone sulfate in the B preparation. The clinical significance of this is unknown.

**ESTROPIPATE** (*Ogen, Ortho-Est*) ►L ♀X ►- $

ADULT - Moderate to severe menopausal vasomotor symptoms, vulvar & vaginal atrophy: 0.75 to 6 mg PO daily. Female hypogonadism, bilateral oophorectomy, or ovarian failure: 1.5–9 mg PO daily. Prevention of osteoporosis: 0.75 mg PO daily.

PEDS - Not approved in children.

FORMS - Generic/Trade: Tabs 0.75, 1.5, 3, 6 mg of estropipate.

NOTES - 6 mg estropipate = 5 mg sodium estrone sulfate.

**TRIEST** (estradiol + estriol + estrone) ►L ♀X ►- $$$

ADULT - Hormone therapy: Apply topically daily to bid as directed.

PEDS - Not approved in children.

FORMS - Must be compounded by a pharmacist. Gel, cream or troches: 10% estradiol/10% estrone/80% estriol.

NOTES - Although compounded bioidentical hormones have been advocated for hormone therapy, these plant-derived, non-FDA approved formulations lack sufficient evidence to support either effectiveness or safety. Further, in the absence of data otherwise, these products should be considered to have the same safety issues raised by the Women's Health Initiative as those associated with hormone therapy agents that are FDA approved.

---

## OB/GYN: GnRH Agents

**NOTE:** Anaphylaxis has occurred with synthetic GnRH agents.

**CETRORELIX ACETATE** (*Cetrotide*) ►Plasma ♀X ►- $$$$$

ADULT - Infertility: Multiple dose regimen: 0.25 mg SC daily during the early to mid follicular phase. Continue treatment daily until the d of hCG administration. Single dose regimen: 3 mg SC × 1 usually on stimulation d 7.

PEDS - Not approved in children.

FORMS - Trade only: Injection 0.25 mg in 1 & 7-dose kits. 3 mg in 1 dose kit.

NOTES - Best sites for SC self-injection are on the abdomen around the navel. Storage in original carton: 0.25 mg refrigerated (36–46F); 3 mg room temperature (77F). Contraindicated with severe renal impairment.

**GANIRELIX** (*Follistim-Antagon Kit, ✦Orgalutran*) ►Plasma ♀X ►? $$$$$

ADULT - Infertility: 250 mcg SC daily during the early to mid follicular phase. Continue treatment daily until the d of hCG administration.

PEDS - Not approved in children.

FORMS - Trade only: Injection 250 mcg/0.5 mL in pre-filled, disposable syringes with 3 vials follitropin beta.

NOTES - Best sites for SC self-injection are on the abdomen around the navel or on the upper thigh. Store at room temperature (77F) for up to 3 mo. Protect from light. Packaging contains natural rubber latex which may cause allergic reactions.

**NAFARELIN** (*Synarel*) ►L ♀X ►- $$$$$

ADULT - Endometriosis: 200 mcg spray into one nostril q am & the other nostril q pm. May be increased to one 200 mcg spray into each nostril bid. Duration of treatment: 6 mo.

**NAFARELIN** (cont.)
PEDS - Central precocious puberty: 2 sprays into each nostril bid for a total of 1600 mcg/d. May be increased to 1800 mcg/d. Allow 30 sec to elapse between sprays.
FORMS - Trade only: Nasal soln 2 mg/mL in 8 mL bottle (200 mcg per spray) about 80 sprays/bottle.

NOTES - Ovarian cysts have occurred in the first 2 mo of therapy. Symptoms of hypoestrogenism may occur. Elevations of phosphorus & eosinophil counts, and decreases in serum calcium & WBC counts have been documented. Consider norethindrone as "addback" therapy to decrease bone loss (see norethindrone).

## OB/GYN: Hormone Combinations

**NOTE:** See also estrogens. Unopposed estrogens increase the risk of endometrial cancer in postmenopausal women. Malignancy should be ruled out in cases of persistent or recurrent abnormal vaginal bleeding. Do not use during pregnancy. May increase the risk of DVT/PE, gallbladder disease. Interactions with oral anticoagulants, phenytoin, rifampin, barbiturates, corticosteroids and St. John's wort. For preparations containing testosterone derivatives, observe women for signs of virilization and lipid abnormalities. In the Women's Health Initiative, the combination of conjugated estrogens and medroxyprogesterone (PremPro) caused an increase in the risk of breast cancer, MI, CVA, & DVT/PE and did not improve overall quality of life. Women >65 yo with 4 yr of therapy had an increased risk of dementia. Estrogen/progestin combinations should be prescribed at the lowest effective doses and for the shortest durations. Patients should be counseled regarding the risks/benefits of hormone replacement.

**ACTIVELLA** (estradiol + norethindrone) ▶L ♀X ▶- $$
ADULT - Moderate to severe menopausal vasomotor symptoms, vulvar & vaginal atrophy, prevention of postmenopausal osteoporosis: 1 tab PO daily.
PEDS - Not approved in children.
FORMS - Trade only: Tab 1/0.5 mg and 0.5/0.1 mg estradiol/norethindrone acetate in calendar dial pack dispenser.

**ANGELIQ** (estradiol + drospirenone) ▶L ♀X ▶- $$$
ADULT - Moderate to severe menopausal vasomotor symptoms, vulvar & vaginal atrophy: 1 tab PO daily.
PEDS - Not approved in children.
FORMS - Trade only: Tabs 1 mg estradiol/0.5 mg drospirenone.
NOTES - May cause hyperkalemia in high-risk patients due to antimineralocorticoid activity of drospirenone. Monitor potassium in patients on ACEIs, ARBs, potassium-sparing diuretics, heparin, aldosterone antagonists, & NSAIDs. Should not be used if renal insufficiency, hepatic dysfunction or adrenal insufficiency.

**CLIMARA PRO** (estradiol + levonorgestrel) ▶L ♀X ▶- $$
ADULT - Moderate to severe menopausal vasomotor symptoms, prevention of postmenopausal osteoporosis: 1 patch weekly.
PEDS - Not approved in children.
FORMS - Trade only: Transdermal 0.045/0.015 estradiol/levonorgestrel in mg/d, 4 patches/box.
NOTES - Rotate application sites; avoid the waistline.

**COMBIPATCH** (estradiol + norethindrone) (✦ Estalis) ▶L ♀X ▶- $$$
ADULT - Moderate to severe menopausal vasomotor symptoms, vulvar & vaginal atrophy, female hypogonadism, bilateral oophorectomy, & ovarian failure, prevention of postmenopausal osteoporosis: 1 patch twice weekly.
PEDS - Not approved in children.

FORMS - Trade only: Transdermal patch 0.05 estradiol/0.14 norethindrone & 0.05 estradiol/0.25 norethindrone in mg/d, 8 patches/box.
NOTES - Rotate application sites, avoid the waistline.

**ESTRATEST** (esterified estrogens + methyltestosterone) ▶L ♀X ▶- $$$$
ADULT - Moderate to severe menopausal vasomotor symptoms: 1 tab PO daily.
PEDS - Not approved in children.
UNAPPROVED ADULT - Menopause-associated decrease in libido: 1 tab PO daily.
FORMS - Trade only: Tabs 1.25 mg esterified estrogens/2.5 mg methyltestosterone.
NOTES - Monitor LFTs and lipids.

**ESTRATEST H.S.** (esterified estrogens + methyltestosterone) ▶L ♀X ▶- $$$
ADULT - Moderate to severe menopausal vasomotor symptoms: 1 tab PO daily.
PEDS - Not approved in children.
UNAPPROVED ADULT - Menopause-associated decrease in libido: 1 tab PO daily.
FORMS - Trade only: Tabs 0.625 mg esterified estrogens/1.25 mg methyltestosterone.
NOTES - HS = half-strength. Monitor LFTs and lipids.

**FEMHRT** (ethinyl estradiol + norethindrone) ▶L ♀X ▶- $$
WARNING - Multiple strengths; see FORMS & write specific product on Rx.
ADULT - Moderate to severe menopausal vasomotor symptoms, prevention of postmenopausal osteoporosis: 1 tab PO daily.
PEDS - Not approved in children.
FORMS - Trade only: Tabs 5/1 and 2.5/0.5 mcg ethinyl estradiol/mg norethindrone, 28/blister card.

**PREFEST** (estradiol + norgestimate) ▶L ♀X ▶- $$$
ADULT - Moderate to severe menopausal vasomotor symptoms, vulvar atrophy, atrophic vaginitis, prevention of postmenopausal osteoporosis:

(cont.)

**PREFEST** (cont.)

1 pink tab PO daily × 3 d followed by 1 white tab PO daily × 3 d, sequentially throughout the mo.
PEDS - Not approved in children.
FORMS - Trade only: Tabs in 30-d blister packs 1 mg estradiol (15 pink) & 1 mg estradiol/0.09 mg norgestimate (15 white).

**PREMPHASE (estrogens conjugated + medroxyprogesterone)** ▶L ♀X ▶- $$$
ADULT - Moderate to severe menopausal vasomotor symptoms, vulvar/vaginal atrophy, & prevention of postmenopausal osteoporosis: 0.625 mg conjugated estrogens PO daily d 1–14 & 0.625 mg conjugated estrogens/5 mg medroxyprogesterone PO daily d 15–28.
PEDS - Not approved in children.
FORMS - Trade only: Tabs in 28-d EZ-Dial dispensers: 0.625 mg conjugated estrogens (14) & 0.625 mg/5 mg conjugated estrogens/medroxyprogesterone (14).

**PREMPRO (estrogens conjugated + medroxyprogesterone) (✦Premplus)** ▶L ♀X ▶- $$$
WARNING - Multiple strengths; see FORMS & write specific product on Rx.
ADULT - Moderate to severe menopausal vasomotor symptoms, vulvar/vaginal atrophy, & prevention of postmenopausal osteoporosis: 1 PO daily.

PEDS - Not approved in children.
FORMS - Trade only: Tabs in 28-d EZ-Dial dispensers: 0.625 mg/5 mg, 0.625 mg/2.5 mg, 0.45 mg/1.5 mg (Prempro low dose), or 0.3 mg/1.5 mg conjugated estrogens/medroxyprogesterone.

**SYNTEST D.S. (esterified estrogens + methyltestosterone)** ▶L ♀X ▶- $$
ADULT - Moderate to severe menopausal vasomotor symptoms: 1 tab PO daily.
PEDS - Not approved in children.
UNAPPROVED ADULT - Menopause-associated decrease in libido: 1 tab PO daily.
FORMS - Trade only: Tabs 1.25 mg esterified estrogens/2.5 mg methyltestosterone.
NOTES - Monitor LFTs and lipids. Same as Estratest.

**SYNTEST H.S. (esterified estrogens + methyltestosterone)** ▶L ♀X ▶- $$
ADULT - Moderate to severe menopausal vasomotor symptoms: 1 tab PO daily.
PEDS - Not approved in children.
UNAPPROVED ADULT - Menopause-associated decrease in libido: 1 tab PO daily.
FORMS - Trade only: Tabs 0.625 mg esterified estrogens/1.25 mg methyltestosterone.
NOTES - H = half-strength. Monitor LFTs and lipids. Same as Estratest HS.

---

**DRUGS GENERALLY ACCEPTED AS SAFE IN PREGNANCY    (selected)**

Analgesics: acetaminophen, codeine*, meperidine*, methadone*. Antimicrobials: penicillins, cephalosporins, erythromycins (not estolate), azithromycin, nystatin, clotrimazole, metronidazole, nitrofurantoin***, Nix. Antivirals: acyclovir, valacyclovir, famciclovir. CV: labetalol, methyldopa, hydralazine, nifedipine. Derm: erythromycin, clindamycin, benzoyl peroxide. Endo: insulin, liothyronine, levothyroxine. ENT: chlorpheniramine, diphenhydramine, dimenhydrinate, dextromethorphan, guaifenesin, nasal steroids, nasal cromolyn. GI: trimethobenzamide, antacids*, simethicone, cimetidine, famotidine, ranitidine, nizatidine, psyllium, metoclopramide, bisacodyl, docusate, doxylamine, meclizine. Heme: Heparin, low molecular weight heparins. Psych: desipramine, doxepin. Pulmonary: short-acting inhaled beta-2 agonists, cromolyn, nedocromil, beclomethasone, budesonide, theophylline, prednisone**.    *Except if used long-term or in high dose at term.    **Except 1st trimester.    ***Contraindicated at term and during labor and delivery.

---

| APGAR SCORE | | | | |
|---|---|---|---|---|
| | Heart rate | 0. Absent | 1. <100 | 2. >100 |
| | Respirations | 0. Absent | 1. Slow/irreg | 2. Good/crying |
| | Muscle tone | 0. Limp | 1. Some flexion | 2. Active motion |
| | Reflex irritability | 0. No response | 1. Grimace | 2. Cough/sneeze |
| | Color | 0. Blue | 1. Blue extremities | 2. Pink |

---

## OB/GYN: Labor Induction/Cervical Ripening

**NOTE:** Fetal well-being should be documented prior to use.

**DINOPROSTONE (PGE2, Prepidil, Cervidil, Prostin E2)** ▶Lung ♀C ▶? $$$$$
ADULT - Cervical ripening: Gel - one syringe via catheter placed into cervical canal below the internal os. May be repeated q6h to a max of 3 doses. Vaginal insert: place in posterior fornix. Evacuation of uterine contents after fetal death up to 28 wk or termination of pregnancy 12–20th gestational wk: 20 mg intravaginal susp; repeat at 3–5 h intervals until abortion occurs. Do not use for >2 d.

PEDS - Not approved in children.
FORMS - Trade only: Gel (Prepidil) 0.5 mg/3 g syringe. Vaginal insert (Cervidil) 10 mg. Vaginal susp (Prostin E2) 20 mg.
NOTES - Patient should remain supine for 15 - 30 min after gel and 2 h after vaginal insert. For hospital use only. Monitor for uterine hyperstimulation & abnormal fetal heart rate. Caution with asthma or glaucoma. Contraindicated in prior C-section or major uterine surgery due to potential for uterine rupture.

**OXYTOCIN (*Pitocin*)** ▶LK ♀? ▶- $
WARNING - Not approved for elective labor induction, although widely used.
ADULT - Induction/stimulation of labor: 10 units in 1000 mL NS, 1–2 milliunits/min IV as a continuous infusion (6–12 mL/h). Increase in increments of 1–2 milliunits/min q30 min until a contraction pattern is established, up to a max of 20 milliunits/min. Postpartum bleeding: 10 units IM after delivery of the placenta. 10–40 units in 1000 mL NS IV infusion, infuse 20–40 milliunits/min.
PEDS - Not approved in children.

UNAPPROVED ADULT - Augmentation of labor: 0.5–2 milliunits/min IV as a continuous infusion, increase by 1–2 milliunits/min q30 min until adequate pattern of labor to a max of 40 milliunits/min.
NOTES - Use a pump to accurately control the infusion while patient is under continuous observation. Continuous fetal monitoring is required. Concurrent sympathomimetics may result in postpartum hypertension. Anaphylaxis and severe water intoxication have occurred. Caution in patients undergoing a trial of labor after c-section.

## OB/GYN: Ovulation Stimulants

**NOTE:** Potentially serious adverse effects include DVT/PE, ovarian hyperstimulation syndrome, adnexal torsion, ovarian enlargement & cysts, & febrile reactions.

**CHORIOGONADOTROPIN ALFA (*hCG, Ovidrel*)** ▶L ♀X ▶? $$$
ADULT - Specialized dosing for ovulation induction.
PEDS - Not approved in children.
FORMS - Trade only: Powder for injection or, pre-filled syringe 250 mcg.
NOTES - Best site for SC self-injection is on the abdomen below the navel. Beware of multiple pregnancy & multiple adverse effects. Store in original package & protect from light. Use immediately after reconstitution.

**CHORIONIC GONADOTROPIN (*hCG, Pregnyl, Profasi*)** ▶L ♀X ▶? $$
ADULT - Specialized dosing for ovulation induction.
PEDS - Not approved in children.
NOTES - Beware of multiple pregnancy & multiple adverse effects. For IM use only.

**CLOMIPHENE (*Clomid, Serophene*)** ▶L ♀D ▶? $$
ADULT - Specialized dosing for infertility.
PEDS - Not approved in children.
FORMS - Generic/Trade: Tabs 50 mg, scored.
NOTES - Beware of multiple pregnancy & multiple adverse effects.

**FOLLITROPIN ALFA (*FSH, Gonal-F, Gonal-F RFF Pen*)** ▶L ♀X ▶? $$$$$
ADULT - Specialized dosing for infertility.
PEDS - Not approved in children.
FORMS - Trade only: Powder for injection, 37.5 IU, 75 IU, & 150 IU FSH activity. 450 & 1200 IU multidose vial. Pre-filled, multiple-dose pen, 300 IU, 450 IU, & 900 IU FSH activity with single-use disposable needles.
NOTES - Best site for SC self-injection is on the abdomen below the navel. Beware of multiple gestation pregnancy & multiple adverse effects. Store in original package & protect from light. Use immediately after reconstitution. Pen may be stored at room temperature for up to 1 mo or expiration, whichever is first.

**FOLLITROPIN BETA (*FSH, Follistim, Follistim AQ*) (✦*Puregon*)** ▶L ♀X ▶? $$$$$
ADULT - Specialized dosing for infertility.
PEDS - Not approved in children.

FORMS - Trade only: Powder for injection, 75 IU FSH activity. Cartridge, for use with the Follistim Pen, 150, 300, 600, 900 IU. Aqueous soln 75 & 150 IU FSH activity.
NOTES - Best site for SC self-injection is on the abdomen below the navel. Beware of multiple pregnancy & multiple adverse effects. Store in original package & protect from light. Use powder for injection immediately after reconstitution. Cartridge may be stored for up to 28 d. Store aqueous soln in refrigerator.

**GONADOTROPINS (*menotropins, FSH and LH, Menopur, Pergonal, Repronex, ✦Propasi HP*)** ▶L ♀X ▶? $$$$$
ADULT - Specialized dosing for infertility.
PEDS - Not approved in children.
FORMS - Trade only: Powder or pellet for injection, 75 IU & 150 IU FSH/LH activity.
NOTES - Best site for SC self-injection is on the abdomen below the navel. Beware of multiple pregnancy & numerous adverse effects. Use immediately after reconstitution.

**LUTROPIN ALFA (*Luveris*)** ▶L ♀X ▶- $$$$$
ADULT - Specialized dosing for infertility.
PEDS - Not approved in children.
FORMS - Trade only: Powder for injection, 75 IU LH activity.
NOTES - For use with follitropin alfa. Best site for SC self-injection is on the abdomen below the navel. Protect from light. Use immediately after reconstitution.

**UROFOLLITROPIN (*Bravelle, FSH, Fertinex*)** ▶L ♀X ▶? $$$$$
ADULT - Specialized dosing for infertility & polycystic ovary syndrome.
PEDS - Not approved in children.
FORMS - Trade only: Powder or pellet for injection, 75 IU & 150 IU (FSH, Fertinex only) FSH activity.
NOTES - Best site for SC self-injection is on the abdomen below the navel. Beware of multiple pregnancy & numerous adverse effects. Use immediately after reconstitution.

## OB/GYN: Progestins

**NOTE:** Do not use in pregnancy. DVT, PE, cerebrovascular disorders, & retinal thrombosis may occur. Effectiveness may be reduced by hepatic enzyme-inducing drugs such as certain anticonvulsants and barbiturates, rifampin, rifabutin, griseofulvin & protease inhibitors. The effects of St John's wort-containing products on progestin only pills is currently unknown. In the Women's Health Initiative, the combination of conjugated estrogens and medroxyprogesterone (PremPro) caused a statistically significant increase in the risk of breast cancer, MI, CVA, & DVT/PE. Additionally, women >65 yo with 4 yr of therapy had an increased risk of dementia. Estrogen/progestin combinations should be prescribed at the lowest effective doses and for the shortest durations. Patients should be counseled regarding the risks/benefits of hormone replacement.

**HYDROXYPROGESTERONE CAPROATE** ▶L ♀X ▶? $

ADULT - Amenorrhea, dysfunctional uterine bleeding, metrorrhagia: 375 mg IM. Production of secretory endometrium and desquamation: 125–250 mg IM on 10th d of the cycle, repeat q7days until suppression no longer desired.

PEDS - Not approved in children.

UNAPPROVED ADULT - Endometrial hyperplasia: 500 mg IM weekly. Prevention of preterm delivery in patients with a history of preterm birth: 250 mg IM weekly starting at 16–20 wk gestation until 36 wk or delivery.

**MEDROXYPROGESTERONE (Provera, Amen)** ▶L ♀X ▶+ $

ADULT - Secondary amenorrhea: 5–10 mg PO daily × 5–10 d. Abnormal uterine bleeding: 5–10 mg PO daily × 5–10 d beginning on the 16th or 21st d of the cycle (after estrogen priming). Withdrawal bleeding usually occurs 3–7 d after therapy ends.

PEDS - Not approved in children.

UNAPPROVED ADULT - Add to estrogen replacement therapy to prevent endometrial hyperplasia: 10 mg PO daily for 10–12 d of mo, or 2.5–5 mg PO daily. Endometrial hyperplasia: 10–30 mg PO daily (long-term); 40–100 mg PO daily (short-term) or 500 mg IM twice/d wk.

FORMS - Generic/Trade: Tabs 2.5, 5, & 10 mg, scored.

NOTES - Breakthrough bleeding/spotting may occur. Amenorrhea usually after 6 mo of continuous dosing.

**MEDROXYPROGESTERONE - INJECTABLE (Depo-Provera, depo-subQ provera 104)** ▶L ♀X ▶+ $

WARNING - Risk of significant bone loss, possibly irreversible, increases with duration of use. Long-term use (>2 yr) only recommended if other methods of birth control are inadequate or symptoms of endometriosis return after discontinuation.

ADULT - Contraception/Endometriosis: 150 mg IM in deltoid or gluteus maximus or 104 mg SC in anterior thigh or abdomen q13 wk. Also used for adjunctive therapy in endometrial & renal carcinoma.

PEDS - Not approved in children.

UNAPPROVED ADULT - Dysfunctional uterine bleeding: 150 mg IM in deltoid or gluteus maximus q13 wk.

NOTES - Breakthrough bleeding/spotting may occur. Amenorrhea usually after 6 mo. Weight gain is common. To be sure that the patient is not pregnant give this injection only during the first 5 d after the onset of a normal menstrual period or after a negative pregnancy test. May be given immediately post-pregnancy termination as well as postpartum, including breastfeeding women. May be given as often as 11 wk apart. If the time between injections is >14 wk, exclude pregnancy before administering. Return to fertility can be variably delayed after last injection, with the median time to pregnancy being 10 mo. Bone loss may occur with prolonged administration. Evaluate bone mineral density if considering retreatment for endometriosis.

**MEGESTROL (Megace, Megace ES)** ▶L ♀D ▶? $$$$$

ADULT - AIDS anorexia: 800 mg (20 mL) susp PO daily or 625 mg (5 mL) ES daily. Palliative treatment for advanced breast carcinoma: 40 mg (tabs) PO qid. Endometrial carcinoma: 40–320 mg/d (tabs) in divided doses.

PEDS - Not approved in children.

UNAPPROVED ADULT - Endometrial hyperplasia: 40–160 mg PO daily × 3–4 mo. Cancer-associated anorexia/cachexia: 80–160 mg PO daily.

FORMS - Generic/Trade: Tabs 20 & 40 mg. Suspension 40 mg/mL in 240 mL. Trade only: Megace ES susp 125 mg/mL (150 mL).

NOTES - In HIV-infected women, breakthrough bleeding/spotting may occur.

**NORETHINDRONE (Aygestin, Micronor, Nor-Q.D., Camila, Errin, Jolivette, Nora-BE)** ▶L ♀D/X ▶See notes $

ADULT - Contraception: 0.35 mg PO daily. Amenorrhea, abnormal uterine bleeding: 2.5–10 mg PO daily × 5–10 d during the 2nd half of the menstrual cycle. Endometriosis: 5 mg PO daily × 2 wk. Increase by 2.5 mg q 2 wk to 15 mg/d.

PEDS - Not approved in children.

UNAPPROVED ADULT - "Addback" therapy with GnRH agonists (eg, leuprolide) to decrease bone loss: 5 mg PO daily.

FORMS - Generic/Trade: Tabs 5 mg, scored. Trade only: 0.35 mg tabs.

NOTES - Contraceptive doses felt compatible with breast feeding, but not higher doses.

**PROGESTERONE GEL (Crinone, Prochieve)** ▶Plasma ♀- ▶? $$$

ADULT - Secondary amenorrhea: 45 mg (4%) intravaginally every other d up to 6 doses. If no response, use 90 mg (8%) intravaginally every other d up to 6 doses. Specialized dosing for infertility.

PEDS - Not approved in children.

FORMS - Trade only: 4%, 8% single-use, prefilled applicators.

NOTES - An increase in dose from the 4% gel can only be accomplished using the 8% gel; doubling the volume of 4% does not increase absorption.

**PROGESTERONE IN OIL** ▶L ♀X ▶? $
WARNING - Contraindicated in peanut allergy since some products contain peanut oil.
ADULT - Amenorrhea, uterine bleeding: 5–10 mg IM daily for 6–8 d.
PEDS - Not approved in children.
NOTES - Discontinue with thrombotic disorders, sudden or partial loss of vision, proptosis, diplopia or migraine.

**PROGESTERONE MICRONIZED** (*Prometrium*) ▶L ♀B ▶+ $$
WARNING - Contraindicated in patients allergic to peanuts since caps contain peanut oil.
ADULT - Hormone therapy to prevent endometrial hyperplasia: 200 mg PO qhs 10–12 d per mo. Secondary amenorrhea: 400 mg PO qhs × 10 d.
PEDS - Not approved in children.
UNAPPROVED ADULT - Hormone therapy to prevent endometrial hyperplasia: 100 mg qhs daily.
FORMS - Trade only: Caps 100 & 200 mg.
NOTES - Breast tenderness, dizziness, headache & abdominal cramping may occur.

**PROGESTERONE MICRONIZED GEL** (*Progest*) ▶L ♀B? ▶? $
ADULT - Hormone therapy: Apply topically daily to bid as directed.
PEDS - Not approved in children.
FORMS - Must be compounded by a pharmacist. Gel - micronized progesterone from wild yams or soybeans 25mg/g, 50mg/g & 100mg/g.
NOTES - Although compounded bioidentical hormones have been advocated for hormone therapy, these plant-derived, non-FDA approved formulations lack sufficient evidence to support effectiveness or safety. Further, absence of data otherwise, these products should be considered to have the same safety issues raised by the Women's Health Initiative as those associated with hormone therapy agents that are FDA approved.

**PROGESTERONE VAGINAL INSERT** (*Endometrin*) ▶Plasma ♀- ▶? $$$$
ADULT - Specialized dosing for infertility.
PEDS - Not approved in children.
FORMS - Trade only: 100 mg vaginal insert.
NOTES - Do not use concomitantly with other vaginal products, such as antifungals, as this may alter absorption.

## OB/GYN: Selective Estrogen Receptor Modulators

**RALOXIFENE** (*Evista*) ▶L ♀X ▶- $$$$
WARNING - Increases the risk of venous thromboembolism & stroke. Do not use during pregnancy.
ADULT - Postmenopausal osteoporosis prevention/treatment, breast cancer prevention: 60 mg PO/d.
PEDS - Not approved in children.
FORMS - Trade only: Tabs 60 mg.
NOTES - Contraindicated with history of venous thromboembolism. Interactions with oral anticoagulants & cholestyramine. May increase risk of DVT/PE. Discontinue use 72 h prior to and during prolonged immobilization because of DVT risk. Does not decrease (and may increase) hot flashes. Leg cramps. Triglyceride levels may increase in women with prior estrogen-associated hypertriglyceridemia (>500 mg/dL).

**TAMOXIFEN** (*Nolvadex, Soltamox, Tamone, ✦Tamofen*) ▶L ♀D ▶- $$$$
WARNING - Uterine malignancies, stroke & pulmonary embolism, sometimes fatal. Visual disturbances, cataracts, hypercalcemia, increased LFTs, bone pain, fertility impairment, hot flashes, menstrual irregularities, endometrial hyperplasia & cancer, alopecia. Do not use during pregnancy.
ADULT - Breast cancer prevention in high-risk women: 20 mg PO daily × 5 yr. Breast cancer: 10–20 mg PO bid × 5 yr.
PEDS - Not approved in children.
UNAPPROVED ADULT - Mastalgia: 10 mg PO daily × 4 mo. Anovulation: 5–40 mg PO bid × 4 d.
FORMS - Generic/Trade: Tabs 10 & 20 mg, Trade only (Soltamox): sugar-free soln 10mg/5mL (150 mL).
NOTES - Reliable contraception is recommended. Monitor CBCs, LFTs. Regular gynecologic & ophthalmologic examinations. Interacts with oral anticoagulants. Does not decrease hot flashes.

## OB/GYN: Uterotonics

**CARBOPROST** (*Hemabate, 15-methyl-prostaglandin F2 alpha*) ▶LK ♀C ▶? $$$
ADULT - Refractory postpartum uterine bleeding: 250 mcg deep IM. If necessary, may repeat at 15–90 min intervals up to a total dose of 2 mg (8 doses).
PEDS - Not approved in children.
NOTES - Caution with asthma. Transient fever, HTN, nausea, bronchoconstriction & flushing. May augment oxytocics.

**METHYLERGONOVINE** (*Methergine*) ▶LK ♀C ▶? $
ADULT - To increase uterine contractions & decrease postpartum bleeding: 0.2 mg IM after delivery of the placenta, delivery of the anterior shoulder, or during the puerperium. Repeat q2–4h prn. 0.2 mg PO tid-qid in the puerperium for a max of 1 wk.
PEDS - Not approved in children.
FORMS - Trade only: Tabs 0.2 mg.
NOTES - Contraindicated in pregnancy-induced hypertension/pre-eclampsia. Avoid IV route due to risk of sudden HTN and stroke. If IV absolutely necessary, give slowly over no less than 1 min, monitor BP.

(cont.)

## OB/GYN: Vaginitis Preparations

**NOTE:** See also STD/vaginitis table in antimicrobial section. Many experts recommend 7 d antifungal therapy for pregnant women w/candida vaginitis. Many of these creams & suppositories are oil-based and may weaken latex condoms & diaphragms. Do not use latex products for 72 h after last dose.

**BORIC ACID ▶NOT ABSORBED ♀? ▶- $**
PEDS - Not approved in children.
UNAPPROVED ADULT - Resistant vulvovaginal candidiasis: 600 mg susp intravaginally qhs × 2 wk.
FORMS - No commercial preparation; must be compounded by pharmacist. Vaginal suppositories 600 mg in gelatin caps.
NOTES - Reported use for azole-resistant non-albicans (C. glabrata) or recurrent albicans failing azole therapy. Do not use if abdominal pain, fever or foul-smelling vaginal discharge is present. Avoid vaginal intercourse during treatment.

**BUTOCONAZOLE (Gynazole, Mycelex-3) ▶LK ♀C ▶? $(OTC), $$$(Rx)**
ADULT - Local treatment of vulvovaginal candidiasis, nonpregnant patients: Mycelex 3: 1 applicatorful (~5g) intravaginally qhs × 3 d, up to 6 d, if necessary. Pregnant patients: (2nd & 3rd trimesters only) 1 applicatorful (~5g) intravaginally qhs × 6 d. Gynazole-1: 1 applicatorful (~5g) intravaginally daily × 1.
PEDS - Not approved in children.
FORMS - OTC: Trade only (Mycelex 3): 2% vaginal cream in 5 g pre-filled applicators (3s) & 20 g tube with applicators. Rx: Trade only (Gynazole-1): 2% vaginal cream in 5 g pre-filled applicator.
NOTES - Do not use if abdominal pain, fever or foul-smelling vaginal discharge is present. Since small amount may be absorbed from the vagina, use during the 1st trimester only when essential. During pregnancy, use of a vaginal applicator may be contraindicated & manual insertion may occur. Vulvar/vaginal burning may occur. Avoid vaginal intercourse during treatment.

**CLINDAMYCIN - VAGINAL (Cleocin, Clindesse, ✦Dalacin) ▶L ♀- ▶+ $$**
ADULT - Bacterial vaginosis: Cleocin: 1 applicatorful (~100 mg clindamycin phosphate in 5g cream) intravaginally qhs × 7 d, or one supp qhs × 3 d. Clindesse: 1 applicatorful cream × 1.
PEDS - Not approved in children.
FORMS - Generic/Trade: 2% vaginal cream in 40 g tube with 7 disposable applicators (Cleocin). Vag supp (Cleocin Ovules) 100 mg (3) w/applicator. 2% vaginal cream in a single-dose prefilled applicator (Clindesse).
NOTES - Clindesse may degrade latex/rubber condoms & diaphragms for 5 d after the last dose (Cleocin for up to 3 d). Not recommended during pregnancy despite B rating, as it does not prevent the adverse effects of bacterial vaginosis (eg, pre-term birth, neonatal infection). Cervicitis, vaginitis, & vulvar irritation may occur. Avoid vaginal intercourse during treatment.

**CLOTRIMAZOLE - VAGINAL (Mycelex 7, Gyne-Lotrimin, ✦Canesten, Clotrimaderm) ▶LK ♀B ▶? $**
ADULT - Local treatment of vulvovaginal candidiasis: 1 applicatorful 1% cream qhs × 7 d. 1 applicatorful 2% cream qhs × 3 d. 100 mg susp intravaginally qhs × 7 d. 200 mg supp qhs × 3 d. Topical cream for external symptoms bid × 7 d.
PEDS - Not approved in children.
FORMS - OTC Generic/Trade: 1% vaginal cream with applicator (some pre-filled). 2% vaginal cream with applicator and 1% topical cream in some combination packs. OTC Trade only (Gyne-Lotrimin): Vaginal suppositories 100 mg (7) & 200 mg (3) with applicators.

**METRONIDAZOLE - VAGINAL (MetroGel-Vaginal, Vandazole) ▶LK ♀B ▶? $$**
ADULT - Bacterial vaginosis: 1 applicatorful (~ 5 g containing ~ 37.5 mg metronidazole) intravaginally qhs or bid × 5 d.
PEDS - Not approved in children.
FORMS - Generic/Trade: 0.75% gel in 70 g tube with applicator.
NOTES - Cure rate same with qhs and bid dosing. Vaginally applied metronidazole could be absorbed in sufficient amounts to produce systemic effects. Caution in patients with CNS diseases due to rare reports of seizures, neuropathy & numbness. Do not administer to patients who have taken disulfiram within the last 2 wk. Interaction with ethanol. Caution with warfarin. Candida cervicitis & vaginitis, & vaginal, perineal or vulvar itching may occur. Avoid vaginal intercourse during treatment.

**MICONAZOLE (Monistat, Femizol-M, M-Zole, Micozole, Monazole) ▶LK ♀+ ▶? $**
ADULT - Local treatment of vulvovaginal candidiasis: 1 applicatorful 2% cream intravaginally qhs × 7 d or 4% cream qhs × 3 d. 100 mg supp intravaginally qhs × 7 d, 400 mg qhs × 3 d, or 1200 mg × 1. Topical cream for external symptoms bid × 7 d.
PEDS - Not approved in children.
FORMS - OTC: Generic/Trade: 2% vaginal cream in 45 g with 1 applicator or 7 disposable applicators. Vaginal suppositories 100 mg (7) OTC: Trade only: 400 mg (3) & 1200 mg (1) with applicator. Generic/Trade: 4% vaginal cream in 25 g tubes or 3 prefilled applicators. Some in combination packs with 2% miconazole cream for external use.
NOTES - Do not use if abdominal pain, fever or foul-smelling vaginal discharge is present. Since small amounts of these drugs may be absorbed from the vagina, use during the 1st trimester only when essential. During pregnancy, use of a vaginal applicator may be contraindicated; manual insertion

**MICONAZOLE** (*cont.*)

of suppositories may be preferred. Vulvovaginal burning, itching, irritation & pelvic cramps may occur. Avoid vaginal intercourse during treatment. May increase warfarin effect.

**NYSTATIN - VAGINAL** (*Mycostatin, + Nilstat, Nyaderm*)
▶Not metabolized ♀A ▶? $$

ADULT - Local treatment of vulvovaginal candidiasis: 100,000 units tab intravaginally qhs × 2 wk.

PEDS - Not approved in children.

FORMS - Generic/Trade: Vaginal Tabs 100,000 units in 15s & 30s with or without applicator(s).

NOTES - Topical azole products more effective. Do not use if abdominal pain, fever or foul-smelling vaginal discharge is present. During pregnancy use of a vaginal applicator may be contraindicated, manual insertion of tabs may be preferred. Avoid vaginal intercourse during treatment.

**TERCONAZOLE** (*Terazol*) ▶LK ♀C ▶- $$

ADULT - Local treatment of vulvovaginal candidiasis: 1 applicatorful 0.4% cream intravaginally qhs × 7 d. 1 applicatorful 0.8% cream intravaginally qhs × 3 d. 80 mg supp intravaginally qhs × 3 d.

PEDS - Not approved in children.

FORMS - All forms supplied with applicators: Generic/Trade: Vag cream 0.4% (Terazol 7) in 45

g tube, 0.8% (Terazol 3) in 20 g tube. Vag supp (Terazol 3) 80 mg (#3).

NOTES - Do not use if abdominal pain, fever or foul-smelling vaginal discharge is present. Since small amounts of these drugs may be absorbed from the vagina, use during the 1st trimester only when essential. During pregnancy, use of a vaginal applicator may be contraindicated; manual insertion of suppositories may be preferred. Avoid vaginal intercourse during treatment. Vulvovaginal irritation, burning, & pruritus may occur.

**TIOCONAZOLE** (*Monistat 1-Day, Vagistat-1*) ▶Not absorbed ♀C ▶- $

ADULT - Local treatment of vulvovaginal candidiasis: 1 applicatorful (~ 4.6 g) intravaginally qhs × 1.

PEDS - Not approved in children.

FORMS - OTC: Trade only: Vaginal ointment: 6.5% (300 mg) in 4.6 g prefilled single-dose applicator.

NOTES - Do not use if abdominal pain, fever or foul-smelling vaginal discharge is present. Since small amounts of these drugs may be absorbed from the vagina, use during the 1st trimester only when essential. During pregnancy, use of a vaginal applicator may be contraindicated. Avoid vaginal intercourse during treatment. Vulvovaginal burning & itching may occur.

**DANAZOL** (*Danocrine, + Cyclomen*) ▶L ♀X ▶- $$$$$

ADULT - Endometriosis: Start 400 mg PO bid, then titrate downward to a dose sufficient to maintain amenorrhea × 3–6 mo, up to 9 mo. Fibrocystic breast disease: 100–200 mg PO bid × 4–6 mo.

PEDS - Not approved in children.

UNAPPROVED ADULT - Menorrhagia: 100–400 mg PO daily × 3 mo. Cyclical mastalgia: 100–200 mg PO bid × 4–6 mo.

FORMS - Generic only: Caps 50, 100, 200 mg.

NOTES - Contraindications: impaired hepatic, renal or cardiac function. Androgenic effects may not be reversible even after the drug is discontinued. May alter voice. Hepatic dysfunction has occurred. Insulin requirements may increase in diabetics. Prolongation of PT/INR has been reported with concomitant warfarin.

**MIFEPRISTONE** (*Mifeprex, RU-486*) ▶L ♀X ▶? $$$$$

WARNING - Rare cases of sepsis and death have occurred. Surgical intervention may be necessary with incomplete abortions. Patients need to be given info on where such services are available & what do in case of an emergency.

ADULT - Termination of pregnancy, up to 49 d: Day 1: 600 mg PO. Day 3: 400 mcg misoprostol (unless abortion confirmed). Day 14: confirmation of pregnancy termination.

PEDS - Not approved in children.

FORMS - Trade only: Tabs 200 mg.

NOTES - Bleeding/spotting & cramping most common side effects. Prolonged heavy bleeding may be

a sign of incomplete abortion. Contraindications: ectopic pregnancy, IUD use, adrenal insufficiency & long-term steroid use, use of anticoagulants, hemorrhagic disorders & porphyrias. CYP3A4 inducers may increase metabolism & lower levels. Available through physician offices only.

**PREMESIS-RX** (pyridoxine + folic acid + cyanocobalamin + calcium carbonate) ▶L ♀A ▶+ $

ADULT - Treatment of pregnancy-induced nausea: 1 tab PO daily.

PEDS - Unapproved in children.

FORMS - Trade only: Tabs 75 mg vitamin B6 (pyridoxine), sustained-release, 12 mcg vitamin B12 (cyanocobalamin), 1 mg folic acid, and 200 mg calcium carbonate.

NOTES - May be taken in conjunction with prenatal vitamins.

**RHO IMMUNE GLOBULIN** (*HyperRHO S/D, MICRhoGAM, RhoGAM, Rhophylac, WinRho SDF*) ▶L ♀C ▶? $$$$$

ADULT - Prevention of hemolytic disease of the newborn if mother Rh- and baby is or might be Rh+: 300 mcg vial IM to mother at 28 wk gestation followed by a 2nd dose ≤72 h of delivery. Doses >1 vial may be needed if large fetal-maternal hemorrhage occurs during delivery (see complete prescribing information to determine dose). Following amniocentesis, miscarriage, abortion or ectopic pregnancy ≥13 wk gestation: 1 vial (300 mcg) IM. <12 wk gestation: 1 vial (50 mcg) microdose IM. Immune thrombocytopenic purpura (ITP), nonsplenectomized (WinRho): 250 units/kg/dose (50

(cont.)

**RHO IMMUNE GLOBULIN** *(cont.)*
mcg/kg/dose) IV × 1 if hemoglobin >10 g/dL or 125–200 units/kg/dose (25–40 mcg/kg/dose) IV × 1 if hemoglobin <10 g/dL. Additional doses of 125–300 units/kg/dose (25–60 mcg/kg/dose) IV may be given as determined by patient's response.
PEDS - Immune thrombocytopenic purpura (ITP), nonsplenectomized (WinRho): 250 units/kg/dose (50 mcg/kg/dose) IV × 1 if hemoglobin >10g/dL or 125–200 units/kg/dose (25–40 mcg/kg/dose) IV × 1 if hemoglobin <10 g/dL. Additional

doses of 125–300 units/kg/dose (25–60 mcg/kg/dose) IV may be given as determined by patient's response.
UNAPPROVED ADULT - Rh-incompatible transfusion: specialized dosing.
NOTES - One 300 mcg vial prevents maternal sensitization to the Rh factor if the fetomaternal hemorrhage is less than 15 mL fetal RBCs (30 mL of whole blood). When the fetomaternal hemorrhage exceeds this (as estimated by Kleihauer-Betke testing), administer more than one 300 mcg vial.

## ONCOLOGY: Alkylating Agents

**ALTRETAMINE (*Hexalen*)** ▶L ♀D ▶- $ varies by therapy
WARNING - Peripheral neuropathy, bone marrow suppression, fertility impairment, N/V, alopecia. Instruct patients to report promptly fever, sore throat, signs of local infection, bleeding from any site, or symptoms suggestive of anemia.
ADULT - Chemotherapy doses vary by indication. Ovarian cancer.
PEDS - Not approved in children.
UNAPPROVED ADULT - Lung, breast, cervical cancer, non-Hodgkin's Lymphoma.
FORMS - Trade only: Cap 50 mg.
NOTES - Reliable contraception is recommended. Monitor CBCs. Cimetidine increases toxicity. MAO inhibitors may cause severe orthostatic hypotension.
**BENDAMUSTINE (*Treanda*)** ▶Plasma ♀D ▶- $ varies by therapy
WARNING - Anaphylaxis, bone marrow suppression, nephrotoxicity, severe rash. Instruct patients to report promptly fever, sore throat, signs of local infection, bleeding from any site, or symptoms suggestive of anemia.
ADULT - Chemotherapy doses vary by indication. CLL.
PEDS - Not approved in children.
NOTES - Reliable contraception is recommended. Monitor CBCs & renal function.
**BUSULFAN (*Myleran, Busulfex*)** ▶LK ♀D ▶- $ varies by therapy
WARNING - Secondary malignancies, bone marrow suppression, adrenal insufficiency, hyperuricemia, pulmonary fibrosis, seizures, cellular dysplasia, hepatic veno-occlusive disease, fertility impairment, alopecia. Instruct patients to report promptly fever, sore throat, signs of local infection, bleeding from any site, symptoms suggestive of anemia, or yellow discoloration of the skin or eyes.
ADULT - Chemotherapy doses vary by indication. Tabs: CML. Injection: conditioning regimen prior to allogeneic hematopoietic progenitor cell transplantation for CML, in combination w/cyclophosphamide.
PEDS - Chemotherapy doses vary by indication. Tablets: CML. Safety of the injection has not been established.
UNAPPROVED ADULT - High dose in conjunction with stem cell transplant for leukemia and lymphoma.

FORMS - Trade only (Myleran) Tab 2 mg. Busulfex injection for hospital/oncology clinic use; not intended for outpatient prescribing.
NOTES - Reliable contraception is recommended. Monitor CBCs & LFTs. Hydration & allopurinol to decrease adverse effects of uric acid. Acetaminophen & itraconazole decrease busulfan clearance. Phenytoin increases clearance.
**CARMUSTINE (*BCNU, BiCNU, Gliadel*)** ▶Plasma ♀D ▶- $ varies by therapy
WARNING - Secondary malignancies, bone marrow suppression, pulmonary fibrosis, nephrotoxicity, hepatotoxicity, ocular nerve fiber-layer infarcts & retinal hemorrhages, fertility impairment, alopecia. Wafer: seizures, brain edema & herniation, intracranial infection. Instruct patients to report promptly fever, sore throat, signs of local infection, bleeding from any site, symptoms suggestive of anemia, or yellow discoloration of the skin or eyes.
ADULT - Chemotherapy doses vary by indication. Injection: glioblastoma, brainstem glioma, medulloblastoma, astrocytoma, ependymoma & metastatic brain tumors, multiple myeloma w/ prednisone; Hodgkin's disease & non-Hodgkin's lymphomas, in combination regimens. Wafer: glioblastoma multiforme, adjunct to surgery. High-grade malignant glioma, adjunct to surgery & radiation.
PEDS - Not approved in children.
UNAPPROVED ADULT - Mycosis fungoides, topical soln.
NOTES - Reliable contraception is recommended. Monitor CBCs, PFTs, LFTs & renal function. May decrease phenytoin & digoxin levels. Cimetidine may increase myelosuppression
**CHLORAMBUCIL (*Leukeran*)** ▶L ♀D ▶- $ varies by therapy
WARNING - Secondary malignancies, bone marrow suppression, seizures, fertility impairment, alopecia. Instruct patients to report promptly fever, sore throat, signs of local infection, bleeding from any site, or symptoms suggestive of anemia.
ADULT - Chemotherapy doses vary by indication. CLL. Lymphomas including indolent lymphoma & Hodgkin's disease.

**CHLORAMBUCIL** (cont.)

PEDS - Not approved in children.

UNAPPROVED ADULT - Uveitis & meningoencephalitis associated with Behcet's disease. Idiopathic membranous nephropathy. Ovarian carcinoma.

FORMS - Trade only: Tab 2 mg.

NOTES - Reliable contraception is recommended. Monitor CBCs. Avoid live vaccines.

**CYCLOPHOSPHAMIDE** (*Cytoxan, Neosar*) ▶L ♀D ▶- $ varies by therapy

WARNING - Secondary malignancies, leukopenia, cardiac toxicity, acute hemorrhagic cystitis, hypersensitivity, fertility impairment, alopecia. Instruct patients to report promptly fever, sore throat, signs of local infection, bleeding from any site, symptoms suggestive of anemia, or yellow discoloration of the skin or eyes.

ADULT - Chemotherapy doses vary by indication. Non-Hodgkin's lymphomas, Hodgkin's disease. Multiple myeloma. Disseminated neuroblastoma. Adenocarcinoma of the ovary. Retinoblastoma. Carcinoma of the breast. CLL. CML. AML. Mycosis fungoides.

PEDS - Chemotherapy doses vary by indication. ALL. "Minimal change" nephrotic syndrome.

UNAPPROVED ADULT - Wegener's granulomatosis, other steroid-resistant vasculitides. Severe progressive RA. Systemic lupus erythematosus. Multiple sclerosis. Polyarteritis nodosa. Lung, testicular and bladder cancer, sarcoma.

FORMS - Generic/Trade: Tabs 25 & 50 mg. Injection for hospital/oncology clinic use; not intended for outpatient prescribing.

NOTES - Reliable contraception is recommended. Monitor CBCs, urine for red cells. Allopurinol may increase myelosuppression. Thiazides may prolong leukopenia. May reduce digoxin levels, reduce fluoroquinolone activity. May increase anticoagulant effects. Coadministration with mesna reduces hemorrhagic cystitis when used in high doses.

**DACARBAZINE** (*DTIC-Dome*) ▶LK ♀C ▶- $ varies by therapy

WARNING - Extravasation associated w/severe necrosis. Secondary malignancies, bone marrow suppression, hepatotoxicity, anorexia, N/V, anaphylaxis, alopecia. Instruct patients to report promptly fever, sore throat, signs of local infection, bleeding from any site, symptoms suggestive of anemia, or yellow discoloration of the skin or eyes.

ADULT - Chemotherapy doses vary by indication. Metastatic melanoma. Hodgkin's disease, in combination regimens.

PEDS - Not approved in children.

UNAPPROVED ADULT - Malignant pheochromocytoma, in combination regimens. Sarcoma.

NOTES - Monitor CBCs & LFTs.

**IFOSFAMIDE** (*Ifex*) ▶L ♀D ▶- $ varies by therapy

WARNING - Secondary malignancies, hemorrhagic cystitis, confusion, coma, bone marrow suppression, hematuria, nephrotoxicity, alopecia. Instruct

patients to report promptly fever, sore throat, signs of local infection, bleeding from any site, symptoms suggestive of anemia, or yellow discoloration of the skin or eyes.

ADULT - Chemotherapy doses vary by indication. Germ cell testicular cancer, in combination regimens.

PEDS - Not approved in children.

UNAPPROVED ADULT - Lung, breast, ovarian, pancreatic & gastric cancer; sarcomas, acute leukemias (except AML), lymphomas.

NOTES - Reliable contraception is recommended. Monitor CBCs, renal function & urine for red cells. Coadministration with mesna reduces hemorrhagic cystitis.

**LOMUSTINE** (*CeeNu, CCNU*) ▶L ♀D ▶- $ varies by therapy

WARNING - Secondary malignancies, bone marrow suppression, hepatotoxicity, nephrotoxicity, pulmonary fibrosis, fertility impairment, alopecia. Instruct patients to report promptly fever, sore throat, signs of local infection, bleeding from any site, symptoms suggestive of anemia, or yellow discoloration of the skin or eyes.

ADULT - Chemotherapy doses vary by indication. Brain tumors. Hodgkin's disease, in combination regimens.

PEDS - Chemotherapy doses vary by indication. Brain tumors. Hodgkin's disease, in combination regimens.

FORMS - Trade only: Caps 10, 40 & 100 mg.

NOTES - Reliable contraception is recommended. Monitor CBCs, LFTs, PFTs & renal function. Avoid alcohol.

**MECHLORETHAMINE** (*Mustargen*) ▶Plasma ♀D ▶- $ varies by therapy

WARNING - Extravasation associated w/severe necrosis. Secondary malignancies, bone marrow suppression, amyloidosis, herpes zoster, anaphylaxis, fertility impairment, alopecia. Instruct patients to report promptly fever, sore throat, signs of local infection, bleeding from any site, or symptoms suggestive of anemia.

ADULT - Chemotherapy doses vary by indication. IV: Hodgkin's disease (Stages III & IV). Lymphosarcoma. Chronic myelocytic or chronic lymphocytic leukemia. Polycythemia vera. Mycosis fungoides. Bronchogenic carcinoma. Intrapleurally, intraperitoneally or intrapericardially: metastatic carcinoma resulting in effusion.

PEDS - Not approved in children.

UNAPPROVED ADULT - Cutaneous mycosis fungoides: topical soln or ointment.

UNAPPROVED PEDS - Hodgkin's disease (Stages III & IV), in combination regimens.

NOTES - Reliable contraception is recommended. Monitor CBCs.

**MELPHALAN** (*Alkeran*) ▶Plasma ♀D ▶- $ varies by therapy

WARNING - Secondary malignancies, bone marrow suppression, anaphylaxis, fertility impairment,

(cont.)

**MELPHALAN** (*cont.*)

alopecia. Instruct patients to report promptly fever, sore throat, signs of local infection, bleeding from any site, or symptoms suggestive of anemia.
ADULT - Chemotherapy doses vary by indication. Multiple myeloma & non-resectable epithelial ovarian carcinoma.
PEDS - Not approved in children.
UNAPPROVED ADULT - Non-Hodgkin's lymphoma in high doses for stem cell transplant, testicular cancer.
FORMS - Trade only: Tabs 2 mg. Injection for hospital/clinic use; not intended for outpatient prescribing.
NOTES - Reliable contraception is recommended. Monitor CBCs. Avoid live vaccines.

**PROCARBAZINE** (*Matulane*) ▶LK ♀D ▶- $ varies by therapy

WARNING - Secondary malignancies, bone marrow suppression, hemolysis & Heinz-Ehrlich inclusion bodies in erythrocytes, hypersensitivity, fertility impairment, alopecia. Peds: tremors, convulsions & coma have occurred. Instruct patients to report promptly fever, sore throat, signs of local infection, bleeding from any site, symptoms suggestive of anemia, black tarry stools or vomiting of blood.
ADULT - Chemotherapy doses vary by indication. Hodgkin's disease (Stages III & IV), in combination regimens.
PEDS - Chemotherapy doses vary by indication. Hodgkin's disease (Stages III & IV), in combination regimens.
FORMS - Trade only: Cap 50 mg.
NOTES - Reliable contraception is recommended. Monitor CBCs. Renal/hepatic function impairment may predispose toxicity. UA, LFTs, & BUN weekly. May decrease digoxin levels. May increase effects of opioids, sympathomimetics, TCAs. Ingestion of foods with high tyramine content may result in a potentially fatal hypertensive crisis. Alcohol may cause a disulfiram-like reaction.

**STREPTOZOCIN** (*Zanosar*) ▶Plasma ♀C ▶- $ varies by therapy

WARNING - Extravasation associated w/severe necrosis. Secondary malignancies, nephrotoxicity, N/V, hepatotoxicity, decrease in hematocrit, hypoglycemia, fertility impairment, alopecia.
ADULT - Chemotherapy doses vary by indication. Metastatic islet cell carcinoma of the pancreas.
PEDS - Not approved in children.
NOTES - Hydration important. Monitor renal function, CBCs & LFTs.

**TEMOZOLOMIDE** (*Temodar*, ✦*Temodal*) ▶Plasma ♀D ▶- $ varies by therapy

WARNING - Secondary malignancies, bone marrow suppression, fertility impairment, alopecia. Instruct patients to report promptly fever, sore throat, signs of local infection, bleeding from any site, or symptoms suggestive of anemia.
ADULT - Chemotherapy doses vary by indication. Anaplastic astrocytoma, glioblastoma multiforme.
PEDS - Not approved in children.
UNAPPROVED ADULT - Metastatic melanoma, renal cell carcinoma.
FORMS - Trade only: Caps 5, 20, 100, 140, 180, 250 mg.
NOTES - Reliable contraception is recommended. Monitor CBCs. Valproic acid decreases clearance.

**THIOTEPA** (*Thioplex*) ▶L ♀D ▶- $ varies by therapy

WARNING - Secondary malignancies, bone marrow suppression, hypersensitivity, fertility impairment, alopecia. Instruct patients to report promptly fever, sore throat, signs of local infection, bleeding from any site, symptoms suggestive of anemia, black tarry stools or vomiting of blood.
ADULT - Chemotherapy doses vary by indication. Adenocarcinoma of the breast or ovary. Control of intracavitary malignant effusions. Superficial papillary carcinoma of the urinary bladder. Hodgkin's disease. Lymphosarcoma.
PEDS - Not approved in children.
NOTES - Reliable contraception is recommended. Monitor CBCs.

## ONCOLOGY:ANTIBIOTICS

**BLEOMYCIN** (*Blenoxane*) ▶K ♀D ▶- $ varies by therapy

WARNING - Pulmonary fibrosis, skin toxicity, nephro/hepatotoxicity, alopecia, & severe idiosyncratic reaction consisting of hypotension, mental confusion, fever, chills, & wheezing.
ADULT - Chemotherapy doses vary by indication. Squamous cell carcinoma of the head & neck. Carcinoma of the skin, penis, cervix, & vulva. Hodgkin's and non-Hodgkin's lymphoma. Testicular carcinoma. Malignant pleural effusion: sclerosing agent.
PEDS - Not approved in children.
NOTES - Reliable contraception is recommended. Frequent chest x-rays. May decrease digoxin & phenytoin levels.

**DACTINOMYCIN** (*Cosmegen*) ▶Not metabolized ♀C ▶- $ varies by therapy

WARNING - Extravasation associated w/severe necrosis. Contraindicated with active chicken pox

or herpes zoster. Erythema & vesiculation (with radiation), bone marrow suppression, alopecia. Instruct patients to report promptly fever, sore throat, signs of local infection, bleeding from any site, or symptoms suggestive of anemia.
ADULT - Chemotherapy doses vary by indication. Wilms' tumor. Rhabdomyosarcoma. Metastatic & nonmetastaticchoriocarcinoma.Nonseminomatous testicular carcinoma. Ewing's sarcoma. Sarcoma botryoides. Most in combination regimens.
PEDS - Chemotherapy doses vary by indication. See adult. Contraindicated in infants <6mo.
NOTES - Monitor CBCs.

**DAUNORUBICIN** (*DaunoXome, Cerubidine*) ▶L ♀D ▶- $ varies by therapy

WARNING - Extravasation associated w/severe necrosis. Cardiac toxicity, more frequent in children. Bone marrow suppression, infusion-related

**DAUNORUBICIN** (*cont.*)

reactions. Instruct patients to report promptly fever, sore throat, signs of local infection, bleeding from any site, or symptoms suggestive of anemia.
ADULT - Chemotherapy doses vary by indication. First line treatment of Advanced HIV-associated Kaposi's sarcoma (DaunoXome). AML, in combination regimens. ALL (Cerubidine).
PEDS - Chemotherapy doses vary by indication. ALL (Cerubidine). DaunoXome not approved in children.
NOTES - Reliable contraception is recommended. Monitor CBCs, cardiac, renal & hepatic function (toxicity increased w/impaired function). Transient urine discoloration (red).

**DOXORUBICIN LIPOSOMAL** (*Doxil, ✦Caelyx, Myocet*) ▶L ♀D ▶- $ varies by therapy
WARNING - Extravasation associated w/severe necrosis. Cardiac toxicity, more frequent in children. Bone marrow suppression, infusion-associated reactions, necrotizing colitis, mucositis, hyperuricemia, palmar-plantar erythrodysesthesia. Secondary malignancies. Instruct patients to report promptly fever, sore throat, signs of local infection, bleeding from any site, or symptoms suggestive of anemia.
ADULT - Chemotherapy doses vary by indication. Advanced HIV-associated Kaposi's sarcoma, multiple myeloma, ovarian carcinoma.
PEDS - Not approved in children.
UNAPPROVED ADULT - Ovarian carcinoma.
NOTES - Heart failure with cumulative doses. Monitor ejection fraction, CBCs, LFTs, uric acid levels, & renal function (toxicity increased w/ impaired function). Reliable contraception is recommended. Transient urine discoloration (red).

**DOXORUBICIN NON-LIPOSOMAL** (*Adriamycin, Rubex*) ▶L ♀D ▶- $ varies by therapy
WARNING - Extravasation associated w/severe necrosis. Cardiac toxicity, more frequent in children. Bone marrow suppression, infusion-associated reactions, necrotizing colitis, mucositis, hyperuricemia, alopecia. Secondary malignancies. Instruct patients to report promptly fever, sore throat, signs of local infection, bleeding from any site, or symptoms suggestive of anemia.
ADULT - Chemotherapy doses vary by indication. ALL. AML. Wilms' tumor. Neuroblastoma. Soft tissue & bone sarcomas. Breast carcinoma. Ovarian carcinoma. Transitional cell bladder carcinoma. Thyroid carcinoma. Hodgkin's & non-Hodgkin's lymphomas. Bronchogenic carcinoma. Gastric carcinoma.
PEDS - Chemotherapy doses vary by indication: see adult.
UNAPPROVED ADULT - Sarcoma, small cell lung cancer.
NOTES - Heart failure with cumulative doses. Monitor ejection fraction, CBCs, LFTs, uric acid levels, & renal function (toxicity increased w/ impaired function). Reliable contraception is recommended. Transient urine discoloration (red).

**EPIRUBICIN** (*Ellence, ✦Pharmorubicin*) ▶L ♀D ▶- $ varies by therapy
WARNING - Extravasation associated w/severe necrosis. Cardiac toxicity, bone marrow suppression, secondary malignancy (AML), hyperuricemia, fertility impairment, alopecia. Instruct patients to report promptly fever, sore throat, signs of local infection, bleeding from any site, or symptoms suggestive of anemia.
ADULT - Chemotherapy doses vary by indication. Adjuvant therapy for breast cancer, axillary-node positive.
PEDS - Not approved in children.
UNAPPROVED ADULT - Neoadjuvant and metastatic breast cancer.
NOTES - Reliable contraception is recommended. Monitor CBCs, cardiac, hepatic & renal function (toxicity increased w/impaired function). Cimetidine increase levels. Transient urine discoloration (red).

**IDARUBICIN** (*Idamycin*) ▶? ♀D ▶- $ varies by therapy
WARNING - Extravasation associated w/severe necrosis. Cardiac toxicity, bone marrow suppression, hyperuricemia, alopecia. Instruct patients to report promptly fever, sore throat, signs of local infection, bleeding from any site, or symptoms suggestive of anemia.
ADULT - Chemotherapy doses vary by indication. AML, in combination regimens.
PEDS - Not approved in children.
UNAPPROVED ADULT - ALL, CML.
NOTES - Reliable contraception is recommended. Monitor CBCs, LFTs, cardiac & renal function (toxicity increased w/impaired function).

**MITOMYCIN** (*Mutamycin, Mitomycin-C*) ▶L ♀D ▶- $ varies by therapy
WARNING - Extravasation associated w/severe necrosis. Bone marrow suppression, hemolytic uremic syndrome, nephrotoxicity, adult respiratory distress syndrome, alopecia. Instruct patients to report promptly fever, sore throat, signs of local infection, bleeding from any site, or symptoms suggestive of anemia.
ADULT - Chemotherapy doses vary by indication. Disseminated adenocarcinoma of stomach, pancreas, or colorectum, in combination regimens.
PEDS - Not approved in children.
UNAPPROVED ADULT - Superficial bladder cancer, intravesical route; pterygia, adjunct to surgical excision: ophthalmic soln.
NOTES - Reliable contraception is recommended. Monitor CBCs & renal function.

**MITOXANTRONE** (*Novantrone*) ▶LK ♀D ▶- $ varies by therapy
WARNING - Secondary malignancies (AML), bone marrow suppression, cardiac toxicity/heart failure, hyperuricemia, increased LFTs. Instruct patients to report promptly fever, sore throat, signs of local infection, bleeding from any site, or symptoms suggestive of anemia.

(cont.)

**MITOXANTRONE** (*cont.*)

ADULT - Chemotherapy doses vary by indication. AML, in combination regimens. Symptomatic patients with hormone refractory prostate cancer. Multiple sclerosis (secondary progressive, progressive relapsing, or worsening relapsing-remitting): 12 mg per square meter of BSA IV q 3 mo.

PEDS - Not approved in children.

UNAPPROVED ADULT - Breast cancer. Non-Hodgkin's lymphoma. ALL, CML, Ovarian carcinoma. Sclerosing agent for malignant pleural effusions.

NOTES - Reliable contraception is recommended. Monitor CBCs & LFTs. Baseline echocardiogram and repeat echoes prior to each dose are recom-

mended. Transient urine & sclera discoloration (blue-green).

**VALRUBICIN** (*Valstar, ＋Valtaxin*) ▶K ♀C ▶- $ varies by therapy

WARNING - Induces complete responses in only 1 in 5 patients. Delaying cystectomy could lead to development of lethal metastatic bladder cancer. Irritable bladder symptoms, alopecia.

ADULT - Chemotherapy doses vary by indication. Bladder cancer, intravesical therapy of BCG-refractory carcinoma in situ.

PEDS - Not approved in children.

NOTES - Reliable contraception is recommended. Transient urine discoloration (red).

## ONCOLOGY: Antimetabolites

**AZACITIDINE** (*Vidaza*) ▶K ♀D ▶- $ varies by therapy

WARNING - Contraindicated with malignant hepatic tumors. Bone marrow suppression. Fertility impairment. Instruct patients to report promptly fever, sore throat, or signs of local infection or bleeding from any site.

ADULT - Chemotherapy doses vary by indication. Myelodysplastic syndrome subtypes.

PEDS - Not approved in children.

NOTES - Reliable contraception is recommended. Men should not father children while on this drug. Monitor CBC, renal & hepatic function.

**CAPECITABINE** (*Xeloda*) ▶L ♀D ▶- $ varies by therapy

WARNING - Increased INR & bleeding with warfarin. Contraindicated in severe renal dysfunction (CrCl <30mL/min). Severe diarrhea, fertility impairment, palmar-plantar erythrodysesthesia or chemotherapy-induced acral erythema, cardiac toxicity, hyperbilirubinemia, neutropenia, alopecia. Instruct patients to report promptly fever, sore throat, or signs of local infection or bleeding from any site.

ADULT - Chemotherapy doses vary by indication. Metastatic breast & colorectal cancer.

PEDS - Not approved in children.

UNAPPROVED ADULT - Stomach, esophageal , pancreatic, hepatocellular carcinoma.

FORMS - Trade only: Tabs 150 & 500 mg.

NOTES - Reliable contraception is recommended. Aluminum hydroxide- & magnesium hydroxide-containing antacids increase levels. May increase phenytoin levels.

**CLADRIBINE** (*Leustatin, chlorodeoxyadenosine*) ▶intracellular ♀D ▶- $ varies by therapy

WARNING - Bone marrow suppression, nephrotoxicity, neurotoxicity, fever, fertility impairment, alopecia. Instruct patients to report promptly fever, sore throat, or signs of local infection, bleeding from any site, or symptoms suggestive of anemia.

ADULT - Chemotherapy doses vary by indication. Hairy cell leukemia.

PEDS - Not approved in children.

UNAPPROVED ADULT - Advanced cutaneous T-cell lymphomas. Chronic lymphocytic leukemia, Non-

Hodgkin's lymphomas. AML. Autoimmune hemolytic anemia. Mycosis fungoides. Sezary syndrome.

NOTES - Reliable contraception is recommended. Monitor CBCs & renal function.

**CLOFARABINE** (*Clolar*) ▶K ♀D ▶- $ varies by therapy

WARNING - Myelodysplastic syndrome, bone marrow suppression, tumor lysis syndrome, hepatotoxicity. Instruct patients to report promptly fever, sore throat, or signs of local infection, bleeding from any site, or symptoms suggestive of anemia.

ADULT - Not approved in adults.

PEDS - 1–21 yo: Chemotherapy doses vary by indication. Relapsed or refractory acute lymphoblastic leukemia.

NOTES - Reliable contraception is recommended. Monitor CBCs, LFTs & renal function.

**CYTARABINE** (*Cytosar-U, Tarabine, Depo-Cyt, AraC*) ▶LK ♀D ▶- $ varies by therapy

WARNING - Bone marrow suppression, hepatotoxicity, N/V/D, hyperuricemia, pancreatitis, peripheral neuropathy, "cytarabine syndrome" (fever, myalgia, bone pain, occasional chest pain, maculopapular rash, conjunctivitis, & malaise), alopecia. Neurotoxicity. Chemical arachnoiditis (N/V, headache, & fever) with Depo-Cyt. Instruct patients to report promptly fever, sore throat, or signs of local infection, bleeding from any site, symptoms suggestive of anemia, or yellow discoloration of the skin or eyes.

ADULT - Chemotherapy doses vary by indication. AML. ALL. CML. Prophylaxis & treatment of meningeal leukemia, intrathecal (Cytosar-U, Tarabine). Lymphomatous meningitis, intrathecal (Depo-Cyt).

PEDS - Chemotherapy doses vary by indication. AML. ALL. Chronic myelocytic leukemia. Prophylaxis & treatment of meningeal leukemia, intrathecal (Cytosar-U, Tarabine). Depo-Cyt not approved in children.

NOTES - Reliable contraception is recommended. Monitor CBCs, LFTs & renal function. Decreases digoxin levels. Chemical arachnoiditis can be reduced by coadministration of dexamethasone. Use dexamethasone eye drops with high doses.

**DECITABINE (*Dacogen*)** ▶L ♀D ▶- $ varies by therapy
WARNING - Bone marrow suppression, pulmonary edema. Instruct patients to report promptly fever, sore throat, or signs of local infection, bleeding from any site, or symptoms suggestive of anemia.
ADULT - Chemotherapy doses vary by indication. Myelodysplastic syndromes.
PEDS - Not approved in children.
NOTES - Reliable contraception is recommended. Men should not father children during and two mo after therapy. Monitor CBCs, baseline LFTs.

**FLOXURIDINE (*FUDR*)** ▶L ♀D ▶- $ varies by therapy
WARNING - Bone marrow suppression, nephrotoxicity, increased LFTs, alopecia. Instruct patients to report promptly fever, sore throat, or signs of local infection, bleeding from any site, or symptoms suggestive of anemia.
ADULT - Chemotherapy doses vary by indication. GI adenocarcinoma metastatic to the liver given by intrahepatic arterial pump.
PEDS - Not approved in children.
NOTES - Reliable contraception is recommended. Monitor CBCs, LFTs & renal function.

**FLUDARABINE (*Fludara*)** ▶Serum ♀D ▶- $ varies by therapy
WARNING - Neurotoxicity (agitation, blindness, & coma), progressive multifocal leukoencephalopathy & death, bone marrow suppression, fertility impairment, hyperuricemia, alopecia. Instruct patients to report promptly fever, sore throat, or signs of local infection, bleeding from any site, or symptoms suggestive of anemia.
ADULT - Chemotherapy doses vary by indication. Chronic lymphocytic leukemia.
PEDS - Not approved in children.
UNAPPROVED ADULT - Non-Hodgkin's lymphoma. Mycosis fungoides. Hairy-cell leukemia. Hodgkin's disease.
NOTES - Reliable contraception is recommended. Monitor CBCs & renal function.

**FLUOROURACIL (*Adrucil, 5-FU*)** ▶L ♀D ▶- $ varies by therapy
WARNING - Increased INR and bleeding with warfarin. Bone marrow suppression, angina, fertility impairment, alopecia, diarrhea, mucositis, hand & foot syndrome (palmar plantar erythrodysesthesia). Instruct patients to report promptly fever, sore throat, signs of local infection, bleeding from any site, or symptoms suggestive of anemia.
ADULT - Chemotherapy doses vary by indication. Colon, rectum, breast, stomach, & pancreatic carcinoma. Dukes' stage C colon cancer with irinotecan or leucovorin after surgical resection.
PEDS - Not approved in children.
UNAPPROVED ADULT - Head & neck, renal cell, prostate, ovarian, esophageal, anal and topical to skin for basal and squamous cell carcinoma.
NOTES - Reliable contraception is recommended. Monitor CBCs.

**GEMCITABINE (*Gemzar*)** ▶intracellular ♀D ▶- $ varies by therapy
WARNING - Bone marrow suppression, fever, rash, increased LFTs, proteinuria, hematuria, alopecia. Instruct patients to report promptly fever, sore throat, signs of local infection, bleeding from any site, or symptoms suggestive of anemia.
ADULT - Chemotherapy doses vary by indication. Adenocarcinoma of the pancreas. Non-small cell lung cancer, in combination regimens. Metastatic breast cancer, in combination regimens. Advanced ovarian cancer.
PEDS - Not approved in children.
NOTES - Reliable contraception is recommended. Monitor CBCs, LFTs & renal function.

**HYDROXYUREA (*Hydrea, Droxia*)** ▶LK ♀D ▶- $ varies by therapy
WARNING - Bone marrow suppression, erythropoiesis, mucositis, nephrotoxicity, rash, alopecia. Instruct patients to report promptly fever, sore throat, signs of local infection, bleeding from any site, or symptoms suggestive of anemia. Cutaneous vasculitic toxicities, including vasculitic ulcerations and gangrene, have been reported most often in patients on interferon therapy.
ADULT - Chemotherapy doses vary by indication. Melanoma. CML. Recurrent, metastatic or inoperable carcinoma of the ovary. Squamous cell carcinoma of the head and neck, acute leukemia. Sickle cell anemia (Droxia): Start 15 mg/kg PO daily while monitoring CBC q 2 wk. If no marrow depression, then increase dose q 12 wk by 5 mg/kg/d (max 35 mg/kg/d). Give concomitant folic acid 1 mg/d.
PEDS - Not approved in children.
UNAPPROVED ADULT - Essential thrombocythemia at high risk for thrombosis: 0.5–1 g PO daily adjusted to keep platelets <400/mm³. Also has been used for HIV, psoriasis, polycythemia vera.
UNAPPROVED PEDS - Sickle cell anemia.
FORMS - Generic/Trade: Cap 500 mg. Trade only: (Droxia) Caps 200, 300, 400 mg.
NOTES - Reliable contraception is recommended. Monitor CBCs & renal function. Elderly may need lower doses. Minimize exposure to the drug by wearing gloves during handling.

**MERCAPTOPURINE (*6-MP, Purinethol*)** ▶L ♀D ▶- $ varies by therapy
WARNING - Bone marrow suppression, hepatotoxicity, hyperuricemia, alopecia. Instruct patients to report promptly fever, sore throat, signs of local infection, bleeding from any site, symptoms suggestive of anemia, or yellow discoloration of the skin or eyes.
ADULT - Chemotherapy doses vary by indication. ALL. AML. CML.
PEDS - Chemotherapy doses vary by indication. ALL. AML.
UNAPPROVED ADULT - Inflammatory bowel disease: Start at 50 mg PO daily, titrate to response. Typical dose range 0.5–1.5 mg/kg PO daily.
UNAPPROVED PEDS - Inflammatory bowel disease: 1.5 mg/kg PO daily.

(cont.)

**MERCAPTOPURINE** *(cont.)*
 FORMS - Generic/Trade: Tab 50 mg
 NOTES - Reliable contraception is recommended. Monitor CBCs, LFTs & renal function. Consider folate supplementation. Allopurinol & trimethoprim/sulfamethoxazole increase toxicity.

**NELARABINE** *(Arranon)* ▶LK ♀D ▶- $ varies by therapy
 WARNING - Peripheral neuropathy, paralysis, demyelination, severe somnolence, convulsions. Bone marrow suppression.
 ADULT - Chemotherapy doses vary by indication. ALL, T-cell lymphoblastic lymphoma.
 PEDS - Chemotherapy doses vary by indication. ALL, T-cell lymphoblastic lymphoma.
 NOTES - Reliable contraception is recommended. Monitor renal function.

**PEMETREXED** *(Alimta)* ▶K ♀D ▶- $ varies by therapy
 WARNING - Bone marrow suppression, rash. Instruct patients to report promptly fever, sore throat, signs of local infection, bleeding from any site, symptoms suggestive of anemia.
 ADULT - Chemotherapy doses vary by indication. Malignant pleural mesothelioma, in combination with cisplatin. Non-small cell lung cancer. Supplement with folic acid and B12.
 PEDS - Not approved in children.
 NOTES - Reliable contraception is recommended. Monitor CBCs & renal function. Do not use in patients with CrCl <45 mL/min. Avoid NSAIDs around the time of administration.

**PENTOSTATIN** *(Nipent)* ▶K ♀D ▶- $ varies by therapy
 WARNING - Bone marrow suppression, nephrotoxicity, hepatotoxicity, CNS toxicity, pulmonary toxicity, severe rash, fertility impairment, alopecia. Instruct patients to report promptly fever, sore throat, signs of local infection, bleeding from any site, symptoms suggestive of anemia, or yellow discoloration of the skin or eyes.
 ADULT - Chemotherapy doses vary by indication. Hairy cell leukemia, refractory to alpha-interferon.
 PEDS - Not approved in children.
 UNAPPROVED ADULT - ALL, CLL, Non-Hodgkin's Lymphoma, Mycosis fungoides.
 NOTES - Reliable contraception is recommended. Monitor CBCs & renal function.

**THIOGUANINE** *(Tabloid, ✦Lanvis)* ▶L ♀D ▶- $ varies by therapy
 WARNING - Bone marrow suppression, hepatotoxicity, hyperuricemia, alopecia. Instruct patients to report promptly fever, sore throat, signs of local infection, bleeding from any site, symptoms suggestive of anemia, or yellow discoloration of the skin or eyes.
 ADULT - Chemotherapy doses vary by indication. Acute nonlymphocytic leukemias.
 PEDS - Chemotherapy doses vary by indication. Acute nonlymphocytic leukemias.
 FORMS - Trade only: Tab 40 mg, scored.
 NOTES - Reliable contraception is recommended. Monitor CBCs & LFTs.

## ONCOLOGY: Cytoprotective Agents

**AMIFOSTINE** *(Ethyol)* ▶plasma ♀C ▶- $ varies by therapy
 WARNING - Hypotension, hypocalcemia, N/V, hypersensitivity.
 ADULT - Doses vary by indication. Reduction of renal toxicity w/cisplatin. Reduction of xerostomia & mucositis w/radiation.
 PEDS - Not approved in children.
 NOTES - Monitor calcium & BP.

**DEXRAZOXANE** *(Zinecard)* ▶plasma ♀C ▶- $ varies by therapy
 WARNING - Additive bone marrow suppression, secondary malignancies, fertility impairment, N/V.
 ADULT - Doses vary by indication. Reduction of cardiac toxicity w/doxorubicin.
 PEDS - Not approved in children.
 NOTES - Monitor CBCs.

**MESNA** *(Mesnex, ✦Uromitexan)* ▶plasma ♀B ▶- $ varies by therapy
 WARNING - Hypersensitivity, bad taste in the mouth.
 ADULT - Doses vary by indication. Reduction of hemorrhagic cystis w/ifosfamide.
 PEDS - Not approved in children.
 UNAPPROVED ADULT - Doses vary by indication. Reduction of hemorrhagic cystis w/high dose cyclophosphamide.
 UNAPPROVED PEDS - Doses vary by indication.
 FORMS - Trade only: Tab 400 mg, scored.
 NOTES - False positive test urine ketones.

**PALIFERMIN** *(Kepivance)* ▶plasma ♀C ▶? $ varies by therapy
 ADULT - Doses vary by indication. Decreases incidence, duration, and severity of severe oral mucositis in patients receiving therapy for hematologic malignancies.
 PEDS - Not approved in children.

## ONCOLOGY: Hormones

**ABARELIX** *(Plenaxis)* ▶plasma ♀X ▶- $ varies by therapy
 WARNING - Immediate-onset of systemic allergic reactions which increases with the duration of treatment. Patients should be observed for at least 30 min following each injection. Physicians

who have enrolled in Plenaxis PLUS Risk Management Program may prescribe. Serum testosterone suppression decreases with continued dosing in some patients. Effectiveness beyond 12 mo has not been established. Treatment failure can be detected by measuring serum total

**ABARELIX** *(cont.)*
testosterone concentrations just prior to administration on d 29 & every 8 wk thereafter.
ADULT - Palliative treatment of prostate cancer, in whom LHRH agonist therapy is not appropriate & who refuse surgical castration & have one or more of the following: risk of neurological compromise due to metastases, ureteral or bladder outlet obstruction due to local encroachment or metastatic disease, or severe bone pain from skeletal metastases persisting on narcotic analgesia. 100 mg IM to the buttock on d 1, 15, 29 (wk 4) & every 4 wk thereafter.
PEDS - Not approved in children.
NOTES - Monitor LFTs and PSA. Avoid use if known hypersensitivity with carboxymethylcellulose. May prolong QT interval. May decrease bone mineral density. Decreases in effectiveness are seen more in patients who weigh >225 pounds. MDs must be enrolled in the Plenaxis Prescribing Program.

**ANASTROZOLE** *(Arimidex)* ▶L ♀D ▶- $ varies by therapy
WARNING - Patients with estrogen receptor-negative disease & patients who do not respond to tamoxifen therapy rarely respond to anastrozole. Fertility impairment, vaginal bleeding, hot flashes, alopecia, decrease in bone mineral density.
ADULT - Chemotherapy doses vary by indication. Locally advanced or metastatic breast cancer. Adjuvant early breast cancer.
PEDS - Not approved in children.
FORMS - Trade only: Tab 1 mg.
NOTES - Reliable contraception is recommended. Monitor CBCs.

**BICALUTAMIDE** *(Casodex)* ▶L ♀X ▶- $ varies by therapy
WARNING - Hypersensitivity, hepatotoxicity, interstitial lung disease, gynecomastia/breast pain, fertility impairment, hot flashes, diarrhea, alopecia.
ADULT - Prostate cancer: 50 mg PO daily in combination with a LHRH analog (eg, goserelin or leuprolide). Not indicated in women.
PEDS - Not approved in children.
UNAPPROVED ADULT - Adjuvant prostate cancer.
FORMS - Trade only: Tab 50 mg.
NOTES - Monitor PSA levels & LFTs. Displaces warfarin, possibly increasing anticoagulant effects. Gynecomastia and breast pain occur.

**CYPROTERONE** *(◆ANDROCUR, ANDROCUR DEPOT)* ▶L ♀X ▶- $ varies by therapy
ADULT - Prostate cancer.
PEDS - Not approved in children.
FORMS - Generic/Trade: Tab 50 mg.
NOTES - Dose-related hepatotoxicity has occurred, monitor LFTs at initiation and during treatment. Monitor adrenocortical function periodically. May impair carbohydrate metabolism; monitor blood glucose, especially in diabetics.

**ESTRAMUSTINE** *(Emcyt)* ▶L ♀X ▶- $ varies by therapy
WARNING - Thrombosis, including MI, glucose intolerance, HTN, fluid retention, increased LFTs, alopecia.
ADULT - Chemotherapy doses vary by indication. Hormone refractory prostate cancer.

PEDS - Not approved in children.
FORMS - Trade only: Cap 140 mg.
NOTES - Reliable contraception is recommended. Monitor LFTs, glucose & BP. Milk, milk products & calcium-rich foods or drugs may impair absorption.

**EXEMESTANE** *(Aromasin)* ▶L ♀D ▶- $ varies by therapy
WARNING - Lymphocytopenia, alopecia.
ADULT - Chemotherapy doses vary by indication. Breast cancer.
PEDS - Not approved in children.
UNAPPROVED ADULT - Chemotherapy doses vary by indication. Prevention of prostate cancer.
FORMS - Trade only: Tab 25 mg.
NOTES - Contraindicated in premenopausal women. Reliable contraception is recommended. Monitor CBCs.

**FLUTAMIDE** *(Eulexin, ◆Euflex)* ▶L ♀D ▶- $ varies by therapy
WARNING - Hepatic failure, methemoglobinemia, hemolytic anemia, breast neoplasms, gynecomastia, fertility impairment, photosensitivity, alopecia.
ADULT - Prostate cancer: 250 mg PO q8h in combination with a LHRH analog (eg, goserelin or leuprolide). Not indicated in women.
PEDS - Not approved in children.
UNAPPROVED ADULT - Hirsutism in women.
FORMS - Generic only: Cap 125 mg.
NOTES - Monitor LFTs, PSA, methemoglobin levels. Transient urine discoloration (amber or yellow-green). Avoid exposure to sunlight/use sunscreen. Increased INR with warfarin. Gynecomastia and breast pain occur.

**FULVESTRANT** *(Faslodex)* ▶L ♀D ▶- $ varies by therapy
WARNING - Contraindicated in pregnancy. Hypersensitivity, N/V/D, constipation, abdominal pain, hot flashes.
ADULT - Chemotherapy doses vary by indication. Breast cancer.
PEDS - Not approved in children.
NOTES - Reliable contraception is recommended.

**GOSERELIN** *(Zoladex)* ▶LK ♀D/X ▶- $ varies by therapy
WARNING - Transient increases in sex hormones, increases in lipids, hypercalcemia, decreases in bone mineral density, vaginal bleeding, fertility impairment, hot flashes, decreased libido, alopecia.
ADULT - Prostate cancer: 3.6 mg implant SC into upper abdominal wall every 28 d, or 10.8 mg implant SC q12 wk. Endometriosis: 3.6 mg implant SC q 28 d or 10.8 mg implant q12 wk × 6 mo. Specialized dosing for breast cancer.
PEDS - Not approved in children.
UNAPPROVED ADULT - Adjuvant prostate cancer. Palliative treatment of breast cancer: 3.6 mg implant SC q28 d indefinitely. Endometrial thinning prior to ablation for dysfunctional uterine bleeding: 3.6 mg SC 4 wk prior to surgery or 3.6 mg SC q4 wk × 2 with surgery 2-4 wk after last dose.
FORMS - Trade only: Implants 3.6, 10.8 mg.

(cont.)

**GOSERELIN** *(cont.)*
NOTES - Transient increases in testosterone and estrogen occur. Hypercalcemia may occur in patients with bone metastases. Vaginal bleeding may occur during the first 2 mo of treatment & should stop spontaneously. Reliable contraception is recommended. Consider norethindrone as "addback" therapy to decrease bone loss (see norethindrone).

**HISTRELIN** *(Vantas, Supprelin LA)* ▶Not metabolized ♀X ▶- $ varies by therapy
WARNING - Worsening of symptoms, especially during the 1st wk of therapy: increase in bone pain, difficulty urinating. Decreases in bone mineral density.
ADULT - Palliative treatment of advanced prostate cancer: Insert 1 implant SC in the inner upper arm q12 mo. May repeat if appropriate after 12 mo.
PEDS - Central precocious puberty (Supprelin LA), >2 yo: Insert 1 implant SC in the inner upper arm. May repeat if appropriate after 12 mo.
FORMS - Trade only: 50 mg implant.
NOTES - Causes transient increase of testosterone level during the first wk of treatment which may create or exacerbate symptoms. Patients with metastatic vertebral lesions and/or urinary tract obstruction should be closely observed during the first few wk of therapy. Avoid wetting arm for 24h after implant insertion and from heavy lifting or strenuous exertion of the involved arm for 7 d after insertion. Measure testosterone levels and PSA periodically. May decrease bone density. Monitor LH, FSH, estradiol or testosterone, height & bone age in children with central precocious puberty at 1 mo post implantation & q6 mo thereafter.

**LETROZOLE** *(Femara)* ▶LK ♀D ▶- $ varies by therapy
WARNING - Fertility impairment, decreases in lymphocytes, increased LFTs, alopecia.
ADULT - Breast cancer: 2.5 mg PO daily.
PEDS - Not approved in children.
FORMS - Trade only: Tab 2.5 mg.
NOTES - Reliable contraception is recommended. Monitor CBCs, LFTs, & lipids.

**LEUPROLIDE** *(Eligard, Lupron, Lupron Depot, Oaklide, Viadur)* ▶L ♀X ▶- $ varies by therapy
WARNING - Worsening of symptoms: increase in bone pain, difficulty urinating. Decreases in bone mineral density. Anaphylaxis, alopecia.
ADULT - Advanced prostate cancer: Lupron: 1 mg SC daily. Eligard: 7.5mg SC q mo, 22.5mg SC q3 mo, 30 mg SC q4 mo, or 45 mg SC q6 mo. Lupron depot: 7.5mg IM q mo, 22.5mg IM q3 mo or 30 mg IM q4 mo. Viadur: 65 mg SC implant q12 mo. Endometriosis or

uterine leiomyomata (fibroids): 3.75 mg IM q mo or 11.25 mg IM q3 mo for total therapy of 6 mo (endometriosis) or 3 mo (fibroids). Administer concurrent iron for fibroid-associated anemia.
PEDS - Central precocious puberty: Injection: 50 mcg/kg/d SC. Increase by 10 mcg/kg/d until total down regulation. Depot-Ped: 0.3 mg/kg q4 wk IM (minimum dose 7.5 mg). Increase by 3.75 mg q4 wk IM until adequate down regulation.
NOTES - For prostate cancer, monitor testosterone, prostatic acid phosphatase & PSA levels. Transient increases in testosterone and estrogen occur. For endometriosis, a fractional dose of the 3-mo depot preparation is not equivalent to the same dose of the monthly formulation. Rotate the injection site periodically. Consider norethindrone as "addback" therapy to decrease bone loss (see norethindrone).

**NILUTAMIDE** *(Nilandron)* ▶L ♀C ▶- $ varies by therapy
WARNING - Interstitial pneumonitis, hepatitis, aplastic anemia (isolated cases), delay in adaptation to the dark, hot flashes, alcohol intolerance, alopecia.
ADULT - Prostate cancer: 300 mg PO daily for 30 d, then 150 mg PO daily. Begin therapy on same d as surgical castration.
PEDS - Not approved in children.
FORMS - Trade only: Tabs 150 mg.
NOTES - Monitor CBCs, LFTs & chest x-rays. Caution patients who experience delayed adaptation to the dark about driving at night or through tunnels; suggest wearing tinted glasses. May increase phenytoin & theophylline levels. Avoid alcohol.

**TOREMIFENE** *(Fareston)* ▶L ♀D ▶- $ varies by therapy
WARNING - Hypercalcemia & tumor flare, endometrial hyperplasia, thromboembolism, hot flashes, vaginal bleeding, fertility impairment, alopecia.
ADULT - Chemotherapy doses vary by indication. Breast cancer.
PEDS - Not approved in children.
FORMS - Trade only: Tab 60 mg.
NOTES - Reliable contraception is recommended. Monitor CBCs, calcium levels & LFTs. May increase effects of anticoagulants.

**TRIPTORELIN** *(Trelstar Depot)* ▶LK ♀X ▶- $ varies by therapy
WARNING - Transient increases in sex hormones, bone pain, neuropathy, hematuria, urethral/bladder outlet obstruction, spinal cord compression, anaphylaxis, hot flashes, impotence, alopecia.
ADULT - Chemotherapy doses vary by indication. Prostate cancer.
PEDS - Not approved in children.

## ONCOLOGY: Immunomodulators

**ALDESLEUKIN** *(Proleukin, interleukin-2)* ▶K ♀C ▶- $ varies by therapy
WARNING - Capillary leak syndrome, resulting in hypotension & reduced organ perfusion. Exacerbation of autoimmune diseases & symptoms of CNS metastases, impaired neutrophil function, hepato/nephrotoxicity, mental status changes, decreased thyroid function,

anemia, thrombocytopenia, fertility impairment, alopecia.
ADULT - Chemotherapy doses vary by indication. Renal-cell carcinoma.
PEDS - Not approved in children.
UNAPPROVED ADULT - Kaposi's sarcoma. Metastatic melanoma. Colorectal cancer. Non-Hodgkin's lymphoma.

**ALDESLEUKIN** (*cont.*)
NOTES - Monitor CBCs, electrolytes, LFTs, renal function & chest x-rays. Baseline PFTs. Avoid iodinated contrast media. Antihypertensives potentiate hypotension.

**ALEMTUZUMAB** (*Campath*, ◆*MabCampath*) ▶? ♀C ▶- $ varies by therapy
WARNING - Idiopathic thrombocytopenic purpura, bone marrow suppression, hemolytic anemia, hypersensitivity, & immunosuppression.
ADULT - Chemotherapy doses vary by indication. B-cell chronic lymphocytic leukemia.
PEDS - Not approved in children.
NOTES - Monitor CBC.

**BCG** (*Bacillus of Calmette & Guerin, Pacis, TheraCys, Tice BCG,* ◆*Oncotice, Immucyst*) ▶Not metabolized ♀C ▶? $ varies by therapy
WARNING - Hypersensitivity, hematuria, urinary frequency, dysuria, bacterial urinary tract infection, flu-like syndrome, alopecia.
ADULT - Chemotherapy doses vary by indication. Carcinoma in situ of the urinary bladder, intravesical.
PEDS - Not approved in children.
NOTES - Bone marrow depressants, immunosuppressants & antimicrobial therapy may impair response. Increase fluid intake after treatments.

**BEVACIZUMAB** (*Avastin*) ▶? ♀C ▶- $ varies by therapy
WARNING - CVA, MI, TIA, angina, GI perforation, wound dehiscence, serious hemorrhage, HTN, heart failure, nephrotic syndrome, reversible posterior leukoencephalopathy syndrome (brain capillary leak syndrome), nasal septum perforation. Tracheoesophageal fistula has been reported. Microangiopathic hemolytic anemia (MAHA) in patients on concomitant sunitinib malate.
ADULT - Chemotherapy doses vary by indication. Metastatic colorectal carcinoma, non-small cell lung cancer.
PEDS - Not approved in children.
NOTES - Monitor BP, and UA for protein. Do not use in combination with sunitinib.

**CETUXIMAB** (*Erbitux*) ▶? ♀C ▶- $ varies by therapy
WARNING - Anaphylaxis, cardiopulmonary arrest/sudden death, pulmonary toxicity, rash, sepsis, renal failure, pulmonary embolus, hypomagnesemia.
ADULT - Chemotherapy doses vary by indication. Metastatic colorectal carcinoma, head & neck squamous cell carcinoma.
PEDS - Not approved in children.
NOTES - Monitor renal function & electrolytes including magnesium. Caution with known coronary artery disease, heart failure, or arrhythmias. Premedication with a H1-antagonist and a 1-h observation period after infusion is recommended due to potential for anaphylaxis.

**DASATINIB** (*Sprycel*) ▶L ♀D ▶- $ varies by therapy
WARNING - Bone marrow suppression, hemorrhage, prolonged QT interval, pleural effusion.
ADULT - Chemotherapy doses vary by indication. CML. ALL.
PEDS - Not approved in children.
FORMS - Trade only: Tabs 20, 50, 70 mg.

NOTES - Reliable contraception is recommended. Monitor LFTs, CBCs, and weight. Monitor for signs and symptoms of fluid retention. Increased by ketoconazole, erythromycin, itraconazole, clarithromycin, ritonavir, atazanavir, indinavir, nelfinavir, saquinavir & telithromycin. Decreased by rifampin, phenytoin, carbamazepine, phenobarbital & dexamethasone. Increases simvastatin. Antacids should be taken at least 2 h pre- or post-dose. Avoid H2 blockers and PPIs.

**DENILEUKIN** (*Ontak*) ▶Plasma ♀C ▶- $ varies by therapy
WARNING - Hypersensitivity, vascular leak syndrome (hypotension, edema, hypoalbuminemia), visual loss, thrombosis, rash, diarrhea, alopecia.
ADULT - Chemotherapy doses vary by indication. Cutaneous T-cell lymphoma.
PEDS - Not approved in children.
NOTES - Monitor CBCs, LFTs & renal function. Visual loss is usually persistent.

**ERLOTINIB** (*Tarceva*) ▶L ♀D ▶- $ varies by therapy
WARNING - Interstitial lung disease, acute renal failure.
ADULT - Chemotherapy doses vary by indication. Non-small cell lung cancer, pancreatic cancer.
PEDS - Not approved in children.
FORMS - Trade only: Tabs 25, 100, 150 mg.
NOTES - Reliable contraception is recommended. CYP3A4 inhibitors such as ketoconazole increase concentrations. CYP3A4 inducers such as rifampin decrease concentrations. Increases INR in patients on warfarin. Monitor LFTs.

**GEMTUZUMAB** (*Mylotarg*) ▶Not metabolized ♀D ▶- $ varies by therapy
WARNING - Bone marrow suppression, infusion-related reactions, pulmonary edema, hepatic veno-occlusive disease.
ADULT - Chemotherapy doses vary by indication. Acute myeloid leukemia.
PEDS - Not approved in children.
NOTES - Reliable contraception is recommended. Monitor CBC, LFTs.

**IBRITUMOMAB** (*Zevalin*) ▶L ♀D ▶- $ varies by therapy
WARNING - Contraindicated in patients with allergy to murine proteins. Fatal infusion reactions, severe cutaneous & mucocutaneous reactions, bone marrow suppression, hypersensitivity.
ADULT - Chemotherapy doses vary by indication. Non-Hodgkin's lymphoma.
PEDS - Not approved in children.
NOTES - Reliable contraception is recommended. Monitor CBCs.

**IMATINIB** (*Gleevec*) ▶L ♀D ▶- $ varies by therapy
WARNING - Bone marrow suppression, increased LFTs, hemorrhage, erythema multiforme, Stevens-Johnson syndrome, N/V, pulmonary edema, CHF, muscle cramps.
ADULT - Chemotherapy doses vary by indication. CML. GI stromal tumors (GIST).
PEDS - Chemotherapy doses vary by indication. CML.
FORMS - Trade only: Tab 100, 400 mg.

(cont.)

**IMATINIB** *(cont.)*
NOTES - Reliable contraception is recommended. Monitor LFTs, CBCs, and weight. Monitor for signs and symptoms of fluid retention. Increased by ketoconazole, erythromycin, itraconazole, clarithromycin. Decreased by phenytoin, carbamazepine, rifampin, phenobarbital, St. John's wort. Increases acetaminophen levels & warfarin effects. Monitor INR.

**INTERFERON ALFA-2A** *(Roferon-A)* ▶Plasma ♀C ▶- $ varies by therapy
WARNING - GI hemorrhage, CNS reactions, leukopenia, increased LFTs, anemia, neutralizing antibodies, depression/suicidal behavior, alopecia.
ADULT - Discontinued by manufacturer February 2008. Chemotherapy doses vary by indication. Hairy cell leukemia. AIDS-related Kaposi's sarcoma. CML.
PEDS - Not approved in children.
UNAPPROVED ADULT - Superficial bladder tumors. Carcinoid tumor. Cutaneous T-cell lymphoma. Essential thrombocythemia. Non-Hodgkin's lymphoma.
UNAPPROVED PEDS - CML
NOTES - Reliable contraception is recommended. Monitor CBCs & LFTs. Hydration important. Decreases clearance of theophylline.

**LAPATINIB** *(Tykerb)* ▶L ♀D ▶- $ varies by therapy
WARNING - Decreased left ventricular ejection fraction, QT prolongation, interstitial lung disease, pneumonitis, severe diarrhea.
ADULT - Chemotherapy doses vary by indication. Advanced or metastatic breast cancer.
PEDS - Not approved in children.
FORMS - Trade only: Tab 250 mg.
NOTES - Reliable contraception is recommended. Monitor LVEF, EKG, and LFTs. Increased by ketoconazole, erythromycin, itraconazole, clarithromycin. Decreased by phenytoin, carbamazepine, rifampin, phenobarbital, St. John's wort. Increases acetaminophen levels & warfarin effects. Must be taken 1 h pre- or post-meals.

**NILOTINIB** *(Tasigna)* ▶L ♀D ▶- $ varies by therapy
WARNING - Prolonged QT interval & sudden death, bone marrow suppression, intracranial hemorrhage, pneumonia, elevated lipase.
ADULT - Chemotherapy doses vary by indication. CML.
PEDS - Not approved in children.
FORMS - Trade only: Caps, 200 mg.
NOTES - Contraindicated with hypokalemia, hypomagnesemia, or long QT syndrome. Reliable contraception is recommended. Monitor EKG, LFTs, CBCs & lipase. Increased by potent CYP450 inhibitors such as ketoconazole and decreased by CYP450 inducers such as rifampin. Avoid food at least 2 h pre- or 1 h post-dose.

**PANITUMUMAB** *(Vectibix)* ▶Not metabolized ♀C ▶- $ varies by therapy
WARNING - Skin exfoliation, severe dermatologic reactions complicated by sepsis & death. Anaphylaxis.
ADULT - Chemotherapy doses vary by indication. Metastatic colorectal carcinoma.

PEDS - Not approved in children.
NOTES - Reliable contraception is recommended. Monitor potassium & magnesium.

**RITUXIMAB** *(Rituxan)* ▶Not metabolized ♀C ▶- $ varies by therapy
WARNING - Contraindicated if allergy to murine proteins. Fatal infusion reactions, tumor lysis syndrome, severe mucocutaneous reactions, cardiac arrhythmias, nephrotoxicity, bowel obstruction/perforation, hypersensitivity, neutropenia, thrombocytopenia, anemia, serious viral infections with death. Hepatitis B virus reactivation with fulminant hepatitis, liver failure and death in patients with hematologic malignancies have been reported; monitor hepatitis B carriers closely. Two cases of fatal progressive multifocal leukoencephalopathy have been reported.
ADULT - RA: 1000 mg IV infusion weekly x2 in combination with methotrexate and methylprednisolone 100 mg IV pretreatment. Chemotherapy doses vary by indication. Non-Hodgkin's lymphoma.
PEDS - Not approved in children.
UNAPPROVED ADULT - Immune thrombocytopenic purpura (ITP), thrombotic thrombocytopenic purpura (TTP), multiple sclerosis.
NOTES - Monitor CBCs.

**SUNITINIB** *(Sutent)* ▶L ♀D ▶- $ varies by therapy
WARNING - Decrease in left ventricular ejection fraction with possible clinical CHF, bone marrow suppression, bleeding, hypertension, yellow skin discoloration, depigmentation of hair or skin.
ADULT - Chemotherapy doses vary by indication. Gastrointestinal stromal tumors, advanced renal cell carcinoma.
PEDS - Not approved in children.
FORMS - Trade only: Caps 12.5, 25, 50 mg.
NOTES - Reliable contraception is recommended. CYP3A4 inhibitors such as ketoconazole increase concentrations. CYP3A4 inducers such as rifampin & St John's wort can decrease concentrations. Increases INR in patients on warfarin. Monitor CBC.

**TEMSIROLIMUS** *(Torisel)* ▶L ♀C ▶- $ varies by therapy
WARNING - Hypersensitivity, interstitial lung disease, bowel perforation, renal failure, hyperglycemia, bone marrow suppression. Avoid live vaccines.
ADULT - Chemotherapy doses vary by indication. Advanced renal cell carcinoma.
PEDS - Not approved in children.
NOTES - Reliable contraception is recommended. Drugs that induce the CYP4503A4 system such as phenytoin, phenobarbital, rifampin may decrease concentrations. Inhibitors such as clarithromycin, itraconazole, ketoconazole and ritonavir may increase concentrations. Avoid live vaccines. Monitor CBC, hepatic & renal function, glucose and lipid profile.

**TOSITUMOMAB** *(Bexxar)* ▶Not metabolized ♀X ▶- $ varies by therapy
WARNING - Contraindicated in patients with allergy to murine proteins. Hypersensitivity, anaphylaxis,

**TOSITUMOMAB** (*cont.*)
infusion reactions, neutropenia, thrombocytopenia, anemia. Hypothyroidism.
ADULT - Chemotherapy doses vary by indication. Follicular, non-Hodgkin's lymphoma unresponsive to rituximab.
PEDS - Not approved in children.
NOTES - This product is a combination of tositumomab + iodine I 131 tositumomab. Reliable contraception is recommended. Monitor CBC, TSH.
**TRASTUZUMAB** (*Herceptin*) ▶Not metabolized ♀B ▶- $ varies by therapy

WARNING - Hypersensitivity, including fatal anaphylaxis, fatal infusion-related reactions, pulmonary events including ARDS & death, ventricular dysfunction & heart failure. Anemia, leukopenia, diarrhea, alopecia.
ADULT - Chemotherapy doses vary by indication. Breast cancer with tumors overexpressing the HER2 NEU protein.
PEDS - Not approved in children.
NOTES - Monitor w/ECG, echocardiogram, or MUGA scan. CBCs.

## ONCOLOGY: Mitotic Inhibitors

**DOCETAXEL** (*Taxotere*) ▶L ♀D ▶- $ varies by therapy
WARNING - Severe hypersensitivity with anaphylaxis, bone marrow suppression, fluid retention, neutropenia, rash, erythema of the extremities, nail hypo- or hyperpigmentation, hepatotoxicity, paresthesia/dysesthesia, asthenia, fertility impairment, alopecia. Instruct patients to report promptly fever, sore throat, or signs of local infection.
ADULT - Chemotherapy doses vary by indication. Breast cancer. Non-small cell lung cancer. Prostate cancer, in combination with prednisone. Advanced gastric adenocarcinoma with cisplatin and fluorouracil. Squamous cell carcinoma of the head & neck.
PEDS - Not approved in children.
UNAPPROVED ADULT - Gastric cancer. Melanoma. Non-Hodgkin's lymphoma. Ovarian cancer. Pancreatic cancer. Prostate cancer. Small-cell lung cancer. Soft-tissue sarcoma. Urothelial cancer. Adjuvant and neoadjuvant breast cancer.
NOTES - Reliable contraception is recommended. Monitor CBCs & LFTs. CYP3A4 inhibitors or substrates may lead to significant increases in blood concentrations.
**ETOPOSIDE** (*VP-16, Etopophos, Toposar, VePesid*) ▶K ♀D ▶- $ varies by therapy
WARNING - Bone marrow suppression, anaphylaxis, hypotension, CNS depression, alopecia. Instruct patients to report promptly fever, sore throat, or signs of local infection.
ADULT - Chemotherapy doses vary by indication. Testicular cancer. Small cell lung cancer, in combination regimens.
PEDS - Not approved in children.
UNAPPROVED ADULT - AML. Hodgkin's disease. Non-Hodgkin's lymphomas. Kaposi's Sarcoma. Neuroblastoma. Choriocarcinoma. Rhabdomyosarcoma. Hepatocellular carcinoma. Epithelial ovarian, non-small & small cell lung, testicular, gastric, endometrial & breast cancers. ALL. Soft tissue sarcoma.
FORMS - Generic/Trade: Cap 50 mg. Injection for hospital/clinic use; not intended for outpatient prescribing.
NOTES - Reliable contraception is recommended. Monitor CBCs, LFTs & renal function. May increase INR w/warfarin.

**IXABEPILONE** (*Ixempra*) ▶L ♀D ▶- $ varies by therapy
WARNING - Contraindicated in patients with AST or ALT ≥ 2.5X or bilirubin $> = 1 \times$ upper limit of normal. Contraindicated in patients with hypersensitivity reactions to products containing Cremophor EL (polyoxyethylated castor oil). Neutropenia. Instruct patients to report promptly fever, sore throat, signs of local infection or anemia.
ADULT - Chemotherapy doses vary by indication. Metastatic or locally advanced breast cancer.
PEDS - Not approved in children.
NOTES - CYP450 inhibitors such as ketoconazole may increase concentration; inducers such as rifampin, phenytoin or carbamazepine may reduce levels.
**PACLITAXEL** (*Taxol, Abraxane, Onxol*) ▶L ♀D ▶- $ varies by therapy
WARNING - Anaphylaxis, bone marrow suppression, cardiac conduction abnormalities, peripheral neuropathy, fertility impairment, alopecia. Contraindicated in patients with hypersensitivity reactions to products containing Cremophor EL (polyoxyethylated castor oil). Instruct patients to report promptly fever, sore throat, signs of local infection or anemia.
ADULT - Chemotherapy doses vary by indication. Ovarian cancer. Metastatic breast cancer. Non-small cell lung cancer, in combination regimens. AIDS-related Kaposi's sarcoma.
PEDS - Not approved in children.
UNAPPROVED ADULT - Advanced head and neck cancer. Small-cell lung cancer. Adenocarcinoma of the upper GI tract. Gastric, esophageal and colon adenocarcinoma. Hormone-refractory prostate cancer. Non-Hodgkin's lymphoma. Transitional cell carcinoma of the urothelium. Adenocarcinoma or unknown primary, adjuvant and neoadjuvant breast cancer, uterine cancer. Pancreatic cancer. Polycystic kidney disease.
NOTES - Abraxane is a form of paclitaxel bound to albumin. Reliable contraception is recommended. Monitor CBCs. Ketoconazole, felodipine, diazepam, & estradiol may increase paclitaxel.
**TENIPOSIDE** (*Vumon, VM-26*) ▶K ♀D ▶- $ varies by therapy
WARNING - Bone marrow suppression, anaphylaxis, hypotension, CNS depression, alopecia. Instruct

(cont.)

**TENIPOSIDE** *(cont.)*
patients to report promptly fever, sore throat, or signs of local infection.
ADULT - Not approved in adult patients.
PEDS - Chemotherapy doses vary by indication. ALL, refractory, in combination regimens.
NOTES - Reliable contraception is recommended. Monitor CBCs, LFTs & renal function.

**VINBLASTINE (*Velban, VLB*)** ▶L ♀D ▶- $ varies by therapy
WARNING - Extravasation associated w/severe necrosis. Leukopenia, fertility impairment, bronchospasm, alopecia. Instruct patients to report promptly fever, sore throat, or signs of local infection.
ADULT - Chemotherapy doses vary by indication. Hodgkin's disease. Non-Hodgkin's' lymphoma. Histiocytic lymphoma. Mycosis fungoides. Advanced testicular carcinoma. Kaposi's sarcoma. Letterer-Siwe disease (histiocytosis X). Choriocarcinoma. Breast cancer.
PEDS - Not approved in children.
UNAPPROVED ADULT - Non small cell lung cancer, renal cancer, CML.
NOTES - Reliable contraception is recommended. May decrease phenytoin levels. Erythromycin/drugs that inhibit CYP450 enzymes may increase toxicity.

**VINCRISTINE (*Oncovin, Vincasar, VCR*)** ▶L ♀D ▶- $ varies by therapy
WARNING - Extravasation associated w/severe necrosis. CNS toxicity, hypersensitivity, bone marrow suppression, hyperuricemia, bronchospasm, fertility impairment, alopecia. Instruct patients to report promptly fever, sore throat, signs of local infection or anemia.
ADULT - Chemotherapy doses vary by indication. ALL. Hodgkin's disease. Non-Hodgkin's lymphomas. Rhabdomyosarcoma. Neuroblastoma. Wilms' tumor. All in combination regimens.
PEDS - Chemotherapy doses vary by indication. Acute leukemia. Sarcoma, multiple myeloma.
UNAPPROVED ADULT - Idiopathic thrombocytopenic purpura. Kaposi's sarcoma. Breast cancer. Bladder cancer.
NOTES - Reliable contraception is recommended. Monitor CBCs. May decrease phenytoin & digoxin levels.

**VINORELBINE (*Navelbine*)** ▶L ♀D ▶- $ varies by therapy
WARNING - Extravasation associated w/severe necrosis. Granulocytopenia, pulmonary toxicity, bronchospasm, peripheral neuropathy, increased LFTs, alopecia. Instruct patients to report promptly fever, sore throat, or signs of local infection.
ADULT - Chemotherapy doses vary by indication. Non-small cell lung cancer, alone or in combination regimens.
PEDS - Not approved in children.
UNAPPROVED ADULT - Breast cancer. Cervical carcinoma. Desmoid tumors. Kaposi's sarcoma. Ovarian, Hodgkin's disease, head & neck cancer.
NOTES - Reliable contraception is recommended. Monitor CBCs. Drugs that inhibit CYP450 enzymes may increase toxicity.

## ONCOLOGY: Platinum-Containing Agents

**CARBOPLATIN (*Paraplatin*)** ▶K ♀D ▶- $ varies by therapy
WARNING - Secondary malignancies, bone marrow suppression, increased in patients with renal insufficiency; emesis, anaphylaxis, nephrotoxicity, peripheral neuropathy, increased LFTs, alopecia. Instruct patients to report promptly fever, sore throat, signs of local infection, bleeding from any site, symptoms suggestive of anemia, or yellow discoloration of the skin or eyes.
ADULT - Chemotherapy doses vary by indication. Ovarian carcinoma.
PEDS - Not approved in children.
UNAPPROVED ADULT - Small cell lung cancer, in combination regimens. Squamous cell carcinoma of the head & neck. Advanced endometrial cancer. Acute leukemia. Seminoma of testicular cancer. Non small cell lung cancer. Adenocarcinoma of unknown primary. Cervical cancer. Bladder carcinoma.
NOTES - Reliable contraception is recommended. Monitor CBCs, LFTs & renal function. May decrease phenytoin levels.

**CISPLATIN (*Platinol-AQ*)** ▶K ♀D ▶- $ varies by therapy
WARNING - Secondary malignancies, nephrotoxicity, bone marrow suppression, N/V, very highly emetogenic, ototoxicity, anaphylaxis, hepatotoxicity, vascular toxicity, hyperuricemia, electrolyte disturbances, optic neuritis, papilledema & cerebral blindness, neuropathies, muscle cramps, alopecia. Amifostine can be used to reduce renal toxicity in patients w/advanced ovarian cancer. Instruct patients to report promptly fever, sore throat, signs of local infection, bleeding from any site, symptoms suggestive of anemia, or yellow discoloration of the skin or eyes.
ADULT - Chemotherapy doses vary by indication. Metastatic testicular & ovarian tumors, bladder cancer.
PEDS - Not approved in children.
UNAPPROVED ADULT - Esophageal cancer, gastric cancer, non small cell lung cancer & small cell lung cancer, head & neck cancer, endometrial cancer, cervical cancer, neoadjuvant bladder sparing chemotherapy, sarcoma.
NOTES - Reliable contraception is recommended. Monitor CBCs, LFTs, renal function & electrolytes. Audiometry. Aminoglycosides potentiate renal toxicity. Decreases phenytoin levels. Patients >65 yo may be more susceptible to nephrotoxicity, bone marrow suppression & peripheral neuropathy.

**OXALIPLATIN (*Eloxatin*)** ▶LK ♀D ▶- $ varies by therapy
WARNING - Anaphylaxis, neuropathy, pulmonary fibrosis, bone marrow suppression, N/V/D, fertility impairment. Instruct patients to report promptly fever, sore throat, signs of local infection, bleeding from any site, or symptoms suggestive of anemia.
ADULT - Chemotherapy doses vary by indication. Colorectal cancer w/5 FU + leucovorin.
PEDS - Not approved in children.
NOTES - Reliable contraception is recommended. Monitor CBCs and renal function.

## ONCOLOGY: Radiopharmaceuticals

**SAMARIUM 153 (*Quadramet*)** ▶Not metabolized ♀C ▶- $ varies by therapy
WARNING - Bone marrow suppression, flare reactions. Instruct patients to report promptly fever, sore throat, signs of local infection or anemia.
ADULT - Chemotherapy doses vary by indication. Osteoblastic metastatic bone lesions, relief of pain.
PEDS - Not approved in children.
UNAPPROVED ADULT - Ankylosing spondylitis. Paget's disease. RA.
NOTES - Reliable contraception is recommended. Monitor CBCs. Radioactivity in excreted urine × 12h after dose.

**STRONTIUM-89 (*Metastron*)** ▶K ♀D ▶- $ varies by therapy
WARNING - Bone marrow suppression, flare reactions, flushing sensation. Instruct patients to report promptly fever, sore throat, signs of local infection or anemia.
ADULT - Chemotherapy doses vary by indication. Painful skeletal metastases, relief of bone pain.
PEDS - Not approved in children.
NOTES - Reliable contraception is recommended. Monitor CBCs. Radioactivity in excreted urine × 12h after dose.

## ONCOLOGY: Miscellaneous

**ARSENIC TRIOXIDE (*Trisenox*)** ▶L ♀D ▶- $ varies by therapy
WARNING - APL differentiation syndrome: fever, dyspnea, weight gain, pulmonary infiltrates & pleural/pericardial effusions, occasionally with impaired myocardial contractility & episodic hypotension, with or w/o leukocytosis. QT prolongation, AV block, torsade de pointes, N/V/D, hyperglycemia, alopecia.
ADULT - Chemotherapy doses vary by indication. Acute promyelocytic leukemia, refractory.
PEDS - Not approved in children <5 yo. Chemotherapy doses vary by indication. Acute promyelocytic leukemia, refractory.
UNAPPROVED ADULT - Chemotherapy doses vary by indication. Chronic myeloid leukemia. ALL.
NOTES - Reliable contraception is recommended. Monitor ECG, electrolytes, renal function, CBCs & PT.

**ASPARAGINASE (*Elspar*, ✦*Kidrolase*)** ▶? ♀C ▶- $ varies by therapy
WARNING - Contraindicated with previous/current pancreatitis. Anaphylaxis, bone marrow suppression, bleeding, hyperglycemia, pancreatitis, hepato/nephrotoxicity, alopecia. Instruct patients to report promptly fever, sore throat, signs of local infection, bleeding from any site, or symptoms suggestive of anemia.
ADULT - Chemotherapy doses vary by indication. ALL, in combination regimens.
PEDS - Chemotherapy doses vary by indication. ALL, in combination regimens.
NOTES - Toxicity greater in children. Monitor CBCs, LFTs, renal function, PT, glucose & amylase. May interfere with interpretation of thyroid function tests.

**BEXAROTENE (*Targretin*)** ▶L ♀X ▶- $ varies by therapy
WARNING - Gel: Rash, pruritus, contact dermatitis. Caps: lipid abnormalities, increased LFTs, pancreatitis, hypothyroidism, leukopenia, cataracts, photosensitivity, alopecia.
ADULT - Chemotherapy doses vary by indication. Cutaneous T-cell lymphoma.
PEDS - Not approved in children.
FORMS - Trade only: 1% gel (60 g). Cap 75 mg.
NOTES - Gel: Do not use with DEET (insect repellant) or occlusive dressings. Caps: Monitor lipids, LFTs, thyroid function tests, CBCs. Multiple drug interactions; consult product insert for info. Reliable contraception is recommended.

**BORTEZOMIB (*Velcade*)** ▶L ♀D ▶- $ varies by therapy
WARNING - Peripheral neuropathy, orthostatic hypotension, heart failure, pneumonia, acute respiratory distress syndrome, thrombocytopenia, neutropenia, N/V/D. Instruct patients to report promptly acute onset of dyspnea, cough and low-grade fever and bleeding from any site.
ADULT - Chemotherapy doses vary by indication. Multiple myeloma, mantle cell lymphoma.
PEDS - Not approved in children.
NOTES - Reliable contraception is recommended. Monitor CBCs.

**DEXRAZOXANE (*Totect*)** ▶K ♀D ▶- $ varies by therapy
ADULT - Treatment of anthracycline extravasation; give ASAP within 6 h of extravasation.
PEDS - Not approved in children.
NOTES - Monitor CBCs & LFTs. Decrease dose by 50% if CrCl <40 mL/min.

**GEFITINIB (*Iressa*)** ▶L ♀D ▶- $ varies by therapy
WARNING - Pulmonary toxicity, corneal erosion, N/V. Instruct patients to report promptly acute onset of dyspnea, cough and low-grade fever.

(cont.)

**GEFITINIB** (cont.)
ADULT - Chemotherapy doses vary by indication. Non-small cell lung cancer.
PEDS - Not approved in children.
FORMS - Trade only: Tab 250 mg.
NOTES - Reliable contraception is recommended. Monitor LFTs. Potent inducers of CYP3A4 (eg, rifampin, phenytoin) decrease concentration; use 500 mg. May increase warfarin effect; monitor INR. Potent inhibitors of CYP3A4 (eg, ketoconazole, itraconazole) increase toxicity. Ranitidine increases concentrations.

**IRINOTECAN** (*Camptosar*) ▶L ♀D ▶- $ varies by therapy
WARNING - Diarrhea & dehydration (may be life-threatening), bone marrow suppression (worse w/radiation), orthostatic hypotension, colitis, hypersensitivity, pancreatitis. Instruct patients to report promptly diarrhea, fever, sore throat, signs of local infection, bleeding from any site, or symptoms suggestive of anemia.
ADULT - Chemotherapy doses vary by indication. Metastatic carcinoma of the colon or rectum, in combination regimens
PEDS - Not approved in children.
UNAPPROVED ADULT - Non small cell lung cancer and small cell lung cancer, ovarian and cervical cancer.
NOTES - Enzyme-inducing drugs such as phenytoin, phenobarbital, carbamazepine, rifampin, & St John's wort decrease concentrations and possibly effectiveness. Ketoconazole is contraindicated during therapy. Atazanavir increases concentrations. Reliable contraception is recommended. Monitor CBCs. May want to withhold diuretics during active N/V. Avoid laxatives. Loperamide/fluids/electrolytes for diarrhea. Consider atropine for cholinergic symptoms during the infusion.

**LENALIDOMIDE** (*Revlimid*) ▶K ♀X ▶- $ varies by therapy
WARNING - Potential for human birth defects, bone marrow suppression, DVT and PE. Instruct patients to report promptly fever, sore throat, signs of local infection, bleeding from any site, or symptoms suggestive of anemia.
ADULT - Chemotherapy doses vary by indication. Transfusion-dependent anemia due to myelodysplastic syndromes. Multiple myeloma.
PEDS - Not approved in children.
FORMS - Trade only: Caps 5, 10, 15, 25 mg.
NOTES - Analog of thalidomide — can cause birth defects or fetal death. Available only through a restricted distribution program. Reliable contraception is mandated; males must use a latex condom. Monitor CBCs. Do not break, chew or open the caps.

**LEUCOVORIN** (*Wellcovorin, folinic acid*) ▶gut ♀C ▶? $ varies by therapy
WARNING - Allergic sensitization.
ADULT - Doses vary by indication. Reduction of toxicity due to folic acid antagonists, ie, methotrexate. Colorectal cancer w/5-FU. Megaloblastic anemias.

PEDS - Not approved in children.
FORMS - Generic only: Tabs 5, 10, 15, 25 mg. Injection for hospital/oncology clinic use; not intended for outpatient prescribing.
NOTES - Monitor methotrexate concentrations & CBCs.

**LEVOLEUCOVORIN** (*Fusilev*) ▶gut ♀C ▶? $ varies by therapy
WARNING - Allergic sensitization.
ADULT - Doses vary by indication. Reduction of toxicity due to high-dose methotrexate for osteosarcoma.
PEDS - Not approved in children.
NOTES - Monitor methotrexate concentrations & CBCs.

**MITOTANE** (*Lysodren*) ▶L ♀C ▶- $ varies by therapy
WARNING - Adrenal insufficiency, depression. Instruct patients to report promptly if N/V, loss of appetite, diarrhea, mental depression, skin rash or darkening of the skin occurs. N/V/D, alopecia.
ADULT - Chemotherapy doses vary by indication. Adrenal cortical carcinoma, inoperable.
PEDS - Not approved in children.
FORMS - Trade only: Tab 500 mg.
NOTES - Hold after shock or trauma; give systemic steroids. Behavioral & neurological assessments at regular intervals when continuous treatment >2 yr. May decrease steroid & warfarin effects. Reliable contraception is recommended.

**PEGASPARGASE** (*Oncaspar*) ▶? ♀C ▶- $ varies by therapy
WARNING - Contraindicated with previous/current pancreatitis. Hypersensitivity, including anaphylaxis. Bone marrow suppression, bleeding, hyperuricemia, hyperglycemia, hepato/nephrotoxicity, CNS toxicity, N/V/D, alopecia.
ADULT - Chemotherapy doses vary by indication. ALL, in combination regimens.
PEDS - Chemotherapy doses vary by indication. ALL, in combination regimens.
NOTES - Monitor CBCs, LFTs, renal function, amylase, glucose & PT. Bleeding potentiated with warfarin, heparin, dipyridamole, aspirin or NSAIDs.

**PORFIMER** (*Photofrin*) ▶? ♀C ▶- $ varies by therapy
WARNING - Photosensitivity, ocular sensitivity, chest pain, respiratory distress, constipation.
ADULT - Chemotherapy doses vary by indication. Esophageal cancer. Endobronchial non-small cell lung cancer (both w/laser therapy).
PEDS - Not approved in children.
NOTES - Avoid concurrent photosensitizing drugs.

**SORAFENIB** (*Nexavar*) ▶L ♀D ▶- $ varies by therapy
ADULT - Chemotherapy doses vary by indication. Advanced renal cell carcinoma. Unresectable hepatocellular carcinoma.
PEDS - Not approved in children.
FORMS - Trade only: Tab 200 mg.
NOTES - Take 1 h before or 2 h after meals for best absorption. Monitor BP. Monitor INR with warfarin. Reliable contraception is recommended. Hepatic impairment may reduce concentrations. Increases docetaxel & doxorubicin.

**THALIDOMIDE (*Thalomid*)** ▶Plasma ♀X ▶? $$$$$
WARNING - Pregnancy category X. Has caused severe, life-threatening human birth defects. Available only through special restricted distribution program. Prescribers and pharmacists must be registered in this program in order to prescribe or dispense.
ADULT - Chemotherapy doses vary by indication. Multiple myeloma, with dexamethasone. Erythema nodosum leprosum: 100–400 mg PO qhs. Use low end of dose range for initial episodes and if <50 kg.
PEDS - Not approved in children.
UNAPPROVED PEDS - Clinical trials show beneficial effects when combined with dexamethasone in multiple myeloma.
FORMS - Trade only: cap 50, 100, 150, 200 mg.

**TOPOTECAN (*Hycamtin*)** ▶Plasma ♀D ▶- $ varies by therapy
WARNING - Bone marrow suppression (primary neutropenia), severe bleeding. Instruct patients to report promptly fever, sore throat, signs of local infection, bleeding from any site, or symptoms suggestive of anemia.
ADULT - Chemotherapy doses vary by indication. Ovarian & cervical cancer. Small cell lung cancer, relapsed.
PEDS - Not approved in children.
FORMS - Trade only: Caps, 0.25 & 1 mg.

NOTES - Reliable contraception is recommended. Monitor CBCs.

**TRETINOIN (*Vesanoid*)** ▶L ♀D ▶- $ varies by therapy
WARNING - Retinoic acid-APL (RA-APL) syndrome: fever, dyspnea, weight gain, pulmonary edema, pulmonary infiltrates & pleural/pericardial effusions, occasionally with impaired myocardial contractility & episodic hypotension, with or w/o leukocytosis. Reversible hypercholesterolemia/hypertriglyceridemia, increased LFTs, alopecia. Contraindicated in paraben-sensitive patients.
ADULT - Chemotherapy doses vary by indication. Acute promyelocytic leukemia.
PEDS - Not approved in children.
UNAPPROVED PEDS - Acute promyelocytic leukemia, limited data.
FORMS - Generic/Trade: Cap 10 mg.
NOTES - Reliable contraception is recommended. Monitor CBCs, coags, LFTs, triglyceride & cholesterol levels. Ketoconazole increases levels.

**VORINOSTAT (*Zolinza*)** ▶L ♀D ▶- $$$$$
WARNING - PE/DVT, anemia, thrombocytopenia, QT prolongation.
ADULT - Chemotherapy doses vary by indication. Cutaneous T-cell lymphoma.
PEDS - Not approved in children.
FORMS - Trade only: Cap 100 mg.
NOTES - Reliable contraception is recommended. Monitor CBCs, electrolytes, renal function, EKG.

## OPHTHALMOLOGY: Antiallergy—Decongestants & Combinations

**NOTE:** Overuse can cause rebound dilation of blood vessels. Do not administer while wearing soft contact lenses. Wait 10 min after use before inserting contact lenses. On average, each mL of eye drop solution contains approximately 20 drops. Reserve ointment formulations for bedtime use due to severe vision blurring. Most eye medications can be administered 1 drop at a time despite common manufacturer recommendations of 1–2 drops concurrently. Even a single drop is typically more than the eye can hold and thus a 2nd drop is both wasteful and increases the possibility of systemic toxicity. If twice the medication is desired separate single drops by at least 5 min.

**NAPHAZOLINE (*Albalon, All Clear, AK-Con, Naphcon, Clear Eyes*)** ▶? ♀C ▶? $
ADULT - Ocular vasoconstrictor/decongestant: 1 gtt qid prn for up to 4 d.
PEDS - <6 yo: not approved. ≥6 yo: 1 gtt qid prn for up to 4 d.
FORMS - OTC Generic/Trade: solution 0.012, 0.03% (15, 30 mL). Rx Generic/Trade: 0.1% (15 mL).
**NAPHCON-A (naphazoline + pheniramine, Visine-A)** ▶L ♀C ▶? $
ADULT - Ocular decongestant: 1 gtt qid prn for up to 4 d.

PEDS - Age ≥6 yo: Use adult dose. <6 yo: Not approved.
FORMS - OTC Trade only: solution 0.025% + 0.3% (15 mL).
**VASOCON-A (naphazoline + antazoline)** ▶L ♀C ▶? $
ADULT - Ocular decongestant: 1 gtt qid prn for up to 4 d.
PEDS - Age ≥6 yo: Use adult dose. <6 yo: Not approved.
FORMS - OTC Trade only: solution 0.05% + 0.5% (15 mL).

## OPHTHALMOLOGY: Antiallergy—Dual Antihistamine & Mast Cell Stabilizer

**NOTE:** Wait ≥10 min after use before inserting contact lenses. On average, each mL of eye drop solution contains approximately 20 drops. Reserve ointment formulations for bedtime use due to severe vision blurring. Most eye medications can be administered 1 drop at a time despite common manufacturer recommendations of 1–2 drops concurrently. Even a single drop is typically more than the eye can hold and thus a 2nd drop is both wasteful and increases the possibility of systemic toxicity. If twice the medication is desired separate single drops by at least 5 min.

**AZELASTINE - OPHTHALMIC (*Optivar*)** ▶L ♀C ▶? $$$
ADULT - Allergic conjunctivitis: 1 gtt bid.
PEDS - Age ≥3 yo: Use adult dose. <3 yo: Not approved.
FORMS - Trade only: solution 0.05% (6 mL).

**EPINASTINE (*Elestat*)** ▶K ♀C ▶? $$$
ADULT - Allergic conjunctivitis: 1 gtt bid.
PEDS - Age <3 yo: not approved. Age ≥3 yo: Use adult dose.
FORMS - Trade only: solution 0.05% (5 mL).

**KETOTIFEN - OPHTHALMIC (*Alaway, Zaditor*)** ▶Minimal absorption ♀C ▶? $
ADULT - Allergic conjunctivitis: 1 gtt in each eye q8–12h.
PEDS - Allergic conjunctivitis children >3yo: 1 gtt in each eye q8–12h.
FORMS - OTC-Generic/Trade: solution 0.025% (5 mL).

**OLOPATADINE (*Pataday, Patanol*)** ▶K ♀C ▶? $$$
ADULT - Allergic conjunctivitis: 1 gtt of 0.1% solution in each eye bid (Patanol) or 1 gtt of 0.2% solution in each eye daily (Pataday).
PEDS - Age ≥3 yo: Use adult dose. <3 yo: Not approved.
FORMS - Trade only: solution 0.1% (5 mL, Patanol), 0.2% (2.5 mL, Pataday).
NOTES - Do not administer while wearing soft contact lenses.

## OPHTHALMOLOGY: Antiallergy—Pure Antihistamines

NOTE: Antihistamines may aggravate dry eye symptoms. Wait 10 min after use before inserting contact lenses. On average, each mL of eye drop solution contains approximately 20 drops. Reserve ointment formulations for bedtime use due to severe vision blurring. Most eye medications can be administered 1 drop at a time despite common manufacturer recommendations of 1–2 drops concurrently. Even a single drop is typically more than the eye can hold and thus a 2nd drop is both wasteful and increases the possibility of systemic toxicity. If twice the medication is desired separate single drops by at least 5 min.

**EMEDASTINE (*Emadine*)** ▶L ♀B ▶? $$$
ADULT - Allergic conjunctivitis: 1 gtt up to qid.
PEDS - Age ≥3 yo: Use adult dose. <3yo: Not approved.
FORMS - Trade only: solution 0.05% (5 mL).
**LEVOCABASTINE - OPHTHALMIC (*Livostin*)** ▶Minimal absorption ♀C ▶? $$$

ADULT - Allergic conjunctivitis: 1 gtt up to qid for 2 wk.
PEDS - Age ≥12 yo: Use adult dose. <12 yo: Not approved.
FORMS - Trade only: susp 0.05% (5,10 mL).
NOTES - Wait 10 min after use before inserting contact lenses.

## OPHTHALMOLOGY: Antiallergy—Pure Mast Cell Stabilizers

NOTE: Works best as preventative agent; use continually during at risk season. Wait 10 min after use before inserting contact lenses. On average, each mL of eye drop solution contains approximately 20 drops. Reserve ointment formulations for bedtime use due to severe vision blurring. Most eye medications can be administered 1 drop at a time despite common manufacturer recommendations of 1–2 drops concurrently. Even a single drop is typically more than the eye can hold and thus a 2nd drop is both wasteful and increases the possibility of systemic toxicity. If twice the medication is desired separate single drops by at least 5 min.

**CROMOLYN - OPHTHALMIC (*Crolom, Opticrom*)** ▶LK ♀B ▶? $$
ADULT - Allergic conjunctivitis: 1–2 gtts 4–6 times/d.
PEDS - Age ≥4 yo: Use adult dose. <4 yo: Not approved.
FORMS - Generic/Trade: solution 4% (10 mL).
NOTES - Response may take up to 6 wk.
**LODOXAMIDE (*Alomide*)** ▶K ♀B ▶? $$$
ADULT - Allergic conjunctivitis: 1–2 gtts in each eye qid for up to 3 mo.
PEDS - Age ≥2 yo: Use adult dose. <2 yo: Not approved.
FORMS - Trade only: solution 0.1% (10 mL).
NOTES - Do not administer while wearing soft contact lenses.

**NEDOCROMIL - OPHTHALMIC (*Alocril*)** ▶L ♀B ▶? $$$
ADULT - Allergic conjunctivitis: 1–2 gtts in each eye bid.
PEDS - Children >3 yo: Allergic conjunctivitis: 1–2 gtts bid. Not approved in children <3yo.
FORMS - Trade only: solution 2% (5 mL).
NOTES - Solution normally appears slightly yellow.
**PEMIROLAST (*Alamast*)** ▶? ♀C ▶? $$$
ADULT - Allergic conjunctivitis: 1–2 gtts in each eye qid.
PEDS - Not approved in children <3 yo. Children >3 yo: 1–2 gtts qid.
FORMS - Trade only: solution 0.1% (10 mL).
NOTES - Decreased itching may be seen within a few d, but full effect may require up to four wk.

## OPHTHALMOLOGY: Antibacterials—Aminoglycosides

NOTE: On average, each mL of eye drop solution contains approximately 20 drops. Reserve ointment formulations for bedtime use due to severe vision blurring. Most eye medications can be administered 1 drop at a time despite common manufacturer recommendations of 1–2 drops concurrently. Even a single drop is typically more than the eye can hold and thus a 2nd drop is both wasteful and increases the possibility of systemic toxicity. If twice the medication is desired separate single drops by at least 5 min.

**GENTAMICIN - OPHTHALMIC (*Garamycin, Genoptic, Gentak, ✦Diogent*)** ▶K ♀C ▶? $
ADULT - Ocular infections: 1–2 gtts q2–4h or ½ inch ribbon of ointment bid- tid.

PEDS - Not approved in children.
UNAPPROVED PEDS - Ocular infections: 1–2 gtts q4h or ½ inch ribbon of ointment bid-tid.

**GENTAMICIN** (*cont.*)
FORMS - Generic/Trade: solution 0.3% (5 ,15 mL), ointment 0.3% (3.5 g tube).
NOTES - For severe infections, use up to 2 gtts every h.
**TOBRAMYCIN - OPHTHALMIC** (*Tobrex*) ▶K ♀B ▶- $
ADULT - Ocular infections, mild to moderate: 1–2 gtts q4h or ½ inch ribbon of ointment bid-tid. Ocular infections, severe: 2 gtts q1h, then taper

to q4h or ½ inch ribbon of ointment q3–4h, then taper to bid-tid.
PEDS - ≥2 mo: 1–2 gtts q1–4h or ½ inch ribbon of ointment q3–4h or bid-tid.
UNAPPROVED PEDS - Ocular infections: 1–2 gtts q4h or ½ inch ribbon of ointment bid-tid.
FORMS - Generic/Trade: solution 0.3% (5 mL). Trade only: ointment 0.3% (3.5 g tube).

## OPHTHALMOLOGY: Antibacterials—Fluoroquinolones

**NOTE:** Avoid the overuse of fluoroquinolones for conjunctivitis. Ocular administration has not been shown to cause arthropathy. On average, each mL of eye drop solution contains approximately 20 drops. Reserve ointment formulations for bedtime use due to severe vision blurring. Most eye medications can be administered 1 drop at a time despite common manufacturer recommendations of 1–2 drops concurrently. Even a single drop is typically more than the eye can hold and thus a 2nd drop is both wasteful and increases the possibility of systemic toxicity. If twice the medication is desired separate single drops by at least 5 min.

**CIPROFLOXACIN - OPHTHALMIC** (*Ciloxan*) ▶LK ♀C ▶? $$
ADULT - Corneal ulcers/keratitis: 2 gtts q15 min × 6 h, then 2 gtts q30 min × 1 d; then, 2 gtts q1h × 1

d, and 2 gtts q4h × 3–14 d. Bacterial conjunctivitis: 1–2 gtts q2h while awake × 2 d, then 1–2 gtts q4h while awake × 5 d; or ½ inch ribbon ointment tid × 2 d, then ½ inch ribbon bid × 5 d.

(cont.)

Hold card in good light 14 inches from eye. Record vision for each eye separately with and without glasses. Presbyopic patients should read through bifocal glasses. Myopic patients should wear glasses only.

**CIPROFLOXACIN** *(cont.)*
PEDS - Bacterial conjunctivitis: use adult dose for age ≥1 yo (solution) and ≥2 yo (ointment). Not approved below these ages.
FORMS - Generic/Trade: solution 0.3% (2.5,5,10 mL). Trade only: ointment 0.3% (3.5 g tube).
NOTES - May cause white precipitate of active drug at site of epithelial defect that may be confused with a worsening infection. Resolves within 2 wk and does not necessitate discontinuation.

**GATIFLOXACIN - OPHTHALMIC** *(Zymar)* ▶K ♀C ▶? $$$
ADULT - Bacterial conjunctivitis: 1–2 gtts q2h while awake up to 8 times/d on d 1&2, then 1–2 gtts q4h up to 4 times/d on d 3–7.
PEDS - >1 yo: Adult dose. <1 yo: Not approved.
FORMS - Trade only: solution 0.3%.

**LEVOFLOXACIN - OPHTHALMIC** *(Iquix, Quixin)* ▶KL ♀C ▶? $$$
ADULT - Bacterial conjunctivitis, Quixin: 1–2 gtts q2h while awake up to 8 times/d on d 1&2, then 1–2 gtts q4h up to 4 times/d on d 3–7. Bacterial conjunctivitis, Iquix: 1–2 gtts q30 min to 2h while awake and q4–6h overnight on d 1–3, then 1–2 gtts q1–4h while awake on d 4 to completion of therapy.

PEDS - Bacterial conjunctivitis, Quixin: =<1 yo: Not approved. >1yo: 1–2 gtts q2h while awake up to 8 times/d on d 1&2, then 1–2 gtts q4h up to 4 times/d on d 3–7. Bacterial conjunctivitis, Iquix: <6 yo: Not approved. ≥6 yo: 1–2 gtts q30 min to 2h while awake and q4–6h overnight on d 1–3, then 1–2 gtts q1–4h while awake on d 4 to completion of therapy.
FORMS - Trade only: solution 0.5% (Quixin, 5 mL), 1.5% (Iquix, 5 mL).

**MOXIFLOXACIN - OPHTHALMIC** *(Vigamox)* ▶LK ♀C ▶? $$$
ADULT - Bacterial conjunctivitis: 1 gtt tid × 7 d.
PEDS - >1 yo: Adult dose. <1 yo: Not approved.
FORMS - Trade only: solution 0.5% (3 mL).

**OFLOXACIN - OPHTHALMIC** *(Ocuflox)* ▶LK ♀C ▶? $$
ADULT - Corneal ulcers/keratitis: 1–2 gtts q30 min while awake and 1–2 gtts 4–6 h after retiring × 2 d, then 1–2 gtts q1h while awake × 5 d, then 1–2 gtts qid × 3 d. Bacterial conjunctivitis: 1–2 gtts q2–4 h × 2 d, then 1–2 gtts qid × 5 d.
PEDS - Bacterial conjunctivitis: age ≥1 yo: Use adult dose. <1 yo: Not approved.
FORMS - Generic/Trade: solution 0.3% (5, 10 mL).

## OPHTHALMOLOGY: Antibacterials—Other

**NOTE:** On average, each mL of eye drop solution contains approximately 20 drops. Reserve ointment formulations for bedtime use due to severe vision blurring. Most eye medications can be administered 1 drop at a time despite common manufacturer recommendations of 1–2 drops concurrently. Even a single drop is typically more than the eye can hold and thus a 2nd drop is both wasteful and increases the possibility of systemic toxicity. If twice the medication is desired separate single drops by at least 5 min.

**AZITHROMYCIN - OPHTHALMIC** *(Azasite)* ▶L ♀B ▶? $$$
ADULT - Ocular infections: 1 gtt bid × 2 d, then 1 gtt daily × 5 more d.
PEDS - Ocular infections, age ≥1 yo: 1 gtt bid × 2 d, then 1 gtt daily × 5 more d.
FORMS - Trade only: solution 1% (2.5 mL).

**BACITRACIN - OPHTHALMIC** *(AK Tracin)* ▶Minimal absorption ♀C ▶? $
ADULT - Ocular infections: apply ¼–½ inch ribbon of ointment q3–4h or bid-qid.
PEDS - Not approved in children.
UNAPPROVED PEDS - Ocular infections: apply ½ inch ribbon of ointment q3–4h or bid-qid.
FORMS - Generic/Trade: ointment 500 units/g (3.5g tube)

**ERYTHROMYCIN - OPHTHALMIC** *(Ilotycin, AK-Mycin)* ▶L ♀B ▶+ $
ADULT - Ocular infections, corneal ulceration: ½ inch ribbon of ointment q3–4h or 2–8 times/d. For chlamydial infections: bid × 2 mo or bid × 5 d/mo for 6 mo.
PEDS - Ophthalmia neonatorum prophylaxis: ½ inch ribbon to both eyes within 1 h of birth.
FORMS - Generic only: ointment 0.5% (1, 3.5 g tube).

**FUSIDIC ACID - OPHTHALMIC,** ◆*FUCITHALMIC* ▶L ♀? ▶? $
ADULT - Canada only. Eye infections: 1 gtt in both eyes q12h × 7 d.

PEDS - Canada only. Children ≥2 yo, eye infections: 1 gtt in both eyes q12h × 7 d.
FORMS - Canada trade only: Drops 1%. Multidose tubes of 3, 5 g. Single dose preservative-free tubes of 0.2 g in a box of 12.

*NEOSPORIN OINTMENT - OPHTHALMIC* (neomycin + bacitracin + polymyxin) ▶K ♀C ▶? $
ADULT - Ocular infections: ½ inch ribbon of ointment q3–4 h × 7–10 d or ½ inch ribbon 2–3 times/d for mild-moderate infection.
PEDS - Not approved in children.
UNAPPROVED PEDS - ½ inch ribbon of ointment q3–4h × 7–10 d.
FORMS - Generic only: ointment. (3.5 g tube).
NOTES - Contact dermatitis can occur after prolonged use.

*NEOSPORIN SOLUTION - OPHTHALMIC* (neomycin + polymyxin + gramicidin) ▶KL ♀C ▶? $$
ADULT - Ocular infections:1–2 gtts q1–6h × 7–10 d.
PEDS - Not approved in children.
UNAPPROVED PEDS - 1–2 gtts q1–6h × 7–10 d.
FORMS - Generic/Trade: solution (10 mL).
NOTES - Contact dermatitis can occur after prolonged use.

*POLYSPORIN - OPHTHALMIC* (polymyxin + bacitracin) ▶K ♀C ▶? $$
ADULT - Ocular infections: ½ inch ribbon of ointment q3–4h × 7–10 d or ½ inch ribbon bid-tid for mild-moderate infection.

**POLYSPORIN** (cont.)
PEDS - Not approved in children.
UNAPPROVED PEDS - Ocular infections: ½ inch ribbon of ointment q3–4h × 7–10 d.
FORMS - Generic only: ointment (3.5 g tube).

***POLYTRIM - OPHTHALMIC* (polymyxin + trimethoprim)** ▶KL ♀C ▶? $
ADULT - Ocular infections: 1–2 gtts q3–6h × 7–10 d. Max 6 gtts/d.
PEDS - Age ≥2 mo: Use adult dose. <2 mo: Not approved.
FORMS - Generic/Trade: solution (10 mL).

**SULFACETAMIDE - OPHTHALMIC** (*Bleph-10, Sulf-10*) ▶K ♀C ▶- $
ADULT - Ocular infections, corneal ulceration: 1–2 gtts q2–3h initially, then taper by decreasing frequency as condition allows × 7- 10 d or ½ inch ribbon of ointment q3–4h initially, then taper × 7–10 d. Trachoma: 2 gtts q2h with systemic antibiotic such as doxycycline or azithromycin.
PEDS - Age ≥2 mo: Use adult dose. <2 mo: Not approved.
FORMS - Generic/Trade: solution 10% (15 mL), ointment 10% (3.5g tube). Generic only: solution 30% (15 mL).
NOTES - Ointment may be used as an adjunct to solution.

## OPHTHALMOLOGY: Antiviral Agents

**NOTE:** On average, each mL of eye drop solution contains approximately 20 drops. Reserve ointment formulations for bedtime use due to severe vision blurring. Most eye medications can be administered 1 drop at a time despite common manufacturer recommendations of 1–2 drops concurrently. Even a single drop is typically more than the eye can hold and thus a 2nd drop is both wasteful and increases the possibility of systemic toxicity. If twice the medication is desired separate single drops by at least 5 min.

**TRIFLURIDINE** (*Viroptic*) ▶Minimal absorption ♀C ▶- $$$
ADULT - HSV keratitis: 1 gtt q2h to max 9 gtts/d. After re-epithelialization, decrease dose to 1 gtt q4–6h while awake × 7–14 d. Max of 21 d of treatment.
PEDS - Age ≥6 yo: Use adult dose. <6 yo: Not approved.
FORMS - Generic/Trade solution 1% (7.5 mL).
NOTES - Avoid continuous use >21 d; may cause keratitis and conjunctival scarring. Urge frequent use of topical lubricants (ie, tear substitutes) to minimize surface damage.

## OPHTHALMOLOGY: Corticosteroid & Antibacterial Combinations

**NOTE:** Recommend that only ophthalmologists or optometrists prescribe due to infection, cataract, corneal/scleral perforation, and glaucoma risk from prolonged use. Monitor intraocular pressure. Gradually taper when discontinuing. Shake suspensions well before using. On average, each mL of eye drop solution contains approximately 20 drops. Reserve ointment formulations for bedtime use due to severe vision blurring. Most eye medications can be administered 1 drop at a time despite common manufacturer recommendations of 1–2 drops concurrently. Even a single drop is typically more than the eye can hold and thus a 2nd drop is both wasteful and increases the possibility of systemic toxicity. If twice the medication is desired separate single drops by at least 5 min.

**BLEPHAMIDE (prednisolone - ophthalmic + sulfacetamide)** ▶KL ♀C ▶? $
ADULT - Steroid-responsive inflammatory condition with bacterial infection or risk of bacterial infection: Start 1–2 gtts q1h during the d and q2h during the night, then 1 gtt q4–8h; or ½ inch ribbon (ointment) tid-qid initially, then daily-bid thereafter.
PEDS - Not approved in children.
FORMS - Generic/Trade: solution/susp (5,10 mL), Trade only: ointment (3.5 g tube).

***CORTISPORIN - OPHTHALMIC* (neomycin + polymyxin + hydrocortisone - ophthalmic)** ▶LK ♀C ▶? $
ADULT - Steroid-responsive inflammatory condition with bacterial infection or risk of bacterial infection: 1–2 gtts or ½ inch ribbon of ointment q3–4h or more frequently prn.
PEDS - Not approved in children.
UNAPPROVED PEDS - 1–2 gtts or ½ inch ribbon of ointment q3–4h.
FORMS - Generic/Trade: susp (7.5 mL). Generic only: ointment (3.5 g tube).

**FML-S LIQUIFILM (prednisolone - ophthalmic + sulfacetamide)** ▶KL ♀C ▶? $$
ADULT - Steroid-responsive inflammatory condition with bacterial infection or risk of bacterial infection: Start 1–2 gtts q1h during the d and q2h during the night, then 1 gtt q4–8h; or ½ inch ribbon (ointment) tid-qid initially, then daily-bid thereafter.
PEDS - Not approved in children.
FORMS - Trade only: susp (10 mL).

***MAXITROL* (dexamethasone - ophthalmic + neomycin + polymyxin)** ▶KL ♀C ▶? $
ADULT - Steroid-responsive inflammatory condition with bacterial infection or risk of bacterial infection: Start 1–2 gtts q1h during the d and q2h during the night, then 1 gtt q4–8h; or ½ -1 inch ribbon (ointment) tid-qid initially, then daily- bid thereafter.
PEDS - Not approved in children.
FORMS - Generic/Trade: susp (5 mL), ointment (3.5 g tube).

**PRED G (prednisolone - ophthalmic + gentamicin)** ▶KL ♀C ▶? $$
ADULT - Steroid-responsive inflammatory condition with bacterial infection or risk of bacterial

(cont.)

**PRED G** *(cont.)*
infection: Start 1–2 gtts q1h during the d and q2h during the night, then 1 gtt q4–8h or ½ inch ribbon of ointment bid-qid.
PEDS - Not approved in children.
FORMS - Trade only: susp (2,5,10 mL), ointment (3.5 g tube).

**TOBRADEX (tobramycin + dexamethasone - ophthalmic)** ▶L ♀C ▶? $$$
ADULT - Steroid-responsive inflammatory condition with bacterial infection or risk of bacterial infection: 1–2 gtts q2h × 1–2 d, then 1–2 gtts q4–6h; or ½ inch ribbon of ointment bid-qid.
PEDS - <2 yo: not approved. ≥2 yo: 1–2 gtts q2h × 1–2 d, then 1–2 gtts q4–6h; or ½ inch ribbon of ointment bid-qid.
FORMS - Trade only: susp (2.5,5,10 mL), ointment (3.5 g tube).

**VASOCIDIN (prednisolone - ophthalmic + sulfacetamide)** ▶KL ♀C ▶? $
ADULT - Steroid-responsive inflammatory condition with bacterial infection or risk of bacterial infection: Start 1–2 gtts q1h during the d and q2h during the night, then 1 gtt q4–8h; or ½ inch ribbon (ointment) tid-qid initially, then daily-bid thereafter.
PEDS - Not approved in children.
FORMS - Generic only: solution (5,10 mL)

**ZYLET (loteprednol + tobramycin)** ▶LK ♀C ▶? $$$
ADULT - 1–2 gtts q1–2h × 1–2 d then 1–2 gtts q4–6h.
PEDS - Not approved in children.
FORMS - Trade only: susp 0.5% loteprednol + 0.3% tobramycin (2.5, 5, 10 mL)

## OPHTHALMOLOGY: Corticosteroids

**NOTE:** Recommend that only ophthalmologists or optometrists prescribe due to infection, cataract, corneal/scleral perforation, and glaucoma risk. Monitor intraocular pressure. Gradually taper when discontinuing. Shake susp well before using. On average, each mL of eye drop solution contains approximately 20 drops. Reserve ointment formulations for bedtime use due to severe vision blurring. Most eye medications can be administered 1 drop at a time despite common manufacturer recommendations of 1–2 drops concurrently. Even a single drop is typically more than the eye can hold and thus a 2nd drop is both wasteful and increases the possibility of systemic toxicity. If twice the medication is desired separate single drops by at least 5 min.

**DIFLUPREDNATE (Durezol)** ▶Not absorbed ♀C ▶? ?
ADULT - 1 gtt into affected eye qid, beginning 24 h after surgery × 2 wk, then 1 gtt into affected eye bid × 1 wk, then taper based on response.
PEDS - Not approved in children.
FORMS - Ophthalmic emulsion 0.05% (2.5, 5 mL) .
NOTES - If used for more than 10 d, monitor IOP.

**FLUOCINOLONE - OPHTHALMIC (Retisert)** ▶Not absorbed ♀C ▶? $$$$$
ADULT - 1 gtt into affected eye qid, beginning 24 h after surgery × 2 wk, then 1 gtt into affected eye bid × 1 wk, then taper based on response.
PEDS - Not approved in children <12 yo.
FORMS - Implantable tab 0.59 mg only available from manufacturer.
NOTES - Releases 0.6 mcg/d decreasing over about 1 mo, then 0.3–0.4 mcg/d over about 30 mo. Within 34 wk 60% require medication to control intraocular pressure and within 2 yr nearly all phakic eyes develop cataracts.

**FLUOROMETHOLONE (FML, FML Forte, Flarex)** ▶L ♀C ▶? $$
ADULT - 1–2 gtts q1–2h or ½ inch ribbon of ointment q4h × 1–2 d, then 1–2 gtts bid-qid or ½ inch of ointment daily-tid.
PEDS - Age ≥2 yo: Use adult dose. <2 yo: Not approved.
FORMS - Trade only: susp 0.1% (5,10,15 mL), 0.25% (2,5,10,15 mL), ointment 0.1% (3.5 g tube)
NOTES - Fluorometholone acetate (Flarex) is more potent than fluorometholone (FML, FML Forte). Use caution in glaucoma.

**LOTEPREDNOL (Alrex, Lotemax)** ▶L ♀C ▶? $$$
ADULT - 1–2 gtts qid, may increase to 1 gtt q1h during first wk of therapy prn. Postoperative inflammation: 1–2 gtts qid.
PEDS - Not approved in children.
FORMS - Trade only: susp 0.2% (Alrex 5,10 mL), 0.5% (Lotemax 2.5, 5,10,15 mL).

**PREDNISOLONE - OPHTHALMIC (Pred Forte, Pred Mild, Inflamase Forte, Econopred Plus, ✦AK Tate, Diopred)** ▶L ♀C ▶? $$
ADULT - Sol.: 1–2 gtts up to q1h during d and q2h at night, when response observed, then 1 gtt q4h, then 1 gtt tid-qid. Suspen.: 1–2 gtts bid-qid.
PEDS - Not approved in children.
FORMS - Generic/Trade: solution & susp 1% (5,10,15 mL). Trade only (Pred Mild): susp 0.12% (5,10 mL), susp (Pred Forte) 1% (1 mL).
NOTES - Prednisolone acetate (Pred Mild, Pred Forte) is more potent than prednisolone sodium phosphate (AK-Pred, Inflamase Forte).

**RIMEXOLONE (Vexol)** ▶L ♀C ▶? $$
ADULT - Post-operative inflammation: 1–2 gtts qid × 2 wk. Uveitis: 1–2 gtts q1h while awake × 1 wk, then 1 gtt q2h while awake × 1 wk, then taper.
PEDS - Not approved in children.
FORMS - Trade only: susp 1% (5,10 mL).
NOTES - Prolonged use associated with corneal/scleral perforation and cataracts.

**TRIAMCINOLONE - VITREOUS (Triesence)** ▶L ♀D ▶? ?
ADULT - Administered intravitreally.
PEDS - Not approved in children.
NOTES - Do not use in patients with systemic fungal infections.

## OPHTHALMOLOGY: Glaucoma Agents—Beta Blockers

**NOTE:** May be absorbed and cause side effects and drug interactions associated with systemic beta-blocker therapy. Use caution in cardiac conditions and asthma. Advise patients to apply gentle pressure over nasolacrimal duct for 5 min after instillation to minimize systemic absorption. On average, each mL of eye drop solution contains approximately 20 drops. Reserve ointment formulations for bedtime use due to severe vision blurring. Most eye medications can be administered 1 drop at a time despite common manufacturer recommendations of 1–2 drops concurrently. Even a single drop is typically more than the eye can hold and thus a 2nd drop is both wasteful and increases the possibility of systemic toxicity. If twice the medication is desired separate single drops by at least 5 min.

**BETAXOLOL - OPHTHALMIC (*Betoptic, Betoptic S*)** ▶LK ♀C ▶? $$
ADULT - Chronic open angle glaucoma or ocular hypertension: 1–2 gtts bid.
PEDS - Chronic open angle glaucoma or ocular hypertension: 1–2 gtts bid.
FORMS - Trade only: susp 0.25% (5,10,15 mL). Generic only: solution 0.5% (5,10,15 mL).
NOTES - Selective beta1-blocking agent. Shake susp before use.

**CARTEOLOL - OPHTHALMIC (*Ocupress*)** ▶KL ♀C ▶? $
ADULT - Chronic open angle glaucoma or ocular hypertension: 1 gtt bid.
PEDS - Not approved in children.
FORMS - Generic only: solution 1% (5,10,15 mL).
NOTES - Nonselective beta-blocker but has intrinsic sympathomimetic activity.

**LEVOBUNOLOL (*Betagan*)** ▶? ♀C ▶- $$
ADULT - Chronic open angle glaucoma or ocular hypertension: 1–2 gtts (0.5%) daily-bid or 1–2 gtts (0.25%) bid.
PEDS - Not approved in children.
FORMS - Generic/Trade: solution 0.25% (5,10 mL) 0.5% (5,10,15 mL - Trade only 2 mL).

NOTES - Nonselective beta blocker.

**METIPRANOLOL (*Optipranolol*)** ▶? ♀C ▶? $
ADULT - Chronic open angle glaucoma or ocular hypertension: 1 gtt bid.
PEDS - Not approved in children.
FORMS - Generic/Trade: solution 0.3% (5,10 mL).
NOTES - Nonselective beta blocker.

**TIMOLOL - OPHTHALMIC (*Betimol, Timoptic, Timoptic XE, Istalol, Timoptic Ocudose*)** ▶LK ♀C ▶+ $$
ADULT - Chronic open angle glaucoma or ocular hypertension: 1 gtt (0.25 or 0.5%) bid or 1 gtt of gel-forming solution (0.25 or 0.5% Timoptic XE) daily or 1 gtt (0.5% Istalol solution) daily.
PEDS - Chronic open angle glaucoma or ocular hypertension: 1 gtt (0.25 or 0.5%) of gel-forming solution daily.
FORMS - solution 0.25 & 0.5% (5,10,15 mL), preservative free solution* 0.25% (0.2 mL), gel forming solution^ 0.25 & 0.5% (2.5, 5 mL). Note: *Timoptic Ocudose ^Timoptic XE.
NOTES - Administer other eye meds ≥10 min before Timoptic XE. Greatest effect if Timoptic XE is administered in the morning. Nonselective beta blocker.

## OPHTHALMOLOGY: Glaucoma Agents—Carbonic Anhydrase Inhibitors

**NOTE:** Sulfonamide derivatives; verify absence of sulfa allergy before prescribing. On average, each mL of eye drop solution contains approximately 20 drops. Reserve ointment formulations for bedtime use due to severe vision blurring. Most eye medications can be administered 1 drop at a time despite common manufacturer recommendations of 1–2 drops concurrently. Even a single drop is typically more than the eye can hold and thus a 2nd drop is both wasteful and increases the possibility of systemic toxicity. If twice the medication is desired separate single drops by at least 5 min.

**BRINZOLAMIDE (*Azopt*)** ▶LK ♀C ▶? $$$
ADULT - Chronic open angle glaucoma or ocular hypertension: 1 gtt tid.
PEDS - Not approved in children.
FORMS - Trade only: susp 1% (5,10,15 mL).
NOTES - Do not administer while wearing soft contact lenses. Wait 10 min after use before inserting contact lenses.

**DORZOLAMIDE (*Trusopt*)** ▶KL ♀C ▶- $$$
ADULT - Chronic open angle glaucoma or ocular hypertension: 1 gtt tid.
PEDS - Chronic open angle glaucoma or ocular hypertension: 1 gtt tid.

FORMS - Trade only: solution 2% (5, 10 mL).
NOTES - Do not administer while wearing soft contact lenses. Keep bottle tightly capped to avoid crystal formation. Wait 10 min after use before inserting contact lenses.

**METHAZOLAMIDE (*Neptazane*)** ▶LK ♀C ▶? $$
ADULT - Glaucoma: 100–200 mg PO initially, then 100 mg PO q 12h until desired response. Maintenance dose: 25–50 mg PO daily-tid.
PEDS - Not approved in children.
FORMS - Generic only: Tabs 25, 50 mg.
NOTES - Mostly metabolized in the liver thus less chance of renal calculi than with acetazolamide.

## OPHTHALMOLOGY: Glaucoma Agents—Miotics

**NOTE:** Observe for cholinergic systemic effects (eg, salivation, lacrimation, urination, diarrhea, gastrointestinal upset, excessive sweating). On average, each mL of eye drop solution contains approximately 20 drops. Reserve ointment formulations for bedtime use due to severe vision blurring. Most eye medications can be administered

(cont.)

1 drop at a time despite common manufacturer recommendations of 1–2 drops concurrently. Even a single drop is typically more than the eye can hold and thus a 2nd drop is both wasteful and increases the possibility of systemic toxicity. If twice the medication is desired separate single drops by at least 5 min.

**ACETYLCHOLINE** (*Miochol-E*) ▶Acetylcholinesterases ♀? ▶? $$
ADULT - Intraoperative miosis or pressure lowering: 0.5 mL to 3 mL injected intraocularly.
PEDS - Not approved in children.

**CARBACHOL** (*Isopto Carbachol, Miostat*) ▶? ♀C ▶? $$
ADULT - Glaucoma: 1 gtt tid. Intraoperative miosis or pressure lowering: 0.5 mL injected intraocularly.
PEDS - Not approved in children.
FORMS - Trade only: solution (Isopto Carbachol) 1.5 & 3% (15 mL). Intraocular solution (Miostat) 0.01%.

**ECHOTHIOPHATE IODIDE** (*Phospholine Iodide*) ▶? ♀C ▶? $$$
ADULT - Glaucoma: 1 gtt bid.
PEDS - Accommodative estropia: 1 gtt daily (0.06%) or 1 gtt qod (0.125%).
FORMS - Trade only: solution 0.125% (5 mL).
NOTES - Use lowest effective dose strength. Use extreme caution if asthma, spastic GI diseases,

GI ulcers, bradycardia, hypotension, recent MI, epilepsy, Parkinson's Disease, history of retinal detachment. Stop 3 wk before general anesthesia as may cause prolonged succinylcholine paralysis. Discontinue if cardiac effects noted.

**PILOCARPINE - OPHTHALMIC** (*Pilopine HS, Isopto Carpine, ✦Diocarpine, Akarpine*) ▶Plasma ♀C ▶? $
ADULT - Glaucoma: 1–2 gtts up to tid-qid up to 6 times/d or ½ inch ribbon (4% gel) qhs.
PEDS - Glaucoma: 1–2 gtts up to tid-qid up to 6 times/d.
FORMS - Generic only: solution 0.5%(15 mL), 1%(2 mL), 2%(2 mL), 3%(15 mL), 4%(2 mL), 6%(15 mL). Generic/Trade: solution 1% (15 mL), 2% (15 mL), 4% (15 mL). Trade only (Pilopine HS): gel 4% (4 g tube).
NOTES - Do not administer while wearing soft contact lenses. Wait ≥15 min after use before inserting contact lenses. Causes miosis. May cause blurred vision and difficulty with night vision.

## OPHTHALMOLOGY: Glaucoma Agents—Prostaglandin Analogs

**NOTE:** Do not administer while wearing soft contact lenses. Wait 10 min after use before inserting contact lenses. May aggravate intraocular inflammation. On average, each mL of eye drop solution contains approximately 20 drops. Reserve ointment formulations for bedtime use due to severe vision blurring. Most eye medications can be administered 1 drop at a time despite common manufacturer recommendations of 1–2 drops concurrently. Even a single drop is typically more than the eye can hold and thus a 2nd drop is both wasteful and increases the possibility of systemic toxicity. If twice the medication is desired separate single drops by at least 5 min.

**BIMATOPROST** (*Lumigan*) ▶LK ♀C ▶? $$$
ADULT - Chronic open angle glaucoma or ocular hypertension: 1 gtt qhs.
PEDS - Not approved in children.
FORMS - Trade only: solution 0.03% (2.5, 5, 7.5 mL).

**LATANOPROST** (*Xalatan*) ▶LK ♀C ▶? $$$
ADULT - Chronic open angle glaucoma or ocular hypertension: 1 gtt qhs.
PEDS - Not approved in children.
FORMS - Trade only: solution 0.005% (2.5 mL).

**TRAVOPROST** (*Travatan, Travatan Z*) ▶L ♀C ▶? $$$
ADULT - Chronic open angle glaucoma or ocular hypertension: 1 gtt qhs.
PEDS - Not approved in children.
FORMS - Trade only: solution (Travatan) & benzalkonium chloride-free (Travatan Z) 0.004% (2.5, 5 mL).
NOTES - Wait 10 min after use before inserting contact lenses. Avoid if prior or current intraocular inflammation.

## OPHTHALMOLOGY: Glaucoma Agents—Sympathomimetics

**NOTE:** Do not administer while wearing soft contact lenses. Wait 10 min after use before inserting contact lenses. On average, each mL of eye drop solution contains approximately 20 drops. Reserve ointment formulations for bedtime use due to severe vision blurring. Most eye medications can be administered 1 drop at a time despite common manufacturer recommendations of 1–2 drops concurrently. Even a single drop is typically more than the eye can hold and thus a 2nd drop is both wasteful and increases the possibility of systemic toxicity. If twice the medication is desired separate single drops by at least 5 min.

**APRACLONIDINE** (*Iopidine*) ▶KL ♀C ▶? $$$$
ADULT - Perioperative IOP elevation: 1 gtt (1%) 1h prior to surgery, then 1 gtt immediately after surgery.
PEDS - Not approved in children.
FORMS - Trade only: solution 0.5% (5,10 mL), 1% (0.1 mL).
NOTES - Rapid tachyphylaxis may occur. Do not use long-term.

**BRIMONIDINE** (*Alphagan P, ✦Alphagan*) ▶L ♀B ▶? $$
ADULT - Chronic open angle glaucoma or ocular hypertension: 1 gtt tid.
PEDS - Glaucoma >2 yo: 1 gtt tid.
FORMS - Trade only: solution 0.1% (5,10,15 mL). Generic/Trade: solution 0.15% (5,10,15 mL). Generic only: 0.2% solution (5,10,15 mL).
NOTES - Contraindicated in patients receiving MAO inhibitors. BID dosing may have similar efficacy.

**DIPIVEFRIN (*Propine*)** ▶Eye/plasma/L ♀B ▶? $
ADULT - Chronic open angle glaucoma or ocular hypertension: 1 gtt bid.

PEDS - Glaucoma: 1 gtt bid.
FORMS - Generic/Trade: solution 0.1% (5,10, 15 mL).

## OPHTHALMOLOGY: Glaucoma Agents—Combinations and Other

**NOTE:** On average, each mL of eye drop solution contains approximately 20 drops. Reserve ointment formulations for bedtime use due to severe vision blurring. Most eye medications can be administered 1 drop at a time despite common manufacturer recommendations of 1–2 drops concurrently. Even a single drop is typically more than the eye can hold and thus a 2nd drop is both wasteful and increases the possibility of systemic toxicity. If twice the medication is desired separate single drops by at least 5 min.

***COMBIGAN* (brimonidine + timolol)** ▶LK ♀C ▶- $$$
ADULT - Chronic open angle glaucoma or ocular hypertension: 1 gtt q12h.
PEDS - Not approved in children <2 yo.
FORMS - Trade only: solution brimonidine 0.2% + timolol 0.5% (5,10 mL).
NOTES - Do not administer while wearing soft contact lenses. Wait 10 min after use before inserting contact lenses. Contraindicated with MAO inhibitors. See beta-blocker warnings.

***COSOPT* (dorzolamide + timolol)** ▶LK ♀D ▶- $$$
ADULT - Chronic open angle glaucoma or ocular hypertension: 1 gtt bid.
PEDS - Not approved in children.
FORMS - Trade only: solution dorzolamide 2% + timolol 0.5% (5, 10 mL).
NOTES - Do not administer while wearing soft contact lenses. Wait 10 min after use before inserting contact lenses. Not recommended if severe renal or hepatic dysfunction. Use caution in sulfa allergy. See beta-blocker warnings.

## OPHTHALMOLOGY: Macular Degeneration

**NOTE:** On average, each mL of eye drop solution contains approximately 20 drops. Reserve ointment formulations for bedtime use due to severe vision blurring. Most eye medications can be administered 1 drop at a time despite common manufacturer recommendations of 1–2 drops concurrently. Even a single drop is typically more than the eye can hold and thus a 2nd drop is both wasteful and increases the possibility of systemic toxicity. If twice the medication is desired separate single drops by at least 5 min.

**PEGAPTANIB (*Macugen*)** ▶Minimal absorption ♀B ▶? $$$$$
ADULT - "Wet" macular degeneration: 0.3 mg intravitreal injection q 6 wk.
PEDS - Not approved in children.
**RANIBIZUMAB (*Lucentis*)** ▶Intravitreal ♀C ▶? $$$$$
ADULT - Treatment of neovascular (wet) macular degeneration: 0.5 mg intravitreal injection once a mo. If monthly injections not feasible, can administer every 3 mo, but this regimen is less effective.

PEDS - Not approved in children.
NOTES - Increased stroke risk noted with higher doses (0.5 mg) and with prior stroke.
**VERTEPORFIN (*Visudyne*)** ▶L/plasma ♀C ▶? $$$$$
ADULT - Treatment of exudative age-related macular degeneration: 6 mg/m² IV over 10 min; laser light therapy 15 min after start of infusion.
PEDS - Not approved in children.
NOTES - Severe risk of photosensitivity × 5 d; must avoid exposure to sunlight.

## OPHTHALMOLOGY: Mydriatics & Cycloplegics

**NOTE:** Use caution in infants. On average, each mL of eye drop solution contains approximately 20 drops. Reserve ointment formulations for bedtime use due to severe vision blurring. Most eye medications can be administered 1 drop at a time despite common manufacturer recommendations of 1–2 drops concurrently. Even a single drop is typically more than the eye can hold and thus a 2nd drop is both wasteful and increases the possibility of systemic toxicity. If twice the medication is desired separate single drops by at least 5 min.

**ATROPINE - OPHTHALMIC (*Isopto Atropine, Atropine Care*)** ▶L ♀C ▶+ $
ADULT - Uveitis: 1–2 gtts (0.5 or 1% solution) up to qid or ¼ inch ribbon (1% ointment) up to tid. Refraction: 1–2 gtts (1% solution) 1 h before procedure or 1/8–1/4 inch ribbon daily-tid.
PEDS - Uveitis: 1–2 gtts (0.5%) up to tid or 1/8–1/4 inch ribbon up to tid. Refraction: 1–2 gtts (0.5%) bid × 1–3 d before procedure or 1/8 inch ribbon (1% ointment) × 1–3 d before procedure.
UNAPPROVED PEDS - Amblyopia: 1 gtt in good eye daily.

FORMS - Generic/Trade: solution 1% (2, 5,15 mL) Generic only: ointment 1% (3.5 g tube).
NOTES - Cycloplegia may last up to 5–10d and mydriasis may last up to 7–14d. Each drop of a 1% solution contains 0.5 mg atropine. Treat atropine overdose with physostigmine 0.25 mg every 15 min until symptoms resolve.
**CYCLOPENTOLATE (*AK-Pentolate, Cyclogyl, Pentolair*)** ▶? ♀C ▶? $
ADULT - Refraction: 1–2 gtts (1–2%), repeat in 5–10 min prn. Give 45 min before procedure.

(cont.)

*CYCLOPENTOLATE (cont.)*
PEDS - May cause CNS disturbances in children. Refraction: 1–2 gtts (0.5,1, or 2%), repeat in 5–10 min prn. Give 45 min before procedure.
FORMS - Generic/Trade: solution 1% (2,15 mL). Trade only (Cyclogyl): 0.5% (15 mL), 1% (5 mL) and 2% (2,5,15 mL)
NOTES - Cycloplegia may last 6–24h; mydriasis may last 1 d.

**HOMATROPINE (*Isopto Homatropine*)** ▶? ♀C ▶? $
ADULT - Refraction: 1–2 gtts (2%) or 1 gtt (5%) in eye(s) immediately before procedure, repeat q5–10 min prn. Max 3 doses. Uveitis: 1–2 gtts (2–5%) bid-tid or as often as q3–4h.
PEDS - Refraction: 1 gtt (2%) in eye(s) immediately before procedure, repeat q10 min prn. Uveitis: 1 gtt (2%) bid-tid.
FORMS - Trade only: solution 2% (5 mL), 5% (15 mL). Generic/Trade: solution 5% (5 mL)
NOTES - Cycloplegia & mydriasis last 1–3 d.

**PHENYLEPHRINE - OPHTHALMIC (*AK-Dilate, Altafrin, Mydfrin, Refresh*)** ▶Plasma, L ♀C ▶? $
ADULT - Ophthalmologic exams: 1–2 gtts (2.5,

10%) before procedure. Ocular surgery: 1–2 gtts (2.5, 10%) before surgery.
PEDS - Not routinely used in children.
UNAPPROVED PEDS - Ophthalmologic exams: 1 gtt (2.5%) before procedure. Ocular surgery: 1 gtt (2.5%) before surgery.
FORMS - Rx Generic/Trade: solution 2.5% (2,3,5,15 mL),10% (5 mL). OTC Trade only (Altafrin & Refresh): solution 0.12% (15 mL).
NOTES - Overuse can cause rebound dilation of blood vessels. No cycloplegia; mydriasis may last up to 5 h. Systemic absorption, especially with 10% solution, may be associated with sympathetic stimulation (eg, increased BP).

**TROPICAMIDE (*Mydriacyl, Tropicacyl*)** ▶? ♀? ▶? $
ADULT - Dilated eye exam: 1–2 gtts (0.5%) in eye(s) 15- 20 min before exam, repeat q30 min prn.
PEDS - Not approved in children.
FORMS - Generic/Trade: solution 0.5% (15 mL), 1% (3,15 mL). Generic only: solution 1% (2mL).
NOTES - Mydriasis may last 6 h and has weak cycloplegic effects.

---

## OPHTHALMOLOGY: Nonsteroidal Anti-Inflammatories

**NOTE:** On average, each mL of eye drop solution contains approximately 20 drops. Reserve ointment formulations for bedtime use due to severe vision blurring. Most eye medications can be administered 1 drop at a time despite common manufacturer recommendations of 1–2 drops concurrently. Even a single drop is typically more than the eye can hold and thus a 2nd drop is both wasteful and increases the possibility of systemic toxicity. If twice the medication is desired separate single drops by at least 5 min.

**BROMFENAC - OPHTHALMIC (*Xibrom*)** ▶Minimal absorption ♀C, D (3rd trimester) ▶? $$$$
ADULT - Post-op inflammation and pain following cataract surgery: 1 gtt bid beginning 24 h after cataract surgery × 2 wk.
PEDS - Not approved in children.
FORMS - Trade only: solution 0.09% (2.5, 5 mL).
NOTES - Not for use with soft contact lenses. Contains sodium sulfite and may cause allergic reactions.

**DICLOFENAC - OPHTHALMIC (*Voltaren, ✦Voltaren Ophtha*)** ▶L ♀B, D (3rd trimester) ▶? $$$
ADULT - Post-op inflammation following cataract surgery: 1 gtt qid × 1–2 wk. Ocular photophobia and pain associated with corneal refractive surgery: 1–2 gtt to operative eye(s) 1 h prior to surgery and 1–2 gtt within 15 min after surgery, then 1 gtt qid prn for ≤3 d.
PEDS - Not approved in children.
FORMS - Generic/Trade: solution 0.1% (2.5, 5 mL).
NOTES - Contraindicated for use with soft contact lenses.

**FLURBIPROFEN - OPHTHALMIC (*Ocufen*)** ▶L ♀C ▶? $
ADULT - Inhibition of intraoperative miosis: 1 gtt q30 min beginning 2h prior to surgery (total of 4 gtts).
PEDS - Not approved in children.

UNAPPROVED ADULT - Treatment of cystoid macular edema, inflammation after glaucoma or cataract laser surgery, uveitis syndromes.
FORMS - Generic/Trade: solution 0.03% (2.5 mL).

**KETOROLAC - OPHTHALMIC (*Acular, Acular LS*)** ▶L ♀C ▶? $$$
ADULT - Allergic conjunctivitis: 1 gtt (0.5%) qid. Post-op inflammation following cataract surgery: 1 gtt (0.5%) qid beginning 24 h after surgery × 1–2 wk. Post-op corneal refractive surgery: 1 gtt (0.4%) prn for up to 4 d.
PEDS - Age ≥3 yo: Use adult dose. <3 yo: Not approved.
FORMS - Trade only: solution Acular LS 0.4% (5 mL), Acular 0.5% (3, 5, 10 mL), preservative free Acular 0.5% unit dose (0.4 mL).
NOTES - Do not administer while wearing soft contact lenses. Wait 10 min after use before inserting contact lenses. Avoid use in late pregnancy.

**NEPAFENAC (*Nevanac*)** ▶Minimal absorption ♀C ▶? $$$
ADULT - Post-op inflammation following cataract surgery: 1 gtt tid beginning 24 h before cataract surgery and continued for 2 wk after surgery.
PEDS - Not approved in children.
FORMS - Trade only: susp 0.1% (3 mL).
NOTES - Not for use with contact lenses. Caution if previous allergy to ASA or other NSAIDs.

## OPHTHALMOLOGY: Other Ophthalmologic Agents

**NOTE:** On average, each mL of eye drop solution contains approximately 20 drops. Reserve ointment formulations for bedtime use due to severe vision blurring. Most eye medications can be administered 1 drop at a time despite common manufacturer recommendations of 1–2 drops concurrently. Even a single drop is typically more than the eye can hold and thus a 2nd drop is both wasteful and increases the possibility of systemic toxicity. If twice the medication is desired separate single drops by at least 5 min.

**ARTIFICIAL TEARS** (*Tears Naturale, Hypotears, Refresh Tears, GenTeal, Systane*) ▶Minimal absorption ♀A ▶ + $
ADULT - Ophthalmic lubricant: 1–2 gtts tid-qid prn.
PEDS - Ophthalmic lubricant: 1–2 gtts tid-qid prn.
FORMS - OTC Generic/Trade: solution (15, 30 mL among others).

**CYCLOSPORINE - OPHTHALMIC** (*Restasis*) ▶Minimal absorption ♀C ▶? $$$$
ADULT - Keratoconjunctivitis sicca (chronic dry eye disease): 1 gtt in each eye q12h.
PEDS - Not approved in children.
FORMS - Trade only: emulsion 0.05% (0.4 mL single-use vials).
NOTES - Wait 10 min after use before inserting contact lenses. May take mo to note clinical improvement.

**FLUORESCEIN** (*Fluor-I-Strip, Fluor-I-Strip AT, Ful-Glo*) ▶Minimal absorption ♀? ▶? $
ADULT - Following ocular anesthetic, apply enough stain to bulbar conjunctiva to assess integrity of cornea.
PEDS - Following ocular anesthetic, apply enough stain to bulbar conjunctiva to assess integrity of cornea.
FORMS - Trade only (Fluor-I-Strip AT): Fluorescein 1 mg in sterile ophthalmic strip. (Fluor-I-Strip): Fluorescein 9 mg in sterile ophthalmic strip.
NOTES - Do not use with soft contact lenses

**HYDROXYPROPYL CELLULOSE** (*Lacrisert*) ▶Minimal absorption ♀+ ▶+ $$$
ADULT - Moderate-severe dry eyes: One insert in each eye daily. Some patients may require bid use.
PEDS - Not approved in children.

FORMS - Trade only: ocular insert 5 mg.
NOTES - Do not use with soft contact lenses.

**PETROLATUM** (*Lacrilube, Dry Eyes, Refresh PM, ✦Duolube*) ▶Minimal absorption ♀A ▶+ $
ADULT - Ophthalmic lubricant: Apply ¼-½ inch ointment to inside of lower lid prn.
PEDS - Ophthalmic lubricant: Apply ¼-½ inch ointment to inside of lower lid prn.
FORMS - OTC Trade only: ointment (3.5 & 7 g) tube.

**PROPARACAINE** (*Ophthaine, Ophthetic, ✦Alcaine*) ▶L ♀C ▶? $
ADULT - Do not prescribe for unsupervised use. Corneal toxicity may occur with repeated use. Local anesthetic: 1–2 gtts before procedure. Repeat q5–10 min × 1–3 doses (suture or foreign body removal) or × 5–7 doses (ocular surgery).
PEDS - Not approved in children.
FORMS - Generic/Trade: solution 0.5% (15 mL).

**TETRACAINE - OPHTHALMIC** (*Pontocaine*) ▶Plasma ♀C ▶? $
ADULT - Do not prescribe for unsupervised use. Corneal toxicity may occur with repeated use. Local anesthetic: 1–2 gtts or ½-1 inch ribbon of ointment before procedure.
PEDS - Not approved in children.
FORMS - Generic only: solution 0.5% (15 mL), unit-dose vials (0.7 & 2 mL).

**TRYPAN BLUE** (*Vision Blue*) ▶Not absorbed ♀C ▶? $$
ADULT - Aid during ophthalmic surgery by staining anterior cap: inject into anterior chamber of eye.
PEDS - Not approved in children.
FORMS - Trade only: 0.06% ophthalmic solution (0.5 mL).

## PSYCHIATRY: Antidepressants—Heterocyclic Compounds

**NOTE:** Gradually taper when discontinuing cyclic antidepressants to avoid withdrawal symptoms. Seizures, orthostatic hypotension, arrhythmias, and anticholinergic side effects may occur. Don't use with MAOIs. Antidepressants increase the risk of suicidal thinking and behavior in children, adolescents, and young adults; carefully weigh the risks and benefits before starting and monitor patients closely.

**AMITRIPTYLINE** (*Elavil*) ▶L ♀D ▶- $$
ADULT - Depression: Start 25–100 mg PO qhs; gradually increase to usual effective dose of 50–300 mg/d.
PEDS - Depression, adolescents: Use adult dosing. Not approved in children <12 yo.
UNAPPROVED ADULT - Migraine prophylaxis and/or chronic pain: 10–100 mg/d. Fibromyalgia: 25–50 mg/d.
UNAPPROVED PEDS - Depression, <12 yo: Start 1 mg/kg/d PO divided tid × 3 d, then increase to 1.5 mg/kg/d. Max 5 mg/kg/d.

FORMS - Generic: Tabs 10, 25, 50, 75, 100,150 mg. Elavil brand name no longer available; has been retained in this entry for name recognition purposes only.
NOTES - Tricyclic, tertiary amine - primarily inhibits serotonin reuptake. Demethylated to nortriptyline, which primarily inhibits norepinephrine reuptake. Usual therapeutic range is 150–300 ng/mL (amitriptyline + nortriptyline).

**AMOXAPINE** ▶L ♀C ▶- $$$
ADULT - Rarely used; other drugs preferred. Depression: Start 25–50 mg PO bid-tid; increase

(cont.)

**AMOXAPINE** *(cont.)*
by 50–100 mg bid-tid after 1 wk. Usual effective dose is 150–400 mg/d. Max 600 mg/d.
PEDS - Not approved in children <16 yo.
FORMS - Generic only: Tabs 25, 50, 100, 150 mg.
NOTES - Tetracyclic - primarily inhibits norepinephrine reuptake. Dose ≤300 mg/d may be given once daily at bedtime.

**CLOMIPRAMINE** *(Anafranil)* ▶L ♀C ▶+ $$$
ADULT - OCD: Start 25 mg PO qhs; gradually increase over 2 wk to usual effective dose of 150–250 mg/d. Max 250 mg/d.
PEDS - OCD, ≥10 yo: Start 25 mg PO qhs, then increase gradually over 2 wk to 3 mg/kg/d or 100 mg/d, max 200 mg/d. Not approved for <10 yo.
UNAPPROVED ADULT - Depression: 100–250 mg/d. Panic disorder: 12.5–150 mg/d. Chronic pain: 100–250 mg/d.
FORMS - Generic/Trade: Caps 25, 50, 75 mg.
NOTES - Tricyclic, tertiary amine - primarily inhibits serotonin reuptake.

**DESIPRAMINE** *(Norpramin)* ▶L ♀C ▶+ $$
ADULT - Depression: Start 25–100 mg PO given once daily or in divided doses. Gradually increase to usual effective dose of 100–200 mg/d, max 300 mg/d.
PEDS - Adolescents: 25–100 mg/d. Not approved in children.
FORMS - Generic/Trade: Tabs 10, 25, 50, 75, 100, 150 mg.
NOTES - Tricyclic, secondary amine - primarily inhibits norepinephrine reuptake. Usual therapeutic range is 125–300 ng/mL. May cause fewer anticholinergic side effects than tertiary amines. Use lower doses in adolescents or elderly.

**DOXEPIN** *(Sinequan)* ▶L ♀C ▶- $$
ADULT - Depression and/or anxiety: Start 75 mg PO qhs. Gradually increase to usual effective dose of 75–150 mg/d, max 300 mg/d.
PEDS - Adolescents: Use adult dosing. Not approved in children <12 yo.
UNAPPROVED ADULT - Chronic pain: 50–300 mg/d. Pruritus: Start 10–25 mg at bedtime. Usual effective dose is 10–100 mg/d.
FORMS - Generic/Trade: Caps 10, 25, 50, 75, 100, 150 mg. Oral concentrate 10 mg/mL.
NOTES - Tricyclic, tertiary amine - primarily inhibits norepinephrine reuptake. Do not mix oral concentrate with carbonated beverages. Some patients with mild symptoms may respond to 25–50 mg/d.

**IMIPRAMINE** *(Tofranil, Tofranil PM)* ▶L ♀D ▶- $$$
ADULT - Depression: Start 75–100 mg PO qhs or in divided doses; gradually increase to max 300 mg/d.
PEDS - Not approved for depression if <12 yo. Enuresis ≥6 yo: 10- 25 mg/d PO given one h before bedtime, then increase in increments of 10–25 mg at 1–2 wk intervals not to exceed 50 mg/d in 6–12 yo children or 75 mg/d in children >12 yo. Do not exceed 2.5 mg/kg/d.

UNAPPROVED ADULT - Panic disorder: Start 10 mg PO qhs, titrate to usual effective dose of 50–300 mg/d. Enuresis: 25–75 mg PO qhs.
UNAPPROVED PEDS - Depression, children: Start 1.5 mg/kg/d PO divided tid; increase by 1–1.5 mg/kg/d q3–4 d to max 5 mg/kg/d.
FORMS - Generic/Trade: Tabs 10, 25, 50 mg. Trade only: Caps 75, 100, 125, 150 mg (as pamoate salt).
NOTES - Tricyclic, tertiary amine - inhibits serotonin and norepinephrine reuptake. Demethylated to desipramine, which primarily inhibits norepinephrine reuptake.

**MAPROTILINE** *(Ludiomil)* ▶KL ♀B ▶? $$$
ADULT - Rarely used; other drugs preferred. Depression: Start 25 mg PO daily, then gradually increase by 25 mg q2 wk to max 225 mg/d. Usual effective dose is 150–225 mg/d. Max 200 mg/d for chronic use.
PEDS - Not approved in children.
FORMS - Generic only: Tabs 25, 50, 75 mg.
NOTES - Tetracyclic - primarily inhibits norepinephrine reuptake.

**NORTRIPTYLINE** *(Aventyl, Pamelor)* ▶L ♀D ▶+ $$$
ADULT - Depression: Start 25 mg PO given once daily or divided bid-qid. Gradually increase to usual effective dose of 75–100 mg/d, max 150 mg/d.
PEDS - Not approved in children.
UNAPPROVED ADULT - Panic disorder: Start 25 mg PO qhs, titrate to usual effective dose of 50–150 mg/d. Smoking cessation: Start 25 mg PO daily 14 d prior to quit date. Titrate to 75 mg/d as tolerated. Continue for ≥6 wk after quit date.
UNAPPROVED PEDS - Depression 6–12 yo: 1–3 mg/kg/d PO divided tid-qid or 10–20 mg/d PO divided tid-qid.
FORMS - Generic/Trade: Caps 10, 25, 50, 75 mg. Oral Solution 10 mg/5 mL.
NOTES - Tricyclic, secondary amine - primarily inhibits norepinephrine reuptake. Usual therapeutic range is 50–150 ng/mL. May cause fewer anticholinergic side effects than tertiary amines. May be used in combination with nicotine replacement for smoking cessation.

**PROTRIPTYLINE** *(Vivactil)* ▶L ♀C ▶+ $$$$
ADULT - Depression: 15–40 mg/d PO divided tid-qid. Max dose is 60 mg/d.
PEDS - Not approved in children.
FORMS - Trade only: Tabs 5, 10 mg.
NOTES - Tricyclic, secondary amine - primarily inhibits norepinephrine reuptake. May cause fewer anticholinergic side effects than tertiary amines. Dose increases should be made in the morning.

**TRIMIPRAMINE** *(Surmontil)* ▶L ♀C ▶? $$$$
ADULT - Depression: Start 25 mg PO qhs; gradually increase to 75–150 mg/d. Max 300 mg/d.
PEDS - Not approved in children.
FORMS - Trade only: Caps 25, 50, 100 mg.
NOTES - Tricyclic, tertiary amine - primarily inhibits norepinephrine reuptake.

## PSYCHIATRY: Antidepressants—Monoamine Oxidase Inhibitors (MAOIs)

**NOTE:** May interfere with sleep; avoid qhs dosing. Must be on tyramine-free diet throughout treatment, and for 2 wk after discontinuation. Numerous drug interactions; risk of hypertensive crisis and serotonin syndrome with many medications, including OTC. Allow ≥2 wk wash-out when converting from an MAOI to an SSRI (6 wk after fluoxetine), TCA, or other antidepressant. Contraindicated with carbamazepine or oxcarbazepine. Antidepressants increase the risk of suicidal thinking and behavior in children, adolescents, and young adults; carefully weigh the risks and benefits before starting and monitor patients closely.

**ISOCARBOXAZID (*Marplan*) ►L ♀C ▶? $$$**
ADULT - Depression: Start 10 mg PO bid; increase by 10 mg q2–4 d. Usual effective dose is 20–40 mg/d. Max 60 mg/d divided bid-qid.
PEDS - Not approved in children <16 yo.
FORMS - Trade only: Tabs 10 mg.
NOTES - Requires MAOI diet.

**MOCLOBEMIDE, ✦*MANERIX* ►L ♀C ▶- $$**
ADULT - Canada only. Depression: Start 300 mg/d PO divided bid after meals. May increase after 1 wk to max 600 mg/d.
PEDS - Not approved in children.
FORMS - Generic/Trade: Tabs 150, 300 mg. Generic only: Tabs 100 mg.
NOTES - No dietary restrictions. Don't use with tricyclic antidepressants; use caution with conventional MAOIs, other antidepressants, epinephrine, thioridazine, sympathomimetics, dextromethorphan, meperidine, and other opiates. Reduce dose in severe hepatic dysfunction.

**PHENELZINE (*Nardil*) ►L ♀C ▶? $$$**
ADULT - Depression: Start 15 mg PO tid. Usual effective dose is 60–90 mg/d in divided doses.
PEDS - Not approved in children <16 yo.
FORMS - Trade only: Tabs 15 mg.
NOTES - Requires MAOI diet. May increase insulin sensitivity. Contraindicated with meperidine.

**SELEGILINE - TRANSDERMAL (*Emsam*) ►L ♀C ▶? $$$$$**
ADULT - Depression: Start 6 mg/24h patch q 24 h. Adjust dose in ≥2 wk intervals to max 12 mg/24hr.
PEDS - Not approved in children.
FORMS - Trade only: Transdermal patch 6 mg/24hr, 9 mg/24hr, 12 mg/24hr.
NOTES - MAOI diet is required for doses ≥9 mg/24 h.

**TRANYLCYPROMINE (*Parnate*) ►L ♀C ▶- $$**
ADULT - Depression: Start 10 mg PO qam; increase by 10 mg/d at 1–3 wk intervals to usual effective dose of 10–40 mg/d divided bid. Max 60 mg/d.
PEDS - Not approved in children <16 yo.
FORMS - Generic/Trade: Tabs 10 mg.
NOTES - Requires MAOI diet.

## PSYCHIATRY: Antidepressants—Selective Serotonin Reuptake Inhibitors (SSRIs)

**NOTE:** Gradually taper when discontinuing SSRIs to avoid withdrawal symptoms. Observe patients for worsening depression or the emergence of suicidality, anxiety, agitation, panic attacks, insomnia, irritability, hostility, impulsivity, akathisia, mania, or hypomania, particularly early in therapy or after increases in dose. Antidepressants increase the risk of suicidal thinking and behavior in children, adolescents, and young adults; carefully weigh the risks and benefits before starting treatment and then monitor patients closely. Use of SSRIs during the third trimester of pregnancy has been associated with neonatal complications including respiratory (including persistent pulmonary hypertension), gastrointestinal, and feeding problems, as well as seizures and withdrawal symptoms. Balance these risks against those of withdrawal and depression for the mother. Paroxetine should be avoided throughout pregnancy. Don't use sibutramine with SSRIs. Increased risk of abnormal bleeding; use caution when combined with NSAIDs or aspirin. Use cautiously and observe closely for serotonin syndrome if SSRI is used with a triptan. SSRIs and SNRIs have been associated with hyponatremia, which is often associated with SIADH. The elderly and those taking diuretics may be at increased risk.

**CITALOPRAM (*Celexa*) ►LK ♀C but - in 3rd trimester ▶- $$$**
ADULT - Depression: Start 20 mg PO daily; increase by 20 mg/d at >1 wk intervals. Usual effective dose is 20–40 mg/d, max 60 mg/d.
PEDS - Not approved in children.
FORMS - Generic/Trade: Tabs 10, 20, 40 mg. Oral solution 10 mg/5 mL. Generic only: Oral disintegrating tab 10, 20, 40 mg.
NOTES - Don't use with MAOIs or tryptophan.

**ESCITALOPRAM (*Lexapro*, ✦*Cipralex*) ►LK ♀C but - in 3rd trimester ▶- $$$**
ADULT - Depression, generalized anxiety disorder: Start 10 mg PO daily; may increase to max 20 mg PO daily after >1 wk.
PEDS - Not approved in children.
UNAPPROVED ADULT - Social anxiety disorder: 5–20 mg PO daily.
FORMS - Generic/Trade: Tabs 5, 10, 20 mg. Trade only: Oral solution 1 mg/mL.
NOTES - Don't use with MAOIs. Doses >20 mg daily have not been shown to be superior to 10 mg daily. Escitalopram is the active isomer of citalopram.

**FLUOXETINE (*Prozac, Prozac Weekly, Sarafem*) ►L ♀C but - in 3rd trimester ▶- $$$**
ADULT - Depression, OCD: Start 20 mg PO q am; may increase after several wk to usual effective dose of 20–40 mg/d, max 80 mg/d. Depression, maintenance therapy: 20–40 mg/d (standard-release) or 90 mg PO once weekly (Prozac Weekly) starting 7 d after last standard-release dose. Bulimia: 60 mg

(cont.)

**FLUOXETINE** (*cont.*)

PO qam; may need to titrate up to this dose slowly over several d. Panic disorder: Start 10 mg PO q am; titrate to 20 mg/d after one wk, max 60 mg/d. Premenstrual Dysphoric Disorder (Sarafem): 20 mg PO daily given continuously throughout the menstrual cycle (continuous dosing) or 20 mg PO daily for 14 d prior to menses (intermittent dosing); max 80 mg daily. Doses >20 mg/d can be divided (q am and q noon).

PEDS - Depression 7–17 yo: 10–20 mg PO q am (10 mg for smaller children), max 20 mg/d. OCD: Start 10 mg PO q am; max 60 mg/d (30 mg/d for smaller children).

UNAPPROVED ADULT - Hot flashes: 20 mg PO daily. Post-traumatic stress disorder: 20–80 mg PO daily. Social anxiety disorder: 10–60 mg PO daily.

FORMS - Generic/Trade: Tabs 10 mg. Caps 10, 20, 40 mg. Oral solution 20 mg/5 mL. Caps (Sarafem) 10, 20 mg. Trade only: Tabs (Sarafem) 10, 15, 20 mg. Caps, delayed-release (Prozac Weekly) 90 mg. Generic only: Tabs 20, 40 mg.

NOTES - Half-life of parent is 1–3 d and for active metabolite norfluoxetine is 6–14 d. Don't use with thioridazine, MAOIs, cisapride, or tryptophan; use caution with lithium, phenytoin, TCAs, and warfarin. Pregnancy exposure has been associated with premature delivery, low birth weight, and lower Apgar scores. Decrease dose with liver disease. Increases risk of mania with bipolar disorder.

**FLUVOXAMINE** (*Luvox, Luvox CR*) ▶L ♀C but - in 3rd trimester ▶- $$$$

ADULT - Start 50 mg PO qhs, then increase by 50 mg/d q4–7 d to usual effective dose of 100–300 mg/d divided bid. Max 300 mg/d. OCD and Social Anxiety Disorder (CR): Start 100 mg PO qhs; increase by 50 mg/d q wk prn to max 300 mg/d.

PEDS - OCD (≥8 yo): Start 25 mg PO qhs; increase by 25 mg/d q4–7 d to usual effective dose of 50–200 mg/d divided bid. Max 200 mg/d (8–11 yo) or 300 mg/d (>11 yo). Therapeutic effect may be seen with lower doses in girls.

FORMS - Generic/Trade: Tabs 25, 50, 100 mg. Trade only: Caps, extended-release 100, 150 mg.

NOTES - Don't use with thioridazine, pimozide, alosetron, cisapride, tizanidine, tryptophan, or MAOIs; use caution with benzodiazepines, theophylline, TCAs, and warfarin. Luvox brand not currently on US market.

**PAROXETINE** (*Paxil, Paxil CR, Pexeva*) ▶LK ♀D ▶? $$$

ADULT - Depression: Start 20 mg PO qam; increase by 10 mg/d at intervals ≥1 wk to usual effective dose of 20–50 mg/d, max 50 mg/d. Depression, controlled-release tabs: Start 25 mg PO qam; may increase by 12.5 mg/d at intervals ≥1 wk to usual effective dose of 25–62.5 mg/d; max 62.5 mg/d. OCD: Start 20 mg PO qam; increase by 10 mg/d at intervals ≥1 wk to usual recommended dose of 40 mg/d; max 60 mg/d. Panic disorder: Start 10 mg PO qam; increase by 10 mg/d at

intervals ≥1 wk to target dose of 40 mg/d; max 60 mg/d. Panic disorder, controlled-release tabs: start 12.5 mg/d; increase by 12.5 mg/d at intervals ≥1 wk to usual effective dose of 12.5–75 mg/d; max 75 mg/d. Social anxiety disorder: Start 20 mg PO qam (which is the usual effective dose); max 60 mg/d. Social anxiety disorder, controlled-release tabs: Start 12.5 mg PO qam; may increase at intervals ≥1 wk to max 37.5 mg/d. Generalized anxiety disorder: Start 20 mg PO qam (which is the usual effective dose); max 50 mg/d. Post-traumatic stress disorder: Start 20 mg PO qam; usual effective dose is 20–40 mg/d; max 50 mg/d. Premenstrual dysphoric disorder (PMDD), continuous dosing: Start 12.5 mg PO qam (controlled-release tabs); may increase dose after 1 wk to max 25 mg qam. PMDD, intermittent dosing (given for 2 wk prior to menses): Start 12.5 mg PO qam (controlled-release tabs), max 25 mg/d.

PEDS - Not recommended for use in children or adolescents due to increased risk of suicidality.

UNAPPROVED ADULT - Hot flashes related to menopause or breast cancer: 20 mg PO daily (tabs), or 12.5–25 mg PO daily (controlled-release tabs).

FORMS - Generic/Trade: Tabs 10, 20, 30, 40 mg. Oral Suspension 10 mg/5 mL. Controlled-release tabs 12.5, 25 mg. Trade only: (Paxil CR) 37.5 mg.

NOTES - Start at 10 mg/d and do not exceed 40 mg/d in elderly or debilitated patients or those with renal or hepatic impairment. Paroxetine is an inhibitor of CYP2D6, and is contraindicated with thioridazine, pimozide, MAOIs, and tryptophan; use caution with barbiturates, cimetidine, phenytoin, theophylline, TCAs, risperidone, atomoxetine, and warfarin. Taper gradually after long-term use; reduce by 10 mg/d q wk to 20 mg/d; continue for 1 wk at this dose, and then stop. If withdrawal symptoms develop, then restart at prior dose and taper more slowly. Pexeva is paroxetine mesylate and is a generic equivalent for paroxetine HCl.

**SERTRALINE** (*Zoloft*) ▶LK ♀C but - in 3rd trimester ▶+ $$$

ADULT - Depression, OCD: Start 50 mg PO daily; may increase after 1 wk. Usual effective dose is 50–200 mg/d, max 200 mg/d. Panic disorder, post-traumatic stress disorder, social anxiety disorder: Start 25 mg PO daily; may increase after 1 wk to 50 mg PO daily. Usual effective dose is 50–200 mg/d; max 200 mg/d. Premenstrual dysphoric disorder (PMDD), continuous dosing: Start 50 mg PO daily; max 150 mg/d. PMDD, intermittent dosing (given for 14 d prior to menses): Start 50 mg PO daily × 3 d, then increase to max 100 mg/d.

PEDS - OCD, 6–12 yo: Start 25 mg PO daily, max 200 mg/d. OCD, ≥13 yo: Use adult dosing.

UNAPPROVED PEDS - Major depressive disorder: Start 25 mg PO daily; usual effective dose is 50–200 mg/d.

**SERTRALINE** *(cont.)*
FORMS - Generic/Trade: Tabs 25, 50, 100 mg. Oral concentrate 20 mg/mL (60 mL).
NOTES - Don't use with cisapride, tryptophan, or MAOIs; use caution with cimetidine, warfarin,

pimozide, or TCAs. Must dilute oral concentrate before administration. Administration during pregnancy has been associated with premature delivery, low birth weight, and lower Apgar scores.

## PSYCHIATRY: Antidepressants—Serotonin-Norepinephrine Reuptake Inhibitors (SNRIs)

**NOTE:** Monitor for the emergence of anxiety, agitation, panic attacks, insomnia, irritability, hostility, impulsivity, akathisia, mania, or hypomania, and for worsening depression or the emergence of suicidality, particularly early in therapy or after increases in dose. Antidepressants increase the risk of suicidal thinking and behavior in children, adolescents, and young adults; carefully weigh the risks and benefits before starting treatment, and then monitor closely. SSRIs and SNRIs have been associated with hyponatremia, which is often associated with SIADH. The elderly and those taking diuretics may be at increased risk. Do not use with MAO inhibitors.

**DESVENLAFAXINE** *(Pristiq)* ►LK ♀C ▶? $$$$
ADULT - 50 mg PO daily. Max 400 mg/d.
PEDS - Not approved for use in children.
FORMS - Trade only: Tabs, extended-release 50, 100 mg.
NOTES - There is no evidence that doses >50 mg/d offer additional benefit. Reduce dose to 50 mg PO qod in severe renal impairment (CrCl <30 mL/min). Caution in cardiovascular, cerebrovascular, or lipid disorders. Gradually taper when discontinuing therapy to avoid withdrawal symptoms after prolonged use. Exposure to SSRIs or SNRIs during the third trimester of pregnancy has been associated with neonatal complications including respiratory, gastrointestinal, and feeding problems, as well as seizures and withdrawal symptoms. Balance these risks against those of withdrawal and depression for the mother.

**DULOXETINE** *(Cymbalta)* ►L ♀C ▶? $$$$
ADULT - Depression: 20 mg PO bid; max 60 mg/d given once daily or divided bid. Generalized anxiety disorder: Start 30–60 mg PO daily, max 120 mg/d. Diabetic peripheral neuropathic pain: 60 mg PO daily, max 60 mg/d. Fibromyalgia: Start 30–60 mg PO daily, max 60 mg/d.
PEDS - Not approved in children.
FORMS - Trade only: Caps 20, 30, 60 mg.
NOTES - Avoid in renal insufficiency (CrCl <30 mL/min), hepatic insufficiency, or substantial alcohol use. Don't use with thioridazine, MAOIs, or potent inhibitors of CYP1A2; use caution with inhibitors of CYP2D6. Small BP increases (2 mm Hg systolic, 0.5 mm Hg diastolic) have been observed. Exposure during the third trimester of pregnancy has been associated with neonatal complications including respiratory, gastrointestinal, and feeding problems, as well as seizures, and withdrawal symptoms; balance these risks against those of withdrawal and depression for the mother.

**VENLAFAXINE** *(Effexor, Effexor XR)* ►LK ♀C but - in 3rd trimester ▶? $$$$
ADULT - Depression: Start 37.5–75 mg PO daily (Effexor XR) or 75 mg/d divided bid-tid (Effexor). Increase in 75 mg increments q4 d to usual effective dose of 150–225 mg/d, max 225 mg/d (Effexor XR) or 375 mg/d (Effexor). Generalized anxiety disorder: Start 37.5–75 mg PO daily (Effexor XR); increase in 75 mg increments q4 d to max 225 mg/d. Social anxiety disorder: 75 mg PO daily (Effexor XR). Panic disorder: Start 37.5 mg PO daily (Effexor XR), may titrate by 75 mg/d at weekly intervals to max 225 mg/d.
PEDS - Not approved in children. May increase the risk of suicidality in children and teenagers.
UNAPPROVED ADULT - Hot flashes (primarily in cancer patients): 37.5–75 mg/d of the extended-release form.
FORMS - Trade only: Caps, extended-release 37.5, 75, 150 mg. Generic/Trade: Tabs 25, 37.5, 50, 75, 100 mg. Generic only: Tabs, extended-release 37.5, 75, 150, 225 mg.
NOTES - Non-cyclic, serotonin-norepinephrine reuptake inhibitor (SNRI). Decrease dose in renal or hepatic impairment. Monitor for increases in BP. Don't give with MAOIs; use caution with cimetidine and haloperidol. Use caution and monitor for serotonin syndrome if used with triptans. Gradually taper when discontinuing therapy to avoid withdrawal symptoms after prolonged use. Hostility, suicidal ideation, and self-harm have been reported when used in children. Exposure during the third trimester of pregnancy has been associated with neonatal complications including respiratory, gastrointestinal, and feeding problems, as well as seizures and withdrawal symptoms. Balance these risks against those of withdrawal and depression for the mother. Mydriasis and increased intraocular pressure can occur; use caution in glaucoma.

## PSYCHIATRY: Antidepressants—Other

**NOTE:** Monitor for the emergence of anxiety, agitation, panic attacks, insomnia, irritability, hostility, impulsivity, akathisia, mania, or hypomania, and for worsening depression or the emergence of suicidality, particularly early in therapy or after increases in dose. Antidepressants increase the risk of suicidal thinking and behavior in children, adolescents, and young adults; carefully weigh the risks and benefits before starting treatment, and then monitor closely.

**BUPROPION** (*Wellbutrin, Wellbutrin SR, Wellbutrin XL, Aplenzin, Zyban, Buproban*) ▶LK ♀C ▶- $$$$
ADULT - Depression: Start 100 mg PO bid (immediate-release tabs); can increase to 100 mg tid after 4–7 d. Usual effective dose is 300–450 mg/d, max 150 mg/dose and 450 mg/d. Depression, sustained-release tabs (Wellbutrin SR): Start 150 mg PO q am; may increase to 150 mg bid after 4–7 d, max 400 mg/d. Give the last dose no later than 5 pm. Depression, extended-release tabs (Wellbutrin XL): Start 150 mg PO q am; may increase to 300 mg q am after 4 d, max 450 mg q am. Depression, extended-release (Aplenzin): Start 174 mg PO q am; increase to target dose of 348 mg/d after ≥4 d. May increase to max dose of 522 mg/d after ≥4 wk. Seasonal affective disorder, extended-release tabs (Wellbutrin XL): Start 150 mg PO q am in autumn; may increase after 1 wk to target dose of 300 mg q am, max 300 mg/d. In the spring, decrease to 150 mg/d for 2 wk and then discontinue. Smoking cessation (Zyban, Buproban): Start 150 mg PO qam × 3 d, then increase to 150 mg PO bid × 7–12 wk. Allow 8 h between doses, with the last dose given no later than 5 pm. Max 150 mg PO bid. Target quit date should be after at least 1 wk of therapy. Stop if there is no progress towards abstinence by the 7th wk. Write "dispense behavioral modification kit" on first script.
PEDS - Not approved in children.
UNAPPROVED ADULT - ADHD: 150–450 mg/d PO.
UNAPPROVED PEDS - ADHD: 1.4–5.7 mg/kg/d PO.
FORMS - Generic/Trade (for depression, bupropion HCl): Tabs 75,100 mg. Sustained release tabs 100, 150, 200 mg. Extended-release tabs 150, 300 mg (Wellbutrin XL). Generic/Trade (smoking cessation): Sustained-release tabs 150 mg (Zyban, Buproban). Trade only: extended release (Aplenzin, bupropion hydrobromide) tabs 174, 348, 522 mg.
NOTES - Weak inhibitor of dopamine reuptake. Don't use with MAOIs. Seizures occur in 0.4% of patients taking 300–450 mg per d. Contraindicated in seizure disorders, eating disorders, or with abrupt alcohol or sedative withdrawal. Wellbutrin SR, Zyban, and Buproban are all the same formulation. Equivalent doses: 174 HBr = 150 mg HCl, 348 mg HBr = 300 mg HCl, 522 mg HBr = 450 mg HCl. Consider dose reductions for hepatic and renal impairment.

**MIRTAZAPINE** (*Remeron, Remeron SolTab*) ▶LK ♀C ▶? $$
ADULT - Depression: Start 15 mg PO qhs, increase after 1–2 wk to usual effective dose of 15–45 mg/d.
PEDS - Not approved in children.
FORMS - Generic/Trade: Tabs 15, 30, 45 mg. Tabs, orally disintegrating (SolTab) 15, 30, 45 mg. Generic only: Tabs 7.5 mg.
NOTES - 0.1% risk of agranulocytosis. May cause drowsiness, increased appetite, and weight gain. Don't use with MAOIs.

**NEFAZODONE** ▶L ♀C ▶? $$$
WARNING - Rare reports of life-threatening liver failure. Discontinue if signs or symptoms of liver dysfunction develop. Brand name product withdrawn from the market in USA and Canada.
ADULT - Depression: Start 100 mg PO bid. Increase by 100–200 mg/d at ≥1 wk intervals to usual effective dose of 150–300 mg PO bid, max 600 mg/d. Start 50 mg PO bid in elderly or debilitated patients.
PEDS - Not approved in children.
FORMS - Generic only: Tabs 50, 100, 150, 200, 250 mg.
NOTES - Don't use with cisapride, MAOIs, pimozide, or triazolam; use caution with alprazolam. Many other drug interactions.

**TRAZODONE** ▶L ♀C ▶- $
ADULT - Depression: Start 50–150 mg/d PO in divided doses, increase by 50 mg/d q3–4 d. Usual effective dose is 400–600 mg/d.
PEDS - Not approved in children.
UNAPPROVED ADULT - Insomnia: 50–100 mg PO qhs, max 150 mg/d.
UNAPPROVED PEDS - Depression, 6–18 yo: Start 1.5–2 mg/kg/d PO divided bid-tid; may increase q3–4 d to max 6 mg/kg/d.
FORMS - Generic only: Tabs 50, 100, 150, 300 mg.
NOTES - May cause priapism. Rarely used as monotherapy for depression; most often used as a sleep aid and adjunct to another antidepressant. Use caution with CYP3A4 inhibitors or inducers.

**TRYPTOPHAN**, *←TRYPTAN* ▶K ♀? ▶? $$
ADULT - Canada only. Adjunct to antidepressant treatment for affective disorders: 8–12 g/d in 3–4 divided doses.
PEDS - Not indicated.
FORMS - Trade only: L-tryptophan tabs 250, 500, 750, 1000 mg.
NOTES - Caution in diabetics; may worsen glycemic control.

## PSYCHIATRY: Antimanic (Bipolar) Agents

**LAMOTRIGINE** (*Lamictal, Lamictal CD*) ▶LK ♀C (see Notes) ▶- $$$$
WARNING - Potentially life-threatening rashes (eg, Stevens-Johnson Syndrome, toxic epidermal necrolysis) have been reported in 0.3% of adults and 0.8% of children, usually within 2–8 wk of initiation; discontinue at first sign of rash. Drug interaction with valproate — see adjusted dosing guidelines. Recent data suggest an increased risk of suicidal ideation or behaviors with antiepileptic drugs. Monitor closely for signs of depression, anxiety, hostility, and hypomania/mania. Symptoms may develop within one wk of initiation and risk continues through at least 24 wk.
ADULT - Bipolar disorder (maintenance): Start 25 mg PO daily, 50 mg PO daily if on carbamazepine or other enzyme-inducing drugs, or 25 mg PO qod if on valproate. Increase for wk 3–4 to 50 mg/d,

**LAMOTRIGINE** (*cont.*)
50 mg bid if on enzyme-inducing drugs, or 25 mg/d if on valproate, then adjust over wk 5–7 to target doses of 200 mg/d, 400 mg/d divided bid if on enzyme-inducing drugs, or 100 mg/d if on valproate. See neurology section for epilepsy dosing.

PEDS - Not approved in children.

FORMS - Generic/Trade: Chewable dispersible tabs 5, 25 mg. Trade only: Tabs 25, 100, 150, 200 mg.

NOTES - Drug interactions with valproate and enzyme-inducing antiepileptic drugs (ie, carbamazepine, phenobarbital, phenytoin, primidone); may need to adjust dose. May increase carbamazepine toxicity. Preliminary evidence suggests that exposure during the first trimester of pregnancy is associated with a risk for cleft palate and/or cleft lip. Please report all fetal exposure to the Lamotrigine Pregnancy Registry (800-336-2176) and the North American Antiepileptic Drug Pregnancy Registry (888-233-2334).

**LITHIUM** (*Eskalith, Eskalith CR, Lithobid, ✦Lithane*) ►K ♀D ▶- $

WARNING - Lithium toxicity can occur at therapeutic levels.

ADULT - Acute mania: Start 300–600 mg PO bid-tid; usual effective dose is 900–1,800 mg/d. Bipolar maintenance usually 900–1,200 mg/d titrated to therapeutic trough level of 0.6–1.2 mEq/L.

PEDS - Adolescents ≥12 yo: Use adult dosing.

UNAPPROVED PEDS - Mania (<12 yo): Start 15–60 mg/kg/d PO divided tid-qid. Adjust weekly to achieve therapeutic levels.

FORMS - Generic/Trade: Caps 300, Extended release tabs 300, 450 mg. Generic only: Caps 150, 600 mg, Tabs 300 mg, Syrup 300/5 mL.

NOTES - Steady state levels occur in 5 d (later in elderly or renally-impaired patients). Usual therapeutic trough levels are 1.0–1.5 mEq/L (acute mania) or 0.6–1.2 mEq/L (maintenance). 300 mg = 8 mEq or mmol. A dose increase of 300 mg/d will increase the level by approx 0.2 mEq/L. Monitor renal and thyroid function, avoid dehydration or salt restriction, and watch closely for polydipsia or polyuria. Diuretics, ACE inhibitors, angiotensin receptor blockers, and NSAIDs may increase lithium levels (ASA & sulindac OK). Dose-related related side effects (eg, tremor, GI upset) may improve by dividing doses tid-qid or using extended-release tabs. Monitor renal function and electrolytes.

**TOPIRAMATE** (*Topamax*) ►K ♀C ▶? $$$$$

WARNING - Recent data suggest an increased risk of suicidal ideation or behaviors with antiepileptic drugs. Monitor closely for signs of depression, anxiety, hostility, and hypomania/mania. Symptoms may develop within one wk of initiation and risk continues through at least 24 wk.

ADULT - See neurology section

PEDS - Not approved for psychiatric use in children; see Neurology section.

UNAPPROVED ADULT - Bipolar disorder: Start 25–50 mg/d PO; titrate prn to max 400 mg/d divided bid.

Alcohol dependence: Start 25 mg/d PO; titrate weekly to max 150 mg bid.

FORMS - Trade only: Tabs 25, 50, 100, 200 mg. Sprinkle caps 15, 25 mg.

NOTES - Give ½ usual adult dose to patients with renal impairment (CrCl <70 mL/min). Cognitive symptoms, confusion, renal stones, glaucoma, and weight loss may occur. Risk of oligohidrosis and hyperthermia, particularly in children; use caution in warm ambient temperatures and/or with vigorous physical activity. Hyperchloremic, non-anion gap metabolic acidosis may occur; monitor serum bicarbonate and reduce dose and taper off if this occurs.

**VALPROIC ACID** (*Depakote, Depakote ER, Stavzor, divalproex, ✦Epiject, Epival, Deproic*) ►L ♀D ▶+ $$$$

WARNING - Fatal hepatic failure has occurred, especially in children <2 yo with multiple anticonvulsants and co-morbidities. Monitor LFTs frequently during first 6 mo. Life-threatening pancreatitis has been reported after initial or prolonged use. Evaluate for abdominal pain, N/V, and/or anorexia and discontinue if pancreatitis occurs. May be more teratogenic than other anticonvulsants (eg, carbamazepine, lamotrigine, and phenytoin). Hepatic failure and clotting disorders have also occurred when used during pregnancy. Recent data suggest an increased risk of suicidal ideation or behaviors with antiepileptic drugs. Monitor closely for signs of depression, anxiety, hostility, and hypomania/mania. Symptoms may develop within one wk of initiation and risk continues through at least 24 wk.

ADULT - Mania: Start 250 mg PO tid (Depakote or Stavzor) or 25 mg/kg once daily (Depakote ER); titrate to therapeutic level. Max 60 mg/kg/d.

PEDS - Not approved for mania in children.

UNAPPROVED PEDS - Bipolar disorder, manic or mixed phase (>2 yo): Start 125–250 mg PO bid or 15 mg/kg/d in divided doses. Titrate to therapeutic trough level of 45–125 mcg/mL, max 60 mg/kg/d.

FORMS - Generic/Trade: Caps 250mg (Depakene), syrup (Depakene, valproic acid) 250 mg/5 mL. Trade only (Depakote): Caps, sprinkle 125 mg, delayed release tabs 125, 250, 500 mg; extended release tabs (Depakote ER) 250, 500mg. Trade only (Stavzor): Delayed release caps 125, 250, 500mg.

NOTES - Contraindicated in urea cycle disorders or hepatic dysfunction. Reduce dose in the elderly. Recommended therapeutic trough level is 50–125 mcg/mL for Depakote and 85–125 mcg/mL for Depakote ER, though higher levels have been used. Many drug interactions. Hyperammonemia, GI irritation, or thrombocytopenia may occur. Depakote ER is about 10% less bioavailable than Depakote. Depakote releases divalproex sodium over 8–12h (daily-qid dosing) and Depakote ER releases divalproex sodium over 18–24h (daily dosing).

## PSYCHIATRY: Antipsychotics—First Generation (Typical)

**NOTE:** Antipsychotic potency is determined by affinity for D2 receptors. Extrapyramidal side effects (EPS) including tardive dyskinesia and dystonia may occur with antipsychotics. High potency agents are more likely to cause EPS and hyperprolactinemia. Can be given in qhs doses, but may be divided initially to decrease side effects and daytime sedation. Antipsychotics have been associated with an increased risk of venous thromboembolism, especially early in therapy. Assess for other risk factors and monitor carefully. Off-label use for dementia-related psychosis in the elderly has been associated with increased mortality.

**CHLORPROMAZINE (***Thorazine***)** ▶LK ♀C ▶- $$$
ADULT - Psychotic disorders: 10- 50 mg PO bid-qid or 25–50 mg IM, can repeat in 1 h. Severe cases may require 400 mg IM q4–6h up to max of 2,000 mg/d IM. Hiccups: 25–50 mg PO/IM tid-qid. Persistent hiccups may require 25–50 mg in 0.5–1 L NS by slow IV infusion.
PEDS - Severe behavioral problems/psychotic disorders age 6 mo-12 yo: 0.5 mg/kg PO q4–6h prn or 1 mg/kg PR q6–8h prn or 0.5 mg/kg IM q6–8h prn.
FORMS - Generic only: Tabs 10, 25, 50, 100, 200 mg. Generic/Trade: Oral concentrate 30 mg/mL, 100 mg/mL. Trade only: Syrup 10 mg/5 mL. Suppositories 25, 100 mg.
NOTES - Monitor for hypotension with IM or IV use.
**FLUPENTHIXOL (***flupentixol***, ✦***Fluanxol***, ***Fluanxol Depot***)** ▶? ♀? ▶- $$
ADULT - Canada only. Schizophrenia/psychosis: Tablets initial dose: 3 mg PO daily in divided doses, maintenance 3–12 mg daily in divided doses. IM initial dose 5–20 mg IM q2–4 wk, maintenance 20–40 mg q 2–4 wk. Higher doses may be necessary in some patients.
PEDS - Not approved in children.
FORMS - Trade only: tabs 0.5, 3 mg.
NOTES - Relatively non-sedating antipsychotic.
**FLUPHENAZINE (***Prolixin***, ✦***Modecate, Modeten***)** ▶LK ♀C ▶? $$$
ADULT - Psychotic disorders: Start 0.5- 10 mg/d PO divided q6–8h. Usual effective dose 1–20 mg/d. Max dose is 40 mg/d PO or 1.25- 10 mg/d IM divided q6–8h. Max dose is 10 mg/d IM. May use long-acting formulations (enanthate/decanoate) when patients are stabilized on a fixed daily dose. Approximate conversion ratio: 12.5- 25 mg IM/SC (depot) q3 wk = 10- 20 mg/d PO.
PEDS - Not approved in children.
FORMS - Generic/Trade: Tabs 1, 2.5, 5, 10 mg. Elixir 2.5 mg/5 mL. Oral concentrate 5 mg/mL.
NOTES - Do not mix oral concentrate with coffee, tea, cola, or apple juice.
**HALOPERIDOL (***Haldol***)** ▶LK ♀C ▶- $$
ADULT - Psychotic disorders/Tourette's: 0.5- 5 mg PO bid-tid. Usual effective dose is 6- 20 mg/d, max dose = 100 mg/d or 2–5 mg IM q1–8h prn. May use long-acting (depot) formulation when patients are stabilized on a fixed daily dose. Approximate conversion ratio: 100- 200 mg IM (depot) q4 wk = 10 mg/d PO haloperidol.
PEDS - Psychotic disorders age 3- 12 yo: 0.05-0.15 mg/kg/d PO divided bid-tid. Tourette's or non-psychotic behavior disorders age 3- 12 yo: 0.05- 0.075 mg/kg/d PO divided bid-tid. Increase

dose by 0.5 mg q wk to max dose of 6 mg/d. Not approved for IM administration in children.
UNAPPROVED ADULT - Acute psychosis and combative behavior: 5–10 mg IV/IM, repeat prn in 10–30 min. IV route associated with QT prolongation, Torsades de Pointes, and sudden death; use ECG monitoring.
UNAPPROVED PEDS - Psychosis 6–12 yo: 1–3 mg/dose IM (as lactate) q4–8h, max 0.15 mg/kg/d.
FORMS - Generic only: Tabs 0.5, 1, 2, 5, 10, 20 mg. Oral concentrate 2 mg/mL.
NOTES - Therapeutic range is 2- 15 ng/mL.
**LOXAPINE (***Loxitane***, ✦***Loxapac***)** ▶LK ♀C ▶- $$$$
ADULT - Psychotic disorders: Start 10 mg PO bid, usual effective dose is 60–100 mg/d divided bid-qid. Max dose is 250 mg/d.
PEDS - Not approved in children.
FORMS - Generic/Trade: Caps 5, 10, 25, 50 mg.
**METHOTRIMEPRAZINE, ✦***NOZINAN***)** ▶L ♀? ▶? $
ADULT - Canada only. Anxiety/analgesia: 6—25 mg PO per d given tid. Sedation: 10–25 mg hs. Psychoses/intense pain: Start 50–75 mg PO per d given in 2–3 doses, max 1000 mg/d. Postoperative pain: 20–40 mg PO or 10–25 mg IM q 8h. Anesthesia premedication: 10–25 mg IM or 20–40 mg PO q 8h with last dose of 25–50 mg IM 1h before surgery. Limit therapy to ≤30 d.
PEDS - Canada only. 0.25 mg/kg/d given in 2–3 doses, max 40 mg/d for child <12 yo.
FORMS - Canada only - Generic/Trade: Tabs 2, 5, 25, 50 mg.
**MOLINDONE (***Moban***)** ▶LK ♀C ▶? $$$$$
ADULT - Psychotic disorders: Start 50- 75 mg/d PO divided tid- qid, usual effective dose is 50- 100 mg/d. Max dose is 225 mg/d.
PEDS - Adolescents: Adult dosing. Not approved in children <12 yo.
FORMS - Trade only: Tabs 5,10,25,50 mg.
**PERPHENAZINE** ▶LK ♀C ▶? $$$
ADULT - Psychotic disorders: Start 4–8 mg PO tid or 8–16 mg PO bid-qid (hospitalized patients), max PO dose is 64 mg/d. Can give 5–10 mg IM q6h, max IM dose is 30 mg/d.
PEDS - Not approved for children <12 yo.
FORMS - Generic only: Tabs 2, 4, 8, 16 mg. Oral concentrate 16 mg/5 mL.
NOTES - Do not mix oral concentrate with coffee, tea, cola, or apple juice.
**PIMOZIDE (***Orap***)** ▶L ♀C ▶- $$$
ADULT - Tourette's: Start 1–2 mg/d PO in divided doses, increase q2 d to usual effective dose of 1–10 mg/d. Max dose is 0.2 mg/kg/d up to 10 mg/d.

**PIMOZIDE** (*cont.*)

PEDS - Tourette's age >12 yo: 0.05 mg/kg PO qhs, increase q3 d to max of 0.2 mg/kg/d up to 10 mg/d.

FORMS - Trade only: Tabs 1, 2 mg.

NOTES - QT prolongation may occur. Monitor ECG at baseline and periodically throughout therapy. Contraindicated with macrolide antibiotics, nefazodone, and sertraline. Use caution with inhibitors of CYP3A4.

**THIORIDAZINE** (*Mellaril, ✦Rideril*) ▶LK ♀C ▶? $$

WARNING - Can cause QTc prolongation, torsade de pointes-type arrhythmias, and sudden death.

ADULT - Psychotic disorders: Start 50—100 mg PO tid, usual effective dose is 200—800 mg/d divided bid-qid. Max dose is 800 mg/d.

PEDS - Behavioral disorders 2- 12 yo: 10- 25 mg PO bid-tid, max dose is 3 mg/kg/d.

FORMS - Generic only: Tabs 10, 15, 25, 50, 100, 150, 200 mg. Oral concentrate 30, 100 mg/mL.

NOTES - Not recommended as first-line therapy. Contraindicated in patients with a history of cardiac arrhythmias, congenital long QT syndrome, or those taking fluvoxamine, propranolol, pindolol, drugs that inhibit CYP 2D6 (eg, fluoxetine, paroxetine), and other drugs that prolong the QTc interval. Only use for patients with schizophrenia who do not respond to other antipsychotics. Monitor baseline ECG and potassium. Pigmentary retinopathy with doses >800 mg/d.

**THIOTHIXENE** (*Navane*) ▶LK ♀C ▶? $$$

ADULT - Psychotic disorders: Start 2 mg PO tid. Usual effective dose is 20—30 mg/d, max dose is 60 mg/d PO.

PEDS - Adolescents: Adult dosing. Not approved in children <12 yo.

FORMS - Generic/Trade: Caps 1, 2, 5, 10. Oral concentrate 5 mg/mL. Trade only: Caps 20 mg.

**TRIFLUOPERAZINE** (*Stelazine*) ▶LK ♀C ▶- $$$

ADULT - Psychotic disorders: Start 2—5 mg PO bid. Usual effective dose is 15- 20 mg/d, some patients may require ≥40 mg/d. Anxiety: 1—2 mg PO bid for up to 12 wk. Max dose is 6 mg/d.

PEDS - Psychotic disorders 6—12 yo: 1 mg PO daily-bid, gradually increase to max dose of 15 mg/d.

FORMS - Generic/Trade: Tabs 1, 2, 5, 10 mg. Trade only: Oral concentrate 10 mg/mL.

NOTES - Dilute oral concentrate just before giving.

**ZUCLOPENTHIXOL** (*✦Clopixol, Clopixol Accuphase, Clopixol Depot*) ▶L ♀? ▶? $$$$

ADULT - Canada only. Antipsychotic. Tablets: Start 10—50 mg PO daily, maintenance 20—60 mg daily. Injectable: Accuphase (acetate) 50—150 mg IM q2—3 d, Depot (decanoate) 150—300 mg IM q2—4 wk.

PEDS - Not approved in children.

FORMS - Trade, Canada-only: Tab 10, 20 mg (Clopixol).

## PSYCHIATRY: Antipsychotics—Second Generation (Atypical)

**NOTE:** Tardive dyskinesia, neuroleptic malignant syndrome, drug-induced parkinsonism, dystonia, and other extrapyramidal side effects may occur with antipsychotic medications. Atypical antipsychotics have been associated with weight gain, dyslipidemia, hyperglycemia, and diabetes mellitus; monitor closely. Off-label use for dementia-related psychosis in the elderly has been associated with increased mortality. Antipsychotics have been associated with an increased risk of venous thromboembolism, particularly early in therapy; assess for other risk factors and monitor carefully.

**ARIPIPRAZOLE** (*Abilify, Abilify Discmelt*) ▶L ♀C ▶? $$$$$

WARNING - Children, adolescents, and young adults taking antidepressants for major depressive disorder and other psychiatric disorders are at increased risk of suicidal thinking or behavior.

ADULT - Schizophrenia: Start 10—15 mg PO daily. Max 30 mg daily. Bipolar disorder (acute and maintenance for manic or mixed episodes, monotherapy or adjunctive to lithium or valproate): Start 15 mg PO daily; . May increase to 30 mg based on response and tolerability. Agitation associated with schizophrenia or bipolar disorder: 9.75 mg IM recommended. May consider 5.25 to 15 mg if indicated. May repeat in >2 h up to max 30 mg/d. Depression, adjunctive therapy: Start 2—5 mg PO daily. Increase by 5 mg/d at intervals ≥1 wk to max of 15 mg/d.

PEDS - Schizophrenia, 13—17 yo: Start 2 mg PO daily. May increase to 5 mg/d at ≥2 d, and to target dose of 10 mg/d after 2 more d. Max 30 mg/d. Bipolar disorder (acute and maintenance for manic or mixed episodes, monotherapy or

adjunctive to lithium or valproate), 10—17 yo: Start 2 mg PO daily. May increase to 5 mg/d at ≥2 d, and to target dose of 10 mg/d after 2 more d. Increase by 5 mg/d to max 30 mg/d.

FORMS - Trade only: Tabs 2, 5, 10, 15, 20, 30 mg. Oral solution 1 mg/mL (150 mL). Orally disintegrating tabs (Discmelt) 10, 15, 20, 30 mg.

NOTES - Low EPS and tardive dyskinesia risk. Increase dose when used with CYP3A4 inducers such as carbamazepine. Decrease usual dose by at least half when used with CYP3A4 or CYP2D6 inhibitors such as ketoconazole, fluoxetine or paroxetine. Increase dose by one-half to 20—30 mg/d when used with CYP3A4 inducers such as carbamazepine. Reduce when inducer is stopped.

**CLOZAPINE** (*Clozaril, FazaClo ODT*) ▶L ♀B ▶- $$$$$

WARNING - Risk of agranulocytosis is 1—2%, monitor WBC and ANC counts q wk × 6 mo, then q2 wk thereafter, and weekly for 4 wk after discontinuation. Contraindicated if WBC <3,500 or ANC <2,000/mm$^3$. Discontinue if WBC <3,000/mm$^3$. May decrease monitoring to q4 wk after 12 mo if WBC >3,500/mm$^3$ and ANC >2,000/mm$^3$. See

**(cont.)**

**CLOZAPINE** (cont.)

package insert for more details. Risk of myocarditis (particularly during the first mo), seizures, orthostatic hypotension, and cardiopulmonary arrest.

ADULT - Severe, medically-refractory schizophrenia or schizophrenia/schizoaffective disorder with suicidal behavior: Start 12.5 mg PO daily or bid; increase by 25–50 mg/d to usual effective dose of 300–450 mg/d, max 900 mg/d. Retitrate if stopped for more than 3–4 d.

PEDS - Not approved in children.

FORMS - Generic/Trade: Tabs 25, 100 mg. Generic only: Tabs 12.5, 50, 200 mg. Trade only: Orally disintegrating tab (Fazaclo ODT) 12.5, 25, 100 mg (scored).

NOTES - Patients rechallenged with clozapine after an episode of leukopenia are at increased risk of agranulocytosis, and must undergo weekly monitoring × 12 mo. Register all occurrences of leukopenia, discontinuation, and/or rechallenge to the Clozaril National Registry at 1-800-448-5938. Much lower risk of EPS and tardive dyskinesia than other neuroleptics. May be effective for treatment-resistant patients who have not responded to conventional agents. May cause significant weight gain, dyslipidemia, hyperglycemia, or new onset diabetes - monitor weight, fasting blood glucose, and triglycerides before initiation and at regular intervals during treatment. Excessive sedation or respiratory depression may occur with CNS depressants, particularly benzodiazepines. If orally-disintegrating tab is split, discard remaining portion.

**OLANZAPINE** (*Zyprexa, Zyprexa Zydis*) ▶L ♀C ▶- $$$$$

ADULT - Agitation in acute bipolar mania or schizophrenia: Start 10 mg IM (2.5–5 mg in elderly or debilitated patients); may repeat in ≥2h to max 30 mg/d. Psychotic disorders, oral therapy: Start 5–10 mg PO daily. Increase weekly to usual effective dose of 10–15 mg/d, max 20 mg/d. Bipolar disorder, maintenance treatment or monotherapy for acute manic or mixed episodes: Start 10–15 mg PO daily. Increase by 5 mg/d at intervals ≥24 h. Clinical efficacy seen at doses of 5–20 mg/d, max 20 mg/d. Bipolar disorder, adjunctive therapy for acute mixed or manic episodes: Start 10 mg PO daily; usual effective dose is 5–20 mg/d, max 20 mg/d.

PEDS - Not approved in children.

UNAPPROVED ADULT - Augmentation of SSRI therapy for OCD: Start 2.5–5.0 mg PO daily, max 20 mg/d. Post-traumatic stress disorder, adjunctive therapy: Start 5 mg PO daily, max 20 mg/d.

UNAPPROVED PEDS - Bipolar disorder, manic or mixed phase: Start 2.5 mg PO daily; increase by 2.5 mg/d every 3 d to max 20 mg/d.

FORMS - Trade only: Tabs 2.5, 5, 7.5, 10, 15, 20 mg. Tabs, orally-disintegrating (Zyprexa Zydis) 5,10,15, 20 mg.

## ANTIPSYCHOTIC RELATIVE ADVERSE EFFECTS[a]

| Generation | Antipsychotic | Anticho-linergic | Sedation | Hypoten-sion | Extrapy-ramidal Symptoms | Weight Gain | Diabetes/ Hyperglycemia | Dyslipi-demia |
|---|---|---|---|---|---|---|---|---|
| 1st | chlorpromazine | +++ | +++ | ++ | ++ | ++ | ? | ? |
| 1st | fluphenazine | ++ | + | + | ++++ | ++ | ? | ? |
| 1st | haloperidol | + | + | + | ++++ | ++ | 0 | ? |
| 1st | loxapine | ++ | + | + | ++ | + | ? | ? |
| 1st | molindone | ++ | ++ | + | ++ | + | ? | ? |
| 1st | perphenazine | ++ | ++ | + | ++ | + | +/? | ? |
| 1st | pimozide | + | + | + | +++ | ? | ? | ? |
| 1st | thioridazine | ++++ | +++ | +++ | + | +++ | +/? | ? |
| 1st | thiothixene | + | ++ | ++ | +++ | ++ | ? | ? |
| 1st | trifluoperazine | ++ | + | + | +++ | ++ | ? | ? |
| 2nd | aripiprazole | ++ | + | 0 | 0 | 0/+ | 0 | 0 |
| 2nd | clozapine | ++++ | +++ | +++ | 0 | +++ | + | + |
| 2nd | olanzapine | +++ | ++ | + | 0b | +++ | + | + |
| 2nd | risperidone | + | ++ | + | +b | ++ | ? | ? |
| 2nd | quetiapine | + | +++ | ++ | 0 | ++ | ? | ? |
| 2nd | ziprasidone | + | + | 0 | 0 | 0/+ | 0 | 0 |

a Risk of specific adverse effects is graded from 0 (absent) to ++++ (high). ? = Limited or inconsistent comparative data. b. EPS (extrapyramidal symptoms) are dose-related and are more likely for risperidone >6-8 mg/d / olanzapine >20 mg/d. Akathisia risk remains unclear and may not be reflected in these ratings. There are limited comparative data for aripiprazole relative to other second generation antipsychotics.

References: Goodman & Gilman 11e p461-500, Applied Therapeutics 8e p78, APA schizophrenia practice guideline, Psychiatry Q 2002; 73:297, Diabetes Care 2004; 27:596.

**OLANZAPINE** *(cont.)*

NOTES - Use for short-term (3–4 wk) acute manic episodes associated with bipolar disorder. May cause significant weight gain, dyslipidemia, hyperglycemia, or new onset diabetes; monitor weight, fasting blood glucose, and triglycerides before initiation and at regular intervals during treatment. Monitor for orthostatic hypotension, particularly when given IM. IM injection can also be associated with bradycardia and hypoventilation especially if used with other drugs that have these effects. Use caution with benzodiazepines.

**PALIPERIDONE** *(Invega, 9-hydroxyrisperidone)* ▶KL ♀C ▶- $$$$$

ADULT - Schizophrenia: Start 6 mg PO qam. 3 mg/d may be sufficient in some. Max 12 mg/d.

PEDS - Not approved in children.

FORMS - Trade only: Extended-release tabs 3, 6, 9 mg. 12 mg strength not available in the USA or Canada.

NOTES - Active metabolite of risperidone. Max 3 mg/d if CrCl is 10–49 mL/min.

**QUETIAPINE** *(Seroquel, Seroquel XR)* ▶LK ♀C ▶- $$$$$

WARNING - Antidepressants including quetiapine when used for bipolar depression increase the risk of suicidal thinking and behavior in children, adolescents, and young adults; carefully weigh the risks and benefits before starting treatment, and then monitor closely.

ADULT - Schizophrenia: Start 25 mg PO bid (regular tabs); increase by 25–50 mg bid-tid on d 2 and 3, and then to target dose of 300–400 mg/d divided bid-tid on d 4. Usual effective dose is 150–750 mg/d, max 800 mg/d. Schizophrenia, extended release tabs: Start 300 mg PO daily in evening, increase by up to 300 mg/d at intervals of >1 d to usual effective range of 400–800 mg/d. Acute bipolar mania, monotherapy or adjunctive: Start 50 mg PO bid on d 1, then increase to no higher than 100 mg bid on d 2, 150 mg bid on d 3, and 200 mg bid on d 4. May increase as needed to 300 mg bid on d 5 and 400 mg bid thereafter. Usual effective dose is 400–800 mg/d,max 800 mg/d. Bipolar depression: 50 mg PO hs on d 1, 100 mg hs d 2, 200 mg hs d 3, and 300 mg hs d 4. May increase prn to 400 mg hs on d 5 and 600 mg hs on d 8. Bipolar maintenance: continue dose required to maintain symptom remisson.

PEDS - Not approved in children.

UNAPPROVED ADULT - Augmentation of SSRI therapy for OCD: Start 25 mg PO bid, max 300 mg/d. Adjunctive for post-traumatic stress disorder: Start 25 mg daily, max 300 mg/d.

UNAPPROVED PEDS - Bipolar disorder (manic or mixed phase): Start 12.5 mg PO bid (children) or 25 mg PO bid (adolescents); max 150 mg PO tid.

FORMS - Trade only: Tabs 25, 50, 100, 200, 300, 400 mg. Extended-release tabs 50, 200, 300, 400 mg.

NOTES - Eye exam for cataracts recommended q 6 mo. Low risk of EPS and tardive dyskinesia. May cause significant weight gain, dyslipidemia, hyperglycemia, or new onset diabetes; monitor weight, fasting blood glucose, and triglycerides before initiation and at regular intervals during treatment. Use lower doses and slower titration in elderly patients or hepatic dysfunction. Extended-release tabs should be taken without food or after light meal.

**RISPERIDONE** *(Risperdal, Risperdal Consta)* ▶LK ♀C ▶- $$$$$

ADULT - Schizophrenia: Start 2 mg/d PO given once daily or divided bid; increase by 1–2 mg/d at intervals ≥24 h. Start 0.5 mg/dose and titrate by ≤0.5 mg bid in elderly, debilitated, hypotensive, or renally or hepatically impaired patients; increases to doses >1.5 mg should occur at intervals ≥1 wk. Usual effective dose is 4–8 mg/d given once daily or divided bid; max 16 mg/d. Long-acting injection (Consta) for schizophrenia: Start 25 mg IM q 2 wk while continuing oral dose × 3 wk. May increase q 4 wk to max 50 mg q 2 wk. Bipolar mania: Start 2–3 mg PO daily; may adjust by 1 mg/d at 24 h intervals to max 6 mg/d.

PEDS - Autistic disorder irritability (5–16 yo): Start 0.25 mg (<20 kg) or 0.5 mg (≥20 kg) PO daily. May increase after ≥4 d to 0.5 mg/d (<20 kg) or 1.0 mg/d (≥20 kg). Maintain ≥14 d. May then increase at ≥14 d intervals by increments of 0.25 mg/d (<20 kg) or 0.5 mg/d (≥20 kg) to max 1.0 mg/d (<20 kg), 2.5 mg/d (20–44 kg) or 3.0 mg/d (>45 kg). Schizophrenia (13–17 yo): Start 0.5 mg PO daily; increase by 0.5–1.0 mg/d at intervals ≥24 h to target dose of 3 mg/d. Max 6 mg/d. Bipolar mania (10–17 yo): Start 0.5 mg PO daily; increase by 0.5–1.0 mg/d at intervals ≥24 h to recommended dose of 2.5 mg/d. Max 6 mg/d.

UNAPPROVED ADULT - Augmentation of SSRI therapy for OCD: Start 1 mg/d PO, max 6 mg/d. Adjunctive therapy for post-traumatic stress disorder: Start 0.5 mg PO qhs, max 3 mg/d.

UNAPPROVED PEDS - Psychotic disorders, mania, aggression: 0.5–1.5 mg/d PO.

FORMS - Trade only: Tabs 0.25, 0.5, 1, 2, 3, 4 mg. Orally disintegrating tabs (M-TAB) 0.5, 1, 2 mg. Oral solution 1 mg/mL (30 mL).

NOTES - Has a greater tendency to produce extrapyramidal side effects (EPS) than other atypical neuroleptics. EPS reported in neonates following use in third trimester of pregnancy. May cause weight gain, hyperglycemia, or new onset diabetes - monitor closely. Patients with Parkinson's disease and dementia have increased sensitivity to side effects such as EPS, confusion, falls, and neuroleptic malignant syndrome. Solution is compatible with water, coffee, orange juice, and low-fat milk; is NOT compatible with cola or tea. Place orally disintegrating tabs on tongue and do not chew. Establish tolerability with oral form before starting long-acting injection. Alternate injections between buttocks.

**ZIPRASIDONE (*Geodon*)** ▶L ♀C ▶- $$$$$
WARNING - May prolong QTc. Avoid with drugs that prolong QTc or in those with long QT syndrome or cardiac arrhythmias.
ADULT - Schizophrenia: Start 20 mg PO bid with food; may increase at >2 d intervals to max 80 mg PO bid. Acute agitation in schizophrenia: 10–20 mg IM. May repeat 10 mg dose q 2 h or 20 mg dose q 4

h, to max 40 mg/d. Bipolar mania: Start 40 mg PO bid with food; may increase to 60–80 mg bid on d 2. Usual effective dose is 40–80 mg bid.
PEDS - Not approved in children.
FORMS - Trade only: Caps 20, 40, 60, 80 mg, Susp 10 mg/mL.
NOTES - Drug interactions with carbamazepine and ketoconazole.

## PSYCHIATRY: Anxiolytics/Hypnotics—Barbiturates

**BUTABARBITAL (*Butisol*)** ▶LK ♀D ▶? ©III $$$
ADULT - Rarely used; other drugs preferred. Sedative: 15–30 mg PO tid-qid. Hypnotic: 50–100 mg PO qhs for up to 2 wk.
PEDS - Pre-op sedation: 2–6 mg/kg PO before procedure, max 100 mg.
FORMS - Trade only: Tabs 30, 50 mg. Elixir 30 mg/5 mL.
**MEPHOBARBITAL (*Mebaral*)** ▶LK ♀D ▶? ©IV $$$
ADULT - Rarely used; other drugs preferred. Sedative: 32–100 mg PO tid-qid, usual dose is 50 mg PO tid-qid.
PEDS - Sedative: 16- 32 mg PO tid-qid.
FORMS - Trade only: Tabs 32, 50, 100 mg.

**SECOBARBITAL (*Seconal*)** ▶LK ♀D ▶+ ©II $
ADULT - Rarely used; other drugs preferred. Hypnotic: 100 mg PO qhs for up to 2 wk.
PEDS - Pre-anesthetic: 2–6 mg/kg PO up to 100 mg.
FORMS - Trade only: Caps 100 mg.
**TUINAL (amobarbital + secobarbital)** ▶LK ♀D ▶? ©II $$
ADULT - Rarely used; other drugs preferred. Hypnotic: 1 cap PO qhs.
PEDS - Not approved in children.
FORMS - Trade only: Caps 100 (50 mg amobarbital + 50 mg secobarbital).

## PSYCHIATRY: Anxiolytics/Hypnotics—Benzodiazepines—Long Half-Life (25–100 h)

**NOTE:** To avoid withdrawal, gradually taper when discontinuing after prolonged use. Use cautiously in the elderly; may accumulate and lead to side effects, psychomotor impairment. Sedative-hypnotics have been associated with severe allergic reactions and complex sleep behaviors including sleep driving. Use caution and discuss with patients.

**BROMAZEPAM, ✦*LECTOPAM*▶**L ♀D ▶- $
ADULT - Canada only. 6–18 mg/d PO in equally divided doses.
PEDS - Not approved in children.
FORMS - Generic/Trade: Tabs 1.5, 3, 6 mg.
NOTES - Do not exceed 3 mg/d initially in the elderly or debilitated. Gradually taper when discontinuing after prolonged use. Half life ~20 h in adults but increased in elderly. Cimetidine may prolong elimination.
**CHLORDIAZEPOXIDE (*Librium*)** ▶LK ♀D ▶- ©IV $$
ADULT - Anxiety: 5–25 mg PO tid- qid or 25–50 mg IM/IV tid-qid (acute/severe anxiety). Acute alcohol withdrawal: 50–100 mg PO/IM/IV, repeat q3–4h prn up to 300 mg/d.
PEDS - Anxiety and >6 yo: 5–10 mg PO bid-qid.
FORMS - Generic/Trade: Caps 5, 10, 25 mg.
NOTES - Half-life 5–30 h.
**CLONAZEPAM (*Klonopin, Klonopin Wafer, ✦Rivotril, Clonapam*)** ▶LK ♀D ▶- ©IV $
ADULT - Panic disorder: 0.25 mg PO bid, increase by 0.125- 0.25 mg q3 d to max dose of 4 mg/d. Akinetic or myoclonic seizures: Start 0.5 mg PO tid. Increase by 0.5–1 mg q3 d prn. Max 20 mg/d.
PEDS - Akinetic or myoclonic seizures, Lennox-Gastaut syndrome (petit mal variant), or absence seizures (≤10 yo or ≤30 kg): 0.01- 0.03 mg/kg PO divided bid-tid. Increase by 0.25- 0.5 mg q3 d prn. Max 0.1- 0.2 mg/kg/d divided tid.

UNAPPROVED ADULT - Neuralgias: 2–4 mg PO daily. Restless legs syndrome: Start 0.25 mg PO qhs. Max 2 mg qhs. REM sleep behavior disorder: 1–2 mg PO qhs.
FORMS - Generic/Trade: Tabs 0.5, 1, 2 mg. Orally disintegrating tabs (approved for panic disorder only) 0.125, 0.25, 0.5, 1, 2 mg.
NOTES - Half-life 18- 50 h. Usual therapeutic range = 20–80 ng/mL. Contraindicated in hepatic failure or acute narrow angle glaucoma.
**CLORAZEPATE (*Tranxene, Tranxene SD*)** ▶LK ♀D ▶- ©IV $
ADULT - Anxiety: Start 7.5–15 mg PO qhs or bid-tid, usual effective dose is 15–60 mg/d. Acute alcohol withdrawal: 60–90 mg/d on first d divided bid-tid, gradually reduce dose to 7.5–15 mg/d over 5 d. Max dose is 90 mg/d. May transfer patients to single-dose Tabs (Tranxene-SD) when dose stabilized.
PEDS - Not approved in children <9 yo.
FORMS - Generic/Trade: Tabs 3.75, 7.5, 15 mg. Trade only (Tranxene SD): Extended release Tabs 11.25, 22.5 mg.
NOTES - Half-life 40–50 h.
**DIAZEPAM (*Valium, Diastat, Diastat AcuDial, ✦Vivol, E Pam, Diazemuls*)** ▶LK ♀D ▶- ©IV $
ADULT - Status epilepticus: 5–10 mg IV. Repeat q10–15 min prn to max 30 mg. Epilepsy, adjunctive therapy: 2–10 mg PO bid-qid. Increased seizure activity: 0.2–0.5 mg/kg PR (rectal gel) to

**DIAZEPAM** (cont.)
max 20 mg/d. Skeletal muscle spasm, spasticity related to cerebral palsy, paraplegia, athetosis, stiff man syndrome: 2–10 mg PO/PR tid-qid. 5–10 mg IM/IV initially, then 5–10 mg q 3–4h prn. Decrease dose in elderly. Anxiety: 2–10 mg PO bid-qid or 2–20 mg IM/IV, repeat dose in 3–4h prn. Alcohol withdrawal: 10 mg PO tid-qid × 24 h then 5 mg PO tid-qid prn.
PEDS - Skeletal muscle spasm: 0.04–0.2 mg/kg/dose IV/IM q2–4h. Max dose 0.6 mg/kg within 8 h. Status epilepticus, age 1 m to 5 yo: 0.2–0.5 mg IV slowly q2–5 min to max 5 mg. Status epilepticus, >5 yo: 1 mg IV slowly q2–5 min to max 10 mg. Repeat q2–4 h prn. Epilepsy, adjunctive therapy, muscle spasm, and anxiety disorders age >6 mo: 1–2.5 mg PO tid-qid; gradually increase as tolerated and needed. Increased seizure activity (rectal gel, age >2 yo): 0.5 mg/kg PR (2–5 yo), 0.3 mg/kg PR (6–11 yo), or 0.2 mg/kg PR (>12 yo). Max 20 mg. May repeat in 4–12 h prn.
UNAPPROVED ADULT - Loading dose strategy for alcohol withdrawal: 10–20 mg PO or 10 mg slow IV in closely monitored setting, then repeat similar or lower doses q1–2 h prn until sedated. Further doses should be unnecessary due to long half-life. Restless legs syndrome: 0.5–4.0 mg PO qhs.
FORMS - Generic/Trade: Tabs 2, 5, 10 mg. Generic only: Oral solution 5 mg/5 mL. Oral concentrate (Intensol) 5 mg/mL. Trade only: Rectal gel (Diastat) 2.5, 5, 10, 15, 20 mg. Rectal gel (Diastat AcuDial) 10, 20 mg.
NOTES - Half-life 20–80h. Respiratory and CNS depression may occur. Caution in liver disease. Abuse potential. Long half-life may increase the risk of adverse effects in the elderly. Cimetidine, oral contraceptives, disulfiram, fluoxetine, isoniazid, ketoconazole, metoprolol, propoxyphene, propranolol, & valproic acid may increase diazepam concentrations. Diazepam may increase digoxin & phenytoin concentrations. Rifampin may increase the metabolism of diazepam. Avoid combination with protease inhibitors. Diastat AcuDial is for home use and allows dosing from 5–20 mg in 2.5 mg increments.

**FLURAZEPAM** (*Dalmane*) ▶LK ♀X ▶- ©IV $
ADULT - Insomnia: 15–30 mg PO qhs.
PEDS - Not approved in children <15 yo.
FORMS - Generic/Trade: Caps 15, 30 mg.
NOTES - Half-life 70–90h. For short term treatment of insomnia.

**NOTE:** To avoid withdrawal, gradually taper when discontinuing after prolonged use. Sedative-hypnotics have been associated with severe allergic reactions and complex sleep behaviors including sleep driving. Use caution and discuss with patients.

**ESTAZOLAM** (*ProSom*) ▶LK ♀X ▶- ©IV $$
ADULT - Insomnia: 1–2 mg PO qhs for up to 12 wk. Reduce dose to 0.5 mg in elderly, small, or debilitated patients.
PEDS - Not approved in children.
FORMS - Generic/Trade: Tabs 1, 2 mg.
NOTES - For short term treatment of insomnia. Avoid with ketoconazole or itraconazole; caution with less potent inhibitors of CYP3A4.

**LORAZEPAM** (*Ativan*) ▶LK ♀D ▶- ©IV $
ADULT - Anxiety: Start 0.5–1 mg PO bid-tid, usual effective dose is 2–6 mg/d. Max dose is 10 mg/d PO. Anxiolytic/sedation: 0.04–0.05 mg/kg IV/IM; usual dose 2 mg, max 4 mg. Insomnia: 2–4 mg PO qhs. Status epilepticus: 4 mg IV over 2 min. May repeat in 10–15 min.
PEDS - Not approved in children.
UNAPPROVED ADULT - Alcohol withdrawal: 1–2 mg PO/IM/IV q 2–4 h prn or 2 mg PO/IM/IV q6h × 24 h then 1 mg q6h × 8 doses. Chemotherapy-induced N/V: 1–2 mg PO/SL/IV/IM q6h.
UNAPPROVED PEDS - Status epilepticus: 0.05–0.1 mg/kg IV over 2–5 min. May repeat 0.05 mg/kg × 1 in 10–15 min. Do not exceed 4 mg as single dose. Anxiolytic/Sedation: 0.05 mg/kg/dose q4–8h PO/IV, max 2 mg/dose. Chemotherapy-induced N/V: 0.05 mg/kg PO/IV q8–12h prn, max 3 mg/dose; or 0.02–0.05 mg/kg IV q6h prn, max 2 mg/dose.
FORMS - Generic/Trade: Tabs 0.5, 1, 2 mg. Generic only: Oral concentrate 2 mg/mL.
NOTES - Half-life 10–20h. No active metabolites. For short term treatment of insomnia.

**NITRAZEPAM,** ✦*MOGADON* ▶L ♀C ▶- $
ADULT - Canada only. Insomnia: 5–10 mg PO qhs.
PEDS - Canada only. Myoclonic seizures: 0.3–1 mg/kg/d in 3 divided doses.
FORMS - Generic/Trade: Tabs 5, 10 mg.
NOTES - Use lower doses in elderly/debilitated patients.

**TEMAZEPAM** (*Restoril*) ▶LK ♀X ▶- ©IV $
ADULT - Insomnia: 7.5- 30 mg PO qhs × 7–10 d.
PEDS - Not approved in children.
FORMS - Generic/Trade: Caps 15, 30 mg. Trade only: Caps 7.5, 22.5 mg.
NOTES - Half-life 8–25h. For short term treatment of insomnia.

**NOTE:** To avoid withdrawal, gradually taper when discontinuing after prolonged use. Sedative-hypnotics have been associated with severe allergic reactions and complex sleep behaviors including sleep driving. Use caution and discuss with patients.

**ALPRAZOLAM (*Xanax, Xanax XR, Niravam*)** ▶LK ♀D ▶- ©IV $
ADULT - Anxiety: Start 0.25- 0.5 mg PO tid, may increase q3–4 d to a max dose of 4 mg/d. Use 0.25 mg PO bid in elderly or debilitated patients. Panic disorder: Start 0.5 mg PO tid (or 0.5–1.0 mg PO daily of Xanax XR), may increase by up to 1 mg/d q3–4 d to usual effective dose of 5–6 mg/d (3–6 mg/d for Xanax XR), max dose is 10 mg/d.
PEDS - Not approved in children.
FORMS - Trade only: Orally disintegrating tab (Niravam) 0.25, 0.5, 1, 2 mg. Generic/Trade: Tabs 0.25, 0.5, 1, 2 mg. Extended release tabs: 0.5, 1, 2, 3 mg. Generic only: Oral concentrate (Intensol) 1 mg/mL.
NOTES - Half-life 12h, but need to give tid. Divide administration time evenly during waking h to avoid interdose symptoms. Don't give with antifungals (ie, ketoconazole, itraconazole); use caution with macrolides, propoxyphene, oral contraceptives, TCAs, cimetidine, antidepressants, anticonvulsants, paroxetine, sertraline, and others that inhibit CYP 3A4.

**OXAZEPAM (*Serax*)** ▶LK ♀D ▶- ©IV $$$
ADULT - Anxiety: 10–30 mg PO tid-qid. Acute alcohol withdrawal: 15–30 mg PO tid-qid.
PEDS - Not approved in children <6 yo.
UNAPPROVED ADULT - Restless legs syndrome: start 10 mg PO qhs. Max 40 mg qhs.
FORMS - Generic/Trade: Caps 10, 15, 30 mg. Trade only: Tabs 15 mg.
NOTES - Half-life 8 h.

**TRIAZOLAM (*Halcion*)** ▶LK ♀X ▶- ©IV $
ADULT - Hypnotic: 0.125- 0.25 mg PO qhs × 7–10 d, max dose is 0.5 mg/d. Start 0.125 mg/d in elderly or debilitated patients.
PEDS - Not approved in children.
UNAPPROVED ADULT - Restless legs syndrome: start 0.125 mg PO qhs. Max 0.5 mg qhs.
FORMS - Generic/Trade: Tabs 0.125, 0.25 mg.
NOTES - Half-life 2–3 h. Anterograde amnesia may occur. Don't use with protease inhibitors, ketoconazole, itraconazole, or nefazodone; use caution with macrolides, cimetidine, and other CYP 3A4 inhibitors.

## PSYCHIATRY: Anxiolytics/Hypnotics—Other

**NOTE:** Sedative-hypnotics have been associated with severe allergic reactions and complex sleep behaviors including sleep driving. Use caution and discuss with patients.

**BUSPIRONE (*BuSpar, Vanspar*)** ▶K ♀B ▶- $$$
ADULT - Anxiety: Start 15 mg "dividose" daily (7.5 mg PO bid), increase by 5 mg/d q2–3 d to usual effective dose of 30 mg/d, max dose is 60 mg/d.
PEDS - Not approved in children.
FORMS - Generic/Trade: Tabs 5, 10, Dividose Tabs 15, 30 mg (scored to be easily bisected or trisected). Generic only: Tabs 7.5 mg.
NOTES - Slower onset than benzodiazepines; optimum effect requires 3–4 wk of therapy. Don't use with MAOIs; caution with itraconazole, cimetidine, nefazodone, erythromycin, and other CYP 3A4 inhibitors.

**CHLORAL HYDRATE (*Aquachloral Supprettes, Somnote*)** ▶LK ♀C ▶+ ©IV $
ADULT - Sedative: 250 mg PO/PR tid after meals. Hypnotic: 500- 1,000 mg PO/PR qhs. Acute alcohol withdrawal: 500- 1,000 mg PO/PR q6h prn.
PEDS - Sedative: 25 mg/kg/d PO/PR divided tid-qid, up to 500 mg tid. Hypnotic: 50 mg/kg PO/PR qhs, up to max of 1 g. Pre-anesthetic: 25- 50 mg/kg PO/PR before procedure.
UNAPPROVED PEDS - Sedative: higher than approved doses 75–100 mg/kg PO/PR.
FORMS - Generic only: Syrup 500 mg/5 mL, rectal suppositories 500 mg. Trade only: Caps 500 mg. Rectal suppositories: 325, 650 mg.
NOTES - Give syrup in ½ glass of fruit juice or water.

**ESZOPICLONE (*Lunesta*)** ▶L ♀C ▶? ©IV $$$$
ADULT - Insomnia: 2 mg PO qhs prn, max 3 mg. Elderly: 1 mg PO qhs prn, max 2 mg.
PEDS - Not approved for children.
FORMS - Trade only: Tabs 1, 2, 3 mg.

NOTES - Half-life = 6 h. Take immediately before bedtime.

**RAMELTEON (*Rozerem*)** ▶L ♀C ▶? $$$
ADULT - Insomnia: 8 mg PO qhs.
PEDS - Not approved for children.
FORMS - Trade only: Tabs 8 mg.
NOTES - Do not take with/after high-fat meal. No evidence of dependence or abuse liability. Inhibitors or CYP 1A2, 3A4, and 2C9 may increase serum level and effect. Avoid with severe liver disease. May decrease testosterone and increase prolactin.

**ZALEPLON (*Sonata, ◆Starnoc*)** ▶L ♀C ▶- ©IV $$$
ADULT - Insomnia: 5–10 mg PO qhs prn, max 20 mg.
PEDS - Not approved in children.
FORMS - Trade only: Caps 5, 10 mg.
NOTES - Half-life = 1 h. Useful if problems with sleep initiation or morning grogginess. For short term treatment of insomnia. Take immediately before bedtime or after going to bed and experiencing difficulty falling asleep. Use 5 mg dose in patients with mild to moderate hepatic impairment, elderly patients, and in patients taking cimetidine. Possible drug interactions with rifampin, phenytoin, carbamazepine, and phenobarbital. Do not use for benzodiazepine or alcohol withdrawal.

**ZOLPIDEM (*Ambien, Ambien CR*)** ▶L ♀B ▶+ ©IV $$$$
ADULT -Insomnia10 mg PO qhs (standard tabs, short-term) or 12.5 mg PO qhs (controlled release tabs). Start with 5 mg (standard tabs) or 6.25 mg (controlled release) in the elderly or debilitated.

**ZOLPIDEM** *(cont.)*
PEDS - Not approved in children.
FORMS - Generic/Trade: Tabs 5, 10 mg. Trade only: Controlled release tabs 6.25, 12.5 mg.
NOTES - Half-life = 2.5 h. Ambien regular release is for short term treatment of insomnia characterized by problems with sleep initiation. CR is useful for problems with sleep initiation and maintenance, and has been studied for up to 24 wk. Do not use for benzodiazepine or alcohol withdrawal.

**ZOPICLONE**, *✦IMOVANE* ▶L ♀D ▶- $
ADULT - Canada only. Short-term treatment of insomnia: 5–7.5 mg PO qhs. In elderly or debilitated, use 3.75 mg qhs initially, and increase prn to 5–7.5 mg qhs. Max 7.5 mg qhs.
PEDS - Not approved in children.
FORMS - Generic/Trade: Tabs 5, 7.5 mg. Generic only: Tabs 3.75 mg.
NOTES - Treatment should usually not exceed 7–10 d without re-evaluation.

## PSYCHIATRY: Combination Drugs

**LIMBITROL** (chlordiazepoxide + amitriptyline, Limbitrol DS) ▶LK ♀D ▶- ⊙IV $$$
ADULT - Rarely used; other drugs preferred. Depression/Anxiety: 1 tab PO tid-qid, may increase up to 6 tabs/d.
PEDS - Not approved in children <12 yo.
FORMS - Generic/Trade: Tabs 5/12.5, 10/25 mg chlordiazepoxide/amitriptyline.
**SYMBYAX** (olanzapine + fluoxetine) ▶LK ♀C ▶- $$$$$
WARNING - Observe patients started on SSRIs for worsening depression or emergence of suicidal thoughts or behaviors especially early in therapy or after increases in dose. Monitor for emergence of anxiety, agitation, panic attacks, insomnia, irritability, hostility, impulsivity, akathisia, mania and hypomania. Antidepressants increase the risk of suicidal thinking and behavior in children, adolescents, and young adults; carefully weigh risks and benefits before starting and then monitor such individuals closely. The use of atypical antipsychotics to treat behavioral problems in patients with dementia has been associated with higher mortality rates. Atypical antipsychotics have been associated with weight gain, dyslipidemia, hyperglycemia, and diabetes mellitus; monitor closely.
ADULT - Bipolar depression: Start 6/25 mg PO qhs. Max 18/75 mg/d.
PEDS - Not approved in children <12 yo.
FORMS - Trade only: Caps (olanzapine/fluoxetine) 3/25, 6/25, 6/50, 12/25, 12/50 mg.
NOTES - Efficacy beyond 8 wk not established. Monitor weight, fasting glucose, and triglycerides before initiation and periodically during treatment. Contraindicated with thioridazine; don't use with cisapride, thioridazine, tryptophan, or MAOIs; caution with lithium, phenytoin, TCAs, ASA, NSAIDs and warfarin. Pregnancy exposure to fluoxetine associated with premature delivery, low birth weight, and lower Apgar scores. Decrease dose with liver disease.
**TRIAVIL** (perphenazine + amitriptyline) ▶LK ♀D ▶? $$
ADULT - Rarely used; other drugs preferred. Depression/Anxiety: 1 tab (2–25 or 4–25) PO tid-qid. Max 8 tabs/d (2–25 or 4–25).
PEDS - Not approved in children.
FORMS - Generic only: Tabs (perphenazine/amitriptyline) 2/10, 2/25, 4/10, 4/25, 4/50 mg.

## PSYCHIATRY: Drug Dependence Therapy

**ACAMPROSATE** *(Campral)* ▶K ♀C ▶? $$$$
ADULT - Maintenance of abstinence from alcohol: 666 mg (2 tabs) PO tid. Start after alcohol withdrawal and when patient is abstinent.
PEDS - Not approved in children.
FORMS - Trade only: delayed-release tabs 333 mg.
NOTES - Reduce dose to 333 mg if CrCl 30–50 mL/min. Contraindicated if CrCl <30 mL/min.
**DISULFIRAM** *(Antabuse)* ▶L ♀C ▶? $$$
WARNING - Never give to an intoxicated patient.
ADULT - Sobriety: 125–500 mg PO daily.
PEDS - Not approved in children.
FORMS - Trade only: Tabs 250, 500 mg.
NOTES - Patient must abstain from any alcohol for ≥12 h before using. Disulfiram-alcohol reaction may occur for up to 2 wk after discontinuing disulfiram. Metronidazole and alcohol in any form (eg, cough syrups, tonics) contraindicated. Hepatotoxicity.
**NALTREXONE** *(ReVia, Depade, Vivitrol)* ▶LK ♀C ▶? $$$$
WARNING - Hepatotoxicity with higher than approved doses.
ADULT - Alcohol dependence: 50 mg PO daily. Extended-release injectable susp: 380 mg IM q 4 wk or monthly. Opioid dependence: Start 25 mg PO daily, increase to 50 mg PO daily if no signs of withdrawal.
PEDS - Not approved in children.
FORMS - Generic/Trade: Tabs 50 mg. Trade only (Vivitrol): extended-release injectable susp kits 380 mg.
NOTES - Avoid if recent (past 7–10 d) ingestion of opioids. Conflicting evidence of efficacy for chronic, severe alcoholism.
**NICOTINE GUM** *(Nicorette, Nicorette DS)* ▶LK ♀C ▶- $$$$$
ADULT - Smoking cessation: Gradually taper 1 piece (2 mg) q1–2h × 6 wk, 1 piece (2 mg) q2–4h × 3 wk, then 1 piece (2 mg) q4–8h × 3 wk. Max 30 pieces/d of 2 mg gum or 24 pieces/d of 4 mg gum. Use 4 mg pieces (Nicorette DS) for high cigarette use (>24 cigarettes/d).
PEDS - Not approved in children.

(cont.)

**NICOTINE GUM** *(cont.)*
FORMS - OTC/Generic/Trade: gum 2, 4 mg.
NOTES - Chew slowly and park between cheek and gum periodically. May cause N/V, hiccups. Coffee, juices, wine, and soft drinks may reduce absorption. Avoid eating/drinking $\times$ 15 min before/during gum use. Available in original, orange, or mint flavor. Do not use beyond 6 mo.

**NICOTINE INHALATION SYSTEM** (*Nicotrol Inhaler,* ◆*Nicorette inhaler*) ▶LK ♀D ▶- $$$$$
ADULT - Smoking cessation: 6–16 cartridges/d $\times$ 12 wk.
PEDS - Not approved in children.
FORMS - Trade only: Oral inhaler 10 mg/cartridge (4 mg nicotine delivered), 42 cartridges/box.

**NICOTINE LOZENGE** (*Commit*) ▶LK ♀D ▶- $$$$$
ADULT - Smoking cessation: In those who smoke <30 min after waking use 4 mg lozenge; others use 2 mg. Take 1–2 lozenges q1–2 h $\times$ 6 wk, then q2–4h in wk 7–9, then q4–8h in wk 10–12. Length of therapy 12 wk.
PEDS - Not approved in children.
FORMS - OTC Generic/Trade: lozenge 2, 4 mg in 48, 72 & 168-count packages
NOTES - Allow lozenge to dissolve and do not chew. Do not eat or drink within 15 min before use. Avoid concurrent use with other sources of nicotine.

**NICOTINE NASAL SPRAY** (*Nicotrol NS*) ▶LK ♀D ▶- $$$$$
ADULT - Smoking cessation: 1–2 doses each h, with each dose = 2 sprays, one in each nostril (1 spray = 0.5 mg nicotine). Minimum recommended: 8 doses/d, max 40 doses/d.
PEDS - Not approved in children.
FORMS - Trade only: nasal solution 10 mg/mL (0.5 mg/inhalation); 10 mL bottles.

**NICOTINE PATCHES** (*Habitrol, NicoDerm CQ, Nicotrol,* ◆*Prostep*) ▶LK ♀D ▶- $$$$
ADULT - Smoking cessation: Start one patch (14- 22 mg) daily and taper after 6 wk. Total duration of therapy is 12 wk.

PEDS - Not approved in children.
FORMS - OTC/Rx/Generic/Trade: patches 11, 22 mg/24 h. 7, 14, 21 mg/24 h (Habitrol & NicoDerm). OTC/Trade: 15 mg/16 h (Nicotrol).
NOTES - Ensure patient has stopped smoking. Dispose of patches safely; can be toxic to kids, pets. Remove opaque NicoDerm CQ patch prior to MRI procedures to avoid possible burns.

**SUBOXONE** (buprenorphine + naloxone) ▶L ♀C ▶- ©III $$$$$
ADULT - Treatment of opioid dependence: Maintenance: 16 mg SL daily. Can individualize to range of 4–24 mg SL daily.
PEDS - Not approved in children.
FORMS - Trade only: SL tabs 2/0.5 and 8/2 mg buprenorphine/naloxone
NOTES - Suboxone preferred over Subutex for unsupervised administration. Titrate in 2–4 mg increments/decrements to maintain therapy compliance and prevent withdrawal. Prescribers must complete training and apply for special DEA number. See www.suboxone.com.

**VARENICLINE** (*Chantix*) ▶K ♀C ▶? $$$$
WARNING - Has been associated with the development of suicidal ideation, changes in behavior, depressed mood and attempted/completed suicides—both during treatment and after withdrawal. Unclear safety in serious psychiatric conditions.
ADULT - Smoking cessation: Start 0.5 mg PO daily for d 1–3, then 0.5 mg bid d 4–7, then 1 mg bid thereafter. Take after meals with full glass of water. Start 1 wk prior to cessation and continue $\times$ 12 wk.
PEDS - Not approved in children.
FORMS - Trade only: Tabs 0.5, 1 mg.
NOTES - For severe renal dysfunction reduce max dose to 0.5 mg bid. For renal failure on hemodialysis may use 0.5 mg once daily if tolerated.

## PSYCHIATRY: Stimulants/ADHD/Anorexiants

**NOTE:** Sudden cardiac death has been reported with stimulants and atomoxetine at usual ADHD doses; carefully assess prior to treatment and avoid if cardiac conditions or structural abnormalities. Amphetamines are associated with high abuse potential and dependence with prolonged administration. Stimulants may also cause or worsen underlying psychosis or induce a manic or mixed episode in bipolar disorder. Problems with visual accommodation have also been reported with stimulants.

**ADDERALL** (dextroamphetamine + amphetamine, Adderall XR) ▶L ♀C ▶- ©II $$$$
ADULT - Narcolepsy, standard-release: Start 10 mg PO q am, increase by 10 mg q wk, max dose is 60 mg/d divided bid-tid at 4–6h intervals. ADHD, extended-release caps (Adderall XR): 20 mg PO daily.
PEDS - ADHD, standard-release tabs: Start 2.5 mg (3–5 yo) or 5 mg (≥6 yo) PO daily-bid, increase by 2.5–5 mg every wk, max 40 mg/d. ADHD, extended-release caps (Adderall XR): If 6–12 yo, then start 5–10 mg PO daily to a max of 30 mg/d.

If 13–17 yo, then start 10 mg PO daily to a max of 20 mg/d. Not recommended if <3 yo. Narcolepsy, standard-release: 6–12 yo: Start 5 mg PO daily, increase by 5 mg q wk. Age >12 yo: Start 10 mg PO daily, increase by 10 mg q wk, max dose is 60 mg/d divided bid-tid at 4–6h intervals.
FORMS - Generic/Trade: Tabs 5, 7.5, 10, 12.5, 15, 20, 30 mg. Trade only: Capsules, extended release (Adderall XR) 5, 10, 15, 20, 25, 30 mg.
NOTES - Capsules may be opened and the beads sprinkled on applesauce; do not chew beads. Adderall XR should be given upon awakening. Avoid

**ADDERALL** (*cont.*)
evening doses. Monitor growth and use drug holidays when appropriate. May increase pulse and BP. May exacerbate bipolar or psychotic conditions.

**ARMODAFINIL (*Nuvigil*)** ▶L ♀C ▶? ©IV ?
ADULT - Obstructive sleep apnea/hypopnea syndrome and narcolepsy: 150–250 mg PO q am. Inconsistent evidence for improved efficacy of 250 mg/d dose. Shift work sleep disorder: 150 mg PO 1 h prior to start of shift.
PEDS - Not approved in children.
FORMS - Trade only: tabs 50, 150, 250 mg.
NOTES - Weak inducer for substrates of CYP3A4/5 (eg, carbamazepine, cyclosporine) which may require dose adjustments. May inhibit metabolism of substrates of CYP2C19 (eg, omeprazole, diazepam, phenytoin). May reduce efficacy of oral contraceptives; consider alternatives during treatment. Reduce dose with severe liver impairment.

**ATOMOXETINE (*Strattera*)** ▶K ♀C ▶? $$$$$
WARNING - Severe liver injury and failure have been reported; discontinue if jaundice or elevated LFTs. Increases risk of suicidal thinking and behavior in children and adolescents; carefully weigh risks/benefits before starting and then monitor such individuals closely for worsening depression or emergence of suicidal thoughts or behaviors especially early in therapy or after increases in dose. Monitor for emergence of anxiety, agitation, panic attacks, insomnia, irritability, hostility, impulsivity, akathisia, mania and hypomania.
ADULT - ADHD: Start 40 mg PO daily, then increase after >3 d to target of 80 mg/d divided daily-bid. Max dose 100 mg/d.
PEDS - ADHD: Children/adolescents ≤70 kg: Start 0.5 mg/kg daily, then increase after >3 d to target dose of 1.2 mg/kg/d divided daily-bid. Max dose 1.4 mg/kg or 100 mg per d whichever is less. If >70 kg use adult dose.
FORMS - Trade only: caps 10, 18, 25, 40, 60, 80, 100 mg.
NOTES - If taking strong CYP2D6 inhibitors, eg, paroxetine or fluoxetine, use same starting dose but only increase if well-tolerated at 4 wk and symptoms unimproved. Caution when co-administered with oral or parenteral albuterol or other beta-2 agonists, as increases in heart rate and BP may occur. May be stopped without tapering. Monitor growth. Give "Patient Medication Guide" when dispensed. Does not appear to exacerbate tics.

**BENZPHETAMINE (*Didrex*)** ▶K ♀X ▶? ©III $$$
WARNING - Chronic overuse/abuse can lead to marked tolerance and psychic dependence; caution with prolonged use.
ADULT - Short-term treatment of obesity: Start with 25–50 mg once daily in the morning and increase if needed to 1–3 times daily.
PEDS - Not approved for children <12 yr of age.
FORMS - Generic/Trade: tabs 50 mg.
NOTES - Tolerance to anorectic effect develops within wk and cross-tolerance to other drugs in class common.

**CAFFEINE (*NoDoz, Vivarin, Caffedrine, Stay Awake, Quick-Pep, Cafcit*)** ▶L ♀B/C ▶? $
ADULT - Fatigue: 100- 200 mg PO q3–4h prn.
PEDS - Not approved in children <12 yo, except apnea of prematurity in infants between 28 & <33 wk gestational age (Cafcit): Load 20 mg/kg IV over 30 min. Maintenance 5 mg/kg PO q 24h. Monitor for necrotizing enterocolitis.
FORMS - OTC Generic/Trade: Tabs/Caps 200 mg. Oral solution caffeine citrate (Cafcit) 20 mg/mL. OTC Trade only: Extended-release tabs 200 mg. Lozenges 75 mg.
NOTES - 2 mg caffeine citrate = 1 mg caffeine base.

**COCAINE** ▶L ♀? ▶? ©II Varies
ADULT - Drug of abuse.
PEDS - Drug of abuse.

**DEXMETHYLPHENIDATE (*Focalin, Focalin XR*)** ▶LK ♀C ▶? ©II $$$
ADULT - ADHD, not already on stimulants: Start 10 mg PO q am (extended release) or 2.5 mg PO bid (immediate release). Max 20 mg/d for both. If taking racemic methylphenidate use conversion of 2.5 mg for each 5 mg of methylphenidate, max 20 mg/d. Doses should be ≥4h apart for immediate release.
PEDS - ADHD and ≥6 yo and not already on stimulants: Start 5 mg PO q am (extended release) or 2.5 mg PO bid (immediate release), max 20 mg/24 h. If already on racemic methylphenidate, use conversion of 2.5 mg for each 5 mg of methylphenidate given bid, max 20 mg/d. Doses should be ≥4h apart.
FORMS - Generic/Trade: Tabs, immediate-release 2.5, 5, 10 mg. Trade only: Extended release caps (Focalin XR) 5, 10, 15, 20 mg.
NOTES - Avoid evening doses. Monitor growth and use drug holidays when appropriate. May increase pulse and BP. 2.5 mg is equivalent to 5 mg racemic methylphenidate. Focalin XR caps may be opened and sprinkled on applesauce, but beads must not be chewed. May exacerbate bipolar or psychotic conditions.

**DEXTROAMPHETAMINE (*Dexedrine, Dextrostat*)** ▶L ♀C ▶- ©II $$$
ADULT - Narcolepsy: Start 10 mg PO qam, increase by 10 mg/d q wk, max 60 mg/d divided daily (sustained release) or bid-tid at 4–6h intervals.
PEDS - Narcolepsy: 6–12 yo: Start 5 mg PO qam, increase by 5 mg/d q wk. Age >12 yo: Start 10 mg PO qam, increase by 10 mg/d q wk, max 60 mg/d divided daily (sustained release) or bid-tid at 4–6h intervals. ADHD: age 3–5 yo: Start 2.5 mg PO daily, increase by 2.5 mg q wk. Age ≥6 yo: Start 5 mg PO daily-bid, increase by 5 mg q wk, usual max 40 mg/d divided daily-tid at 4–6h intervals. Not recommended for patients <3 yo. Extended-release caps not recommended < 6 yo.
FORMS - Generic/Trade: Caps, extended-release 5, 10, 15 mg. Generic only: Tabs 5, 10 mg. Oral soln 5 mg/5 mL.

(cont.)

**DEXTROAMPHETAMINE** *(cont.)*
NOTES - Avoid evening doses. Monitor growth and use drug holidays when appropriate. May exacerbate bipolar or psychotic conditions.

**DIETHYLPROPION** *(Tenuate, Tenuate Dospan)* ▶K ♀B ▶? ©IV $
WARNING - Chronic overuse/abuse can lead to marked tolerance and psychic dependence; caution with prolonged use.
ADULT - Short-term treatment of obesity: 25 mg PO tid 1 h before meals and mid evening if needed or 75 mg sustained-release daily at midmorning.
PEDS - Not approved for children <12 yr of age.
FORMS - Generic/Trade: Tabs 25 mg, Tabs, extended-release 75 mg.
NOTES - Tolerance to anorectic effect develops within wk and cross-tolerance to other drugs in class common.

**LISDEXAMFETAMINE** *(Vyvanse)* ▶L ♀C ▶- ©II $$$$
ADULT - Start 30 mg PO q am. May increase weekly by 10–20 mg/d to max 70 mg/d.
PEDS - ADHD ages 6–12 yo: Start 30 mg PO q am. May increase weekly by 10–20 mg/d to max 70 mg/d. Adolescents use adult dosing.
FORMS - Trade: Caps 20, 30, 40, 50, 60, 70 mg.
NOTES - May open cap and place contents in water for administration. Avoid evening doses. Monitor growth and use drug holidays when appropriate.

**METHAMPHETAMINE** *(Desoxyn)* ▶L ♀C ▶- ©II $$$$
ADULT - Obesity: 5 mg PO prior to meals. Short-term use only.
PEDS - ADHD (≥6 yo): Start 5 mg PO daily-bid. May increase by 5 mg/dose at weekly intervals to usual effective dose of 20–25 mg/d. Obesity (>12 yo): use adult dosing.
FORMS - Trade only: Tabs 5 mg.
NOTES - Should not be used for more than a few wk for obesity.

**METHYLPHENIDATE** *(Ritalin, Ritalin LA, Ritalin SR, Methylin, Methylin ER, Metadate ER, Metadate CD, Concerta, Daytrana, ✦Biphentin)* ▶LK ♀C ▶? ©II $$
ADULT - Narcolepsy: 10 mg PO bid-tid before meals. Usual effective dose is 20–30 mg/d, max 60 mg/d. Use sustained release Tabs when the 8-h dosage corresponds to the titrated 8-h dosage of the conventional tabs. ADHD (Concerta): Start 18–36 mg PO qam, usual dose range 18–72 mg/d.
PEDS - ADHD ≥6 yo: Start 5 mg PO bid before breakfast and lunch, increase gradually by 5–10 mg/d at weekly interval to max 60 mg/d. Sustained and extended release: start 20 mg PO daily, max 60 mg daily. Concerta (extended release) start 18 mg PO qam; titrate in 9–18 mg increments at weekly intervals to max 54 mg/d (6–12 yo) or 72 mg/d (13–17 yo). Consult product labeling for dose conversion from other methylphenidate regimens. Discontinue after 1 mo if no improvement observed. Transdermal patch 6–12 yo: Start 10 mg/9 h, may increase at weekly intervals to max dose of 30 mg/9 h. Apply 2 h prior to desired onset and remove 9 h

later. Effect may last up to 12 h after application. Must alternate sites daily.
FORMS - Trade only: tabs 5, 10, 20 mg (Ritalin, Methylin, Metadate). Extended release tabs 10, 20 mg (Methylin ER, Metadate ER). Extended release tabs 18, 27, 36, 54 mg (Concerta). Extended release caps 10, 20, 30, 40, 50, 60 mg (Metadate CD) May be sprinkled on food. Sustained-release tabs 20 mg (Ritalin SR). Extended release caps 10, 20, 30, 40 mg (Ritalin LA). Chewable tabs 2.5, 5, 10 mg (Methylin). Oral solution 5 mg/5ml, 10 mg/5 mL (Methylin). Transdermal patch (Daytrana) 10 mg/9 h, 15 mg/9 h, 20 mg/9 h, 30 mg/9 h. Generic only: tabs 5, 10, 20 mg, extended release tabs 10, 20 mg, sustained-release tabs 20 mg.
NOTES - Avoid evening doses. Monitor growth and use drug holidays when appropriate. May increase pulse and BP. Ritalin LA may be opened and sprinkled on applesauce. Apply transdermal patch to hip below beltline to avoid rubbing it off. May exacerbate bipolar or psychotic conditions.

**MODAFINIL** *(Provigil, ✦Alertec)* ▶L ♀C ▶? ©IV $$$$$
WARNING - Associated with serious, life-threatening rashes in adults and children; discontinue immediately if unexplained rash.
ADULT - Narcolepsy and sleep apnea/hypopnea: 200 mg PO qam. Shift work sleep disorder: 200 mg PO one h before shift.
PEDS - Not approved in children <16 yo.
FORMS - Trade only: Tabs 100, 200 mg.
NOTES - May increase levels of diazepam, phenytoin, TCAs, warfarin, or propranolol; may decrease levels of cyclosporine, oral contraceptives, or theophylline. Reduce dose in severe liver impairment.

**PHENDIMATRIZINE** *(Bontril, Bontril Slow Release)* ▶K ♀C ▶? ©III $$
WARNING - Chronic overuse/abuse can lead to marked tolerance and psychic dependence; caution with prolonged use.
ADULT - Short-term treatment of obesity: Start 35 mg 2 or 3 times daily 1 h before meals. Sustained-release 105 mg once in the morning before breakfast.
PEDS - Not approved in children <12 yo.
FORMS - Generic/Trade: Tabs/Caps 35 mg, Caps, sustained-release 105 mg.
NOTES - Tolerance to anorectic effect develops within wk and cross-tolerance to other drugs in class common.

**PHENTERMINE** *(Adipex-P, Ionamin, Pro-Fast)* ▶KL ♀C ▶- ©IV $$
WARNING - Chronic overuse/abuse can lead to marked tolerance and psychic dependence; caution with prolonged use.
ADULT - Obesity: 8 mg PO tid before meals or 1–2 h after meals. May give 15–37.5 mg PO q am or 10–14 h before bedtime.
PEDS - Not approved in children <16 yo.
FORMS - Generic/Trade: Caps 15, 30, 37.5 mg. Tabs 37.5 mg. Trade only: Caps, extended release 15, 30 mg (Ionamin). Generic only (Pro-Fast): Caps 18.75 mg, Tabs 8 mg.

| BODY MASS INDEX* | | Heights are in feet and inches; weights are in pounds | | | | | |
|---|---|---|---|---|---|---|---|
| BMI | Classification | 4' 10" | 5' 0" | 5' 4" | 5' 8" | 6' 0" | 6' 4" |
| <19 | Underweight | <91 | <97 | <110 | <125 | <140 | <156 |
| 19–24 | Healthy Weight | 91–119 | 97–127 | 110–144 | 125–163 | 140–183 | 156–204 |
| 25–29 | Overweight | 120–143 | 128–152 | 145–173 | 164–196 | 184–220 | 205–245 |
| 30–40 | Obese | 144–191 | 153–204 | 174–233 | 197–262 | 221–293 | 246–328 |
| >40 | Very Obese | >191 | >204 | >233 | >262 | >293 | >328 |

*BMI = kg/m² = (weight in pounds)(703)/(height in inches)². Anorectants appropriate if BMI ≥30 (with comorbidities ≥27); surgery an option if BMI >40 (with comorbidities 35–40). www.nhlbi.nih.gov

**PHENTERMINE** (*cont.*)
NOTES - Indicated for short term (8–12 wk) use only. Contraindicated for use during or within 14 d of MAOIs (hypertensive crisis).
**SIBUTRAMINE** (*Meridia*) ▶KL ♀C ▶- ©IV $$$$
WARNING - Chronic overuse/abuse can lead to marked tolerance and psychic dependence; caution with prolonged use.
ADULT - Obesity: Start 10 mg PO q am, may titrate to 15 mg/d after one mo. Max dose is 15 mg/d.
PEDS - Not approved in children <16 yo.

FORMS - Trade only: Caps 5, 10, 15 mg.
NOTES - Indicated for BMI >30 kg/m² or >27 kg/m² with risk factors for cardiovascular disease or diabetes. Monitor pulse and BP. Don't use if uncontrolled HTN, heart disease, or severe renal impairment or end-stage renal disease. Caution using with SSRIs or other antidepressants, sumatriptan, ergotamine and other serotonin agents to avoid development of serotonin syndrome. Contraindicated for use during or within 14 d of MAOIs (hypertensive crisis).

## PULMONARY: Beta Agonists—Short Acting

**NOTE:** Palpitations, tachycardia, tremor, lightheadedness, nervousness, headache, & nausea may occur; these effects may be more pronounced with systemic administration. Decreases in serum potassium can occur, rarely leading to adverse cardiovascular effects; monitor accordingly. Potential for tolerance with continued use of short-acting beta agonists.

**ALBUTEROL** (*AccuNeb, Ventolin HFA, Proventil, Proventil HFA, ProAir HFA, VoSpire ER, ♣Airomir, Asmavent, salbutamol*) ▶L ♀C ▶? $$
ADULT - Acute asthma: MDI: 2 puffs q4–6h prn. Soln for inhalation: 2.5 mg nebulized tid-qid. Dilute 0.5 mL 0.5% soln with 2.5 mL NS. Deliver over ~ 5–15 min. One 3 mL unit dose (0.083%) nebulized tid-qid. Caps for inhalation: 200–400 mcg inhaled q4–6h via a Rotahaler device. Asthma: 2–4 mg PO tid-qid or extended release 4–8 mg PO q12h up to 16 mg PO q12h.
PEDS - Acute asthma: MDI: ≥4 yo: 1–2 puffs q4–6 h prn. Soln for inhalation (0.5%): 2–12 yo: 0.1–0.15 mg/kg/dose not to exceed 2.5 mg tid-qid, diluted with NS to 3 mL. Caps for inhalation: ≥4 yo 200–400 mcg inhaled q4–6h via a Rotahaler device. Asthma: Tabs, syrup 6–12 yo: 2–4 mg PO tid-qid, max dose 24 mg/d in divided doses or extended release 4 mg PO q12h. Syrup 2–5 yo: 0.1–0.2 mg/kg/dose PO tid up to 4 mg tid. Prevention of exercise-induced bronchospasm ≥4 yo (Proventil HFA, Ventolin HFA): 2 puffs 15–30 min before exercise.
UNAPPROVED ADULT - COPD: MDI, soln for inhalation: use asthma dose. Acute asthma: MDI, soln for inhalation: dose as above q20 min × 3 or until improvement. Continuous nebulization: 10–15

mg/h until improvement. Emergency hyperkalemia: 10–20 mg via MDI or soln for inhalation.
UNAPPROVED PEDS - Acute asthma: soln for inhalation: 0.15 mg/kg (minimum dose = 2.5 mg) q 20 min × 3 doses then 0.15–0.3 mg/kg up to 10 mg q1–4 h as needed, or 0.5 mg/kg/h continuous nebulization. MDI: 4–8 puffs q 20 min for 3 doses then every 1–4 h prn. Asthma for inhalation (0.5%): <2 yo: 0.05 - 0.15 mg/kg/dose q4–6h. Syrup <2 yo: 0.3 mg/kg/24h PO divided tid, max dose 12 mg/24h. Prevention of exercise-induced bronchospasm: MDI: ≥4 yo 2 puffs 15–30 min before exercise.
FORMS - Generic/Trade: MDI 90 mcg/actuation, 200 metered doses/canister. "HFA" inhalers use hydrofluoroalkane propellant instead of CFCs but are otherwise equivalent. Soln for inhalation 0.042% (AccuNeb) and 0.083% (Proventil) in 3 mL vial, 0.5% (5 mg/mL) in 20 mL with dropper (Proventil). Tabs extended-release 4, 8 mg (VoSpire ER). Soln for inhalation 0.021% in 3 mL vial (AccuNeb). Generic only: Syrup 2 mg/5 mL. Tabs immediate-release 2, 4 mg.
NOTES - Do not crush or chew extended release tabs. Use with caution in patients on MAO inhibitors or cyclic antidepressants—may increase cardiovascular side effects.

**FENETEROL (←BEROTEC)** ▶L ♀C ▶? $
ADULT - Canada only. Acute asthma: MDI: 1–2 puffs tid-qid; max 8 puffs/d. Soln for nebulization: up to 2.5 mg q6 h.
PEDS - Not approved in children.
FORMS - Trade only: MDI 100 mcg/actuation. Soln for inhalation: 20 mL bottles of 1 mg/mL (with preservatives that may cause bronchoconstriction in those with hyperreactive airways).

**LEVALBUTEROL (Xopenex, Xopenex HFA)** ▶L ♀C ▶? $$$
ADULT - Acute asthma: MDI 2 puffs q4–6h prn. Soln for inhalation: 0.63–1.25 mg nebulized q6–8h.
PEDS - Acute asthma: MDI ≥4 yo: 2 puffs q4–6h prn. Soln for inhalation ≥12 yo: Use adult dose. 6–11 yo: 0.31 mg nebulized tid.
FORMS - Generic/Trade: Soln for inhalation 0.31, 0.63, 1.25 mg in 3 mL and 1.25mg in 0.5 mL unit-dose vials.Trade only: HFA MDI 45 mcg/actuation, 15g 200/canister. "HFA" inhalers use hydrofluoroalkane propellant.
NOTES - R-isomer of albuterol. Dyspepsia may occur. Use with caution in patients on MAO inhibitors or cyclic antidepressants - may increase cardiovascular side effects.

**METAPROTERENOL (Alupent, ←Orciprenaline)** ▶L ♀C ▶? $$
ADULT - Acute asthma: MDI: 2–3 puffs q3–4h; max dose 12 puffs/d. Soln for inhalation: 0.2–0.3 mL of the 5% soln in 2.5 mL NS. 20 mg PO tid-qid.
PEDS - Acute asthma: soln for inhalation: >6 yo 0.1–0.3 mL of the 5% soln in 2.5 mL NS. Tabs or syrup: >9 yo or >60 lbs: 20 mg PO tid-qid. 6–9 yo or <60 lbs: 10 mg PO tid-qid. 2–5 yo: 1.3–2.6 mg/kg/d PO in divided doses tid-qid.
UNAPPROVED PEDS - Acute asthma: MDI: >6 yo 2–3 puffs q3–4h; max dose 12 puffs/d. Soln for inhalation: 0.1–0.3 mL of the 5% soln in 2.5 mL

NS q4–6h prn or q20 min until improvement. Tabs or syrup: <2 yo: 0.4 mg/kg/dose PO tid-qid.
FORMS - Trade only: MDI 0.65 mg/actuation, 14g 200/canister. Generic/Trade: Soln for inhalation 0.4% & 0.6% in 2.5 mL unit-dose vials. Generic only: Syrup 10 mg/5 mL, Tabs 10 & 20 mg.

**PIRBUTEROL (Maxair Autohaler)** ▶L ♀C ▶? $$$$
ADULT - Acute asthma: MDI: 1–2 puffs q4–6h. Max dose 12 puffs/d.
PEDS - Not approved in children.
UNAPPROVED PEDS - Acute asthma ≥12 yo: Use adult dose.
FORMS - Trade only: MDI 200 mcg/actuation, 14g 400/canister.
NOTES - Breath-actuated autohaler.

**TERBUTALINE (Brethine, ←Bricanyl Turbuhaler)** ▶L ♀B ▶- $$
ADULT - Asthma: 2.5–5 mg PO q6h while awake. Max dose 15 mg/24h. Acute asthma: 0.25 mg SC into lateral deltoid area; may repeat x1 within 15–30 min. Max dose 0.5 mg/4h.
PEDS - Not approved in children.
UNAPPROVED ADULT - Preterm labor: 0.25 mg SC q30 min up to 1 mg in 4 h. Infusion: 2.5–10 mcg/min IV, gradually increased to effective max doses of 17.5–30 mcg/min.
UNAPPROVED PEDS - Asthma, >12 yo: Use adult dose, max 7.5 mg/24h. If ≤12 yo: 0.05 mg/kg/dose PO tid, increase to max of 0.15 mg/kg/dose tid, max 5 mg/d. Acute asthma: 0.01 mg/kg SC q 20 min × 3 doses then q 2–6 h as needed.
FORMS - Generic/Trade: Tabs 2.5 & 5 mg (Brethine scored). Canada only (Bricanyl): DPI 0.5 mg/actuation, 200 per DPI.
NOTES - Give 50% normal dose in renal insufficiency; avoid in renal failure. Concomitant use with magnesium sulfate may lead to fatal pulmonary edema.

## PULMONARY: Beta Agonists—Long Acting

**NOTE:** Long-acting beta agonists may increase the risk of asthma-related death; it is unclear if this also applies to COPD. Use only as a 2nd agent if inadequate control with an optimal dose of inhaled corticosteroids. Do not use for rescue therapy. Palpitations, tachycardia, tremor, lightheadedness, nervousness, headache, & nausea may occur. Decreases in serum potassium can occur, rarely leading to adverse cardiovascular effects; monitor accordingly.

**ARFORMOTEROL (Brovana)** ▶L ♀C ▶? $$$$$
ADULT - COPD: 15 mcg nebulized bid.
PEDS - Not approved in children.
FORMS - Trade only: Solution for inhalation 15 mcg in 2mL vial.
NOTES - Not for acute COPD exacerbations.

**FORMOTEROL (Foradil, Perforomist, ←Oxeze Turbuhaler)** ▶L ♀C ▶? $$$
ADULT - Chronic asthma, COPD: 1 puff bid. Prevention of exercise-induced bronchospasm: 1 puff 15 min prior to exercise. COPD: 20 mcg nebulized q12h.
PEDS - Chronic asthma ≥5 yo: 1 puff bid. Prevention of exercise-induced bronchospasm ≥12 yo: Use adult dose.
FORMS - Trade only: DPI 12 mcg, 12 & 60 blisters/pack (Foradil). Soln for inhalation: 20 mcg in 2

mL vial (Perforomist). Canada only (Oxeze): DPI 6 & 12 mcg 60 blisters/pack.
NOTES - Do not use additional doses for exercise if on maintenance.

**SALMETEROL (Serevent Diskus)** ▶L ♀C ▶? $$$$
ADULT - Chronic asthma/COPD: 1 puff bid. Prevention of exercise-induced bronchospasm: 1 puff 30 min before exercise.
PEDS - Chronic asthma ≥4 yo: 1 puff bid. Prevention of exercise-induced bronchospasm: 1 puff 30 min before exercise.
FORMS - Trade only: DPI (Diskus): 50 mcg, 60 blisters.
NOTES - Do not use additional doses for exercise if on maintenance. Concomitant ketoconazole increases levels and prolongs QT interval. Do not use with strong CYP3A4 inhibitors such as ritonavir, itraconazole, clarithromycin, nefazodone, etc.

**PREDICTED PEAK EXPIRATORY FLOW** (liters/min)

| Age (yr) | Women (height in inches) | | | | | Men (height in inches) | | | | | Child (height in inches) | |
|---|---|---|---|---|---|---|---|---|---|---|---|---|
| | 55" | 60" | 65" | 70" | 75" | 60" | 65" | 70" | 75" | 80" | | |
| 20 yr | 390 | 423 | 460 | 496 | 529 | 554 | 602 | 649 | 693 | 740 | 44" | 160 |
| 30 yr | 380 | 413 | 448 | 483 | 516 | 532 | 577 | 622 | 664 | 710 | 46" | 187 |
| 40 yr | 370 | 402 | 436 | 470 | 502 | 509 | 552 | 596 | 636 | 680 | 48" | 214 |
| 50 yr | 360 | 391 | 424 | 457 | 488 | 486 | 527 | 569 | 607 | 649 | 50" | 240 |
| 60 yr | 350 | 380 | 412 | 445 | 475 | 463 | 502 | 542 | 578 | 618 | 52" | 267 |
| 70 yr | 340 | 369 | 400 | 432 | 461 | 440 | 477 | 515 | 550 | 587 | 54" | 293 |

*Am Rev Resp Dis* 1963; 88:644

## PULMONARY: Combinations

***ADVAIR*** (fluticasone—inhaled + salmeterol) (Advair HFA) ▶L ♀C ▶? $$$$$
WARNING - Long-acting beta agonists may increase the risk of asthma-related death; use as an adjunct only if inadequate control with an optimal dose of inhaled corticosteroids. Avoid in significantly worsening or acute asthma. Do not use for rescue therapy. Do not stop abruptly.
ADULT - Chronic asthma: DPI: 1 puff bid (all strengths). MDI: 2 puffs bid (all strengths). COPD maintenance: DPI: 1 puff bid (250/50 only).
PEDS - Chronic asthma ≥12 yo: DPI: Use adult dose. 4–11 yo: 1 puff bid (100/50 only).
FORMS - Trade only: DPI: 100/50, 250/50, 500/50 mcg fluticasone/salmeterol per actuation; 60 doses/DPI. Trade only (Advair HFA): MDI 45/21, 115/21, 230/21 mcg fluticasone/salmeterol per actuation; 120 doses/canister.
NOTES - See individual components for additional information. Ritonavir & other CYP3A4 inhibitors such as ketoconazole significantly increase both salmeterol and fluticasone concentrations, resulting in prolongation of QT interval (salmeterol) and systemic effects, including adrenal suppression (fluticasone). Very rare anaphylactic reaction in patients with severe milk protein allergy.

***COMBIVENT*** (albuterol + ipratropium) ▶L ♀C ▶? $$$$
ADULT - COPD: MDI: 2 puffs qid. Max 12 puffs/24 h.
PEDS - Not approved in children.
FORMS - Trade only: MDI: 90 mcg albuterol/18 mcg ipratropium per actuation, 200/canister.
NOTES - Contraindicated with soy or peanut allergy. Refer to components.

***DUONEB*** (albuterol + ipratropium) (*＋Combivent inhalation solution*) ▶L ♀C ▶? $$$$$
ADULT - COPD: One unit dose nebulized qid; may add 2 doses/d prn to max of 6 doses/d.
PEDS - Not approved in children.
FORMS - Generic/Trade: Unit dose: 2.5 mg albuterol/0.5 mg ipratropium per 3 mL vial, premixed; 30 & 60 vials/carton.
NOTES - Refer to components

***DUOVENT UDV*** (ipratropium + fenoterol) ▶L ♀? ▶? $$$$$
ADULT - Canada only. Bronchospasm associated with asthma/COPD: 1 vial (via nebulizer) q6h prn.
PEDS - Canada only. Children ≥12 yo: 1 vial (via nebulizer) q6h prn.
FORMS - Canada trade only: unit dose vial (for nebulization) 0.5 mg ipratropium & 1.25 mg fenoterol in 4 mL of saline.

***SYMBICORT*** (budesonide + formoterol) ▶L ♀C ▶? $$$$
WARNING - Long-acting beta agonists may increase risk of asthma-related death; use as adjunct only if inhaled corticosteroids inadequate. Avoid in significantly worsening acute asthma. Not for rescue therapy. Do not stop abruptly.
ADULT - Chronic asthma: 2 puffs bid (both strengths).
PEDS - Chronic asthma ≥12 yo: Use adult dose.
FORMS - Trade only: MDI: 80/4.5 & 160/4.5 mcg budesonide/formoterol per actuation; 120 doses/canister.
NOTES - See individual components for additional information. Ritonavir & other CYP3A4 inhibitors such as ketoconazole significantly increase budesonide concentrations, resulting in systemic effects, including adrenal suppression.

**INHALER COLORS** (Body then cap—Generics may differ)

| | | | | | |
|---|---|---|---|---|---|
| Advair: | purple | Combivent: | clear/orange | Pulmicort: | white/brown |
| Advair HFA: | purple/light purple | Flovent HFA: | orange/peach | QVAR 40 mcg: | beige/grey |
| Aerobid: | grey/purple | Foradil: | grey/beige | QVAR 80 mcg: | mauve/grey |
| Aerobid-M: | grey/green | Intal: | white/blue | Serevent Diskus: | green |
| Alupent: | clear/blue | Maxair: | white/white | Spiriva: | grey |
| Asmanex: | white/white | Maxair Autohaler: | white/white | Tilade: | white/white |
| Atrovent HFA: | clear/green | ProAir HFA: | red/white | Ventolin HFA: | light blue/navy |
| Azmacort: | white/white | Proventil HFA: | yellow/orange | Xopenex HFA: | blue/red |

## PULMONARY: Inhaled Steroids

**NOTE:** See Endocrine; Corticosteroids when oral steroids necessary. Beware of adrenal suppression when changing from systemic to inhaled steroids. Inhaled steroids are not for treatment of acute asthma; higher doses may be needed for severe asthma and exacerbations. Adjust to lowest effective dose for maintenance. Use of a DPI, a spacing device, & rinsing the mouth with water after each use may decrease the incidence of thrush & dysphonia. Pharyngitis & cough may occur with all products. Use with caution in patients with active or quiescent TB, untreated systemic fungal, bacterial, viral or parasitic infections or in patients with ocular HSV. Inhaled steroids produce small, transient reductions in growth velocity in children. Prolonged use may lead to decreases in bone mineral density & osteoporosis, thereby increasing fracture risk .

**BECLOMETHASONE - INHALED (QVAR)** ▶L ♀C ▶? $$$
ADULT - Chronic asthma: 40 mcg: 1–4 puffs bid. 80 mcg: 1–2 puffs bid.
PEDS - Chronic asthma in 5–11 yo: 40 mcg 1–2 puffs bid.
UNAPPROVED ADULT - Chronic asthma: NHLBI dosing schedule (puffs/d divided bid): Low dose: 2–6 puffs of 40 mcg or 1–3 puffs of 80 mcg. Medium dose: 6–12 puffs of 40 mcg or 3–6 puffs of 80 mcg. High dose: >12 puffs of 40 mcg or >6 puffs 80 mcg.
UNAPPROVED PEDS - Chronic asthma (5–11 yo): NHLBI dosing schedule (puffs/d divided bid): Low dose: 2–4 puffs of 40 mcg or 1–2 puffs of 80 mcg. Medium dose: 4–8 puffs of 40 mcg or 2–4 puffs of 80 mcg. High dose: >8 puffs of 40 mcg or >4 puffs of 80 mcg.
FORMS - Trade only: HFA MDI: 40 mcg & 80 mcg/actuation, 7.3g 100 actuations/canister.

**BUDESONIDE - INHALED (Pulmicort Respules, Pulmicort Flexhaler)** ▶L ♀B ▶? $$$$
ADULT - Chronic asthma: DPI: 1–2 puffs daily-bid up to 4 puffs bid.
PEDS - Chronic asthma 6–12 yo: DPI: 1–2 puffs daily-bid. 12 mo - 8 yo: Suspension for inhalation (Respules). 0.5 mg - 1 mg daily or divided bid.
UNAPPROVED ADULT - Chronic asthma: NHLBI dosing schedule (puffs/d daily or divided bid): DPI: Low dose: 1–3 puffs of 180 mcg or 2–6 puffs of 90 mcg. Medium dose: 3–7 puffs of 180 mcg or 6–13 puffs of 90 mcg. High dose: >7 puffs of 180 mcg or >13 puffs of 90 mcg.
UNAPPROVED PEDS - Chronic asthma (5–11 yo): NHLBI dosing schedule (puffs/d daily or divided bid) DPI: Low dose: 1–2 puffs of 180 mcg or 2–4 puffs of 90 mcg. Medium dose: 2–4 puffs of 180 mcg or 4–9 puffs of 90 mcg. High dose: >4 puffs of 180 mcg or > 9 puffs of 90 mcg. Suspension for inhalation (daily or divided bid): Low dose: up to 4 yo : 0.25–0.5 mg; 5–11 yo: 0.5 mg. Medium dose: up to 4 yo: > 0.5–1 mg; 5–11 yo: 1 mg. High dose: up to 4 yo: > 1mg; 5–11 yo: 2 mg.
FORMS - Trade only: DPI: (Flexhaler) 90 & 180mcg powder/actuation 60 & 120 doses respectively/ canister. Respules: 0.25, 0.5, & 1 mg/2 mL unit dose.
NOTES - Respules should be delivered via a jet nebulizer with a mouthpiece or face mask. CYP3A4 inhibitors such as ketoconazole, erythromycin, ritonavir, etc. may significantly increase systemic concentrations, possibly causing adrenal suppression. Flexhaler contains trace amounts of milk proteins; caution with severe milk protein hypersensitivity.

**CICLESONIDE - INHALED (Alvesco)** ▶L ♀C ▶? $$$$
ADULT - Chronic asthma MDI: 80 mcg/puff: 1–4 puffs bid. 160 mcg/puff: 1–2 puffs bid.
PEDS - Chronic asthma ≥12 yo: Use adult dose.
FORMS - Trade only: 80 mcg/actuation, 60 per canister. 160 mcg/actuation, 60 & 120 per canister.
NOTES - CYP3A4 inhibitors such as ketoconazole may significantly increase systemic concentrations, possibly causing adrenal suppression.

**FLUNISOLIDE (AeroBid, AeroBid-M, Aerospan)** ▶L ♀C ▶? $$$
ADULT - Chronic asthma: MDI: 2 puffs bid up to 4 puffs bid.
PEDS - Chronic asthma: 6–15 yo: MDI: 2 puffs bid.
UNAPPROVED ADULT - Chronic asthma: NHLBI dosing schedule (puffs/d divided bid): Low dose: 2–4 puffs. Medium dose: 4–8 puffs. High dose: >8 puffs.
UNAPPROVED PEDS - Chronic asthma (5–11 yo): NHLBI dosing schedule (puffs/d divided bid): Low dose: 2–3 puffs. Medium dose: 4–5 puffs. High dose: >5 puffs (≥8 puffs for 80 mcg HFA).
FORMS - Trade only: MDI: 250 mcg/actuation, 100 metered doses/canister. AeroBid-M (AeroBid + menthol flavor). Aerospan HFA MDI: 80 mcg/actuation, 60 & 120 metered doses/canister.

**FLUTICASONE - INHALED (Flovent HFA, Flovent Diskus)** ▶L ♀C ▶? $$$$
ADULT - Chronic asthma: MDI: 2 puffs bid up to 4 puffs bid. Max dose 880 mcg bid.
PEDS - Chronic asthma: >12 yo: Use adult dose. 4–11 yo: 2 puffs bid of 44 mcg/puff.
UNAPPROVED ADULT - Chronic asthma: NHLBI dosing schedule (puffs/d divided bid): Low dose: 2–6 puffs of 44 mcg MDI. Medium dose: 2–4 puffs of 110 mcg MDI. 2 puffs of 220 mcg MDI. High dose: >4 puffs 110 mcg MDI. > 2 puffs 220 mcg MDI.
UNAPPROVED PEDS - Chronic asthma (≤11 yo): NHLBI dosing schedule (puffs/d divided bid): Low dose: 2–4 puffs of 44 mcg MDI. Medium dose: 4–8 puffs of 44 mcg MDI. 2–3 puffs of 110 mcg MDI. High dose: ≥4 puffs 110 mcg MDI. ≥2 puffs 220 mcg MDI.
FORMS - Trade only: HFA MDI: 44, 110, 220 mcg/ actuation 120/canister. DPI (Diskus): 50, 100, 250 mcg/actuation delivering 44, 88, 220 mcg respectively.

**FLUTICASONE** (*cont.*)
NOTES - Ritonavir & other CYP3A4 inhibitors such as ketoconazole significantly increase fluticasone concentrations, resulting in systemic effects, including adrenal suppression.

**MOMETASONE - INHALED (*Asmanex Twisthaler*)** ▶L ♀C ▶? $$$$
ADULT - Chronic asthma: 1–2 puffs q pm or 1 puff bid. If prior oral corticosteroid therapy: 2 puffs bid.
PEDS - Chronic asthma: ≥ 12 yo: Use adult dose.
UNAPPROVED ADULT - Chronic asthma: NHLBI dosing schedule (puffs/d divided bid): Low dose: 1 puff. Medium dose: 2 puffs. High dose: >2 puffs.
FORMS - Trade only: DPI: 220 mcg/actuation, 30, 60 & 120/canister.
NOTES - CYP3A4 inhibitors such as ketoconazole may significantly increase concentrations.

**TRIAMCINOLONE - INHALED (*Azmacort*)** ▶L ♀D ▶? $$$$
ADULT - Chronic asthma: MDI: 2 puffs tid-qid or 4 puffs bid. Max dose 16 puffs/d. Severe asthma: 12–16 puffs/d and adjust downward.
PEDS - Chronic asthma >12 yo: Use adult dose. 6–12 yo: 1–2 puffs tid-qid or 2–4 puffs bid. Max dose 12 puffs/d.
UNAPPROVED ADULT - Chronic asthma (5–11 yo): NHLBI dosing schedule (puffs/d divided bid): Low dose: 4–8 puffs. Medium dose: 8–12 puffs. High dose: >12 puffs.
UNAPPROVED PEDS - Chronic asthma: NHLBI dosing schedule (puffs/d divided bid): Low dose: 4–8 puffs. Medium dose: 8–12 puffs. High dose: >12 puffs.
FORMS - Trade only: MDI: 75 mcg/actuation, 240/canister. Built-in spacer.

## INHALED STEROIDS: ESTIMATED COMPARATIVE DAILY DOSES*

| ADULTS | | | | |
| --- | --- | --- | --- | --- |
| Drug | Form | Low Dose | Medium Dose | High Dose |
| beclomethasone MDI | 40 mcg/puff | 2–6 puffs/d | 6–12 puffs/d | >12 puffs/d |
| | 80 mcg/puff | 1–3 puffs/d | 3–6 puffs/d | >6 puffs/d |
| budesonide DPI | 200 mcg/dose | 1–3 inhalations/d | 3–6 inhalations/d | >6 inhalations/d |
| flunisolide MDI | 250 mcg/puff | 2–4 puffs/d | 4–8 puffs/d | >8 puffs/d |
| fluticasone MDI | 44 mcg/puff | 2–6 puffs/d | 6–15 puffs/d | >15 puffs/d |
| | 110 mcg/puff | 1–2 puffs/d | 3–6 puffs/d | >6 puffs/d |
| | 220 mcg/puff | 1 puff/d | 2–3 puffs/d | >3 puffs/d |
| fluticasone DPI | 50 mcg/dose | 2–6 inhalations/d | 6–12 inhalations/d | >12 inhalations/d |
| | 100 mcg/dose | 1–3 inhalations/d | 3–6 inhalations/d | >6 inhalations/d |
| | 250 mcg/dose | 1 inhalation/d | 2 inhalations/d | >2 inhalations/d |
| triamcinolone MDI | 100 mcg/puff | 4–10 puffs/d | 10–20 puffs/d | >20 puffs/d |
| CHILDREN (≤ 12 yo) | | | | |
| Drug | Form | Low Dose | Medium Dose | High Dose |
| beclomethasone MDI | 40 mcg/puff | 2–4 puffs/d | 4–8 puffs/d | >8 puffs/d |
| | 80 mcg/puff | 1–2 puffs/d | 2–4 puffs/d | >4 puffs/d |
| budesonide DPI | 200 mcg/dose | 1–2 inhalations/d | 2–4 inhalations/d | >4 inhalations/d |
| flunisolide MDI | 250 mcg/puff | 2–3 puffs/d | 4–5 puffs/d | >5 puffs/d |
| fluticasone MDI | 44 mcg/puff | 2–4 puffs/d | 4–10 puffs/d | >10 puffs/d |
| | 110 mcg/puff | 1 puff/d | 1–4 puffs/d | >4 puffs/d |
| | 220 mcg/puff | use less concentrated form | 1–2 puffs/d | >2 puffs/d |
| fluticasone DPI | 50 mcg/dose | 2–4 inhalations/d | 4–8 inhalations/d | >8 inhalations/d |
| | 100 mcg/dose | 1–2 inhalations/d | 2–4 inhalations/d | >4 inhalations/d |
| | 250 mcg/dose | use less concentrated form | 1 inhalation/d | >1 inhalation/d |
| triamcinolone MDI | 100 mcg/puff | 4–8 puffs/d | 8–12 puffs/d | >12 puffs/d |

*MDI = metered dose inhaler. DPI = dry powder inhaler. Reference: http://www.nhlbi.nih.gov/guidelines/asthma/execsumm.pdf

## PULMONARY: Leukotriene Inhibitors

**NOTE:** Not for treatment of acute asthma. Abrupt substitution for corticosteroids may precipitate Churg-Strauss syndrome.

**MONTELUKAST (*Singulair*)** ▶L ♀B ▶? $$$$
ADULT - Chronic asthma, allergic rhinitis: 10 mg PO daily. Prevention of exercise-induced bronchoconstriction: 10 mg PO 2 h before exercise.

PEDS - Chronic asthma, allergic rhinitis: 6–14 yo: 5 mg PO daily. 2–5 yo: 4 mg (chew tab or oral granules) PO daily. Asthma 12–23 mo: 4 mg (oral granules) PO daily. Allergic rhinitis 6–23 mo: **(cont.)**

**MONTELUKAST** (cont.)
4 mg (oral granules) PO daily. Prevention of exercise-induced bronchoconstriction: ≥ 15 yo: Use adult dose.

FORMS - Trade only: Tabs 10 mg. Oral granules 4 mg packet, 30/box. Chewable tabs (cherry flavored) 4 & 5 mg.

NOTES - Chew tabs contain phenylalanine. Oral granules may be placed directly into the mouth or mixed with a spoonful of breast milk, baby formula, applesauce, carrots, rice or ice cream. If mixed with food, must be taken within 15 min. Do not mix with liquids. Levels decreased by phenobarbital & rifampin. Dyspepsia may occur. Do not take an additional dose for exercise-induced bronchospasm if already taking chronically.

**ZAFIRLUKAST** (Accolate) ▶L ♀B ▶- $$$
WARNING - Hepatic failure has been reported.
ADULT - Chronic asthma: 20 mg PO bid, 1h ac or 2h pc.

PEDS - Chronic asthma ≥12 yo: use adult dose. 5–11 yo: 10 mg PO bid, 1h ac or 2h pc.

UNAPPROVED ADULT - Allergic rhinitis: 20 mg PO bid, 1h ac or 2h pc.

FORMS - Trade only: Tabs 10, 20 mg.

NOTES - Potentiates warfarin & theophylline. Levels decreased by erythromycin & increased by high-dose aspirin. Nausea may occur. If liver dysfunction is suspected, discontinue drug & manage accordingly. Consider monitoring LFTs.

**ZILEUTON** (Zyflo CR) ▶L ♀C ▶? $$$$$
WARNING - Contraindicated in active liver disease.
ADULT - Chronic asthma: 1200 mg PO bid.
PEDS - Chronic asthma ≥12 yo: use adult dose.
FORMS - Trade only: Tabs, extended release 600 mg.
NOTES - Monitor LFTs for elevation. Potentiates warfarin, theophylline, & propranolol. Dyspepsia & nausea may occur.

## PULMONARY: Other Pulmonary Medications

**ACETYLCYSTEINE - INHALED** (Mucomyst) ▶L ♀B ▶? $
ADULT - Mucolytic nebulization: 3–5 mL of the 20% soln or 6–10 mL of the 10% soln tid-qid. Instillation, direct or via tracheostomy: 1–2 mL of a 10% to 20% soln q1–4h; via percutaneous intratracheal catheter: 1–2 mL of the 20% soln or 2–4 mL of the 10% soln q1–4h.
PEDS - Mucolytic nebulization: Use adult dosing.
FORMS - Generic/Trade: Soln for inhalation 10 & 20% in 4, 10 & 30 mL vials.
NOTES - Increased volume of liquefied bronchial secretions may occur; maintain an open airway. Watch for bronchospasm in asthmatics. Stomatitis, N/V, fever, & rhinorrhea may occur. A slight disagreeable odor may occur & should soon disappear. A face mask may cause stickiness on the face after nebulization; wash with water. The 20% solution may be diluted with NaCl or sterile water.

**ALPHA-1 PROTEINASE INHIBITOR** (alpha-1 antitrypsin, Aralast, Prolastin, Zemaira) ▶Plasma ♀C ▶? $
WARNING - Possible transmission of viruses and Creutzfeldt-Jakob disease.
ADULT - Congenital alpha-1 proteinase inhibitor deficiency with emphysema: 60 mg/kg IV once weekly.
PEDS - Not approved in children.
NOTES - Contraindicated in selected IgA deficiencies with known antibody to IgA. Hepatitis B vaccine recommended in preparation for Prolastin use.

**AMINOPHYLLINE** (+Phyllocontin) ▶L ♀C ▶? $
ADULT - Acute asthma: loading dose if currently not receiving theophylline: 6 mg/kg IV over 20–30 min. Maintenance IV infusion 1g in 250 mL D5W (4 mg/mL) at 0.5–0.7 mg/kg/h (70 kg: 0.7 mg/kg/h = 11 mL/h). In patients with cor pulmonale, heart failure, liver failure, use 0.25 mg/kg/h. If currently on theophylline, each 0.6 mg/kg aminophylline will increase the serum

theophylline concentration by approximately 1 mcg/mL. Maintenance: 200 mg PO bid-qid.
PEDS - Acute asthma: loading dose if currently not receiving theophylline: 6 mg/kg IV over 20–30 min. Maintenance >6 mo: 0.8–1 mg/kg/h IV infusion. >1 yo: 3–4 mg/kg/dose PO q6h.
UNAPPROVED PEDS - Neonatal apnea of prematurity: loading dose 5–6 mg/kg IV/PO. Maintenance: 1–2 mg/kg/dose q6–8 h IV/PO.
FORMS - Generic only: Tabs 100 & 200 mg. Oral liquid 105 mg/5 mL. Canada Trade only: Tabs controlled release (12 h) 225, 350 mg, scored.
NOTES - Aminophylline is 79% theophylline. Administer IV infusion ≤25 mg/min. Multiple drug interactions (especially ketoconazole, rifampin, carbamazepine, isoniazid, phenytoin, macrolides, zafirlukast & cimetidine). Review meds before initiating treatment. Irritability, nausea, palpitations & tachycardia may occur. Overdose may be life-threatening.

**BERACTANT** (Survanta) ▶Lung ♀? ▶? $$$$$
PEDS - RDS (hyaline membrane disease) in premature infants: Specialized dosing.

**CALFACTANT** (Infasurf) ▶Lung ♀? ▶? $$$$$
PEDS - RDS (hyaline membrane disease) in premature infants: Specialized dosing.
FORMS - Trade only: Oral susp: 35 mg/mL in 3 & 6 mL vials. Preservative-free.

**CROMOLYN - INHALED** (Intal, Gastrocrom, +Nalcrom) ▶LK ♀B ▶? $$$
ADULT - Chronic asthma: MDI: 2–4 puffs qid. Soln for inhalation: 20 mg qid. Prevention of exercise-induced bronchospasm: MDI: 2 puffs 10–15 min prior to exercise. Soln for nebulization: 20 mg 10–15 min prior. Mastocytosis: 200 mg PO qid, 30 min ac & qhs.
PEDS - Chronic asthma >5 yo: MDI: 2 puffs qid. >2 yo: soln for nebulization: 20 mg qid. Prevention of exercise-induced bronchospasm >5 yo: MDI: 2

**CROMOLYN** *(cont.)*

     puffs 10–15 min prior to exercise. >2 yo soln for nebulization: 20 mg 10–15 min prior. Mastocytosis: 2–12 yo: 100 mg PO qid 30 min ac & qhs.

FORMS - Trade only: MDI 800 mcg/actuation, 112 & 200/canister. Oral concentrate 100 mg/5 mL in 8 amps/foil pouch (Gastrocrom). Generic/Trade: Soln for nebs: 20 mg/2 mL.

NOTES - Not for treatment of acute asthma. Pharyngitis may occur. Directions for oral concentrate: 1) Break open and squeeze liquid contents of ampule(s) into a glass of water. 2) Stir soln. 3) Drink all of the liquid.

**DORNASE ALFA** *(Pulmozyme)* ▶L ♀B ▶? $$$$$

ADULT - Cystic fibrosis: 2.5 mg nebulized daily-bid.

PEDS - Cystic fibrosis ≥6 yo: 2.5 mg nebulized daily-bid.

UNAPPROVED PEDS - Has been used in a small number of children as young as 3 mo w/similar efficacy & side effects.

FORMS - Trade only: soln for inhalation: 1 mg/mL in 2.5 mL vials.

NOTES - Voice alteration, pharyngitis, laryngitis, & rash may occur. Do not dilute or mix with other drugs.

**DOXAPRAM** *(Dopram)* ▶L ♀B ▶? $$$

ADULT - Acute hypercapnia due to COPD: 1–2 mg/min IV, max 3 mg/min. Max infusion time: 2 h.

PEDS - Not approved in children.

UNAPPROVED PEDS - Apnea of prematurity unresponsive to methylxanthines: Load 2.5–3 mg/kg over 15 min, then 1 mg/kg/h titrated to lowest effective dose. Max: 2.5 mg/kg/h. Contains benzyl alcohol; caution in neonates.

NOTES - Monitor arterial blood gases at baseline and q30 min during infusion. Do not use with mechanical ventilation. Contraindicated with seizure disorder, severe hypertension, CVA, head injury, CAD and severe heart failure.

**EPINEPHRINE RACEMIC** *(S-2, ✦Vaponefrin)* ▶Plasma ♀C ▶- $

ADULT - See cardiovascular section

PEDS - Severe croup: soln for inhalation: 0.05 mL/kg/dose diluted to 3 mL w/NS over 15 min prn not to exceed q1–2h dosing. Max dose 0.5 mL.

FORMS - Trade only: soln for inhalation: 2.25% epinephrine in 15 & 30 mL.

NOTES - Cardiac arrhythmias and hypertension may occur.

**IPRATROPIUM - INHALED** *(Atrovent, Atrovent HFA)* ▶Lung ♀B ▶? $$$

ADULT - COPD: MDI (Atrovent, Atrovent HFA): 2 puffs qid; may use additional inhalations not to exceed 12 puffs/d. Soln for inhalation: 500 mcg nebulized tid-qid.

PEDS - Not approved in children <12 yo.

UNAPPROVED PEDS - Acute asthma: MDI (Atrovent, Atrovent HFA): >12 yo: use adult dose. ≤12 yo: 1–2 puffs tid-qid. Soln for inhalation: >12 yo: 250–500 mcg/dose tid-qid; ≤12 yo: 250 mcg/dose tid-qid. Acute asthma: 2–18yo: 500 mcg nebulized with 2nd & 3rd doses of albuterol.

FORMS - Trade only: Atrovent HFA MDI: 17 mcg/actuation, 200/canister. Generic/Trade: Soln for nebulization: 0.02% (500 mcg/vial) in unit dose vials.

NOTES - Atrovent MDI is contraindicated with soy or peanut allergy; HFA not contraindicated. Caution with glaucoma; myasthenia gravis, BPH, or bladder neck obstruction. Cough, dry mouth & blurred vision may occur.

**KETOTIFEN** *(✦Zaditen)* ▶L ♀C ▶- $$

ADULT - Not approved.

PEDS - Canada only. Chronic asthma: 6 mo to 3 yo: 0.05 mg/kg PO bid. Children >3 yo: 1 mg PO bid.

FORMS - Generic/Trade: Tabs 1 mg. Syrup 1mg/5 mL.

NOTES - Several wk may be necessary before therapeutic effect. Full clinical effectiveness is generally reached after 10 wk.

**METHACHOLINE** *(Provocholine)* ▶Plasma ♀C ▶? $$

WARNING - Life-threatening bronchoconstriction can result; have resuscitation capability available.

ADULT - Diagnosis of bronchial airway hyperreactivity in non-wheezing patients with suspected asthma: 5 breaths each of ascending serial concentrations, 0.025 mg/mL to 25 mg/mL, via nebulization. The procedure ends when there is a ≥20% reduction in the FEV1 compared with baseline.

PEDS - Diagnosis of bronchial airway hyperreactivity: use adult dose.

NOTES - Avoid with epilepsy, bradycardia, peptic ulcer disease, thyroid disease, urinary tract obstruction or other conditions that could be adversely affected by a cholinergic agent. Hold beta-blockers. Do not inhale powder.

**NEDOCROMIL - INHALED** *(Tilade)* ▶L ♀B ▶? $$$

ADULT - Chronic asthma: MDI: 2 puffs qid. Reduce dose to bid-tid as tolerated.

PEDS - Chronic asthma >6 yo: MDI: 2 puffs qid.

FORMS - Trade only: MDI: 1.75 mg/actuation, 112/canister.

NOTES - Not for treatment of acute asthma. Unpleasant taste & dysphonia may occur.

**NITRIC OXIDE** *(INOmax)* ▶Lung, K ♀C ▶? $$$$

PEDS - Respiratory failure with pulmonary hypertension in infants >34 wk old: Specialized dosing.

NOTES - Risk of methemoglobinemia increases with concomitant nitroprusside or nitroglycerin.

**OMALIZUMAB** *(Xolair)* ▶Plasma, L ♀B ▶? $$$$$

WARNING - Anaphylaxis may occur within 2 h of administration; monitor closely and be prepared to treat.

ADULT - Moderate to severe asthma with perennial allergy when symptoms not controlled by inhaled steroids: 150–375 mg SC q 2–4 wk, based on pretreatment serum total IgE level & body weight.

PEDS - Moderate to severe asthma with perennial allergy: ≥12 yo: use adult dose.

NOTES - Not for treatment of acute asthma. Divide doses >150 mg over more than 1 injection site. Monitor for signs of anaphylaxis including bronchospasm, hypotension, syncope, urticaria, angioedema.

**PORACTANT (*Curosurf*)** ▶Lung ♀? ▶? $$$$$
  PEDS - RDS (hyaline membrane disease) in premature infants: Specialized dosing.
**THEOPHYLLINE (*Elixophyllin, Uniphyl, Theo-24,
T-Phyl, →Theo-Dur, Theolair*)** ▶L ♀C ▶+ $
  ADULT - Chronic asthma: 5–13 mg/kg/d PO in
  divided doses. Max dose 900 mg/d.
  PEDS - Chronic asthma, initial: >1 yo & <45 kg:
  12–14 mg/kg/d PO divided q4–6h to max of
  300 mg/24h. Maintenance: 16–20 mg/kg/d PO
  divided q4–6h to max of 600 mg/24h. >1 yo &
  ≥45 kg: Initial: 300 mg/24h PO divided q6–8h.
  Maintenance: 400–600 mg/24h PO divided
  q6–8h. Infants 6–52 wk: [(0.2 × age in wk) +
  5] × kg = 24hr dose in mg PO divided q6–8h.
  UNAPPROVED ADULT - COPD: 10 mg/kg/d PO in
  divided doses.
  UNAPPROVED PEDS - Apnea & bradycardia of
  prematurity: 3–6 mg/kg/d PO divided q6–8h.
  Maintain serum concentrations 3–5 mcg/mL.
  FORMS - Generic/Trade: Elixir 80 mg/15 mL. Trade
  only: Caps - Theo-24: 100, 200, 300, 400 mg.

T-Phyl - 12 Hr SR tabs 200 mg. Theolair - tabs
125, 250 mg. Generic only: 12 h tabs 100, 200,
300, 450 mg, 12 Hr caps 125, 200, 300 mg.
  NOTES - Multiple drug interactions (especially
  ketoconazole, rifampin, carbamazepine, isonia-
  zid, phenytoin, macrolides, zafirlukast & cimetidine). Review meds before initiating treatment.
  Overdose may be life-threatening.
**TIOTROPIUM (*Spiriva*)** ▶K ♀C ▶- $$$$
  ADULT - COPD: Handihaler: 18 mcg inhaled daily.
  PEDS - Not approved in children.
  FORMS - Trade only: Capsule for oral inhalation 18
  mcg. To be used with "Handihaler" device only.
  Packages of 5, 30, 90 caps with Handihaler device.
  NOTES - Not for acute bronchospasm. Administer at
  the same time each d. Use with caution in narrow-angle glaucoma, myasthenia gravis, BPH, or
  bladder-neck obstruction. Avoid touching opened
  cap. Glaucoma, eye pain, or blurred vision may
  occur if powder enters eyes. May increase dosing
  interval in patients with CrCl <50 mL/min. Avoid
  if severe lactose allergy.

## TOXICOLOGY

**ACETYLCYSTEINE (*N-acetylcysteine, Mucomyst,
Acetadote, →Parvolex*)** ▶L ♀B ▶? $$$$
  ADULT - Acetaminophen toxicity: Mucomyst – loading dose 140 mg/kg PO or NG, then 70 mg/kg q4h
  × 17 doses. May be mixed in water or soft drink
  diluted to a 5% solution. Acetadote (IV) – loading
  dose 150 mg/kg in 200 mL of D5W infused over
  60 min; maintenance dose 50 mg/kg in 500 mL
  of D5W infused over 4 h followed by 100 mg/kg in
  1000 mL of D5W infused over 16 h.
  PEDS - Acetaminophen toxicity: same as adult
  dosing.
  UNAPPROVED ADULT - Prevention of contrast-induced
  nephropathy: 600–1200 mg PO bid for 2 doses
  before procedure and 2 doses after procedure.
  FORMS - Generic/Trade: solution 10%, 20%. Trade
  only: IV (Acetadote)
  NOTES - May be diluted with water or soft drink to
  a 5% solution; use diluted solution within 1 h.
  Repeat loading dose if vomited within 1 h. Critical
  ingestion-treatment interval for maximal protection against severe hepatic injury is between
  0–8 h. Efficacy diminishes after 8 h & treatment
  initiation between 15 & 24 h post ingestion yields
  limited efficacy. However, treatment should not be
  withheld, since the reported time of ingestion may
  not be correct. Anaphylactoid reactions usually
  occurs 30–60 min after initiating infusion. Stop
  infusion, administer antihistamine or epinephrine,
  restart infusion slowly. If anaphylactoid reactions
  return or severity increases, then stop treatment.
**CHARCOAL (*activated charcoal, Actidose-Aqua,
CharcoAid, EZ-Char, →Charcodate*)** ▶Not absorbed
♀+ ▶+ $
  ADULT - Gut decontamination: 25–100 g (1–2 g/
  kg or 10 times the amount of poison ingested)

PO or NG as soon as possible. May repeat q1–4h
prn at doses equivalent to 12.5g/h. When sorbitol
is coadministered, use only with the first dose if
repeated doses are to be given.
  PEDS - Gut decontamination: <1 yo - 1 g/kg; 15–30
  g or 1–2 g/kg if 1–12 yo PO or NG as soon as
  possible. Repeat doses in children have not been
  established, but half the initial dose is recommended. Repeat q 2–6h prn. When sorbitol is
  coadministered, use only with the first dose if
  repeated doses are to be given.
  FORMS - OTC/Generic/Trade: Powder 15,30,40,120,240
  g. Solution 12.5 g/60 mL, 15 g/75 mL, 15g/120
  mL, 25 g/120 mL, 30 g/120 mL, 50 g/240 mL.
  Suspension 15g/120 mL, 25g/120ml, 30g/150 mL,
  50g/240 mL. Granules 15g/120 mL.
  NOTES - Some products may contain sorbitol
  to improve taste and reduce GI transit time.
  Chocolate milk/powder may enhance palatability
  for pediatric use. Not usually effective for toxic
  alcohols (methanol, ethylene glycol, isopropa-
  nol), heavy metals (lead, iron, bromide), arsenic,
  lithium, potassium, hydrocarbons, and caustic
  ingestions (acids, alkalis). Mix powder with 8 oz
  water. Greatest effect when administered <1 h
  of ingestion.
***CYANIDE ANTIDOTE KIT* (amyl nitrite + sodium nitrite
+ sodium thiosulfate)** ▶? ♀- ▶? $$$$$
  ADULT - Cyanide toxicity: Induce methemoglobinemia with inhaled amyl nitrite 0.3 mL followed
  by sodium nitrite 300 mg IV over 2–4 min. Then
  administer sodium thiosulfate 12.5 g IV.
  PEDS - Induce methemoglobinemia with inhaled
  amyl nitrite followed by sodium nitrite 240 mg/m²
  (max 300 mg) IV over 2–4 min. Then administer
  sodium thiosulfate 7 g/m² (max 12.5 g) IV.

**CYANIDE ANTIDOTE KIT** (*cont.*)
FORMS - Package contains amyl nitrite inhalant (0.3mL), sodium nitrite (300 mg/10 mL), sodium thiosulfate (12.5 g/50 mL).
NOTES - Risk of excessive methemoglobinemia with both nitrite components; monitor closely.

**DEFERASIROX** (*Exjade*) ▶L ♀B ▶? $$$$$
ADULT - Chronic iron overload: 20 mg/kg PO daily; adjust dose q3–6 mo based on ferritin trends. Max 30 mg/kg/d.
PEDS - Chronic iron overload: ≥2 yo: 20 mg/kg PO daily; adjust dose q3–6 mo based on ferritin trends. Max 30 mg/kg/d.
FORMS - Trade only: Tabs for dissolving into oral susp 125, 250, 500 mg.
NOTES - Assess creatinine in duplicate before therapy and monthly thereafter; renal failure has been reported. Fatal hepatic failure has been reported; monitor LFTs monthly. Perform auditory and ophthalmic testing before initiation of therapy and yearly thereafter. Do not take with aluminum-containing antacids.

**DEFEROXAMINE** (*Desferal*) ▶K ♀C ▶? $$$$$
ADULT - Chronic iron overload: 500 mg- 1000 mg IM daily and 2 g IV infusion (≤15 mg/kg/h) with each unit of blood or 1–2 g SC daily (20–40 mg/kg/d) over 8–24 h via continuous infusion pump. Acute iron toxicity: IV infusion up to 15 mg/kg/h (consult poison center).
PEDS - Acute iron toxicity: IV infusion up to 15 mg/kg/h (consult poison center).
NOTES - Contraindicated in renal failure/anuria unless undergoing dialysis.

**DIMERCAPROL** (*BAL in oil*) ▶KL ♀C ▶? $$$$$
ADULT - Specialized dosing for arsenic, mercury, gold, and lead toxicity. Consult poison center. Mild arsenic or gold toxicity: 2.5 mg/kg IM qid × 2 d, then bid × 1 d, then daily × 10 d. Severe arsenic or gold toxicity: 3 mg/kg IM q4h × 2 d, then qid × 1 d, then bid × 10 d. Mercury toxicity: 5 mg/kg IM initially, then 2.5 mg/kg daily-bid × 10 d. Begin therapy within 1–2 h of toxicity. Acute lead encephalopathy: 4 mg/kg IM initially, then q4h in combination (separate syringe) with calcium edetate × 2–7 d. May reduce dose to 3 mg/kg IM for less severe toxicity. Deep IM injection needed.
PEDS - Not approved in children.
UNAPPROVED PEDS - Same as adult dosing. Consult poison center.

*DUODOTE* (atropine + pralidoxime) ▶K ♀C ▶? $
ADULT - Organophosphate insecticide/nerve agent poisoning, mild symptoms: 1 injection in thigh. Severe symptoms: 3 injections in rapid succession (may administer through clothes).
PEDS - Not approved in children.
FORMS - Each auto-injector dose delivers atropine 2.1 mg + pralidoxime 600 mg.

**EDETATE** (*EDTA, Endrate, versenate*) ▶K ♀C ▶- $$$
WARNING - Beware of elevated intracranial pressure in lead encephalopathy.
ADULT - Consult poison center. Use calcium disodium form only for lead indications. Non-calcium

form (eg, Endrate) is not interchangeable and is rarely used anymore. Lead toxicity: 1000 mg/m²/d IM (divided into equal doses q8–12h) or IV (infuse total dose over 8–12h) × 5 d. Interrupt therapy for 2–4 d, then repeat same regimen. Two courses of therapy are usually necessary. Acute lead encephalopathy: edetate alone or in combination with dimercaprol. Lead nephropathy: 500 mg/m²/dose q24h × 5 doses (creat 2–3 mg/dl), q48h × 3 doses (creat 3–4 mg/dl), or once weekly (creat >4 mg/dl). May repeat at 1 mo intervals.
PEDS - Specialized dosing for lead toxicity; same as adult dosing also using calcium form. Consult poison center.
FORMS - Calcium disodium formulation used for lead poisoning, other form without calcium (eg, Endrate) is not interchangeable and rarely used anymore.

**ETHANOL** (*alcohol*) ▶L ♀D ▶+ $
PEDS - Not approved in children.
UNAPPROVED ADULT - Consult poison center. Specialized dosing for methanol, ethylene glycol toxicity if fomepizole is unavailable or delayed: 1000 mg/kg (10 mL/kg) of 10% ethanol (100 mg/mL) IV over 1–2h then 100 mg/kg/h (1 mL/kg/h) to keep ethanol level approximately 100 mg/dl.

**FLUMAZENIL** (*Romazicon*) ▶LK ♀C ▶? $$$
WARNING - Do not use in chronic benzodiazepine use or acute overdose with tricyclic antidepressants due to seizure risk.
ADULT - Benzodiazepine sedation reversal: 0.2 mg IV over 15 sec, then 0.2 mg q1 min prn up to 1 mg total dose. Usual dose is 0.6- 1 mg. Benzodiazepine overdose reversal: 0.2 mg IV over 30 sec, then 0.3–0.5 mg q30 sec prn up to 3 mg total dose.
PEDS - Benzodiazepine sedation reversal: 0.01 mg/kg up to 0.2 mg IV over 15 sec; repeat q min to max 4 additional doses.
UNAPPROVED PEDS - Benzodiazepine overdose reversal: 0.01 mg/kg IV. Benzodiazepine sedation reversal: 0.01 mg/kg IV initially (max 0.2 mg), then 0.005–0.01 mg/kg (max 0.2 mg) q1 min to max total dose 1 mg. May repeat doses in 20 min, max 3 mg in 1 h.
NOTES - Onset of action 1–3 min, peak effect 6–10 min. For IV use only, preferably through an IV infusion line into a large vein. Local irritation may occur following extravasation.

**FOMEPIZOLE** (*Antizol*) ▶L ♀C ▶? $$$$$
ADULT - Consult poison center. Ethylene glycol or methanol toxicity: 15 mg/kg IV (load), then 10 mg/kg IV q12h × 4 doses, then 15 mg/kg IV q12h until ethylene glycol or methanol level <20 mg/dl. Administer doses as slow IV infusions over 30 min. Increase frequency to q4h during hemodialysis.
PEDS - Not approved in children.

**HYDROXOCOBALAMIN** (*Cyanokit*) ▶K ♀C ▶? $$$$$
ADULT - Cyanide poisoning: 5 g IV over 15 min; may repeat prn.
PEDS - Not approved in children.

**IPECAC SYRUP** ▶GUT ♀C ▶? $
ADULT - Emesis: 15- 30 mL PO, then 3–4 glasses of water.
PEDS - AAP no longer recommends home ipecac for poisoning. Emesis, <1 yo: 5- 10 mL, then ½ - 1 glass of water (controversial in children <1 yr). Emesis, 1- 12 yo: 15 mL, then 1–2 glasses of water. May repeat dose (15 mL) if vomiting does not occur within 20- 30 min.
FORMS - Generic only (OTC): syrup.
NOTES - Many believe ipecac to be contraindicated in infants <6 mo of age. Do not use if any potential for altered mental status (eg, seizure, neurotoxicity), strychnine, beta blocker, calcium channel blocker, clonidine, digitalis glycoside, corrosive, petroleum distillate ingestions, or if at risk for GI bleeding (coagulopathy).

**METHYLENE BLUE (Methblue 65, Urolene blue)** ▶K ♀C ▶? $$
ADULT - Methemoglobinemia: 1- 2 mg/kg IV over 5 min. Dysuria: 65–130 mg PO tid after meals with liberal water.
PEDS - Not approved in children.
UNAPPROVED PEDS - Methemoglobinemia: 1–2 mg/kg/dose IV over 5 min; may repeat in 1 h prn.
FORMS - Trade only: Tab 65 mg.
NOTES - Avoid in G6PD deficiency. May turn urine, stool, skin, contact lenses, and undergarments blue-green.

**PENICILLAMINE (Cuprimine, Depen)** ▶K ♀D ▶- $$$$$
WARNING - Fatal drug-related adverse events have occurred, caution if penicillin allergy.
ADULT - Consult poison center: Specialized dosing for copper toxicity: 750 mg- 1.5 g/d PO × 3 mo based on 24-h urinary copper excretion, max 2 g/d. May start 250 mg/d PO in patients unable to tolerate.
PEDS - Specialized dosing for copper toxicity. Consult poison center.
FORMS - Trade only: Caps 125, 250 mg; Tabs 250 mg.
NOTES - Patients may require supplemental pyridoxine 25–50 mg/d PO. Promotes excretion of heavy metals in urine.

**PHYSOSTIGMINE (Antilirium)** ▶LK ♀D ▶? $
WARNING - Discontinue if excessive salivation, emesis, frequent urination, or diarrhea. Rapid administration can cause bradycardia, hypersalivation, respiratory difficulties and seizures. Atropine should be available as an antagonist.
ADULT - Life-threatening anticholinergic toxicity: 2 mg IV/IM, administer IV slowly, ≤1 mg/min. May repeat q 10–30 min for severe toxicity.
PEDS - Life-threatening anticholinergic toxicity: 0.02 mg/kg IM/IV injection, administer IV slowly, ≤0.5 mg/min. May repeat q15–30 min until a therapeutic effect or max 2 mg dose.
UNAPPROVED ADULT - Postanesthesia reversal of neuromuscular blockade: 0.5 - 1 mg IV/IM, administer IV slowly, ≤1mg/min. May repeat q 10–30 min prn.
FORMS - Generic/Trade: 1mg/mL in 2ml ampules

**PRALIDOXIME (Protopam, 2-PAM)** ▶K ♀C ▶? $$$
ADULT - Consult poison center: Specialized dosing for organophosphate toxicity: 1–2 g IV infusion over 15–30 min or slow IV injection ≥5 min (max rate 200 mg/min). May repeat dose after 1 h if muscle weakness persists.
PEDS - Not approved in children.
UNAPPROVED ADULT - Consult poison center: 20–40 mg/kg/dose IV infusion over 15–30 min.
UNAPPROVED PEDS - Consult poison center. 25 mg/kg load then 10–20 mg/kg/h or 25–50 mg/kg load followed by repeat dose in 1–2 h then q10–12h.
NOTES - Administer <36h of exposure when possible. Rapid administration may worsen cholinergic symptoms. Give in conjunction with atropine. IM or SC may be used if IV access is not available.

**PRUSSIAN BLUE (Radiogardase)** ▶Fecal ♀C ▶+ $$$$$
ADULT - Internal contamination with radioactive cesium/thallium: 3 g PO tid.
PEDS - Internal contamination with radioactive cesium/thallium, 2–12 yo: 1 g PO tid.
FORMS - Trade only: Caps 500 mg.

**SUCCIMER (Chemet)** ▶K ♀C ▶? $$$$$
PEDS - Lead toxicity ≥1 yo: Start 10 mg/kg PO or 350 mg/m² q8h × 5 d, then reduce the frequency to q12h × 2 wk. Not approved in children <12 mo.

## ANTIDOTES

| Toxin | Antidote/Treatment | Toxin | Antidote/Treatment |
|---|---|---|---|
| acetaminophen | N-acetylcysteine | ethylene glycol | fomepizole |
| antidepressants | bicarbonate | heparin | protamine |
| arsenic, mercury | dimercaprol (BAL) | iron | deferoxamine |
| benzodiazepine | flumazenil | lead | EDTA, succimer |
| beta blockers | glucagon | methanol | fomepizole |
| calcium channel | calcium chloride, | methemoglobin | methylene blue |
| blockers | glucagon | narcotics | naloxone |
| cyanide | Lilly cyanide kit | organophosphates | atropine + pralidoxime |
| digoxin | dig immune Fab | warfarin | vitamin K, FFP |

**SUCCIMER** (*cont.*)
FORMS - Trade only: Caps 100 mg.
NOTES - Manufacturer recommends doses of 100 mg
(8–15 kg), 200 mg (16–23 kg), 300 mg (24–34
kg), 400 mg (35–44 kg), and 500 mg (≥45 kg).

Can open cap and sprinkle medicated beads over
food, or give them in a spoon and follow with fruit
drink. Indicated for blood lead levels >45 mcg/
dl. Allow at least 4 wk between edetate disodium
and succimer treatment.

## UROLOGY: Benign Prostatic Hyperplasia

**ALFUZOSIN** (*UroXatral*, *+Xatral*) ▶KL ♀B ▶- $$$
WARNING - Postural hypotension with or with-
out symptoms may develop within a few h after
administration. Avoid in moderate or severe
hepatic insufficiency. Avoid co-administration
with potent CYP3A4 inhibitors.
ADULT - BPH: 10 mg PO daily after a meal.
PEDS - Not approved in children.
UNAPPROVED ADULT - Promotes spontaneous pas-
sage of ureteral calculi: 10 mg PO daily usually
combined with an NSAID, antiemetic and opioid
of choice.
FORMS - Trade only: Extended-release tab 10 mg
NOTES - Do not use in moderate to severe hepatic
insufficiency. Caution in congenital or acquired
QT prolongation & severe renal insufficiency.
Intraoperative floppy iris syndrome has been
observed during cataract surgery.
**DUTASTERIDE** (*Avodart*) ▶L ♀X ▶- $$$$
ADULT - BPH: 0.5 mg PO daily with/without tamsu-
losin 0.4 mg PO daily.
PEDS - Not approved in children.
FORMS - Trade only: Cap 0.5 mg.
NOTES - 6 mo therapy may be needed to assess
effectiveness. Pregnant or potentially pregnant
women should not handle caps due to fetal risk
from absorption. Caution in hepatic insuffi-
ciency. Dutasteride will decrease PSA by 50%;
new baseline PSA should be established after
3–6 mo to assess potentially cancer-related PSA
changes. Capsule should be swallowed whole
and not chewed or opened to avoid oropharyngeal
irritation.
**FINASTERIDE** (*Proscar, Propecia*) ▶L ♀X ▶- $$$
ADULT - Proscar: 5 mg PO daily alone or in combina-
tion with doxazosin to reduce the risk of symptomatic progression of BPH. Propecia: Androgenetic
alopecia in men: 1 mg PO daily.
PEDS - Not approved in children.
UNAPPROVED ADULT - Androgenetic alopecia in
postmenopausal women (no evidence of efficacy):
1 mg PO daily.
FORMS - Generic/Trade: Tabs 1 mg (Propecia), 5 mg
(Proscar).
NOTES - Therapy for 6–12 mo may be needed to
assess effectiveness for BPH and ≥3 mo for alopecia. Pregnant or potentially pregnant women
should not handle crushed tabs because of possible absorption and fetal risk. Use with caution in
hepatic insufficiency. Monitor PSA before therapy;
finasteride will decrease PSA by 50% in patients
with BPH, even with prostate cancer. Does not
appear to alter detection of prostate cancer.
**TAMSULOSIN** (*Flomax*) ▶LK ♀B ▶- $$$
ADULT - BPH: 0.4 mg PO daily 30 min after the
same meal each d. If an adequate response is
not seen after 2–4 wk, may increase dose to 0.8
mg PO daily. If therapy is interrupted for several
d, restart at the 0.4 mg dose.
PEDS - Not approved in children.
UNAPPROVED ADULT - Promotes spontaneous passage
of ureteral calculi: 0.4 mg PO daily usually combined
with an NSAID, antiemetic and opioid of choice.
FORMS - Trade only: Cap 0.4 mg.
NOTES - Dizziness, headache, abnormal ejaculation.
Alpha blockers are generally considered to be first
line treatment in men with more than minimal
obstructive urinary symptoms. Caution in serious
sulfa allergy – rare allergic reactions reported.
Intraoperative floppy iris syndrome with cataract
surgery reported. Caution with strong inhibitors of
CYP450 2D6 (fluoxetine) or 3A4 (ketoconazole).

## UROLOGY: Bladder Agents—Anticholinergics & Combinations

**B&O SUPPRETTES** (belladonna + opium) ▶L ♀C ▶?
©II $$$
ADULT - Bladder spasm: 1 susp PR daily-bid, max
4 doses/d.
PEDS - Not approved in children <12 yo.
FORMS - Generic/Trade: suppositories 30 mg opium
(15A), 60 mg opium (16A).
NOTES - Store at room temperature. Contraindicated
in narrow-angle glaucoma, obstructive conditions
(eg, pyloric, duodenal or other intestinal obstructive
lesions, ileus, achalasia, and obstructive uropathies).
**DARIFENACIN** (*Enablex*) ▶LK ♀C ▶- $$$$
ADULT - Overactive bladder with symptoms of urinary urgency, frequency and urge incontinence

7.5 mg PO daily. May increase to max dose
15 mg PO daily in 2 wk. Max dose 7.5 mg PO
daily with moderate liver impairment or when
coadministered with potent CYP3A4 inhibitors
(ketoconazole, itraconazole, ritonavir, nelfinavir,
clarithromycin & nefazodone).
PEDS - Not approved in children.
FORMS - Trade only: Extended-release tabs 7.5, 15
mg.
NOTES - Contraindicated with uncontrolled narrow-
angle glaucoma, urinary & gastric retention.
Avoid use in severe hepatic impairment. May
increase concentration of medications metabolized by CYP2D6.

**FLAVOXATE (*Urispas*)** ▶K ♀B ▶? $$$$
ADULT - Bladder spasm: 100 or 200 mg PO tid-qid. Reduce dose when improved.
PEDS - Not approved in children <12 yo.
FORMS - Trade only: Tab 100 mg.
NOTES - May cause dizziness, drowsiness, blurred vision, dry mouth, N/V, urinary retention. Contraindicated in glaucoma, obstructive conditions (eg, pyloric, duodenal or other intestinal obstructive lesions, ileus, achalasia, GI hemorrhage, and obstructive uropathies).

**OXYBUTYNIN (*Ditropan, Ditropan XL, Oxytrol, ＋Oxybutyn, Uromax*)** ▶LK ♀B ▶? $
ADULT - Bladder instability: 2.5–5 mg PO bid-tid, max 5 mg PO qid. Extended release tabs: 5–10 mg PO daily same time each d, increase 5 mg/d q wk to 30 mg/d. Oxytrol: 1 patch twice weekly on abdomen, hips or buttocks.
PEDS - Bladder instability >5 yo: 5 mg PO bid, max dose: 5 mg PO tid. Extended release, >6 yo: 5 mg PO daily, max 20 mg/d. Transdermal patch not approved in children.
UNAPPROVED ADULT - Case reports of use for hyperhidrosis.
UNAPPROVED PEDS - Bladder instability ≤5 yo: 0.2 mg/kg/dose PO bid-qid.
FORMS - Generic/Trade: Tab 5 mg. Syrup 5 mg/5 mL. Extended release tabs 5, 10, 15 mg. Trade only: Transdermal (Oxytrol) 3.9 mg/d.
NOTES - May cause dizziness, drowsiness, blurred vision, dry mouth, urinary retention. Contraindicated with glaucoma, obstructive GU or GI disease, unstable cardiovascular status, and myasthenia gravis. Transdermal patch causes less dry mouth than oral form; avoid dose reduction by cutting.

***PROSED/DS* (methenamine + phenyl salicylate + methylene blue + benzoic acid + hyoscyamine)** ▶KL ♀C ▶? $$$
ADULT - Bladder spasm: 1 tab PO qid with liberal fluids.
PEDS - Not approved in children
FORMS - Trade only: Tab (methenamine 81.6 mg/ phenyl salicylate 36.2 mg/methylene blue 10.8 mg/benzoic acid 9.0 mg/hyoscyamine sulfate 0.12 mg). Prosed EC = enteric coated form.
NOTES - May cause dizziness, drowsiness, blurred vision, dry mouth, N/V, urinary retention. May turn urine/contact lenses blue.

**SOLIFENACIN (*VESIcare*)** ▶LK ♀C ▶- $$$$
ADULT - Overactive bladder with symptoms of urinary urgency, frequency or urge incontinence: 5 mg PO daily. Max dose: 10 mg PO daily (5 mg PO daily if CrCl<30 mL/min, moderate hepatic impairment, or concurrent ketoconazole or other potent CYP3A4 inhibitors).
PEDS - Not approved in children.
FORMS - Trade only: Tabs 5, 10 mg
NOTES - Contraindicated with uncontrolled narrow-angle glaucoma, urinary & gastric retention. Avoid use in severe hepatic impairment. Hallucinations have been reported.

**TOLTERODINE (*Detrol, Detrol LA, ＋Unidet*)** ▶L ♀C ▶- $$$$
ADULT - Overactive bladder: 2 mg PO bid (Detrol) or 4 mg PO daily (Detrol LA). Decrease dose to 1 mg PO bid (Detrol) or 2 mg PO daily (Detrol LA) if adverse symptoms, hepatic insufficiency or specific coadministered drugs (see notes).
PEDS - Not approved in children.
FORMS - Trade only: Tabs 1, 2 mg. Caps, extended release 2, 4 mg.
NOTES - Contraindicated with urinary or gastric retention, or uncontrolled glaucoma. High doses may prolong the QT interval. Drug interactions with CYP3A4 inhibitors (eg, erythromycin, ketoconazole, itraconazole); decrease dose to 1 mg PO bid or 2 mg PO daily (Detrol LA).

**TROSPIUM (*Sanctura, Sanctura XR, ＋Trosec*)** ▶LK ♀C ▶? $$$$
ADULT - Overactive bladder with urge incontinence: 20 mg PO bid; give 20 mg qhs if CrCl <30 mL/min. If ≥75 yo may taper down to 20 mg daily. Extended release: 60 mg PO q am, 1 h before food.
PEDS - Not approved in children.
FORMS - Trade only: Tab 20 mg, Cap, extended release, 60 mg.
NOTES - Contraindicated with uncontrolled narrow-angle glaucoma, urinary retention, gastroparesis. May cause heat stroke due to decreased sweating. Take on an empty stomach. Improvement in signs & symptoms may be seen in a wk. Causes minimum CNS side effects.

***URISED* (methenamine + phenyl salicylate + atropine + hyoscyamine + benzoic acid + methylene blue) (Usept)** ▶K ♀C ▶? $$$$
ADULT - Dysuria: 2 Tabs PO qid.
PEDS - Dysuria >6 yo: reduce dose based on age and weight. Not recommended for children <6 yo.
FORMS - Trade only: Tab (methenamine 40.8 mg/ phenyl salicylate 18.1 mg/atropine 0.03 mg/hyoscyamine 0.03 mg/4.5 mg benzoic acid/5.4 mg methylene blue).
NOTES - Take with food to minimize GI upset. May precipitate urate crystals in urine. Avoid use with sulfonamides. May turn urine/contact lenses blue.

***UTA* (methenamine + sodium phosphate + phenyl salicylate + methylene blue + hyoscyamine)** ▶KL ♀C ▶? $$$
ADULT - Treatment of irritative voiding/relief of inflammation, hypermotility & pain with lower urinary tract infection/relief of urinary tract symptoms caused by diagnostic procedures: 1 cap PO qid with liberal fluids.
PEDS - <6 yo: not recommended. >6 yo: dosing must be individualized by physician.
FORMS - Trade only: Cap (methenamine 120 mg/ sodium phosphate 40.8 mg/phenyl salicylate 36 mg/methylene blue 10 mg/hyoscyamine 0.12 mg).
NOTES - May turn urine/feces blue to blue-green. Take 2 h apart from ketoconazole. May decrease absorption of thiazide diuretics. Antacids and

**UTA** (cont.)

antidiarrheals may decrease effectiveness of methenamine.

**UTIRA-C (methenamine + sodium phosphate + phenyl salicylate + methylene blue + hyoscyamine)** ▶KL ♀C ▶? $$

ADULT - Treatment of irritative voiding/relief of inflammation, hypermotility & pain with lower urinary tract infection/relief of urinary tract symptoms caused by diagnostic procedures: 1 cap PO qid with liberal fluids.

PEDS - <6 yo: not recommended. >6 yo: dosing must be individualized by physician.

FORMS - Trade only: Tab (methenamine 81.6 mg/sodium phosphate 40.8 mg/phenyl salicylate 36.2 mg/methylene blue 10.8 mg/hyoscyamine 0.12 mg).

NOTES - May turn urine/feces blue to blue-green. Take 2 h apart from ketoconazole. May decrease absorption of thiazide diuretics. Antacids and antidiarrheals may decrease effectiveness of methenamine.

**BETHANECHOL (Urecholine, Duvoid, ✦Myotonachol)** ▶L ♀C ▶? $

ADULT - Urinary retention: 10–50 mg PO tid-qid or 2.5–5 mg SC tid-qid. Take 1 h before or 2 h after meals to avoid N/V. Determine the minimum effective dose by giving 5–10 mg PO initially and repeat at hourly intervals until response or to a max of 50 mg.

PEDS - Not approved in children.

UNAPPROVED PEDS - Urinary retention/abdominal distention: 0.6 mg/kg/d PO divided q6–8h or 0.12–0.2 mg/kg/d SC divided q6–8h.

FORMS - Generic/Trade: Tabs 5, 10, 25, 50 mg.

NOTES - May cause drowsiness, lightheadedness, and fainting. Not for obstructive urinary retention. Avoid with cardiac disease, hyperthyroidism, parkinsonism, peptic ulcer disease, and epilepsy.

**DIMETHYL SULFOXIDE (DMSO, Rimso-50)** ▶KL ♀C ▶? $$$

ADULT - Interstitial cystitis: Instill 50 mL solution into bladder by catheter & allow to remain for 15 min; expelled by spontaneous voiding. Repeat q2 wk until symptomatic relief is obtained; thereafter, may increase time intervals between treatments.

PEDS - Not approved in children.

NOTES - Apply analgesic lubricant gel to urethra prior to inserting the catheter to avoid spasm. May administer oral analgesics or suppositories containing belladonna & opium prior to instillation to reduce spasms. May give anesthesia in patients with severe interstitial cystitis and very sensitive bladders during the 1st, 2nd & 3rd treatment. May cause lens opacities & changes in refractive index; perform eye exams before & periodically during treatment. May cause a hypersensitivity reaction by liberating histamine. Monitor liver & renal function tests & CBC q6 mo. May be harmful in patients with urinary tract

malignancy; can cause DMSO-induced vasodilation. Peripheral neuropathy may occur when used with sulindac. Garlic-like taste may occur within a few min of administration; odor on breath & skin may be present & remain for up to 72 h.

**PENTOSAN (Elmiron)** ▶LK ♀B ▶? $$$$$

ADULT - Interstitial cystitis: 100 mg PO tid 1h before or 2h after a meal.

PEDS - Not approved in children.

FORMS - Trade only: Caps 100 mg.

NOTES - Pain relief usually occurs at 2–4 mo and decreased urinary frequency takes 6 mo. May increase risk of bleeding, especially with NSAID use. Use with caution in hepatic or splenic dysfunction.

**PHENAZOPYRIDINE (Pyridium, Azo-Standard, Urogesic, Prodium, Pyridiate, Urodol, Baridium, UTI Relief, ✦Phenazo)** ▶K ♀B ▶? $

ADULT - Dysuria: 200 mg PO tid after meals × 2 d.

PEDS - Dysuria in children 6–12 yo: 12 mg/kg/d PO divided tid × 2 d.

FORMS - OTC Generic/Trade: Tabs 95, 97.2 mg. Rx Generic/Trade: Tabs 100, 200 mg.

NOTES - May turn urine/contact lenses orange. Contraindicated with hepatitis or renal insufficiency.

**UROQUID-ACID NO. 2 (methenamine + sodium phosphate)** ▶K ♀C ▶? $

ADULT - Chronic/recurrent UTIs: Initial: 2 tabs PO qid with full glass of water. Maintenance: 2–4 tabs PO daily, in divided doses with full glass of water.

PEDS - Not approved in children.

FORMS - Trade only: Tabs methenamine mandelate 500 mg/sodium acid phosphate 500 mg.

NOTES - 83 mg sodium/tab. Thiazide diuretics, carbonic anhydrase inhibitors, antacids & urinary alkalinizing agents may decrease effectiveness. Caution with concurrent salicylates, may increase levels.

**ALPROSTADIL (Muse, Caverject, Caverject Impulse, Edex, Prostin VR Pediatric, prostaglandin E1, ✦Prostin VR)** ▶L ♀- ▶- $$$$

ADULT - Erectile dysfunction: 1.25–2.5 mcg intracavernosal injection over 5–10 sec initially using a ½ inch, 27 or 30 gauge needle. If no response,

may give next higher dose after 1 h, max 2 doses/d. May increase by 2.5 mcg and then 5–10 mcg incrementally on separate occasions. Dose range = 1–40 mcg. Alternative: 125–250 mcg intraurethral pellet (Muse). Increase or decrease dose on separate occasions until erection

**(cont.)**

**ALPROSTADIL** *(cont.)*
achieved. Max intraurethral dose 2 pellets/24h. The lowest possible dose to produce an acceptable erection should be used.

PEDS - Temporary maintenance of patent ductus arteriosus in neonates: Start 0.1 mcg/kg/min IV infusion. Reduce dose to minimal amount that maintains therapeutic response. Max dose 0.4 mcg/kg/min.

UNAPPROVED ADULT - Erectile dysfunction intracorporeal injection: Specially formulated mixtures of alprostadil, papaverine and phentolamine. 0.10–0.50 mL injection.

FORMS - Trade only: Syringe system (Edex) 10, 20, 40 mcg. (Caverject) 5, 10, 20 mcg. (Caverject Impulse) 10, 20 mcg. Pellet (Muse) 125, 250, 500, 1000 mcg. Intracorporeal injection of locally-compounded combination agents (many variations): "Bi-mix" can be 30 mg/mL papaverine + 0.5 to 1 mg/mL phentolamine, or 30 mg/mL papaverine + 20 mcg/mL alprostadil in 10 mL vials. "Tri-mix" can be 30 mg/mL papaverine + 1 mg/mL phentolamine + 10 mcg/mL alprostadil in 5, 10 or 20 mL vials.

NOTES - Contraindicated in patients at risk for priapism, with penile fibrosis (Peyronie's disease), with penile implants, in women or children, in men for whom sexual activity is inadvisable, and for intercourse with a pregnant woman. Onset of effect is 5–20 min.

**SILDENAFIL** *(Viagra, Revatio)* ▶LK ♀B ▶- $$$$
WARNING - Contraindicated in patients taking nitrates within prior/subsequent 24 h. Caution with alpha blockers due to potential for symptomatic hypotension. There have been a few reports of sudden vision loss due to non-arteritic ischemic optic neuropathy (NAION). Patients with prior NAION are at higher risk. Sudden hearing loss, with or without tinnitus, vertigo or dizziness, has been reported.

ADULT - Erectile dysfunction: 50 mg PO approximately 1h (range 0.5–4h) before sexual activity. Usual effective dose range: 25–100 mg. Max 1 dose/d. Use lower dose (25 mg) if >65 yo, hepatic/renal impairment, or certain coadministered drugs (see notes). Pulmonary hypertension: 20 mg PO tid.

PEDS - Not approved in children.

UNAPPROVED ADULT - Antidepressant-associated sexual dysfunction: Same dosing as above.

FORMS - Trade only (Viagra): Tabs 25, 50, 100 mg. Unscored tab but can be cut in half. Revatio: Tabs 20 mg.

NOTES - Drug interactions with cimetidine, erythromycin, ketoconazole, itraconazole, saquinavir, ritonavir and other CYP3A4 inhibitors; use 25 mg dose. Do not exceed 25 mg/48 h with ritonavir. Doses >25 mg should not be taken <4h after an alpha-blocker. Caution if stroke, MI or other cardiovascular event within last 6 mo.

**TADALAFIL** *(Cialis)* ▶L ♀B ▶- $$$$
WARNING - Contraindicated with nitrates. Caution with alpha blockers due to potential for symptomatic hypotension. There have been a few reports

of sudden vision loss due to non-arteritic ischemic optic neuropathy (NAION). Patients with prior NAION are at higher risk. Retinal artery occlusion has been reported. Sudden hearing loss, with or without tinnitus, vertigo or dizziness, has been reported.

ADULT - Erectile dysfunction: 2.5–5 mg PO daily without regard to timing of sexual activity. As needed dosing: 10 mg PO prn prior to sexual activity. Optimal timing of administration unclear, but should be ≥30–45 min before sexual activity. May increase to 20 mg or decrease to 5 mg. Max 1 dose/d. Start 5 mg (max 1 dose/d) if CrCl 31–50 mL/min. Max 5 mg/d if CrCl <30 mL/min on dialysis. Max 10 mg/d if mild to moderate hepatic impairment; avoid in severe hepatic impairment. Max 10 mg once in 72 h if concurrent potent CYP3A4 inhibitors.

PEDS - Not approved in children.

FORMS - Trade only: Tabs 2.5, 5, 10, 20 mg.

NOTES - If nitrates needed give ≥48 h after the last tadalafil dose. Improves erectile function for up to 36 h. Not FDA-approved for women. Not recommended if MI in prior 90 d, angina during sexual activity, NYHA Class ≥II in prior 6 mo, hypotension (<90/50), hypertension (>170/100) or stroke in prior 6 mo. Rare reports of prolonged erections.

**VARDENAFIL** *(Levitra)* ▶LK ♀B ▶- $$$$
WARNING - Contraindicated with nitrates (time interval for safe administration unknown). Caution with alpha blockers due to potential for symptomatic hypotension. There have been a few reports of sudden vision loss due to non-arteritic ischemic optic neuropathy (NAION). Patients with prior NAION are at higher risk. Sudden hearing loss, with or without tinnitus, vertigo or dizziness, has been reported. Seizures and seizure recurrence have been reported.

ADULT - Erectile dysfunction: 10 mg PO 1 h before sexual activity. Usual effective dose range: 5–20 mg. Max 1 dose/d. Use lower dose (5 mg) if ≥65 yo or moderate hepatic impairment (max 10 mg); 2.5 mg when coadministered with certain drugs (see notes). Not FDA-approved in women.

PEDS - Not approved in children.

FORMS - Trade only: Tabs 2.5, 5, 10, 20 mg

NOTES - See the following parenthetical vardenafil dose adjustments when taken with ritonavir (max 2.5 mg/72 h); indinavir, saquinavir, atazanavir, clarithromycin, ketoconazole 400 mg daily, or itraconazole 400 mg daily (max 2.5mg/24 h); ketoconazole 200 mg daily, itraconazole 200 mg daily, or erythromycin (max 5 mg/24 h). Avoid with alpha blockers & antiarrhythmics, and in congenital QT prolongation. Caution if stroke, MI or other cardiovascular event within last 6 mo, unstable angina, severe liver impairment, end stage renal disease or retinitis pigmentosa.

**YOHIMBINE** *(Yocon, Yohimex)* ▶L ♀- ▶- $
ADULT - No approved indications.
PEDS - No approved indications.

**YOHIMBINE** (*cont.*)
  UNAPPROVED ADULT - Erectile dysfunction: 1 tab PO tid. If side effects (eg, tremor, tachycardia, nervousness) occur, reduce to ½ tab tid, followed by gradual increases to 1 tab tid.
  FORMS - Generic/Trade: Tab 5.4 mg.
  NOTES - Prescription yohimbine and yohimbine bark extract (see Herbal section) are not interchangeable. Contraindicated with renal disease. Avoid with antidepressant use, psychiatric disorders, the elderly, women, or ulcer history. Efficacy of therapy >10 wk unclear. Amer Urological Assoc does not recommend as a standard treatment due to unproven efficacy.

## UROLOGY: Nephrolithiasis

**ACETOHYDROXAMIC ACID (*Lithostat*)** ▶K ♀X ▶? $$$
  ADULT - Chronic UTI, adjunctive therapy: 250 mg PO tid-qid for a total dose of 10–15 mg/kg/d. Max dose is 1.5 g/d. Decrease dose in patients with renal impairment to no more than 1 g/d.
  PEDS - Adjunctive therapy in chronic urea-splitting UTI (eg, Proteus): 10 mg/kg/d PO divided bid-tid.
  FORMS - Trade only: Tab 250 mg.
  NOTES - Do not use if CrCl <20 mL/min. Administer on an empty stomach.

**CELLULOSE SODIUM PHOSPHATE (*Calcibind*)** ▶Fecal ♀C ▶+ $$$$
  WARNING - Avoid in heart failure or ascites due to high sodium content.
  ADULT - Absorptive hypercalciuria Type 1 (>16 yo): Initial dose with urinary calcium >300 mg/d (on moderate calcium-restricted diet): 5 g with each meal. Decrease dose to 5 g with supper, 2.5 g with each remaining meal when calcium declines to <150 mg/d. Initial dose with urinary calcium 200–300 mg/d (controlled calcium-restricted diet): 5 g with supper, 2.5 g with each remaining meal. Mix with water, soft drink or fruit juice. Ingest within 30 min of meal.
  PEDS - Do not use if <16 yo.
  FORMS - Trade only: bulk powder 300 mg.
  NOTES - Give concomitant supplement of 1.5 g magnesium gluconate with 15 g/d. 1 g magnesium gluconate with 10 g/d. Take magnesium supplement ≥1h before or after each dose to avoid binding. May cause hyperparathyroidism. Long-term use may cause hypomagnesemia, hyperoxaluria, hypomagnesuria, depletion of trace metals (copper, zinc, iron); monitor calcium, magnesium, trace metals and CBC q3–6 mo; monitor parathyroid hormone once between the first 2 wk and 3 mo, then q3–6 mo thereafter. Adjust or stop treatment if PTH rises above normal. Stop when inadequate hypocalciuric response (urinary calcium of <30 mg/5 g of cellulose sodium phosphate) occurs while patient is on moderate calcium restriction. Avoid Vitamin C supplementation since metabolized to oxalate.

**CITRATE (*Polycitra-K, Urocit-K, Bicitra, Oracit, Polycitra, Polycitra-LC*)** ▶K ♀C ▶? $$$
  ADULT - Prevention of calcium and urate kidney stones: 1 packet in water/juice PO tid-qid with meals. 15–30 mL PO solution tid-qid with meals. Tabs 10–20 mEq PO tid-qid with meals. Max 100 mEq/d.
  PEDS - Urinary alkalinization: 5–15 mL PO qid with meals.
  FORMS - Trade only: Polycitra-K packet (potassium citrate): 3300 mg. Oracit oral solution: 5 mL = sodium citrate 490 mg. Generic/Trade: Urocit-K wax (potassium citrate) Tabs 5, 10 mEq. Generic only: Polycitra-K oral solution (5 mL = potassium citrate 1100 mg), Bicitra oral solution (5 mL = sodium citrate 500 mg), Polycitra-LC oral solution (5 mL = potassium citrate 550 mg/sodium citrate 500 mg), Polycitra oral syrup (5 mL = potassium citrate 550 mg/sodium citrate 550 mg).
  NOTES - Contraindicated in renal insufficiency, PUD, UTI, and hyperkalemia.

**TIOPRONIN (*Thiola*)** ▶K ♀C ▶- $$$$$
  ADULT - Prevention of kidney stone in severe homozygous cystinuria with urinary cystine >500 mg/d: Start 800 mg/d PO. Average dose in clinical trials is 1000 mg/d, although some patients may require less. A conservative treatment program should be attempted first prior to tiopronin: See NOTES.
  PEDS - ≥9 yo: Start 15 mg/kg/d PO divided tid 1 h before or 2 h after meals. Measure urinary cystine 1 mo after treatment & every 3 mo thereafter. Dosage should be readjusted depending on the urinary cystine value. A conservative treatment program should be attempted first prior to tiopronin: See NOTES.
  FORMS - Trade only: Tab 100 mg
  NOTES - A conservative treatment program should be attempted first before starting tiopronin: 3 L of fluid should be provided, including 2 glasses with each meal & at bedtime. The patients should be expected to awake at night to urinate, they should drink 2 or more glasses of fluids before returning to bed. Additional fluids should be consumed if there is excessive sweating or intestinal fluid loss. A minimum urine output of 2 L/d on a consistent basis should be sought. Provide a modest amount of alkali in order to maintain urinary pH at high normal range (6.5–7). Avoid use in patients with history of agranulocytosis, aplastic anemia or thrombocytopenia. Monitor blood counts, platelets, serum albumin, LFTs, 24-h urinary protein & routine analysis at 3–6 mo during treatment. Monitor urinary cystine analysis frequently during the 1st 6 mo when optimum dose is being determined, then q6 mo thereafter. Abdominal x-ray is advised yearly. Patients who had adverse reactions with d-penicillamine are more likely to have adverse reactions to tiopronin. A close supervision with close monitoring of potential side effects is mandatory.

**AMINOHIPPURATE (*PAH*)** ▶K ♀C ▶? $$$$
ADULT - Estimation of effective renal plasma flow & measurement of functional capacity of renal tubular secretory mechanism: Specialized infusion dosing available.
PEDS - Not approved in children.

NOTES - May precipitate heart failure. Patients receiving sulfonamides, procaine or thiazolsulfone may interfere with chemical color development essential for analysis. Concomitant use of probenecid my result in erroneously low effective renal plasma flow.

# APPENDIX

## DRUG THERAPY REFERENCE WEBSITES (selected)

### Professional societies or governmental agencies with drug therapy guidelines

| | | |
|---|---|---|
| AHRQ | Agency for Healthcare Research and Quality | www.ahcpr.gov |
| AAP | American Academy of Pediatrics | www.aap.org |
| ACC | American College of Cardiology | www.acc.org |
| ACCP | American College of Chest Physicians | www.chestnet.org |
| ACCP | American College of Clinical Pharmacy | www.accp.com |
| AHA | American Heart Association | www.americanheart.org |
| ADA | American Diabetes Association | www.diabetes.org |
| AMA | American Medical Association | www.ama-assn.org |
| ATS | American Thoracic Society | www.thoracic.org |
| ASHP | Amer. Society Health-Systems Pharmacists | www.ashp.org |
| CDC | Centers for Disease Control & Prevention | www.cdc.gov |
| CDC | CDC bioterrorism and radiation exposures | www.bt.cdc.gov |
| IDSA | Infectious Diseases Society of America | www.idsociety.org |
| MHA | Malignant Hyperthermia Association | www.mhaus.org |
| NHLBI | National Heart, Lung, & Blood Institute | www.nhlbi.nih.gov |

### Other therapy reference sites

| | |
|---|---|
| Cochrane library | www.cochrane.org |
| Emergency Contraception Website | www.not-2-late.com |
| Immunization Action Coalition | www.immunize.org |
| Int'l Registry for Drug-Induced Arrhythmias | www.qtdrugs.org |
| Managing Contraception | www.managingcontraception.com |
| Nephrology Pharmacy Associates | www.nephrologypharmacy.com |

## THERAPEUTIC DRUG LEVELS

| Drug | Level | Optimal Timing |
|---|---|---|
| amikacin peak | 20-35 mcg/mL | 30 min after infusion |
| amikacin trough | <5 mcg/mL | Just prior to next dose |
| carbamazepine trough | 4-12 mcg/mL | Just prior to next dose |
| cyclosporine trough | 50-300 ng/mL | Just prior to next dose |
| digoxin | 0.8-2.0 ng/mL | Just prior to next dose |
| ethosuximide trough | 40-100 mcg/mL | Just prior to next dose |
| gentamicin peak | 5-10 mcg/mL | 30 min after infusion |
| gentamicin trough | <2 mcg/mL | Just prior to next dose |
| lidocaine | 1.5-5 mcg/mL | 12-24 h after start of infusion |
| lithium trough | 0.6-1.2 mEq/L | Just prior to first morning dose |
| NAPA | 10-30 mcg/mL | Just prior to next procainamide dose |
| phenobarbital trough | 15-40 mcg/mL | Just prior to next dose |
| phenytoin trough | 10-20 mcg/mL | Just prior to next dose |
| primidone trough | 5-12 mcg/mL | Just prior to next dose |
| procainamide | 4-10 mcg/mL | Just prior to next dose |
| quinidine | 2-5 mcg/mL | Just prior to next dose |
| theophylline | 5-15 mcg/mL | 8-12 h after once daily dose |
| tobramycin peak | 5-10 mcg/mL | 30 min after infusion |
| tobramycin trough | <2 mcg/mL | Just prior to next dose |
| valproate trough (epilepsy) | 50-100 mcg/mL | Just prior to next dose |
| valproate trough (mania) | 45-125 mcg/mL | Just prior to next dose |
| vancomycin trough | 5-20 mcg/mL | Just prior to next dose |

| PEDIATRIC DRUGS | Age Kg Lbs | | 2 mo 5 11 | 4 mo 6½ 15 |
|---|---|---|---|---|
| med | strength | freq | | |
| Tylenol (mg) | | q4h | 80 | 80 |
| Tylenol (tsp) | 160/tab | q4h | ½ | ½ |
| ibuprofen (mg) | | q6h | - | - |
| ibuprofen (tsp) | 100/tab | q6h | - | - |
| amoxicillin or | 125/tab | bid | 1 | 1¼ |
| Augmentin (not otitis media) | 200/tab | bid | ½ | ¾ |
| | 250/tab | bid | ½ | ½ |
| | 400/tab | bid | ¼ | ½ |
| amoxicillin (otitis media)‡ | 200/tab | bid | 1 | 1¼ |
| | 250/tab | bid | ¾ | 1¼ |
| | 400/tab | bid | ½ | ¾ |
| Augmentin ES‡ | 600/tab | bid | ⅜ | ½ |
| azithromycin*§ (5-d Rx) | 100/tab | qd | ¼† | ½† |
| | 200/tab | qd | — | ¼† |
| Bactrim/Septra | — | bid | ½ | ¾ |
| cefaclor* | 125/tab | bid | 1 | 1 |
| | 250/tab | bid | ½ | ½ |
| cefadroxil | 125/tab | bid | ½ | ¾ |
| | 250/tab | bid | ¼ | ½ |
| cefdinir | 125/tab | qd | — | ¾† |
| cefixime | 100/tab | qd | ½ | ½ |
| cefprozil* | 125/tab | bid | — | ¾† |
| | 250/tab | bid | — | ½† |
| cefuroxime | 125/tab | bid | — | ¾ |
| cephalexin | 125/tab | qid | — | ½ |
| | 250/tab | qid | — | ¼ |
| clarithromycin | 125/tab | bid | ½† | ½† |
| | 250/tab | bid | — | — |
| dicloxacillin | 62½/tab | qid | ½ | ¾ |
| nitrofurantoin | 25/tab | qid | ¼ | ½ |
| Pediazole | — | tid | ½ | ½ |
| penicillin V** | 250/tab | bid-tid | — | 1 |
| cetirizine | 5/tab | qd | - | - |
| Benadryl | 12.5/tab | q6h | ½ | ½ |
| prednisolone | 15/tab | qd | ¼ | ½ |
| prednisone | 5/tab | qd | 1 | 1¼ |
| Robitussin | — | q4h | - | - |
| Tylenol w/codeine | | q4h | - | - |

\* Dose shown is for otitis media only; see dosing in text for alternative indications.
† Dosing at this age/weight not recommended by manufacturer.
‡ AAP now recommends high dose (80-90 mg/kg/d) for all otitis media in children; with Augmentin used as ES only.
§Give a double dose of azithromycin the first day.
\*\*AHA dosing for streptococcal pharyngitis. Treat for 10 d.

| 6 mo | 9 mo | 12 mo | 15 mo | 2 yr | 3 yr | 5 yr |
|---|---|---|---|---|---|---|
| 8 | 9 | 10 | 11 | 13 | 15 | 19 |
| 17 | 20 | 22 | 24 | 28 | 33 | 42 |
| teaspoons of liquid per dose (1 tsp = 5 mL) | | | | | | |
| 120 | 120 | 160 | 160 | 200 | 240 | 280 |
| ¾ | ¾ | 1 | 1 | 1¼ | 1½ | 1¾ |
| 75† | 75† | 100 | 100 | 125 | 150 | 175 |
| ¾† | ¾† | 1 | 1 | 1¼ | 1½ | 1¾ |
| 1½ | 1¾ | 1¾ | 2 | 2¼ | 2¾ | 3½ |
| 1 | 1 | 1¼ | 1¼ | 1½ | 1¾ | 2¼ |
| ¾ | ¾ | 1 | 1 | 1¼ | 1¼ | 1¾ |
| ½ | ½ | ¾ | ¾ | ¾ | 1 | 1 |
| 1¾ | 2 | 2 | 2¼ | 2¾ | 3 | 4 |
| 1½ | 1½ | 1¾ | 1¾ | 2¼ | 2½ | 3¼ |
| ¾ | 1 | 1 | 1¼ | 1½ | 1½ | 2 |
| ½ | ¾ | ¾ | ¾ | 1 | 1¼ | 1½ |
| ½ | ½ | ½ | ½ | ¾ | ¾ | 1 |
| ¼ | ¼ | ¼ | ¼ | ½ | ½ | ½ |
| 1 | 1 | 1 | 1¼ | 1½ | 1½ | 2 |
| 1¼ | 1½ | 1½ | 1¾ | 2 | 2½ | 3 |
| ¾ | ¾ | ¾ | 1 | 1 | 1¼ | 1½ |
| 1 | 1 | 1¼ | 1¼ | 1½ | 1¾ | 2¼ |
| ½ | ½ | ¾ | ¾ | ¾ | 1 | 1 |
| 1 | 1 | 1 | 1¼ | 1½ | 1¾ | 2 |
| ¾ | ¾ | ¾ | 1 | 1 | 1¼ | 1½ |
| 1 | 1 | 1¼ | 1½ | 1½ | 2 | 2¼ |
| ½ | ½ | ¾ | ¾ | ¾ | 1 | 1¼ |
| ¾ | 1 | 1 | 1 | 1½ | 1¾ | 2¼ |
| ¾ | ¾ | 1 | 1 | 1¼ | 1½ | 1¾ |
| ¼ | ½ | ½ | ½ | ¾ | ¾ | 1 |
| ½ | ½ | ¾ | ¾ | ¾ | 1 | 1¼ |
| — | ¼ | ½ | ½ | ½ | ½ | ¾ |
| 1 | 1 | 1¼ | 1¼ | 1½ | 1¾ | 2 |
| ½ | ½ | ½ | ¾ | ¾ | ¾ | 1 |
| ¾ | ¾ | 1 | 1 | 1 | 1¼ | 1½ |
| 1 | 1 | 1 | 1 | 1 | 1 | 1 |
| ½ | ½ | ½ | ½ | ½ | ½ | ½ |
| ¾ | ¾ | 1 | 1 | 1¼ | 1½ | 2 |
| ½ | ¾ | ¾ | ¾ | 1 | 1 | 1¼ |
| 1½ | 1¾ | 2 | 2¼ | 2½ | 3 | 3¾ |
| ¼† | ¼† | ½ | ½ | ¾ | ¾ | 1 |
| - | - | - | - | - | 1 | 1 |

| PEDIATRIC VITAL SIGNS AND INTRAVENOUS DRUGS | | | | | |
|---|---|---|---|---|---|
| Age | | Premature | Newborn | 2 mo | 4 mo |
| Weight | (Kg) | 2 | 3½ | 5 | 6½ |
| | (Lbs) | 4½ | 7½ | 11 | 15 |
| Maint fluids | (mL/h) | 8 | 14 | 20 | 26 |
| ET tube | (mm) | 2½ | 3/3½ | 3½ | 3½ |
| Defib | (Joules) | 4 | 7 | 10 | 13 |
| Systolic BP | (high) | 70 | 80 | 85 | 90 |
| | (low) | 40 | 60 | 70 | 70 |
| Pulse rate | (high) | 145 | 145 | 180 | 180 |
| | (low) | 100 | 100 | 110 | 110 |
| Resp rate | (high) | 60 | 60 | 50 | 50 |
| | (low) | 35 | 30 | 30 | 30 |
| adenosine | (mg) | 0.2 | 0.3 | 0.5 | 0.6 |
| atropine | (mg) | 0.1 | 0.1 | 0.1 | 0.13 |
| Benadryl | (mg) | - | - | 5 | 6½ |
| bicarbonate | (mEq) | 2 | 3½ | 5 | 6½ |
| dextrose | (g) | 1 | 2 | 5 | 6½ |
| epinephrine | (mg) | .02 | .04 | .05 | .07 |
| lidocaine | (mg) | 2 | 3½ | 5 | 6½ |
| morphine | (mg) | 0.2 | 0.3 | 0.5 | 0.6 |
| mannitol | (g) | 2 | 3½ | 5 | 6½ |
| naloxone | (mg) | .02 | .04 | .05 | .07 |
| diazepam | (mg) | 0.6 | 1 | 1.5 | 2 |
| fosphenytoin* | (PE) | 40 | 70 | 100 | 130 |
| lorazepam | (mg) | 0.1 | 0.2 | 0.3 | 0.35 |
| phenobarb | (mg) | 30 | 60 | 75 | 100 |
| phenytoin* | (mg) | 40 | 70 | 100 | 130 |
| ampicillin | (mg) | 100 | 175 | 250 | 325 |
| ceftriaxone | (mg) | - | - | 250 | 325 |
| cefotaxime | (mg) | 100 | 175 | 250 | 325 |
| gentamicin | (mg) | 5 | 8 | 12 | 16 |

*Loading doses; fosphenytoin dosed in "phenytoin equivalents."

| 6 mo | 9 mo | 12 mo | 15 mo | 2 yr | 3 yr | 5 yr |
|------|------|-------|-------|------|------|------|
| 8 | 9 | 10 | 11 | 13 | 15 | 19 |
| 17 | 20 | 22 | 24 | 28 | 33 | 42 |
| 32 | 36 | 40 | 42 | 46 | 50 | 58 |
| 3½ | 4 | 4 | 4½ | 4½ | 4½ | 5 |
| 16 | 18 | 20 | 22 | 26 | 30 | 38 |
| 95 | 100 | 103 | 104 | 106 | 109 | 114 |
| 70 | 70 | 70 | 70 | 75 | 75 | 80 |
| 180 | 160 | 160 | 160 | 150 | 150 | 135 |
| 110 | 100 | 100 | 100 | 90 | 90 | 65 |
| 50 | 46 | 46 | 30 | 30 | 25 | 25 |
| 24 | 24 | 20 | 20 | 20 | 20 | 20 |
| 0.8 | 0.9 | 1 | 1.1 | 1.3 | 1.5 | 1.9 |
| 0.16 | 0.18 | 0.2 | 0.22 | 0.26 | 0.30 | 0.38 |
| 8 | 9 | 10 | 11 | 13 | 15 | 19 |
| 8 | 9 | 10 | 11 | 13 | 15 | 19 |
| 8 | 9 | 10 | 11 | 13 | 15 | 19 |
| .08 | .09 | 0.1 | 0.11 | 0.13 | 0.15 | 0.19 |
| 8 | 9 | 10 | 11 | 13 | 15 | 19 |
| 0.8 | 0.9 | 1 | 1.1 | 1.3 | 1.5 | 1.9 |
| 8 | 9 | 10 | 11 | 13 | 15 | 19 |
| .08 | .09 | 0.1 | 0.11 | 0.13 | 0.15 | 0.19 |
| 2.5 | 2.7 | 3 | 3.3 | 3.9 | 4.5 | 5 |
| 160 | 180 | 200 | 220 | 260 | 300 | 380 |
| 0.4 | 0.5 | 0.5 | 0.6 | 0.7 | 0.8 | 1.0 |
| 125 | 125 | 150 | 175 | 200 | 225 | 275 |
| 160 | 180 | 200 | 220 | 260 | 300 | 380 |
| 400 | 450 | 500 | 550 | 650 | 750 | 1000 |
| 400 | 450 | 500 | 550 | 650 | 750 | 1000 |
| 400 | 450 | 500 | 550 | 650 | 750 | 1000 |
| 20 | 22 | 25 | 27 | 32 | 37 | 47 |

## INHIBITORS, INDUCERS, AND SUBSTRATES OF CYTOCHROME P450 ISOZYMES

The cytochrome P450 (CYP) inhibitors and inducers below do not necessarily cause clinically important interactions with substrates listed. Underlined drugs have shown potential for important interactions in human case reports or clinical studies. We exclude in vitro data which can be inaccurate. Refer to the Tarascon Pocket Pharmacopoeia drug interactions database (PDA edition) or other resources for more information if an interaction is suspected based on this chart. A drug that inhibits CYP subfamily activity can block the metabolism of substrates of that enzyme and substrate accumulation and toxicity may result. CYP inhibitors are classified by how much they increase the area-under-the-curve (AUC) of a substrate: weak (1.25-2 fold), moderate (2-5 fold), or strong (≥5 fold). A drug is considered a sensitive substrate if a CYP inhibitor increases the AUC of that drug by ≥5-fold. While AUC increases of >50% often do not affect patient response, smaller increases can be important if the therapeutic range is narrow (eg, theophylline, warfarin, cyclosporine). A drug that induces CYP subfamily activity increases substrate metabolism and reduced substrate efficacy may result. This table may be incomplete since new evidence about drug interactions is continually being identified.

### CYP 1A2

**Inhibitors.** *Strong*: fluvoxamine. *Moderate*: ciprofloxacin, mexiletine, propafenone, zileuton. *Weak*: acyclovir, cimetidine, famotidine, norfloxacin, verapamil. *Unclassified*: amiodarone, atazanavir, citalopram, clarithromycin, erythromycin, estradiol, ipriflavone, isoniazid, paroxetine, peginterferon alfa-2a, tacrine, ziprasidone.
**Inducers**: barbiturates, carbamazepine, charcoal-broiled foods, phenytoin, rifampin, ritonavir, smoking.
**Substrates.** *Sensitive*: alosetron, duloxetine, tizanidine. *Unclassified*: acetaminophen, amitriptyline, bortezomib, caffeine, cinacalcet, clomipramine, clozapine, cyclobenzaprine, estradiol, fluvoxamine, haloperidol, imipramine, lidocaine, mexiletine, mirtazapine, naproxen, olanzapine, ondansetron, propranolol, ramelteon, rasagiline, riluzole, ropinirole, ropivacaine, R-warfarin, tacrine, theophylline, verapamil, zileuton, zolmitriptan.

### CYP 2C8

**Inhibitors.** *Strong*: gemfibrozil. *Weak*: trimethoprim.
**Inducers**: barbiturates, carbamazepine, rifabutin, rifampin.
**Substrates.** *Sensitive*: repaglinide. *Unclassified*: amiodarone, carbamazepine, ibuprofen, isotretinoin, loperamide, paclitaxel, pioglitazone, rosiglitazone, tolbutamide.

### CYP 2C9

**Inhibitors.** *Moderate*: amiodarone, fluconazole, oxandrolone. *Weak*: ketoconazole. Unclassified: atazanavir, capecitabine, chloramphenicol, cimetidine, cotrimoxazole, delavirdine, disulfiram, etravirine, fenofibrate, fluorouracil, fluvoxamine, imatinib, isoniazid, leflunomide, metronidazole, sulfamethoxazole, voriconazole, zafirlukast.
**Inducers**: aprepitant, barbiturates, bosentan, carbamazepine, phenytoin, rifampin, rifapentine, St John's wort.
**Substrates.** *Sensitive*: Flurbiprofen. *Unclassified*: alosetron, bosentan, celecoxib, chlorpropamide, diclofenac, etravirine, fluoxetine, flurbiprofen, fluvastatin, formoterol, glimepiride, glipizide, glyburide, ibuprofen, irbesartan, isotretinoin, losartan, mefenamic acid, meloxicam, montelukast, naproxen, nateglinide, phenytoin, piroxicam, ramelteon, rasagiline, rosiglitazone, rosuvastatin, sildenafil, tolbutamide, torsemide, valsartan, vardenafil, voriconazole, S-warfarin, zafirlukast, zileuton.

### CYP 2C19

**Inhibitors.** *Strong*: omeprazole. *Weak*: citalopram. *Unclassified*: armodafinil, delavirdine, esomeprazole, etravirine, felbamate, fluconazole, fluoxetine, fluvoxamine, isoniazid, letrozole, modafinil, oxcarbazepine, telmisartan, voriconazole.
**Inducers**: rifampin, St John's wort.
**Substrates.** *Sensitive*: omeprazole. *Unclassified*: ambrisentan, amitriptyline, arformoterol, bortezomib, carisoprodol, cilostazol, citalopram, clomipramine, desipramine, diazepam, escitalopram, esomeprazole, etravirine, formoterol, imipramine, lansoprazole, nelfinavir, pantoprazole, phenytoin, progesterone, proguanil, propranolol, rabeprazole, thioridazine, voriconazole, R-warfarin.

## CYP 2D6

**Inhibitors.** *Strong*: cinacalcet, fluoxetine, paroxetine, quinidine. *Moderate*: duloxetine, terbinafine. *Weak*: amiodarone, citalopram, escitalopram, sertraline. *Unclassified*: bupropion, chloroquine, cimetidine, clomipramine, delavirdine, diphenhydramine, fluphenazine, fluvoxamine, haloperidol, hydroxychloroquine, imatinib, perphenazine, propafenone, propoxyphene, ritonavir, tolterodine, thioridazine, venlafaxine.

**Inducers:** None

**Substrates.** *Sensitive*: desipramine. *Unclassified*: almotriptan, amitriptyline, arformoterol, aripiprazole, atomoxetine, carvedilol, cevimeline, chlorpheniramine, chlorpromazine, cinacalcet, clomipramine, clozapine, codeine*, darifenacin, delavirdine, dextromethorphan, dihydrocodeine*, dolasetron, donepezil, doxepin, duloxetine, flecainide, fluoxetine, formoterol, galantamine, haloperidol, hydrocodone*, imipramine, loratadine, maprotiline, methadone, methamphetamine, metoprolol, mexiletine, mirtazapine, morphine, nebivolol, nortriptyline, ondansetron, oxycodone, palonosetron, paroxetine, perphenazine, procainamide, promethazine, propafenone, propoxyphene, propranolol, quetiapine, risperidone, ritonavir, tamoxifen, thioridazine, timolol, tolterodine, tramadol*, trazodone, venlafaxine.

## CYP 3A4

**Inhibitors.** *Strong*: atazanavir, clarithromycin, indinavir, itraconazole, ketoconazole, nefazodone, nelfinavir, ritonavir, saquinavir, telithromycin, voriconazole. *Moderate*: amprenavir, aprepitant, diltiazem, erythromycin, fluconazole, fosamprenavir, grapefruit juice (variable), verapamil. *Weak*: cimetidine. *Unclassified*: amiodarone, conivaptan, cyclosporine, danazol, darunavir, delavirdine, ethinyl estradiol, fluoxetine, fluvoxamine, imatinib, miconazole, posaconazole, sertraline, quinupristin/dalfopristin, troleandomycin, zafirlukast.

**Inducers.** armodafinil, barbiturates, bexarotene, bosentan, carbamazepine, dexamethasone, ✦efavirenz, ethosuximide, etravirine, griseofulvin, modafinil, nafcillin, ✦nevirapine, oxcarbazepine, phenytoin, primidone, rifabutin, ✦rifampin, rifapentine, ritonavir, St Johns wort.

**Substrates.** *Sensitive*: budesonide, buspirone, eletriptan, eplerenone, felodipine, fluticasone, lovastatin, midazolam, saquinavir, sildenafil, simvastatin, triazolam, vardenafil. *Unclassified*: acetaminophen, alfentanil, alfuzosin, aliskiren, almotriptan, alosetron, alprazolam, amiodarone, amlodipine, amprenavir, aprepitant, argatroban, aripiprazole, atazanavir, atorvastatin, bexarotene, bortezomib, bosentan, bromocriptine, buprenorphine, carbamazepine, cevimeline, cilostazol, cinacalcet, cisapride, citalopram, clarithromycin, clomipramine, clonazepam, clopidogrel, colchicine, clozapine, corticosteroids, cyclophosphamide, cyclosporine, dapsone, darifenacin, darunavir, dasatinib, delavirdine, desogestrel, dexamethasone, diazepam, dihydroergotamine, diltiazem, disopyramide, docetaxel, dofetilide, dolasetron, domperidone, donepezil, doxorubicin, dutasteride, efavirenz, ergotamine, erlotinib, erythromycin†, escitalopram, esomeprazole, eszopiclone, ethinyl estradiol, etoposide, etravirine, fentanyl, finasteride, galantamine, gefitinib, glyburide, haloperidol, hydrocodone, ifosfamide, imatinib, imipramine, indinavir, irinotecan, isotretinoin, isradipine, itraconazole, ixabepilone, ketoconazole, lansoprazole, lapatinib, letrozole, lidocaine, loperamide, lopinavir, loratadine, losartan, maraviroc, methadone, methylergonovine, mifepristone, mirtazapine, modafinil, mometasone, montelukast, nateglinide, nefazodone, nelfinavir, nevirapine, nicardipine, nifedipine, nimodipine, nisoldipine, ondansetron, oxybutynin, oxycodone, paclitaxel, pantoprazole, paricalcitol, pimozide, pioglitazone, praziquantel, quetiapine, quinidine, quinine, ranolazine, repaglinide, rifabutin, risperidone, ritonavir, ropivacaine, sertraline, sibutramine, sirolimus, solifenacin, sorafenib, sufentanil, sunitinib, tacrolimus, tadalafil, tamoxifen, telithromycin, temsirolimus, testosterone, theophylline, tiagabine, tinidazole, tipranavir, tolterodine, toremifene, tramadol, trazodone, venlafaxine, verapamil, vinblastine, vincristine, vinorelbine, voriconazole, R-warfarin, zaleplon, zileuton, ziprasidone, zolpidem, zonisamide.

✦ potent inducer

* Metabolism by CYP2D6 required to convert to active analgesic metabolite; analgesia may be impaired by CYP2D6 inhibitors.

† Risk of sudden death may be increased in patients receiving erythromycin concurrently with CYP 3A4 inhibitors like ketoconazole, itraconazole, fluconazole, diltiazem, verapamil, and troleandomycin (NEJM 2004;351:1089).

# INDEX

## U

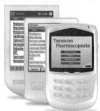

**Jones and Bartlett Publishers**
Phone: 1-800-832-0034 | Web: www.jbpub.com

# Tarascon Publishing
A Jones and Bartlett Company

**Online:**
Order online at:
www.tarascon.com

**Mail Payment to:**
Tarascon Publishing
c/o Jones and Bartlett Publishers
40 Tall Pine Drive
Sudbury, MA 01776

**Fax:**
Fax orders to:
1-978-443-8000

**Phone:**
Order by phone or to speak
to a Customer Service
Representative, call:
1-800-832-0034

## Please provide the information requested below

Name:

Address:

City: State: Zip: Country:

| Title | Quantity | Price |
|---|---|---|
| Tarascon Pocket Pharmacopoeia, Classic Shirt-Pocket Edition | | |
| Tarascon Pocket Pharmacopoeia, Deluxe Lab-Coat Pocket Edition | | |
| Tarascon Pharmacopoeia Professional Desk Reference Edition | | |
| Tarascon Pocket Pharmacopoeia Classic Nursing Edition | | |
| Tarascon Pocket Pharmacopoeia Mobile 12-month subscription | | |
| Tarascon Pocket Pharmacopoeia Mobile CD | | |
| Tarascon Pocket Pharmacopoeia Web Subscription | | |
| Tarascon Pocket Pharmacopoeia Web/Mobile Bundle | | |
| Tarascon Pediatric Outpatient Pocketbook | | |
| Tarascon Primary Care Pocketbook | | |
| Tarascon Internal Medicine & Critical Care Pocketbook | | |
| Tarascon Pediatric Emergency Pocketbook | | |
| Tarascon Adult Emergency Pocketbook | | |
| Tarascon Pocket Orthopaedica | | |
| How to be a Truly Excellent Junior Medical Student | | |
| Tarascon Pocket Rheumatologica | | |
| Tarascon Sports Medicine Pocketbook | | |
| Tarascon Pocket Rheumatologica Mobile | | |
| Tarascon Primary Care Pocketbook Mobile | | |
| Tarascon Adult Emergency Pocketbook Mobile | | |
| Fresnel Magnifying Lens with Ruler | | |
| Tarascon Rapid Reference Cards | | |

❏ **Payment Enclosed**
Make Checks Payable to Jones and Bartlett Publishers

❏ **Charge My:**
❏ MasterCard  ❏ Visa  ❏ American Express  ❏ Discover

Card Number:

Exp. Date:               Security Code:

Signature:

Subtotal: $

Tax: $

Tax is applied to orders purchased in or shipping to: CA
7.25%, FL 6%, IL 6.25%, MA 5%, MD 6%, MI 6%, NY 4%,
PA 6%, SC 6%, TX 6.25%, WA 8.8%, GST 5%

Shipping: $
See previous page for shipping

TOTAL: $